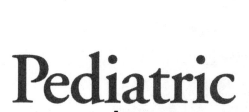

Pediatric
Issues
IN OCCUPATIONAL THERAPY

A Compendium of
Leading Scholarship

Pediatric
Issues
IN OCCUPATIONAL THERAPY

EDITED BY
CHARLOTTE BRASIC ROYEEN,
PHD, OTR, FAOTA

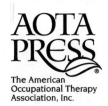

AOTA
PRESS

The American
Occupational Therapy
Association, Inc.

Mission Statement

The American Occupational Therapy Association advances the quality, availability, use, and support of occupational therapy through standard-setting, advocacy, education, and research on behalf of its members and the public.

AOTA Staff

Karen C. Carey, CAE, Associate Executive Director, Membership, Marketing, and Communications
Audrey Rothstein, Group Leader, Communications

Chris Davis, Managing Editor, Books
Barbara Dickson, Production Editor

Robert A. Sacheli, Manager, Creative Services
Sarah E. Ely, Book Production Coordinator

Marge Wasson, Marketing Manager

The American Occupational Therapy Association, Inc.
4720 Montgomery Lane
PO Box 31220
Bethesda, MD 20824-1220
Phone: 301-652-AOTA (2682)
TDD: 800-377-8555
Fax: 301-652-7711
www.aota.org
To order: 1-877-404-AOTA (2682)

Disclaimers

This publication is designed to provide accurate and authoritative information in regard to the subject matter covered. It is sold or distributed with the understanding that the publisher is not engaged in rendering legal, accounting, or other professional service. If legal advice or other expert assistance is required, the services of a competent professional person should be sought.
—*From the Declaration of Principles jointly adopted by the American Bar Association and a Committee of Publishers and Associations*

It is the objective of The American Occupational Therapy Association to be a forum for free expression and interchange of ideas. The opinions expressed by the contributors to this work are their own and not necessarily those of either the editors or The American Occupational Therapy Association.

ISBN: 1-56900-189-8

Library of Congress Control Number: 2003117077

Design by Sarah E. Ely
Composition by Circle Graphics, Columbia, MD
Printed by Victor Graphics, Inc., Baltimore, MD

Contents

Introduction xi
Writing for Success
Charlotte Brasic Royeen, PhD, OTR, FAOTA

Part I. Scholarship of Application

CHAPTER 1 3
Feeding the Infant With Congenital Heart Disease:
An Occupational Performance Challenge
Christine Imms, BAppScOT, MSc

CHAPTER 2 15
Occupational Therapy in Early Intervention:
Applying Concepts From Infant Mental Health
Winifred Schultz-Krohn, MA, OTR, BCP, FAOTA, and
Elizabeth Cara, MA, OTR, MFCC

CHAPTER 3 23
Multisensory Approach to Handwriting Remediation:
Perceptions of School-Based Occupational Therapists
Sara Woodward, MOT, OTR/L, and Yvonne Swinth, PhD, OTR/L

Part II. Scholarship of Integration

CHAPTER 4 37
Eliciting Children's Voices in Qualitative Research
Clare Curtin, PhD, OTR

CHAPTER 5 49
Traumatic Brain Injury in Children:
Issues in Community Function
Anne Frances Cronin, PhD, OTR, BCP

CHAPTER 6 60
Young Children's Occupations:
Explicating the Dynamics of Developmental Processes
Ruth Humphry, PhD, OTR/L

Part III. Scholarship of Assessment

CHAPTER 7 75
Grip Form and Graphomotor Control in Preschool Children
Allen W. Burton, PhD, and Michael J. Dancisak, MA

CHAPTER 8 88
Classroom-Based Assessment:
Validation for the School AMPS
Pat Fingerhut, MSc, OTR; Helen Madill, PhD; Johanna Darrah, PhD;
Megan Hodge, PhD; and Sharon Warren, PhD

CHAPTER 9 94
The Evaluation of Sensory Processing:
A Validity Study Using Contrasting Groups
Cheryl L. Johnson-Ecker, MA, OTR/L, BCP, and
L. Diane Parham, PhD, OTR, FAOTA

CHAPTER 10 108
Construct-Related Validity of the Toglia Category Assessment
and the Deductive Reasoning Test With Children
Who Are Typically Developing
Naomi Josman, PhD, and Tal Jarus, PhD, OTR

CHAPTER 11 118
Prediction of School Performance Using the Miller Assessment
for Preschoolers (MAP):
A Validity Study
Shula Parush, PhD, OTR; Monica Winokur, MSc, OTR;
Sarina Goldstand, OTR/L; and Lucy Jane Miller, PhD, OTR

CHAPTER 12 130
Comparison of Sensory Profile Scores of Young Children
With and Without Autism Spectrum Disorders
Renee L. Watling, MS, OTR; Jean Deitz, PhD, OTR, FAOTA; and Owen White, PhD

CHAPTER 13 141
Reliability and Validity of a Parent Questionnaire
on Childhood Motor Skills
Brenda N. Wilson, MS, OT(C); Bonnie J. Kaplan, PhD; Susan G. Crawford, MSc;
Anne Campbell, BSc, OT(C); and Deborah Dewey, PhD

Part IV. Scholarship of Discovery: Intervention Outcomes

CHAPTER 14 159
Implicit Learning in Children With and Without
Developmental Coordination Disorder
Catherine Candler, PhD, OTR, BCP, and Harry Meeuwsen, PhD

CHAPTER 15 168
Effects of Occupational Therapy Services on Fine Motor
and Functional Performance in Preschool Children
Jane Case-Smith, EdD, OTR/L, BCP

CHAPTER 16 182
Occupational Therapy Effects on Visual–Motor Skills
in Preschool Children
Heather L. Dankert, MS, OTR; Patricia L. Davies, PhD, OTR; and
William J. Gavin, PhD

CHAPTER 17 194
Powered Mobility and Preschoolers With Complex
Developmental Delays
Jean Deitz, PhD, OTR/L, FAOTA; Yvonne Swinth, PhD, OTR/L; and
Owen White, PhD

CHAPTER 18 209
A Comparison of Consultative Model and Direct–Indirect
Intervention With Preschoolers
Diann S. Dreiling, MS, OTR, and Anita C. Bundy, ScD, OTR

CHAPTER 19 215
Effects of a Weighted Vest on Attention to Task and Self-Stimulatory
Behaviors in Preschoolers With Pervasive Developmental Disorders
Doreen Fertel-Daly, MA, OT, BCP; Gary Bedell, PhD, OT; and
Jim Hinojosa, PhD, OT, FAOTA

CHAPTER 20 230
The Effects of Hands-on Occupation Versus Demonstration
on Children's Recall Memory
Beth A. Hartman, MOT; Barbara Kopp Miller, PhD; and
David L. Nelson, PhD, OTR/L, FAOTA

CHAPTER 21 240
Children With Burn Injuries:
Purposeful Activity Versus Rote Exercise
Kim Melchert-McKearnan, MS, OTR/L; Jean Deitz, PhD, OTR, FAOTA;
Joyce M. Engel, PhD, OTR, FAOTA; and Owen White, PhD

CHAPTER 22 254
Playfulness in Children With and Without Disability:
Measurement and Intervention
Ann Mari Okimoto, MS, OTR; Anita Bundy, ScD, OTR; and Jodie Hanzlik, PhD, OTR

CHAPTER 23 268
Classroom Seating for Children With Attention
Deficit Hyperactivity Disorder:
Therapy Balls Versus Chairs
Denise Lynn Schilling, MS, PT; Kathleen Washington, PhD, PT;
Felix F. Billingsley, PhD; and Jean Deitz, PhD, OTR/L, FAOTA

CHAPTER 24 278
Testing the Effect of Kinesthetic Training on Handwriting
Performance in First-Grade Students
Pimjai Sudsawad, ScD, OTR; Catherine A. Trombly, ScD, OTR;
Ann Henderson, PhD, OTR; and Linda Tickle-Degnen, PhD, OTR

CHAPTER 25 289
The Use of a Weighted Vest to Increase On-Task Behavior
in Children With Attention Difficulties
Nancy L. VandenBerg, MS, OTR

CHAPTER 26 301
Outcomes of an Occupational Therapy Program for Mothers
of Children With Disabilities:
Impact on Satisfaction With Time Use and Occupational Performance
Betsy VanLeit, PhD, OTR/L, and Terry K. Crowe, PhD, OTR/L, FAOTA

**Part V. Scholarship of Discovery:
New Information for Application to Practice**

CHAPTER 27 315
Sensory-Processing Correlates of Occupational Performance
in Children With Fragile X Syndrome:
Preliminary Findings
Grace T. Baranek, PhD, OTR/L; Yuki H. Chin, MS, OTR; Laura M. Greiss Hess, MS, OTR;
Jann G. Yankee, MS, OTR/L; Deborah D. Hatton, PhD; and Stephen R. Hooper, PhD

CHAPTER 28 328
Toddlers' Persistence in the Emerging Occupations
of Functional Play and Self-Feeding
Sally J. Bober, MS, OTR/L; Ruth Humphry, PhD, OTR/L;
Heather West Carswell, MS, OTR/L; and Amanda J. Core, MS, OTR/L

CHAPTER 29 339
Pencil Grasp and Children's Handwriting Legibility
During Different-Length Writing Tasks
Julie L. Dennis, MOTR/L, and Yvonne Swinth, PhD, OTR/L

CHAPTER 30 351
Sensory-Processing Issues Associated With Asperger Syndrome:
A Preliminary Investigation
Winnie Dunn, PhD, OTR, FAOTA; Brenda Smith Myles, PhD; and Stephany Orr, MSEd

CHAPTER 31 360
Time Use and Leisure Occupations of Young Offenders
Louise Farnworth, OT, MA, PhD

CHAPTER 32 376
Effects of Billing Medicaid for Occupational Therapy Services
in the Schools:
A Pilot Study
Charlotte Brasic Royeen, PhD, OTR, FAOTA; Maureen Duncan, OTD, OTR; Jeffrey Crabtree,
OTD, FAOTA; Jeannette Richards, OTD, OTR; and Gloria Frolek Clark, MS, OTR/L, FAOTA

CHAPTER 33 384
Relationships Between Handwriting and Keyboarding Performance
of Sixth-Grade Students
Janet Rogers, MS, OTR/L, BCP, and Jane Case-Smith, EdD, OTR/L, BCP, FAOTA

CHAPTER 34 391
The School as Social Context:
Social Interaction Patterns of Children With Physical Disabilities
Pamela K. Richardson, PhD, OTR

CHAPTER 35 404
Perceptual–Motor Function of School-Age Children
With Slow Handwriting Speed
Mei Hui Tseng, ScD, OTR, and Susanna M. K. Chow, BSc, MSc, MA

**Part VI. Scholarship of Discovery: Parental Hopes,
Experiences, Perspectives, Routines, and Shifts**

CHAPTER 36 415
Parental Hopes for Therapy Outcomes:
Children With Sensory Modulation Disorders
Ellen Cohn, ScD, OTR/L, FAOTA; Lucy Jane Miller, PhD, OTR; and
Linda Tickle-Degnen, PhD, OTR/L

CHAPTER 37 428
From Waiting to Relating:
Parents' Experiences in the Waiting Room of an Occupational Therapy Clinic
Ellen S. Cohn, ScD, OTR/L, FAOTA

CHAPTER 38 441
Parent Perspectives of Occupational Therapy Using
a Sensory Integration Approach
Ellen S. Cohn, ScD, OTR/L, FAOTA

CHAPTER 39 455
Mothers' Perceptions of Child Care Assistance:
The Impact of a Child's Disability
Terry K. Crowe, PhD, OTR/L, FAOTA; Betsy VanLeit, MPA, OTR/L; and
Kirsten K. Berghmans, MS, OTR/L

CHAPTER 40 465
Shifts in Parent–Therapist Partnerships:
Twelve Years of Change
Jim Hinojosa, PhD, OT, FAOTA; Christine T. Sproat, MA, OT;
Supawadee Mankhetwit, PhD, OT; and Jill Anderson, MS, OT

CHAPTER 41 476
Constructing Daily Routines:
A Qualitative Examination of Mothers With Young Children With Disabilities
Diane Hammon Kellegrew, PhD, OTR

CHAPTER 42 488
The Orchestration of Occupation:
The Dance of Mothers
Elizabeth A. Larson, PhD, OTR

CHAPTER 43 506
Mothering Young Children With Disabilities
in a Challenging Urban Environment
Judith Olson, PhD, OTR, and Susan Esdaile, PhD, OTR, SROT

CHAPTER 44 518
Maternal Management of the Home as a
Developmental Play Space for Infants and Toddlers
Doris Pierce, PhD, OTR/L

CHAPTER 45 532
Stigma and Its Management:
A Pilot Study of Parental Perceptions of the Experiences of
Children With Developmental Coordination Disorder
*Ruth Segal, PhD, OTR; Angela Mandich, PhD, OT (reg); Helene Polatajko, PhD, OT (reg);
and Joanne Valiant Cook, PhD, OT (reg)*

CHAPTER 46 541
Adaptive Strategies of Mothers With Children With
Attention Deficit Hyperactivity Disorder:
Enfolding and Unfolding Occupations
Ruth Segal, PhD, OTR

Index 551

About the Editor 559

Writing for Success

What is *success?*[1] For parenting, it may be defined as raising a happy, healthy, and productive child. For gardening, it may be growing flowers from spring to fall. For dog training, it might be having the dog come each time a command is given. For these roles, success is relatively easy to define. But defining success for occupational therapy is more difficult.

Success for occupational therapy has meaning at different levels. First, success may be that the goals of the profession, or the services that practitioners provide to consumers, are available, paid for at fair market value, and provided in a culturally sensitive manner. Recently, the American Occupational Therapy Association (AOTA) Board of Directors initiated bold new strategic directions for AOTA, and these provide the foundation for comment and discussion by important professional and related constituent groups:

1. Unity of all in the field of occupational therapy;
2. Readiness of occupational therapy to continue in service to society as new challenges arise, based on the *International Classification of Functioning, Disability, and Health* (World Health Organization, 2001); and
3. Quality of life and participation for all.[2]

These strategic directions chart an exciting course of action for success of the profession in terms of the individuals and populations served by occupational therapy.

Second, it may be that the goals for the profession are ongoing. Goals may include

1. A professional association,
2. A code of ethics, and
3. A body of knowledge.

---

[1] With acknowledgment of the origin of this term by Elizabeth Tournquist (2003).

[2] Kramer, Hinojosa, and Royeen (2003) presented summaries of the theories of occupation explaining human participation in life authored by the pertinent theorists.

With its new strategic directions, AOTA is engaged in activities required to build and sustain occupational therapy. The profession uses the *Occupational Therapy Code of Ethics* (see Scott, 2003) and procedures for handling ethics complaints within the AOTA to appropriately monitor its members. Both AOTA and the *Code of Ethics* may be considered to be essential to the success of the profession.

Most important, however, for the development of full professional status of any field is the rigorous development of a body of knowledge. This success is accomplished through writing—hence the name of this introduction, "Writing for Success." A profession, as well as a discipline, requires that members participate in sharing their knowledge for others to use, build on, and apply. The professional and scholarly way to communicate knowledge is through writing and publishing in a journal. The critical elements of scholarship presented in this manner are that it is based on discipline-related expertise, is innovative, repeatable, documented, public, peer reviewed or systematically evaluated, and has significance for the body of knowledge.

Thus, it is my pleasure and honor to bring you this compendium of leading scholarship in pediatric occupational therapy, an important and growing area in the profession. This compilation of related articles selected from the *American Journal of Occupational Therapy* (AJOT) published from 2000 through the first quarter of 2003 reflects the commitment of many of our colleagues to build scholarship within the profession.

These authors are the heroes of our profession, for by their act of publishing in AJOT, they are participating in the formation of knowledge for use, which is the hallmark of professional and scholarly conduct. They are writing for success not only as individuals but also for our profession. For ease of use, I have

selected Boyer's model of scholarship (Boyer, 1970; Glassick, Huber, & Maeroff, 1997), which is recognized within most U.S. universities and colleges today, as the method for organizing this compilation. For the purposes of this book, I have made some minor modifications to this method.

Dimensions of Scholarship

The dimensions of scholarship are critical to occupational therapy because they broaden the notion of scholarship beyond the traditional idea of research of discovery. This revised model includes other forms of scholarship just as important for service to society. These include the scholarship of application and of integration, in addition to that of discovery. I have taken the liberty of adding the scholarship of assessment in a manner that transcends its typical use in the scholarship of teaching and learning, to include assessment as occupational therapy professionals use it in the clinical sense.

Scholarship of Application

The chapters related to the scholarship of application (Imms; Schultz-Krohn and Cara; Woodward and Swinth) all have to do with taking some degree of existing knowledge and exploring how it applies in practice. Hence, this part of the book deals with the application of knowledge and understanding about pediatric occupational therapy. Those who are studying to be pediatric occupational therapists will learn about the scholarship of application. Those who are new pediatric occupational therapists will learn to sort out what application to practice means in a clinical, school, or community-based setting. We can no longer afford to use knowledge that has been transmitted only by modeling and must incorporate what scholarship tells us is important to apply in practice, challenging ourselves to change our practice based on scholarship.

Scholarship of Integration

The chapters categorized under the scholarship of integration (Curtin, Cronin, Humphry) relate to combining knowledge and theory from distinct disciplines or professions to create a new level of understanding. This reflects an interdisciplinary perspective that is a hallmark of change and innovation. Occupational science and occupational therapy will develop more successfully if we continue to integrate our knowledge and practice with others. The classical literature in sensory integration and occupational therapy is the first such example of the scholarship of integration of two bodies of knowledge—neuroscience and occupation. Current emphasis of pediatric practice on environmental settings, functional outcomes, and family considerations reflects newer integration of scholarship from other fields into pediatric occupational therapy.

Scholarship of Assessment

The practice of occupational therapy is made possible through the use of tools, instruments, and tests that assess or measure the performance of an individual or population in reference to some standard as part of the evaluation process. The authors who wrote chapters on assessment (Burton and Dancisak; Fingerhut, Madill, Darrah, Hodge, and Warren; Johnson-Ecker and Parham; Josman and Jarus; Parush, Winokur, Goldstand, and Miller; Watling, Deitz, and White; Wilson, Kaplan, Crawford, Campbell, and Dewey) are participating in the essential production of knowledge about assessments and their validity, reliability, and appropriate use. *Validity* refers to how well an instrument measures what it is supposed to measure, and *reliability* refers to the consistency of its measurements. Pediatric occupational therapy has long been challenged to develop and refine assessment tools that meet the unique needs of evaluating a child in context considering occupational performance. This compendium contains a comforting range of assessment-related scholarship that demonstrates continuing growth in this area.

Scholarship of Discovery

The traditional notion of research is most commonly associated with the discovery or uncovering of new knowledge. In a field such as occupational therapy, the line between what constitutes scholarship of application and that of discovery is not as clear and distinct as it would be in a basic science discipline. Therefore, I have further categorized chapters into the following categories:

1. Intervention outcomes (Candler and Meeuwsen; Case-Smith; Dankert, Davies, and Gavin; Dietz, Swinth, and White; Dreiling and Bundy; Fertel-Daley, Bedell, and Hinojosa; Hartman, Miller, and Nelson; Melchert-McKearnan, Deitz, Engel, and White; Okimoto, Bundy, and Hanzlik; Schilling, Washington, Billingsley, and Dietz; Sudsawad, Trombly, Henderson, and Tickle-Degnen; Vandenberg; VanLeit and Crowe),

2. New information for application to practice (Baranek, Chin, Hess, Yankee, Hatton, and Hooper; Bober, Humphry, Carswell, and Core; Dennis and Swinth; Dunn, Myles, and Orr; Farnworth; Royeen, Duncan, Crabtree, Richards, and Clark; Rogers and Case-Smith; Richardson; Tseng and Chow), and

3. Parental hopes, experiences, perspectives, routines, and shifts (Cohn, Miller, and Tickle-Degnen; Cohn; Crowe,

VanLeit, and Berghmans; Hinojosa, Sproat, Mankhetwh, and Anderson; Kellegrew; Larson; Olson and Esdaile; Pierce; Segal, Mandich, Polatajko, and Cook).

These authors provide considerable evidence about the process of occupational therapy and its outcomes. Given current emphasis on evidence-based practice, the need for scholarship in this area is critical and the importance of the findings even more so.

Writing for Success

This collection of chapters in *Pediatric Issues in Occupational Therapy: A Compendium of Leading Scholarship* is a hallmark of the success of the authors involved and also success of the occupational therapy profession in furthering a body of knowledge in service to society. Pediatric occupational therapy makes up about one-third of all practice in the field. This compendium of scholarship, therefore, is most important in providing updated information for this large area of occupational therapy. I hope it inspires you, readers, to think about what you might be able to contribute to scholarship in pediatric occupational therapy.

—**Charlotte Brasic Royeen, PhD, OTR, FAOTA**
Dean, Edward and Margaret Doisy School of Allied Health Professions
Saint Louis University
St. Louis, MO

References

Boyer, E. L. (1970). *Scholarship reconsidered: Priorities of the professoriate.* New York: Carnegie Foundation for the Advancement of Teaching.

Glassick, C. E., Huber, M. T., & Maeroff, G. I. (1997). *Scholarship assessed: Evaluation of the professoriate.* New York: Carnegie Foundation for the Advancement of Teaching.

Kramer, P., Hinojosa, J., & Royeen, C. B. (2003). *Perspectives in human occupation: Participation in life.* Philadelphia: Lippincott Williams & Wilkins.

Scott, J. B. (Ed.). (2003). *Reference guide to the occupational therapy code of ethics.* Bethesda, MD: American Occupational Therapy Association.

Tournquist, E. (2003, November). *Writing to succeed.* Presented during the Doisy School of Allied Health's First Friday Series, Saint Louis University, St. Louis, MO.

World Health Organization. (2001). *International classification of functioning, disability, and health.* Geneva: Author.

I

Scholarship of Application

CHAPTER 1

Feeding the Infant With Congenital Heart Disease

An Occupational Performance Challenge

Christine Imms

Christine Imms, BAppScOT, MSc, *is lecturer, Occupational Therapy (Pediatrics), La Trobe University, Bundoora, Victoria 3083 Australia; c.imms@latrobe.edu.au.*

The purpose of this chapter is to review the complexities of infant feeding from an occupational performance perspective using the Canadian Model of Occupational Performance (CMOP) (Canadian Association of Occupational Therapists [CAOT], 1997) as the theoretical framework. The CMOP is a dynamic model that defines the interactions between the person and environment through occupation. The role of infant feeding in supporting infant development within various components of this theoretical model provides a background against which to view the experiences of infants with congenital heart disease (CHD). Many infants with CHD experience feeding difficulties that affect their growth and development (Combs & Marino, 1993; Lobo & Michel, 1995; Schwarz et al., 1990). Feeding the infant with CHD has also been shown to provide special challenges for caregivers (Goldberg, Simmons, Newman, Campbell, & Fowler, 1991; Svavarsdottir & McCubbin, 1996). The literature reviewed here highlights the need for further research, using the CMOP as a method of clarifying the impact of difficult feeding on the infant and family. "Infant feeding is not simply a biological process in response to the metabolic demands of a baby. It is also a complex web of behaviours involving actions and reactions of other people" (Popkin, Lasky, Litvin, Spicer, & Yamamoto, 1986, p. 2).

Theoretical Framework

The CMOP provides a way of looking at human occupation across the life span. It embodies a client-centered approach to understanding the complexity of what people need to do to participate in "life activities" (Baum & Law, 1997, p. 279), using their personal strengths and the resources of their respective environments. The model also provides a way for occupational therapists to consider the impact of disability or illness on specific occupational performance tasks, such as feed-

Originally published 2001 in *American Journal of Occupational Therapy,* 55, 277–284.

ing; of the challenges of adaptation for the person; and of the environment. In infants, viewing the occupation of feeding from a client-centered perspective ensures that occupational therapy interventions go beyond facilitating infant development of oral-motor skills to addressing the myriad complexities that contribute to successful feeding. A client-centered approach to infant feeding ensures active engagement of infants and family members in a therapeutic process that respects diversity, promotes partnership, and shares and celebrates knowledge and experience from all participants. In a client-centered approach, the therapeutic focus is on those occupations that the infant or family members need to, want to, or are expected to perform. As a multilayered framework, the CMOP assists in teasing out the complex interactions and behaviors that characterize infant feeding.

The CMOP and Infant Feeding

Occupational performance, or the ability of a person to perform an activity in a satisfactory way, is influenced by factors in three domains: the person, his or her environment, and the occupation itself. The inner spiritual person is the core of the individual and of the model. The three-dimensional figure (see Figure 1.1) represents the dynamic interaction among all levels of the CMOP. Opti-

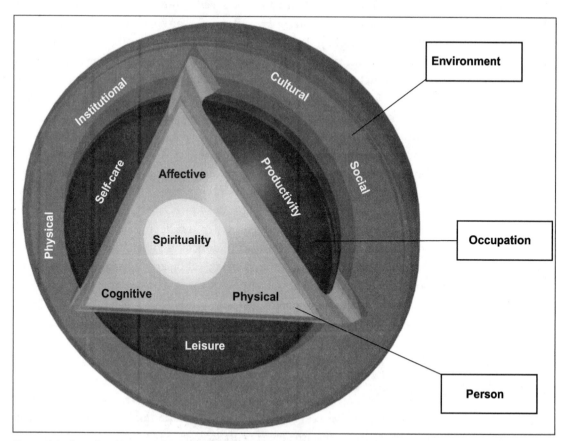

Figure 1.1. Canadian Model of Occupational Performance. *Note.* From *Enabling Occupation: An Occupational Therapy Perspective,* p. 32, by the Canadian Association of Occupational Therapists, 1997, Ottawa, Canada: CAOT Publications ACE. Copyright © 1997 Canadian Association of Occupational Therapists. Reprinted with permission.

mal occupational performance occurs when there is congruence between and across all levels of the model. With regard to feeding, the model allows exploration of the impact that the occupation of feeding can have at each level as well as the impact that the environment, the person, and other occupations can have on infant feeding.

The Person

At the person level, consideration is given to the physical, affective, and cognitive components of the person. These three performance components describe the skills and attributes the person uses to engage in occupational performance tasks. At this level, the performance components of infant feeding can be examined. Both the infant and caregiver bring cognitive, physical, and affective skills and abilities to the feeding process. Physical skills include those required to sense and satisfy hunger and to initiate and participate in the reciprocal interaction that is necessary in infant feeding. Not only do the infant and caregiver bring physical skills to the occupation of feeding, but also development of the physical skills of the infant are affected when feeding difficulties exist. The negative effect of inadequate nutritional intake on growth and physical development has been studied extensively and is known to affect a child's physical functioning, particularly neurodevelopmental status, regardless of the disorder's origin (Bithoney & Dubowitz, 1985).

Cognitive skills include communication of hunger, satiation, pleasure, and displeasure during feeding interactions. These interactive experiences result in the infant learning cause-and-effect processes and lead to an increased understanding that he or she is a participant in the manipulation and control of the environment. Chronic undernutrition and eating irregularities place children at risk for poor social and cognitive functioning (Bremner, Slater, & Butterworth, 1997;

Galler, 1984a; Rudolph, 1994) and disrupt normal parent–child interactions such as cuddling, visual attention, and vocalizations during mealtimes (Galler, 1984b).

Interactions between the infant and caregiver during feeding and the emotional bonding that can occur in successful feeding experiences provide rich opportunity for early development of the infant's affective abilities (Brazelton & Cramer, 1990; Stern, 1985, 1995) and promote the development of a relationship between the caregiver and infant. All aspects of the person level of the CMOP can and must be engaged for satisfactory occupational performance of infant feeding to occur.

The Environment

The outer sphere of the CMOP portrays the elements of the environment, including cultural, institutional, and physical and social resources that can be used to develop strategies to resolve occupational performance issues or that may contribute to occupational performance difficulties. The social context within which an infant and caregiver experience the occupation of feeding has been shown to influence infant development at the person level of the model (Hammer, 1992; Popkin et al., 1986). For example, sources and supplies of infant foods, which are related to household resources (Popkin et al., 1986), may influence feeding, which in turn may affect physical and cognitive development. In addition, the social context in which feeding occurs is important to the development of attachment, an "enduring relationship between a young child and his [or her] mother" (Ainsworth, Blehar, & Waters, 1978), and for learning social and culturally based skills (Brazelton & Cramer, 1990; Hammer, 1992; Stern, 1985, 1995). Affective development at the person level of the model is influenced by early attachment patterns that develop as the person interacts with his or her environment (Brazelton & Cramer, 1990; Stern, 1985, 1995).

Attachment patterns are not present at birth but are mediated in the first year of life through attachment behaviors (Ainsworth et al., 1978; Zeanah, Boris, & Larrieu, 1997) and are linked with the development of a reciprocal caregiving system in the caregiver (George & Solomon, 1996). As the caregiver and infant interact, social and affective exchanges occur. In early infancy, many of these interactions occur during routine tasks of feeding and sleep–wake regulation (Stern, 1995). Indeed, various authors (Lobo, 1992; Ulrey & Rogers, 1982) have used feeding as a "clinical window" (Stern, 1995, p. 70) for viewing attachment and infant–caregiver relationships, thus highlighting infant feeding as a critical occupation. The formation of secure attachment depends on the infant eliciting behavior from the caregiver and receiving reciprocal responses from the environment (George & Solomon, 1996; Zeanah et al., 1997). Research has shown that children who do not establish secure attachment are more prone to psychological or psychiatric ill health (Zeanah et al., 1997), exhibit emotional and behavioral problems in school (Lyons-Ruth, Easterbrooks, & Cibelli, 1997), and have more difficulty in their own relationships as adults (Adams & Cotgrove, 1995).

The social and cultural contexts of the feeding experience gradually give meaning to the routines and behaviors specific to the infant and the caregiver (Frank, Huecker, Segal, Forwell, & Bagatell, 1991; Hammer, 1992; Stern, 1995) and provide a key place for learning social and cultural mores (Waxler-Morrison, Anderson, & Richardson, 1990). The physical environment influences feeding methods and equipment (Popkin et al., 1986), and when infants experience ill health or developmental difficulties, they and their caregivers may encounter feeding within an institutional health care environment. Infants in the hospital may receive food by tube on schedule rather than by mouth on demand, and they and their caregivers may not experience close human contact while feeding.

In addition to the effect that the environment may have on the infant's feeding experience, infant feeding will also affect components of the environment in which it occurs. This effect may be as simple as the introduction of infant feeding equipment in the home or as complex as changing and developing the social, cultural and, perhaps, institutional experiences and roles of the caregivers.

The Occupation

The CMOP also facilitates an understanding of the complexities of occupation itself, of the intricacies of the activities of self-care or looking after personal needs, of productivity whether as a child or an adult, and of leisure or those activities that restore and refresh the person. The model defines occupation as a basic human need that is culturally defined and age related. In infancy, feeding and behavioral regulation are the key occupations (Brazelton & Cramer, 1990). Although feeding is typically classified as a self-care task throughout the rest of the life span, in infancy it can have meaning within each occupational classification. As a daily occupation, feeding is a self-care task that maintains health and well-being. Feeding is also a component of the infant's productive role. Feeding is complex and effortful, and the infant must actively engage in its dynamic process. Feeding is work and provides routine opportunity for behavioral organization. Because feeding influences the social and interactive development of the infant (Brazelton & Cramer, 1990; Popkin et al., 1986; Ulrey & Rogers, 1982), it is also implicated in the leisure component of the model.

Good nutrition and successful feeding interactions play a significant role in the development of the occupational roles of infancy and childhood, such as infant play and social interactions. In addition, infant feeding is a contributor to the development of the caregiver's parenting role (Fosson & Wilson, 1987) and may be affected by or affect other occupations, such as participation in paid employment or leisure pursuits. Recognition of the multiple occupational purposes of infant feeding highlights its importance both to infant development and to the practice of occupational therapy.

Spirituality

Spirituality, as the core of the CMOP, is seen as "the experience of meaning in everyday life" (Urbanowski & Vargo, 1994, p. 89). The model portrays spirituality as including concepts of will, drive, motivation, and self-determination. Spirituality encompasses the "innate essence of self" (CAOT, 1997, p. 43) and leads to an appreciation of the uniqueness of every person within the therapeutic context. The person's spirit is expressed through engagement in occupation (Egan & DeLaat, 1994). It is beyond the scope of this chapter to explore the developmental stages of expressed spirituality. However, Stern's (1985, 1995) portrayal of the interpersonal world of the infant lends some insight into the development of "self" in infancy and suggests a schema that represents "acts of meaning" (Stern, 1995, p. 89). Theoretically, spirituality can be influenced by the infant's early experiences as he or she negotiates daily routines. Meanings attributed to feeding experiences may be an early step in the development and expression of self for the infant and part of an ongoing search for meaning in life for the infant's caregiver.

Traditionally, occupational therapists have evaluated the physical components of feeding, including the motor control of the oral phase, physiology and safety of the swallow, and the behavioral components of the meal experience (Evans-Morris & Klein, 1987; Wolf

& Glass, 1992). The CMOP demands a holistic approach to occupational performance, encompassing broader environmental and occupational components. The model focuses attention on what the mother (or primary caregiver) provides for the infant and on the impact the infant has on his or her environment, including immediate family members. The model clearly acknowledges the dynamic and reciprocal nature of human interaction in this critical occupation.

With the use of the CMOP, feeding can be conceptualized as the interactive process between a caregiver and infant that ensures nutritional intake and provides social and emotional experiences to support development of the infant's physical, cognitive, and affective performance components. In turn, this interactive process may enable successful engagement in a variety of infant and childhood occupations. The process also affects the caregiver's occupational choices and performance. Optimal occupational performance in infant feeding will occur when all levels of the model interact with harmony.

Infants With CHD

It is common for infants to change their feeding behavior and take smaller feeds over a longer period when they become acutely ill (Conway, 1989). This change in feeding behavior may not affect the long-term development of the typical infant when the illness is short term. For infants with CHD and cardiorespiratory compromise, however, the severity and longevity of the feeding difficulty may have a significant long-term effect on both the infant and the family. The literature describing the role of feeding in supporting infant development at the person and occupation levels of the CMOP and the impact of the environment emphasizes the importance of identifying the needs of infants with CHD and their caregivers when feeding difficulties are present.

CHD is a "structural or functional heart disease that is present at birth" (Hoffman, 1990). The incidence of CHD is between 0.7% and 1.0% of live births; 85% of children born with CHD now survive into adulthood (Sparacino, 1994). Congenital heart defects range from minor anomalies, such as small atrial or ventricular septal defects, to complex conditions, such as transposition of the great arteries, tetralogy of Fallot, or univentricular heart (Le Blanc & Williams, 1993). The infant's growth may influence the timing of the surgical management of a heart defect. That is, as infants grow, complications of surgery are likely to be reduced and chances of survival increased (Le Blanc & Williams, 1993). Infants who have complex heart defects may require multiple surgical interventions spanning several years and may experience incomplete repair and cardiovascular compromise either in the interim or as a long-term outcome (Driscoll et al., 1991).

The clinical signs and symptoms of an infant with severe CHD may include cyanosis, respiratory distress, or congestive heart failure. Cyanosis results from reduced hemoglobin and arterial oxygen saturation. Respiratory distress may include an increase in respiratory rate or effort. Congestive heart failure may result in an increased heart rate, changes in cardiac rhythm and output, tachypnea, reduced activity or exercise tolerance, and early fatigue (Daberkow & Washington, 1989). Each of these symptoms may affect the infant's immediate ability to participate in the occupation of feeding (Seer, 1996).

Feeding the Infant With CHD

Indicators of the Prevalence of Feeding Difficulties

Thommessen, Heiberg, and Kase (1991) studied 40 children with CHD between 0.9 years and 13.0 years of age and found that refusal to eat or poor appetite was a significant problem for almost 50% of the children in their study. Limperopoulos et al. (1999) studied a consecutive series of 56 infants with CHD before surgery and reported that more than 53% were fed parenterally and that 5 of the 26 who were fed orally required nasogastric supplementation. Of those infants who received only oral feeds, 34% demonstrated decreased feeding efficiency characterized by longer feeding time and more frequent feeds. Varan, Tokel, and Yilmaz (1999) studied malnutrition and growth failure in 89 children with CHD and found that 65% were below the 5th percentile for weight and 41% below the 5th percentile for height. These studies provide some evidence that feeding difficulties occur for a considerable number of children with heart disease.

Indicators of the Range of Feeding Difficulties

Infants with complex CHD may experience feeding difficulties while awaiting surgical repair of their heart defect, after surgery due to complications, or in association with a congenital syndrome or anomaly, such as cleft palate (Clare, 1985; Daberkow & Washington, 1989; Park & Neches, 1993). Feeding difficulties include those related to increased respiratory effort and congestive heart failure, resulting in fatigue and inadequate caloric intake (Schwarz et al., 1990; Thommessen et al., 1991; Varan et al., 1999). Postsurgically, some infants sustain damage to the left recurrent laryngeal nerve (Park & Neches, 1993), resulting in inadequate airway protection during swallow and a high risk of aspiration. Infants with complex CHD may spend a considerable amount of time with poor oxygenation because of their heart defect and may require slow, frequent feeds. This prolonged reduction in oxygenation has been postulated to affect weight gain in these infants (Combs & Marino, 1993).

In addition, some infants with CHD present with significant oral aversion. Oral aversion may be triggered by oral intubation or surgery (Rudolph, 1994) and results in feeding refusal behaviors that are distressing for both the infant and the caregiver (Dunbar, Jarvis, & Breyer, 1991). Each of these difficulties affects the infant's performance at the person level of the CMOP, with a corresponding effect on the environment and other infant or caregiver occupations.

Feeding Strategies

Attempts to ensure that the infant receives adequate nutrition can result in an altered feeding environment. These strategies might include frequent and prolonged feeding periods, caloric supplementation by bottle or tube rather than by breast, or nasogastric tube feeds for those infants who are unable to meet their nutritional requirements orally (Thommessen et al., 1991). Because malnutrition and growth failure put infants at increased risk during surgery (Le Blanc & Williams, 1993), many studies have focused on methods of improving nutritional intake with the aim of improving surgical outcome. These studies have focused on the physiology or the physical performance components of the infant (Thommessen et al., 1991; Varan et al., 1999). For example, Schwarz et al. (1990) conducted a prospective, randomized study to compare 19 infants with CHD who were fed either by nasogastric tube continuously for 24 hours per day, by nasogastric tube for 12 hours overnight and by mouth during the day, or by mouth only. This was a well-designed and analyzed study, with data drawn from a small sample. Acting on the recommendation that continuous 24-hour nasogastric feeding is effective and safe for children with CHD would result in a significant alteration of the feeding environment and, thus, occupational performance of both the infant and the caregiver. Schwarz et al.

did not address the environmental or occupational impact of their recommendation.

Breast-Feeding and Bottle-Feeding

Recently, there has been a growing interest in the breast-feeding experiences of infants with CHD. Traditionally, breast-feeding was thought to be more stressful for the infant than bottle-feeding, and many mothers were encouraged to feed by bottle (Combs & Marino, 1993; Lambert & Watters, 1998). In a comparison of growth patterns in bottle-fed and breast-fed infants with CHD, Combs and Marino (1993) found that both breast-fed and bottle-fed infants lost weight over 5 months. Bottle-fed infants, however, lost more weight than did breast-fed infants. This descriptive, correlational study, which compared 45 mother–infant dyads, also gave insight into the person–environment interactions that occur as mothers choose their infant-feeding method. The institutional environment (i.e., length of hospital stay) was found to be positively and significantly related to the mothers' decisions to change from breast-feeding to bottle-feeding.

In a later study, Marino, O'Brien, and LoRe (1995) compared seven infants with CHD who were both breast-fed and bottle-fed and found that when the infants were breast-fed, they had greater physiological stability with fewer oxygen desaturations and a more stable postfeed period. A number of limitations existed for this study, including the very small sample size and the disparity in bottle nipple flow rates. However, both of these studies suggest potential improvement of the physiology and physical performance of the infant during breast-feeding compared with bottle-feeding. In addition, the findings suggest a positive impact of breast-feeding on the infant's social environment through the mother–infant interaction.

The positive impact of breast-feeding on the mother–infant environment is supported by the results of an informal breast-feeding survey of 12 parents of children with CHD (Lambert & Watters, 1998). These authors found that institutional barriers, fasting protocols, and infant factors, such as respiratory distress or congestive heart failure, were obstacles to breast-feeding. This self-selected group of parents, however, also reported emotional benefits for themselves and health, growth, and emotional benefits for their infants from breast-feeding. Successful breast-feeding may provide many of the social and emotional opportunities that hospitalized infants appear to be at risk for missing (Combs & Marino, 1993; Gaskin, 1987; Lobo, 1992; Lobo & Michel, 1995).

Mother–Infant Interactions During Feeding

Lobo (1992) reported on a study that investigated the dynamic interactions between mothers and infants during feeding. She compared infants with CHD ($n = 10$) with a healthy control group ($n = 10$). The Nursing Child Assessment Feeding Scale (Barnard, 1978) was used to assess maternal and infant behavior. The findings suggest that infants with CHD gave fewer clear cues and were less responsive to their mothers during feeds than infants without CHD. Mothers of children with CHD also provided less social and emotional growth opportunities while feeding, such as smiling, making eye contact, touching, or singing, than mothers of infants without CHD. Whether the differences in maternal behavior developed in response to infant cues or to maternal fear and stress related to infant fragility remained unclear at the end of this study. Lobo and Michel (1995) analyzed the same data for behavioral and physiological responses during feeding. They found no relationship between physiological response and behavioral cues. However, infants with CHD gave significantly more subtle disengagement cues, such as finger splaying or hand-to-head actions,

than did the healthy infants. This finding suggests that the affective cues of infants with CHD are more difficult to interpret. Small sample sizes and multiple statistical analyses limit these studies; however, the findings suggest that there may be difficulties in the interaction dynamic between the person and environment during the occupation of feeding when the infant has CHD.

Caregiver Stress Related to Feeding

The impact of feeding on the infant's social environment has also been studied in relation to parent stress and time spent in caregiving tasks. Caregivers of children with CHD felt significantly more stress than those of children with other chronic illnesses, and they identified feeding as a key contributor to their stress (Goldberg, Morris, Simmons, Fowler, & Levison, 1990; Svavarsdottir & McCubbin, 1996; Thommessen et al., 1991). Thommessen et al. (1991) found that 65% ($n = 40$) of the parents they studied described feeding children with CHD as difficult, time consuming, and anxiety producing. While studying the information needs of 30 mothers of infants with CHD, Stinson and McKeever (1995) found that more feeding information was the second most frequent request made, supporting Pinelli's (1981) earlier findings. Svavarsdottir and McCubbin (1996) investigated parenthood transitions for 70 parents of infants with CHD younger than 12 months of age. The mothers reported feeding to be the most time consuming and the third most difficult task of their day. The mothers in Combs and Marino's (1993) study supported the finding of increased time spent feeding, with anecdotal evidence suggesting that they were spending 1 hour out of every 2 or 3 hours feeding their infants. The impact of time spent feeding on the occupational choices of the caregivers was not reported in these studies.

These studies of caregiver time use related to feeding are limited by their lack of comparative control group data. However, in other research, families of healthy infants were found to spend only 2.3 hours per day if they had one child and up to 2.9 hours per day if they had four children on all food preparation tasks (Walker & Woods, 1976). Other studies of the challenges of caregiving in relation to time use have not specifically looked at the impact of difficult feeding on time spent caring for a child, and they do not address children with CHD. However, the studies do indicate that families who have a child with a disability spend more time on caregiving tasks than families who do not have children with disabilities (Breslau, 1983; Brust, Leonard, & Sielaff, 1992; Crowe, 1993; Johnson & Deitz, 1985).

Discussion

The literature suggests that feeding in infancy is a complex, multifaceted, and highly critical occupation that is vital to health and well-being. To date, these highly complex feeding processes have been studied in a piecemeal fashion, thus challenging health professionals and family members to determine what "successful feeding" is and how best to facilitate it. The CMOP provides a framework that enables clarification of the multiple factors involved in infant feeding. The dynamic nature of the CMOP means that disturbances at any level of the model will affect other levels. Success in this critical occupation of feeding can influence and be influenced by factors in the infant, the environment, and other occupational areas.

According to the model, successful occupational performance in feeding in infancy will support appropriate development of physical, affective, and cognitive skills at the person level. Environmental variations in physical, cultural, and social contexts may alter the method, style, and specific activities that each infant experiences around feeding. Consequently, each infant will

gradually learn varying behaviors, values, and beliefs on the basis of his or her social and cultural experiences (Waxler-Morrison et al., 1990). These in turn may contribute to the infant's experience of meaning in everyday life (Urbanowski & Vargo, 1994), once again illustrating the interaction among the levels of the CMOP.

The negative effect of inadequate nutrition on each component of the person level of the CMOP supports a medical focus on ensuring optimal nutritional input to infants and the emergence of alternative methods of feeding when oral intake is not sufficient. However, few studies address the broader implications of changing how an infant's nutritional needs are met as the change relates to the ability of either the infant or caregiver to participate successfully in occupational performance tasks.

A causal relationship between occupational performance difficulties in infant feeding and social–emotional difficulties in early or late childhood has not been established. However, feeding is an important component in the early affective development of the child and may have later consequences in the child's ability to participate successfully in their chosen or required occupations. The relationship between early feeding difficulties and later occupational performance, however, requires further investigation.

For the caregiver, feeding provides an opportunity to confirm and develop the parenting role (Fosson & Wilson, 1987) as well as a reciprocal opportunity to develop a relationship with the infant (Brazelton & Cramer, 1990; Stern, 1985, 1995). Caregivers of infants with CHD were found to experience some of the occupational challenges of caregiving, including feeding, as stressful and time consuming (Stinson & McKeever, 1995; Svavarsdottir & McCubbin, 1996; Thommessen et al., 1991). It is not yet clear, however, which components of feeding contribute to this stress or which interventions are effective in promoting the development of the caregiving role as well as infant feeding skills.

Occupational research based on the CMOP could combine ethnographic methodology and quantitative measurement to uncover the complexity of the infant-feeding experience when the infant has CHD. Exploration of caregivers' needs and hopes might be gathered through caregiver narrative. Information on the impact of feeding on the infant's occupational opportunities, such as the frequency of shared social and cultural experiences within the family mealtime environment, could be gathered through participant observation or diary recordings. The influence of difficult feeding on caregiver and infant patterns of occupation and time use could also be measured through participant observation or direct measurement of time use.

Identifying the scope and multiple effects of difficult feeding is unlikely to be simple. Use of the CMOP allows for multiple factors to be exposed, thus facilitating the negotiation of interventions with caregivers that support both infants and caregivers in their quest for meaningful and satisfying feeding experiences.

Acknowledgment

I thank Margaret McCuaig, OT(c), MA, for her helpful comments on the original draft of this chapter.

References

Adams, L., & Cotgrove, A. (1995). Promoting secure attachment patterns in infancy and beyond. *Professional Care of Mother and Child, 5*(6), 158–160.

Ainsworth, M. D. S., Blehar, M., & Waters, E. (1978). *Patterns of attachment: Psychological study of the strange situation.* Hillsdale, NJ: Erlbaum.

Barnard, K. (1978). *Nursing child assessment feeding scales.* Seattle: University of Washington, School of Nursing.

Baum, C. M., & Law, M. (1997). Occupational therapy practice: Focusing on occupational performance. *American Journal of Occupational Therapy, 51,* 277–288.

Bithoney, W. G., & Dubowitz, H. (1985). Organic concomitants of nonorganic failure to thrive: Implications for research. In D. Drotar (Ed.), *New directions in failure to thrive: Implications for research and practice* (pp. 47–68). New York: Plenum.

Brazelton, T. B., & Cramer, B. G. (1990). *The earliest relationship: Parents, infants and the drama of early attachment.* Reading, MA: Addison-Wesley.

Bremner, G., Slater, A., & Butterworth, G. (1997). *Infant development: Recent advances.* Sussex, UK: Psychology Press.

Breslau, N. (1983). Care of disabled children and women's time use. *Medical Care, 21,* 620–629.

Brust, J. D., Leonard, B., & Sielaff, B. H. (1992). Maternal time and the care of disabled children. *Public Health Nursing, 9*(3), 177–184.

Canadian Association of Occupational Therapists. (1997). *Enabling occupation: An occupational therapy perspective.* Ottawa, Ontario: Author.

Clare, M. D. (1985). Home care of infants and children with cardiac disease. *Heart and Lung, 14,* 218–222.

Combs, V., & Marino, B. (1993). A comparison of growth patterns in breast and bottle-fed infants with congenital heart disease. *Pediatric Nursing, 19,* 175–179.

Conway, A. (1989). Young infants' feeding patterns when sick and well. *Maternal–Child Nursing Journal, 18,* 296–339.

Crowe, T. (1993). Time use of mothers with young children: The impact of a child's disability. *Developmental Medicine and Child Neurology, 35,* 621–630.

Daberkow, E., & Washington, R. (1989). Cardiovascular diseases and surgical interventions. In A. Merenstein & J. Gardner (Eds.), *Handbook of neonatal intensive care* (2nd ed., pp. 427–464). St. Louis, MO: Mosby.

Driscoll, D. J., Offord, K., Feldt, R., Schaff, H. V., Puga, F. J., & Danielson, G. K. (1991). Five to fifteen year follow-up after Fontan operation. *Circulation, 85,* 469–495.

Dunbar, S. B., Jarvis, A. H., & Breyer, M. (1991). The transition from nonoral to oral feeding in children. *American Journal of Occupational Therapy, 45,* 402–408.

Egan, M., & DeLaat, D. (1994). Considering spirituality in occupational therapy practice. *Canadian Journal of Occupational Therapy, 61,* 95–101.

Evans-Morris, S., & Klein, M. D. (1987). *Pre-feeding skills.* Tucson, AZ: Therapy SkillBuilders.

Fosson, A., & Wilson, J. (1987). Family interactions surrounding feedings of infants with nonorganic failure to thrive. *Clinical Pediatrics, 26,* 518–523.

Frank, G., Huecker, E., Segal, R., Forwell, S., & Bagatell, N. (1991). Assessment and treatment of a pediatric patient in chronic care: Ethnographic methods applied to occupational therapy practice. *American Journal of Occupational Therapy, 45,* 252–263.

Galler, J. R. (1984a). The behavioral consequences of malnutrition in early life. In J. Galler (Ed.), *Nutrition and behavior* (Vol. 5, pp. 63–111). New York: Plenum.

Galler, J. R. (Ed.). (1984b). *Nutrition and behavior* (Vol. 5). New York: Plenum.

Gaskin, I. M. (1987). *Babies, breastfeeding and bonding.* South Hadley, MA: Bergin & Garvey.

George, C., & Solomon, J. (1996). Representational models of relationships: Links between caregiving and attachment. *Infant Mental Health Journal, 17,* 198–216.

Goldberg, S., Morris, P., Simmons, R. J., Fowler, R., & Levison, H. (1990). Chronic illness in infancy and parenting stress: A comparison of three groups of parents. *Journal of Pediatric Psychology, 15,* 347–358.

Goldberg, S., Simmons, R., Newman, J., Campbell, K., & Fowler, R. (1991). Congenital heart disease, parental stress, and infant–mother relationships. *Journal of Pediatrics, 119,* 661–666.

Hammer, L. (1992). The development of eating behavior in childhood. *Pediatric Clinics of North America, 39,* 379–393.

Hoffman, J. I. E. (1990). Congenital heart disease: Incidence and inheritance. *Pediatric Clinics of North America, 37,* 25–43.

Johnson, C. B., & Deitz, J. C. (1985). Time use of mothers with preschool children: A pilot study. *American Journal of Occupational Therapy, 39,* 578–583.

Lambert, J., & Watters, N. (1998). Breastfeeding the infant/child with a cardiac defect: An informal survey. *Journal of Human Lactation, 14,* 151–155.

Le Blanc, J. G., & Williams, W. G. (1993). *The operative and perioperative management of congenital heart defects.* New York: Academic Press.

Limperopoulos, C., Majnemer, A., Shevell, M. I., Rosenblatt, B., Rohlicek, C., & Tchervenkov, C. (1999). Neurologic status of newborns with congenital heart defects before open heart surgery. *Pediatrics, 103,* 402–408.

Lobo, M. (1992). Parent–infant interaction during feeding when the infant has congenital heart disease. *Journal of Pediatric Nursing, 7,* 97–105.

Lobo, M., & Michel, Y. (1995). Behavioral and physiological response during feeding in infants with congenital heart disease: A naturalistic study. *Progress in Cardiovascular Nursing, 10*(3), 26–34.

Lyons-Ruth, K., Easterbrooks, M. A., & Cibelli, C. D. (1997). Infant attachment strategies, infant mental lag, and maternal depressive symptoms: Predictors of internalizing and externalizing problems at age 7. *Developmental Psychology, 33,* 681–692.

Marino, B., O'Brien, P., & LoRe, H. (1995). Oxygen saturations during breast and bottle feedings in infants with congenital heart disease. *Journal of Pediatric Nursing, 10,* 360–364.

Park, S. C., & Neches, W. H. (1993). The neurologic complications of congenital heart disease. *Neurology Clinics, 11,* 441–462.

Pinelli, J. (1981). A comparison of mothers' concerns regarding the care-taking of newborns with congenital heart disease before and after assuming their care. *Journal of Advanced Nursing, 6,* 261–270.

Popkin, B., Lasky, T., Litvin, J., Spicer, D., & Yamamoto, M. (1986). *The infant-feeding triad: Infant, mother and household* (Vol. 5). New York: Gordon and Breach Science.

Rudolph, C. (1994). Feeding disorders in infants and children. *Journal of Pediatrics, 125*(6), S116–S124.

Schwarz, S., Gewitz, M., See, C., Berezin, S., Glassman, M., Medow, C., et al. (1990). Enteral nutrition in infants with congenital heart disease and growth failure. *Pediatrics, 86,* 386–373.

Seer, M. (1996). Nutrition. In J. G. Le Blanc & W. G. Williams (Eds.), *The operative and perioperative management of congenital heart defects* (pp. 383–400). New York: Futura.

Sparacino, P. (1994). Adult congenital heart disease: An emerging population. *Nursing Clinics of North America, 29,* 213–219.

Stern, D. (1985). *The interpersonal world of the infant: A view from psychoanalysis and developmental psychology.* New York: Basic.

Stern, D. (1995). *The motherhood constellation: A unified view of parent–infant psychotherapy.* New York: Basic.

Stinson, J., & McKeever, P. (1995). Mother's information needs related to caring for infants at home following cardiac surgery. *Journal of Pediatric Nursing, 10,* 48–57.

Svavarsdottir, E. K., & McCubbin, M. (1996). Parenthood transition for parents of an infant diagnosed with a congenital heart condition. *Journal of Pediatric Nursing, 11,* 207–216.

Thommessen, M., Heiberg, A., & Kase, B. F. (1991). Feeding problems in children with congenital heart disease: The impact on energy intake and growth outcome. *European Journal of Clinical Nutrition, 46,* 457–464.

Ulrey, G., & Rogers, S. (1982). *Psychological assessment of handicapped infants and young children.* New York: Thieme-Stratton.

Urbanowski, R., & Vargo, J. (1994). Spirituality, daily practice, and the occupational performance model. *Canadian Journal of Occupational Therapy, 61,* 88–94.

Varan, B., Tokel, K., & Yilmaz, G. (1999). Malnutrition and growth failure in cyanotic and acyanotic congenital heart disease with and without pulmonary hypertension. *Archives of Diseases in Childhood, 81,* 49–52.

Walker, K. E., & Woods, M. (1976). *Time use: A measure of household production of family goods and services.* Washington, DC: American Home Economics Association.

Waxler-Morrison, N., Anderson, J., & Richardson, E. (1990). *Cross cultural caring.* Vancouver, BC: UBC Press.

Wolf, L., & Glass, R. (1992). *Feeding and swallowing disorders in infancy.* Tucson, AZ: Therapy Skill-Builders.

Zeanah, C. H., Boris, N. W., & Larrieu, J. A. (1997). Infant development and developmental risk: A review of the past 10 years. *Journal of American Academy of Child and Adolescent Psychiatry, 36,* 165–178.

CHAPTER 2

Occupational Therapy in Early Intervention

Applying Concepts From Infant Mental Health

Winifred Schultz-Krohn and Elizabeth Cara

Winifred Schultz-Krohn, MA, OTR, BCP, FAOTA, *is assistant professor, Occupational Therapy, San Jose State University, One Washington Square, San Jose, CA 95192-0059; winifred@email.sjsu.edu.*

Elizabeth Cara, MA, OTR, MFCC, *is assistant professor, Occupational Therapy, San Jose State University, San Jose, CA.*

A family-centered approach has been promoted for several years in the practice arena of early intervention and occupational therapy (Anderson & Hinojosa, 1984; Day, 1982; Friedman, 1982). Lawlor and Mattingly (1998) recently discussed various problems embedded in family-centered care, such as defining the client, the professional role, and the nature of work within a family-centered approach. Problems involving collaboration, trust, and equality of decision making can occur when the therapist shifts from an intervention that focuses on the child to one that incorporates the family. Lawlor and Mattingly also presented concerns regarding cultural conflicts and service fragmentation. Hence, the occupational therapist working within early intervention is required to shift focus on many levels: intrapersonal, interpersonal, cultural, and theoretical.

This article focuses on the challenges of shifting to a family-centered approach. Current problems in early intervention from an occupational therapy perspective are discussed. The field of infant mental health has much to offer early intervention occupational therapy. A therapeutic approach that incorporates concepts from infant mental health practice into early intervention occupational therapy is proposed (Emde, 1987; Lieberman & Pawl, 1993; Zeanah, 1993). A description of infant mental health practice that illustrates how ideas from this approach can be blended into early intervention occupational therapy practice is provided. Finally, a case study is presented to demonstrate the application of this blended approach in practice.

Current Occupational Therapy Practice in Early Intervention

Originally published 2000 in *American Journal of Occupational Therapy, 54,* 550–554.

Occupational therapists in pediatric practice demonstrate a wide but disparate range of family-centered care practices (Brown, Humphry, & Taylor, 1997; Humphry, Gonzales, & Taylor, 1993). Brown et al. (1997) identified a seven-level hierarchy of family–therapist involvement. These levels represent a progressive shift in therapeutic intervention from defining the client as an individual to defining the client as a member of a family. At the same time, the levels also shift from the clinician acting as the director of the intervention plan to the family serving as the coordinator of the intervention plan. Although this hierarchy identifies a means to engage the family as an active member of the intervention plan, the focus of occupational therapy service continues to be on the individual client rather than on the family.

Overall, the delivery of family-centered practice within the field of occupational therapy lacks coherence (Lawlor & Mattingly, 1998). Even when occupational therapy literature embraces the concepts of family-centered intervention, the presumed outcome is still identified in terms of the individual child and not in terms of the family function (Brown et al., 1997; Humphry et al., 1993). This is in contrast to a family systems approach that identifies the recipient of service as the family in total (DeMuth, 1994; Dunst, Trivette, & Thompson, 1994). The family systems approach focuses on the changing roles of the family as an evolving entity (Bronfenbrenner, 1986). Several authors have suggested the need to adopt a family systems approach in pediatric occupational therapy intervention (Crowe, VanLeit, Berghmans, & Mann, 1997; Humphry, 1989). Humphry (1989) called for pediatric occupational therapists to consider not only the child's developmental skills, but also the parent–child relationship as part of the intervention plan. Contemporary infant mental health practice provides a framework for occupational therapy to incorporate a family systems model into an intervention plan (Emde, 1987).

Infant Mental Health Practice Concepts

Infant mental health is a field composed of various professionals, such as developmental psychologists, psychiatrists, social workers, and early intervention educators (Bretherton, 1992; Emde, 1987; Zeanah, 1993). The goal of infant mental health practice is to assist an infant under 3 years of age to achieve the necessary socioemotional skills and psychological development to function in his or her immediate environment (Lieberman & Pawl, 1993). Historically, infant mental health intervention was directed toward an infant when the parents had a mental illness. Currently, infant mental health practice focuses on the dynamic relationship between the child and parents or caregivers, who may or may not have a mental illness.

The evaluation process in infant mental health requires the clinician to use observational skills and introspection (Lieberman & Pawl, 1993). Information on the parent–infant relationship is gathered by observing how the parent and child interact, how the child functions developmentally and emotionally, and how the parent experiences the child. At the same time, the infant mental health therapist must assess his or her own threshold for forming an alliance with parents who may have a mental illness or who may have been rejected by a bureaucratic system. Families seen in an infant mental health program often have a history of dysfunction and frequently are disadvantaged economically and socially. Parents may have had prior negative experiences with health services, and these experiences may be transferred to the therapist, clouding perceptions of the current treatment program.

Infant mental health practice consists of three core interventions operating simultaneously: infant–parent psychotherapy or psychoanalytic intervention, nondidactic developmental guidance, and direct support and advocacy (Fraiberg, 1980, 1982; Fraiberg, Adelson, & Shapiro, 1975; Lieberman & Pawl, 1993; Seligman, 1994). These interventions integrate psychoanalysis, developmental psychology, and social work.

Psychoanalytic intervention consists of two strategies for intervention (Lieberman & Pawl, 1993; Seligman, 1994). First, the therapist provides comments that help parents become aware of how they may be reenacting their own traumatic childhood experiences with their infants. Questions posed to a parent such as "Why is it important for the infant to eat an entire bowl of cereal?" may reveal a traumatic experience that a parent had regarding eating. Explicitly identifying these experiences allows the parents to examine the child's behavior in a new light. Second, a therapeutic relationship is established between the therapist and parent to disrupt the negative influence the parent's prior relationships has on current parent–child interaction. The therapist mirrors positive aspects of parent–child interaction back to the parent in the form of comments. For example, a therapist will remark that a child's glances at the parent are signals of love.

Nondidactic developmental guidance is a method of providing developmental information that assumes parents are best able to use information about their children when the relational aspects and affective dynamics are considered (Lieberman & Pawl, 1993; Seligman, 1994). Instead of giving advice, a therapist might ask the parent what he or she thinks or observes about a child's experience. The therapist encourages the parent to view the infant's behavior from alternate perspectives, thus interrupting the current view of the behavior that stems from the parent's own prior negative experiences. This approach supports parental self-exploration and a change in behavior. A change in parental behavior may pro-

duce a change in the infant and, consequently, in the parent–child interaction. An example may be an infant who has eaten enough but has also dropped food on the floor around the high chair. The parent is convinced that the infant rejects the food and does not eat enough. The therapist might ask the parent how much food a 16-month-old infant needs or might remark on the ability of the child to distinguish what he wants to eat while learning to use utensils. The reframing of parental observations does not negate the original observations but provides an alternate explanation for the parent to consider.

Direct support and advocacy includes any activity that directly bolsters the caregiving relationship (Lieberman & Pawl, 1993; Seligman, 1994). Direct support provides a model of a caring relationship that can be translated into a caring parent–child dyad. It can include referrals to public housing agencies or social services or practical assistance with everyday tasks such as shopping or laundry. Often, these concrete interventions provide needed relief and supply some measure of hope to the family.

Providing these core interventions simultaneously in the home can be a challenge for the therapist because the usual professional boundaries of a clinical environment are nonexistent. However, providing family-centered care requires working on these complex levels.

Early Intervention Occupational Therapy and Infant Mental Health

Infant mental health practice has core intervention strategies that can be adapted for use in pediatric occupational therapy (Fraiberg, 1980, 1982; Fraiberg et al., 1975; Lieberman & Pawl, 1993; Seligman, 1994). By adapting these intervention strategies, many of the recently acknowledged challenges to providing family-centered occupational therapy may be resolved (Lawlor & Mattingly, 1998). Additionally, a new model of pediatric occupational therapy can be formed that will clarify the role and the delivery of occupational therapy service using a family-centered approach.

The goal of pediatric occupational therapy, like the goal of infant mental health practice, is to assist the client to achieve satisfactory function socially, emotionally, and psychologically in a natural environment (Lieberman & Pawl, 1993). However, infant mental health practice is focused on the infant's impact on the parent and their relationship; the "client" is identified as the parent and child and their relationship. Although pediatric occupational therapists do not typically address the issue of transference, they use clinical reasoning skills to observe and actively search for ways to enter into alliances or "develop rapport" (Fleming, 1991; Mattingly, 1991; Neistadt, 1996; Rogers, 1982).

An infant mental health approach offers a framework for identifying the strengths and vulnerabilities of the parents and infants and provides a focus for treatment (Lieberman & Pawl, 1993). The treatment observations, along with the desires and needs of the parents, dictate the structure and place of treatment or who is present for the sessions (Cara, 1997). Clearly, pediatric occupational therapy contributes special skills regarding child evaluation, but the parent does not always direct how those skills will be used. Therefore, by adapting the infant mental health framework and responding to the wishes of the parent about structure, direction, and place of treatment, the issue of treatment collaboration is addressed (Lawlor & Mattingly, 1998). This framework also addresses the interacting cultural worlds of the practitioner and family. The occupational therapist is quickly able to learn about the everyday life of the family—their habits, routines, values,

idiosyncrasies, or unique rituals embedded in daily encounters.

Recognizing that both child and caregiver are recipients of service expands the concept of what constitutes early intervention occupational therapy service. Applying intervention strategies from the field of infant mental health practice equips occupational therapists with the tools to meet the demands of this expanded practice. Nondidactic developmental guidance supports a self-righting tendency of the parent–child system (Seligman, 1994). This strategy supports the idea that the caregiver and child have strengths and attributes that can be used for positive change along with the special expertise of the therapist. Use of direct support and advocacy strategies enables the therapist to address multiple dimensions of therapy (Lawlor & Mattingly, 1998). This aspect of service includes activities that directly bolster the parent–child relationship and, therefore, the services provided for the child. These concrete interventions often provide needed relief so that parents will be able to devote other time and emotional sustenance toward the child.

In summary, adapting the interventions of infant mental health to early intervention occupational therapy offers practical strategies that address the challenges of using a family-centered approach (Lawlor & Mattingly, 1998). The use of interventions based on clinical reasoning, nondidactic guidance, and concrete support may ameliorate the problems faced by the occupational therapist providing family-centered intervention.

Case Illustration

The following case illustrates the use of infant mental health care approaches in home-based early intervention occupational therapy. The occupational therapist, one of the authors, speaks limited Spanish.

The family consisted of a 19-year-old mother, whom we will refer to as Maria, a 2 1/2-year-old daughter, and a 16-month-old son. Maria, originally from a Caribbean island but now living in Connecticut, spoke Spanish and English. Maria's family had returned to the place of birth, but she chose to remain in Connecticut with her children. Although an aunt lived in Connecticut, Maria had limited contact with her. Maria was unemployed, living in a subsidized housing project, and unable to attend school because of her children's needs.

Both children had been identified as eligible for early intervention services under the Individuals With Disabilities Education Act of 1990 (P.L. 101–476). Her daughter had developmental delays in the area of language and received home-based services from an early intervention educator weekly. The interventionist who provided services for the daughter said that Maria would often leave the room during the weekly visits and did not appear interested in completing the suggested home exercises. Maria's son had cerebral palsy and a seizure disorder. He had been evaluated by an early intervention identification team and referred for weekly occupational therapy and physical therapy services.

At the time that occupational therapy services were initiated, Maria had a limited understanding of the role of occupational therapy services for her son. The therapist reviewed the focus of occupational therapy with Maria and asked her to help develop the treatment plan for her son. Maria responded by indicating that the therapist was the expert and should develop the care plan. Maria appeared both intimidated by the therapist and resistant to participating in the development of an intervention plan. When asked how other medical professionals interacted with her, Maria reported that the physicians gave her pills for her son and the nurse told her how to feed him. Her past experiences with medical professionals gave her the impression that they were authorities, and she believed that they acted disrespectfully toward her. As a teenage mother, Maria seemed angry that the medical professionals did not approach her as an adult. She appeared to transfer that anger to the therapist and assumed that the therapist would act in a similarly disrespectful manner.

Although the son was the identified client, a family systems approach was used to engage Maria in the decision-making process for her son's care. The focus of the occupational therapy services was to foster developmental gains in the boy through the endorsement of Maria's role as an authority in the care of her children. This represents a shift from defining the client as the child to defining the client as the family.

During the initial visit to the home, two of Maria's friends were present and were overheard asking her for advice regarding boyfriends, family issues, and pregnancy. Maria apparently had a position of authority in her peer group because of her life experiences and her demonstrated ability to care for two children with special needs. There was an apparent discrepancy in her occupational roles: a voice of authority with her friends and a passive recipient of authority with early interventionists.

An attempt was made to engage Maria in developing the care plan for her son by acknowledging her as the expert regarding what activities her son could and could not perform. Maria was then asked to prioritize which activities were most important within the context of her family life. The occupational therapist elicited Maria's perceptions of her son's strengths and challenges, engaging her through the process of interactive and narrative clinical reasoning (Mattingly, 1991). Essentially, the therapist asked Maria to tell her own story about her son and did not rely solely on previous medical evaluations. The treatment plan was developed by asking Maria to evaluate her son's function and role within the family system rather than using a standardized instrument that would compare her son's skills with typical development. The therapist chose not to ask Maria what parenting tasks were difficult for her, a question that would have placed her in a position of admitting lacking parenting skills instead of developing her role as an authority regarding her children. Maria identified difficulties her son had in eating and moving his arms. He was only able to eat pureed foods because of poor oral-motor control. Maria's unique knowledge of her son was used to develop the care plan, and her concerns dictated the course of therapy.

Toward the end of the first home visit, specific feeding techniques were presented in a framework similar to home exercises but with a distinct difference. The techniques were not prescribed; instead, nondidactic developmental guidance was used in first providing suggested feeding methods and then asking the mother to evaluate the effectiveness of these methods.

At the second appointment, Maria reported how successful the suggested techniques had been to promote feeding skills with her son. Maria then asked the therapist to watch how well her son was eating. Maria said that she wanted to introduce textured foods to her son and asked for additional techniques that were then provided by the occupational therapist. These new techniques represented direct support toward Maria's goal of improving her son's feeding skills. Maria was developing her role as the director of the care plan for her son. She, herself, had identified additional needs for her son instead of relying on the therapist.

During subsequent home appointments, Maria was very engaged in activities with her son and appeared eager to learn new techniques to help him develop functional skills. Activities were designed to meet Maria's needs in caring for her children and the children's need to interact with each other. These needs, addressed through support and advocacy, were identified by Maria as a priority for family function. Specific support was provided by informing her of parenting groups held without cost, connecting her with parental support groups in the area, and discussing respite care as an option. The therapist did not make the arrangements for these services but encouraged Maria to use them. In this role, the therapist facilitated Maria's directive role within the family. The other early interventionists commented that she had begun to take a more active role with her son and daughter. Services were continued for an additional 8 weeks, and then Maria decided to move back to her birthplace to be with her family.

Discussion

Occupational therapy services were provided to foster developmental abilities in the son using a family-centered approach that recognized both child and caregiver as recipients of therapy. Instead of the occupational therapist serving as the expert, the strengths of the mother were facilitated. It was evident that this mother had begun to establish a position of expertise with her peers regarding child care; those already established skills were incorporated into the intervention plan. The occupational therapist demonstrated an ability to enter the cultural world of this family. Instead of delegating the mother to a role of helping in the occupational therapy program, she directed the program. The focus of occupational therapy intervention was on strengthening family roles. The mother's developing role as an expert in the care of her children was recognized and fostered within the intervention plan. The family system, particularly the mother–infant relationship and the mother's role in the family, appeared to be strengthened by this approach, which then facilitated changes in the son.

The goal of occupational therapy intervention was to improve the son's developmental skills and was achieved through the use of a family-as-client approach. In this case report, we attempted to illustrate the effectiveness of a family-as-client approach even though an individual family member was the designated client. Strategies adapted from infant mental health practice were demonstrated. Knowledge of bureaucratic transference enabled the therapist to view this mother's initial resistant response to early interventionists from an alternate perspective and to reframe the interaction between the mother and therapist. Use of nondidactic developmental guidance promoted the directive role this young mother was beginning to develop within the family system. Finally, direct support was provided to assist this family with daily function. This article suggests a useful theory and practice model from which occupational therapists may address problems encountered in early intervention and expand intervention techniques in their roles with pediatric clients and their families.

References

Anderson, J., & Hinojosa, J. (1984). Parents and therapists in a professional partnership. *American Journal of Occupational Therapy, 38,* 452–461.

Bretherton, I. (1992). The origins of attachment theory: John Bowlby and Mary Ainsworth. *Developmental Psychology, 28,* 759–775.

Bronfenbrenner, U. (1986). Ecology of the family as a context for human development: Research perspectives. *Developmental Psychology, 22,* 723–742.

Brown, S. M., Humphry, R., & Taylor, E. (1997). A model of the nature of family–therapist relationships: Implications for education. *American Journal of Occupational Therapy, 51,* 597–603.

Cara, E. (1997). *Infant mental health.* Unpublished manuscript, San Jose State University, San Jose, CA.

Crowe, T. K., VanLeit, B., Berghmans, K. K., & Mann, P. (1997). Role perceptions of mothers with young children: The impact of a child's disability. *American Journal of Occupational Therapy, 51,* 651–661.

Day, S. (1982). Mother–infant activities as providers of sensory stimulation. *American Journal of Occupational Therapy, 36,* 579–585.

DeMuth, D. H. (1994). A global paradigm for family therapists in the 21st century. In B. B. Gould & D. H. DeMuth (Eds.), *The global family therapist* (pp. 3–21). Needham Heights, MA: Allyn & Bacon.

Dunst, C. J., Trivette, C. M., & Thompson, R. B. (1994). Supporting and strengthening family functioning: Towards a congruence between principle and practice. In C. J. Dunst, C. M. Trivette, & A. G. Deal (Eds.), *Supporting and strengthening families: Methods, strategies, and practices* (pp. 49–59). Cambridge, MA: Brookline Books.

Emde, R. (1987). Infant mental health: Clinical dilemmas, the expansion of meaning and opportunities. In J. Osofsky (Ed.), *Handbook of infant development* (pp. 1297–1320). New York: Wiley.

Fleming, M. (1991). The therapist with the three-track mind. *American Journal of Occupational Therapy, 45,* 1007–1014.

Fraiberg, S. (1980). *Clinical studies in infant mental health: The first year of life.* New York: Basic Books.

Fraiberg, S. (1982). Pathological defenses in infancy. *Psychoanalytic Quarterly, 51,* 612–635.

Fraiberg, S., Adelson, E., & Shapiro, V. (1975). Ghosts in the nursery: A psychoanalytic approach to the problem of impaired infant–mother relationships. *Journal of American Academy of Child Psychiatry, 14,* 387–422.

Friedman, B. (1982). A program for parents of children with sensory integrative dysfunction. *American Journal of Occupational Therapy, 36,* 586–589.

Humphry, R. (1989). Early intervention and the influence of the occupational therapist on the parent–child relationship. *American Journal of Occupational Therapy, 43,* 738–742.

Humphry, R., Gonzales, S., & Taylor, E. (1993). Family involvement in practice: Issues and attitudes. *American Journal of Occupational Therapy, 47,* 587–593.

Individuals With Disabilities Education Act. (1990). Pub. L. 101–476, 20 U.S.C., Ch 33.

Lawlor, M. C., & Mattingly, C. F. (1998). The complexities embedded in family-centered care. *American Journal of Occupational Therapy, 52,* 259–267.

Lieberman, A. F., & Pawl, J. H. (1993). Infant parent psychotherapy. In C. Zeanah (Ed.), *Handbook of infant mental health* (pp. 427–442). New York: Guilford.

Mattingly, C. (1991). The narrative nature of clinical reasoning. *American Journal of Occupational Therapy, 45,* 998–1005.

Neistadt, M. (1996). Teaching strategies for the development of clinical reasoning. *American Journal of Occupational Therapy, 50,* 676–684.

Rogers, J. C. (1982). Teaching clinical reasoning for practice in geriatrics. *Physical and Occupational Therapy in Geriatrics, 1*(4), 29–60.

Seligman, S. (1994). Applying psychoanalysis in an unconventional context. *Psychoanalytic Study of the Child, 49,* 481–500.

Zeanah, C. (Ed.). (1993). *Handbook of infant mental health.* New York: Guilford.

CHAPTER 3

Multisensory Approach to Handwriting Remediation

Perceptions of School-Based Occupational Therapists

Sara Woodward and Yvonne Swinth

Sara Woodward, MOT, OTR/L, *is occupational therapist, Puyallup School District, 214 West Main Street, Puyallup, WA 98371. At the time of this study, she was graduate student, School of Occupational Therapy and Physical Therapy, University of Puget Sound, Tacoma, WA.*

Yvonne Swinth, PhD, OTR/L, *is associate professor, School of Occupational Therapy and Physical Therapy, University of Puget Sound, Tacoma, WA. She also is occupational therapist, University Place School District, University Place, WA.*

Originally published 2002 in *American Journal of Occupational Therapy,* 56, 305–312.

One of the most important and complex childhood occupations is learning to transmit thoughts and information through written language (Amundson, 1992). Even with recent technological advances that have reduced the need for handwritten communication, handwriting continues to be important throughout a student's elementary school education (Amundson, 1992; Lindsay & McLennan, 1983). Without legible handwriting, children are denied a mode of communication that is still heavily relied on within our society. At school, children are required to write for a variety of academic purposes, including in-class assignments and tests. At home, children may be required to take phone messages, complete homework assignments, or write letters to family members. Given these requirements, it is no wonder that children spend a considerable amount of time in the first few years of school practicing fine motor paper–pencil skills, such as drawing and writing (Laszlo & Bairstow, 1984).

In a study of the relationship between visuomotor and handwriting skills, Weil and Amundson (1994) concluded that most children who are typically developing will be ready for standard handwriting instruction in the latter part of their kindergarten year. Although students who are typically developing are fairly competent at printed writing tasks by 6 or 7 years of age, students with learning disabilities, developmental delays, or neurological impairments may struggle with a standard handwriting curriculum and the task of writing legibly (Bergman & McLaughlin, 1988). Services that go beyond the scope of a standard handwriting curriculum are needed if these children are to become proficient at the task of handwriting.

Children are frequently referred to school-based occupational therapists for handwriting difficulties in the classroom (Clark-Wentz, 1997; Oliver, 1990). Amundson and Weil (1996) stated that the therapist is responsible for identifying underlying motor, sensory, cognitive, or psychosocial deficits that may interfere with the development of legible handwriting and for selecting intervention strategies to overcome those deficits. Although classroom teachers are primarily responsible for the instruction of handwriting, school-based occupational therapists often support teachers by identifying and treating deficits interfering with the development of this skill (Dennis & Swinth, 2001; Reisman, 1991; Tseng & Cermak, 1993). Through classroom observation and examination of work samples, a therapist is able to identify related performance components and administer assessments designed to determine whether deficits in the identified components exist and to what extent (Amundson & Weil, 1996).

Cornhill and Case-Smith (1996) found that students with poor handwriting, as identified by teacher report, scored significantly lower on three assessments of sensorimotor performance components (eye–hand coordination, visuomotor integration, in-hand manipulation) than students with good handwriting. They also found that scores on assessments of these performance components could be used to predict scores in handwriting performance. Weil and Amundson (1994) also found a significant relationship between visuomotor skills and handwriting performance. These findings are consistent with those of Tseng and Cermak (1993). They also suggest that the assessment of suspected performance component deficits is an important part of a comprehensive handwriting assessment.

When deficits in sensorimotor performance components are identified, a multisensory approach often is taken to remediate handwriting problems (Amundson, 1992; Reis, 1990; Rutherford, 1991; Vickery & Cochran, 1987). However, research on the effectiveness of a multisensory approach has been sparse, and findings have been inconsistent (Harris & Livesey, 1992; Lockhart & Law, 1994; Oliver, 1990). Humphries, Wright, Snider, and McDougall (1992) compared sensory integration therapy and perceptual–motor training in treating children

with learning disabilities. They found motor gains in children from both experimental conditions but no group differences or improvements in handwriting performance. As can be seen, previous studies appear to provide support for the use of a multisensory approach for children with learning disabilities, but findings are preliminary.

From the literature, writing tools and surfaces appear to be an important part of a multisensory approach to handwriting. Several studies have examined the effects of different traditional writing materials, such as writing paper and writing tools, on handwriting performance. Lindsay and McLennan (1983) and Weil and Amundson (1994) reported that for beginning writers, lined paper may add an element of confusion and compromise legibility. Krzesni (1971) found the opposite to be true for older children—legibility improved with lined paper in 9-year-old children. Halpin and Halpin (1976) compared handwriting quality in kindergarten children with 1-in.-spaced paper and 1.5-in.-spaced paper and found no significant differences. In a study of writing tools, Lamme and Ayris (1983) found that writing tools did not affect legibility. Krzesni, on the other hand, found a significant increase in writing performance with a felt pen.

Although traditional writing instruction involves sitting at a desk with paper and a no. 2 pencil, a multisensory approach to handwriting uses a plethora of modalities and activities (Amundson, 1992). Appendix 3.1 lists the modalities and activities that have been indicated in the literature. Although studies have provided preliminary support for the effectiveness of a multisensory approach in children with handwriting readiness and handwriting problems (Harris & Livesey, 1992; Lockhart & Law, 1994; Oliver, 1990), no attempt has been made to document systematically the multisensory modalities and activities that school-based occupational therapists use. Studies have compared a multisensory approach with nonmultisensory approaches without documenting the effectiveness of the specific multisensory modalities and activities. Further, these studies have not defined consistently the meaning of a multisensory approach.

Therefore, the purpose of the present study was to determine by national survey what multisensory modalities and activities U.S. school-based occupational therapists currently use in the remediation of handwriting problems in school-age children and to compare these practices to current literature on the subject. Specifically, the study attempted to answer the following questions:

1. What are the most frequently used multisensory modalities and activities in the remediation of handwriting problems, and how many different modalities and activities do therapists use per student?
2. Is there consensus among school-based therapists about which sensory systems the modalities and activities address?
3. Is there a difference in the multisensory modalities and activities used on the basis of demographic variables?

For the purpose of this study, a multisensory approach to handwriting remediation involves using a variety of sensory experiences, media, and instructional materials to control the sensory input and tap into the child's sensory systems, including the proprioceptive, vestibular, tactile, visual, auditory, olfactory, and gustatory senses (Amundson & Weil, 1996).

Method

Sample

A sample of 313 occupational therapists out of approximately 5,000 was randomly selected by the American Occupational Therapy Association's (AOTA's) direct mail service. Therapists eligible for selection were those members who identified themselves as working in a school system as their primary employment setting, recognizing, however, that their employer may be a hospital or private clinic, they may be an independent contractor with the school system, or both. According to the 1996 AOTA Member Data Survey, 17.9% of all registered occupational therapists indicated working in a school system as their primary employment setting (AOTA Research Department, personal communication, November 4, 1997). Because approximately 35,500 registered occupational therapists are members of AOTA, our sample represents approximately 1% of all members and approximately 5% of all school-based occupational therapist members.

Instrument

Each therapist in the sample received a three-part survey by mail. The first part focused on demographic information, such as years of experience as an occupational therapist, last year completed working as a school therapist, age group of children with which the therapist primarily works, employment status within the school, caseload, service delivery model used by the school setting, current position of employment, certification or training status, and geographic setting. The second part consisted of a list of 25 multisensory modalities and activities and a 5-point Likert scale (1 = *never*, 5 = *very often*) for respondents to indicate the frequency of use of each modality and activity. Respondents also were asked to indicate the primary sensory systems they believed each modality and activity addressed. Three closed-ended questions asked them to indicate (a) their top-five modalities and activities used most often, (b) the average number of modalities and activities used per student, and (c) the frames of reference used in handwriting remediation. An open-ended question provided respondents the opportunity to explore what they might say to a school administrator who inquired about the rationale behind a multisensory approach. The third part of the survey was a comment section, inviting respondents to clarify, add to, or comment on any of the survey's contents.

The survey was designed for one-time use; therefore, reliability and validity are unknown. Content of the survey was based on an extensive literature review and feedback from the researcher's faculty advisor and five pilot study participants with extensive experience in schools, research, or handwriting remediation. Recommendations for changes primarily focused on organization and wording rather than on survey content. After these changes were made, the survey was reviewed once more by two therapists who have worked in public schools.

Data Collection

Questionnaires were sent to the sample, with a follow-up mailing at 3 weeks to increase the response rate (Salant & Dillman, 1994). A stamped return envelope was included with each questionnaire. Mailing labels were coded for confidentiality.

Data Analysis

Data from returned surveys were analyzed with the Statistical Package for the Social Sciences (SPSS, 1995). Frequency distributions were used to describe the sample demographics, the use of each of the 25 modalities and activities and the primary sensory systems the respondents believe each modality and activity addresses, the number of modalities and activities used per student, and the characteristics of the rationale described in response to the open-ended question. Measures of central tendency were used to describe mean years of experience and mean caseload. Chi-square analysis was used to compare the responses received from the first mailing with those received

from the second mailing to detect possible response bias. Chi-square analysis also was used to assess the relationship between modalities and activities used and demographic information.

Results

Of the 313 surveys in the first mailing and the 208 in the second mailing to school-based occupational therapists, 207 were returned. Of these, 198 were analyzed, resulting in a 63.3% response rate. Eight surveys were returned blank, and 1 survey from the second mailing had a matching identification number to 1 from the first mailing. Three returned surveys were missing only demographic information, but they were included in this study to increase the number of respondents included in the descriptive statistics on multisensory modality and activity use.

Question 1 asked whether respondents use a multisensory approach in treating children with handwriting problems. The majority (92.1%) indicated yes. Those responding no were asked to stop and return the survey without completing the rest, and these were not used in the analysis.

The frequency distributions for the demographic variables are presented in Table 3.1. The majority of respondents reported working in public schools (83.9%), of which 60.0% were full-time employees. Suburban schools was the most frequently reported setting (48.6%). Respondents primarily served the kindergarten to junior high school age group (6–15 years) (74.7%) under the service delivery model of individual or small group pull-out (49.2%). Respondents reported having the most years of experience as occupational therapists in the public schools ($M = 9.14$ years, $SD = 5.87$), with a mean caseload of 38.13 students ($SD = 21.83$). Respondents working in schools often work with students across a variety of ages and may be employed by a facility other than the school. These demographic variables

Table 3.1. Frequency Distributions for
Demographic Variables[a]

Variable	*n*	%
Employment status directly in school setting (*n* = 180)		
Full-time	108	60.0
Part-time	59	32.8
Not at all	13	7.2
Current position of employment (*n* = 180)[b]		
Public school	151	83.9
Other[c]	68	37.8
Geographic setting (*n* = 179)		
Suburban	87	48.6
Rural	51	28.5
Urban	41	22.9
Primary age group (*n* = 162)		
Early intervention (0–3 years)	5	3.1
Preschool (3–5 years)	36	22.2
K to junior high (6–15 years)	121	74.7
High school (16–21 years)	0	0.0
Service delivery model (*n* = 177)		
Individual or paired pull-out	87	49.2
Student in classroom	47	26.6
Small group pull-out	12	6.8
Classroom consultation	12	6.8
Small group in classroom	10	5.6
Set up and monitor intervention	7	4.0
Entire classroom	2	1.1

[a]Participants who responded yes to working in a school system.
[b]Respondents were allowed to indicate more than one current position of employment.
[c]Other positions of employment respondents indicated included private contracted services, private school, hospital, and private practice.

were not used to exclude respondents as long as they answered yes to Question 1.

Frequency distributions of respondents reporting using each of the 25 modalities and activities often or very often and the primary sensory system indicated for each modality and activity are shown in Table 3.2. A majority of respondents reported using chalk and chalkboard (87.3%), magic markers or felt pens (76.0%), verbal description while student writes (71.2%), finger writing in viscous substances (64.8%), and copying and tracing on regular lined paper (63.2%) and colored or embossed lined paper (61.0%) often or very often. Only 7.6% used bags of hair gel for finger tracing often or very often.

The primary sensory system reported ranges from 64.1% agreement for design copying on paper strips and masking tape on the floor (visual) to 100.0% agreement for wrist weights (proprioceptive) (see Table 3.2).

The most frequently reported number of multisensory modalities and activities used per student was five or more (36.9%), whereas 8.9% reported using two and none using only one. Respondents using three multisensory modalities and activities per student were 32.4%, and 21.8% used four per student.

Questions 10 and 11 of the survey allowed respondents to add additional multisensory modalities and activities to the list. Respondents added 114, 13 of which were mentioned five or more times. These modalities and activities are forming letters with pipe cleaners or Wikki Stix®[1] (*n* = 30); forming letters with play dough, clay, or putty (*n* = 16); using vibrating pens (*n* = 13); writing with water on chalkboard with sponges or paint brushes (*n* = 11); Handwriting Without Tears™[2] (*n* = 11); finger writing with vision occluded (*n* = 9); Callirobics™[3] or writing to music (*n* = 8); combining activities with therapy ball or scooter (*n* = 8); drawing on student's back or hand (*n* = 7); using body to form letters (*n* = 5); weight bearing on forearms in prone (*n* = 5); tracing tactile letters with fingers (*n* = 5); and using computer activities (*n* = 5). Of the 114 different modalities and activities included in the returned surveys, 72 are mentioned only once. None of the 114 modalities and activities were included in the data analyses.

Chi-square tests of independence revealed no significant differences in multisensory modality

[1]Omnicor, Inc., 2432 West Peoria #1188, Phoenix, AZ 85029; www.wikkistix.com.

[2]Jan Olsen, OTR, 8802 Quiet Stream Court, Potomac, MD 20854; www.hwtears.com.

[3]Callirobics™, PO Box 6634, Charlottesville, VA 22906; www.callirobics.com.

Table 3.2. Frequency Distributions[a] of Therapists Reporting Modality and Activity Use as Often or Very Often and Primary Sensory Systems

Modality and Activity	n	%	Primary Sensory System (PSS)		
			PSS	n	%
Chalk and chalkboard	157	87.3	P	149	85.6
Magic markers or felt pens	139	76.0	I	138	80.7
Verbal description of letter shapes while student writes	129	71.2	A	156	95.1
Viscous substances, such as shaving cream, for finger writing	118	64.8	T	159	95.2
Copying and tracing letters on regular lined paper	115	63.2	I	140	84.8
Colored or embossed lined paper	111	61.0	I	131	79.4
Forming letters in a tray of rice or sand with a finger	87	48.1	T	158	95.8
Letter forming with a finger or dowel in clay	85	46.9	T	136	82.9
Tracing or copying letters over a rough surface	82	45.1	T	148	89.2
"Sky writing" letters in the air	78	43.3	P	155	91.7
Block design	70	39.1	I	141	87.6
Bead stringing	65	35.7	T	122	73.9
"Rainbow writing" using different colors to copy the same letter	60	33.0	I	137	87.8
Colored writing lines that represent the sky, grass, and dirt	56	30.7	I	131	89.7
Grease pencils on a plastic template over letters	50	27.6	I	107	70.4
Carpet squares and chalk	47	26.2	T	128	85.9
Dried glue for writing lines	47	25.8	T	145	92.9
Parquetry	43	23.7	I	126	85.1
Wrist weights	43	23.7	P	153	100.0
Paper folding	40	21.9	T	98	64.9
Design copying on paper strips and masking tape on the floor	25	14.0	I	84	64.1
Shape tracing behind a masking box with vision occluded	21	11.5	P	99	75.6
Tracing letters with a magic marker over cellophane	20	10.9	I	85	65.4
Black construction paper covered with salt	18	10.0	T	125	88.0
Bags of hair gel for finger tracing	14	7.6	T	131	92.9

Note. P = proprioceptive; I = visual; A = auditory; T = tactile.
[a]Respondents who left these questions blank were not included.

and activity use based on the demographic variables of service delivery model, primary age group of students served, employment status, and geographic setting. For years of practice in public schools, a significant difference was found for 1 of the 25 modalities and activities: design copying on paper strips and masking tape on the floor, $\chi^2(6, 176) = 23.9$, $p < .001$, that is, more respondents with 5 to 9 years of experience reported a frequent use of this modality than expected. For caseload, a significant difference also was found for 1 of the 25 modalities and activities: bags of hair gel for finger tracing, $\chi^2(4, 177) = 19.5$, $p < .001$, that is, more respondents with caseloads of greater than 50 reported the frequent use of this modality than expected.

When provided with a hypothetical scenario involving explaining the rationale for the use of multisensory modalities and activities to a school administrator, at least 50% of the respondents provided explanations. The explanations most often addressed a particular modality or activity that the respondent reported using, as in the following example:

I often have the child form letters on the blackboard to promote wrist extension and use small pieces of chalk to promote good pencil grasp. We draw letters on the board, trace them, say how to draw the lines, [and] draw with eyes closed, so many sensory systems are alerted, and the letter pattern becomes part of the muscle memory.

Common themes identified in the explanations were making learning fun, tapping into as many senses as possible, and stressing the importance of exploring and finding the ways that students learn best. All of these themes are reflected in the following statement by one respondent:

> The more sensory pathways stimulated during a learning task for both children and adults, the more success we have and the greater our memory for the task will be. Also, the more interesting I make the activity, the more likely the child/children are to participate, enjoy, and remember.

Discussion

A multisensory approach to treating children with handwriting problems is an important and frequent area of practice for school-based occupational therapists as indicated by the significantly large percentage of respondents (92.1%) reporting use of this approach. Descriptive statistics revealed that the highest percentage of respondents work with preschool-age through junior high school–age students on handwriting. The fact that the greatest percentage work with these age groups could be explained partly by well-known theories of neural plasticity. These theories suggest that younger children may benefit greatly from therapy because of their rapidly developing and changing nervous systems (Parham & Mailloux, 1996). For younger and older groups, other skills may be more of a focus than handwriting skills. Because there was no way for therapists not working on handwriting to indicate this on the survey, the very few respondents who indicated working in early intervention or high school settings may have found the survey to be irrelevant to their practice and, thus, may have contributed to the rate of nonrespondents.

In addressing the study's first question of which multisensory modalities and activities are used most often in the remediation of handwriting problems, results indicate that of the 25 presented, 6 are used often or very often by at least 60% of the respondents (see Table 3.2). It was expected that therapists would have reported using more of the 25 often or very often because they were cited in the literature (Amundson, 1998; Harris & Livesey, 1992; Lockhart & Law, 1994; Oliver, 1990; Weiser, 1986) and, therefore, assumed to be used frequently. The fact that respondents reported 114 additional modalities and activities and that 36.9% indicated using 5 or more per student indicates a wide range of multisensory modalities and activities used in the remediation of handwriting problems and that therapists are creative when implementing a multisensory approach.

Multisensory modalities and activities appear to fall into four general categories. As stated in the literature review, writing tools and writing surfaces are an important part of a multisensory approach to handwriting. The results of this survey support this statement. Three of the modalities and activities used most often involve adaptations to standard writing tools and surfaces (e.g., magic markers, vertical or slanted writing surfaces). Commercially available writing programs (e.g., Callirobics, Handwriting Without Tears) also emerged in the results. Many respondents mentioned specific performance components, including intrinsic muscle development and eye tracking. Finally, many modalities and activities involved the use of common children's toys (e.g., Play-Doh™, Etch-a-Sketch®[4]).

Results for the second research question of whether consensus exists among school-based therapists about which sensory systems they believe the modalities and activities address are inconclusive. Some respondents indicated only one sensory system for each modality and activity, whereas others indicated anywhere from one to

---

[4]The Ohio Art Company, One Toy Street, PO Box 111, Bryan, OH 43506-0111; www.world-of-toys.com.

six. This pattern of responses does not demonstrate whether those who indicated only one sensory system made their selection on the basis of their understanding of the question or because they believe it to be the only sensory system affected. Because many of the modalities and activities address more than one sensory system, respondents may have found it difficult to determine which sensory systems are "primarily" stimulated. Additionally, although different respondents may be using the same modalities and activities, they may be doing so for the purpose of stimulating different sensory systems.

In addressing the study's third research question, no differences in modality and activity use appeared to be based on demographic variables. Exceptions are noted for only 1 of the 25 both for years of practice in public schools and for caseload. For the most part, these general results indicate that school-based therapists across the United States are using similar multisensory modalities and activities no matter the service delivery model, size of caseload, primary age group of students, years of school-based practice, geographic setting, or employment status. It appears that many students receiving occupational therapy services for handwriting problems are being exposed to a wide range of multisensory modalities and activities, but demographic variables are not related to the modalities and activities used. This survey did not gather data related to the clinical reasoning behind the respondents' choices, which may be worth exploring in future studies.

Responses to the open-ended question that asked respondents to explore what they might say to a school administrator who inquired about the rationale behind the use of a multisensory approach indicate that therapists believe in the importance of a multisensory approach to handwriting. This belief, as well as the belief in the importance of selecting modalities and activities based on the student's individual needs, is reflected in the following statement from a respondent: "It is very important to use a variety of modalities/activities in the remediation of handwriting. The stimulation, fun, interest, and motivational factors play a part in the activities chosen for each child." It may be that the high number and variety of modalities and activities indicated by respondents make it possible to meet a variety of student needs.

Implications for Occupational Therapy

The results of this study indicate that approximately 90% of school-based occupational therapists responding to this survey use a multisensory approach when treating students identified as having handwriting difficulties. Through existing research and the results of this study, more than 130 different multisensory modalities and activities have been identified as being used in the remediation of handwriting problems. The use of these modalities and activities does not appear to be related to demographic variables. The results of this study suggest that therapists are imaginative in devising and have a wide range from which to choose of multisensory modalities and activities for use in handwriting remediation.

Limitations

Limitations of this study include unclear wording of certain survey questions, all respondents being members of AOTA, and missing data. As stated earlier, some of the survey respondents indicated one sensory system when asked to identify the primary sensory systems for each modality and activity, whereas others indicated up to six, which may be due to potential unclear wording of the survey. It is unclear whether some respondents thought that they should indicate only one "primary" sensory system or whether they believed that only one sensory system is stimulated by the modality and activity. Several respondents did not complete the demographic sections of the survey, whereas others did not respond to some of the items regarding multisensory modalities and activities, resulting in some item-wise exclusions during data analysis.

Directions for Future Research

This research was a pilot study. Suggestions for further research are to examine the effectiveness of those modalities and activities used most often in the remediation of handwriting problems, modify the survey item regarding primary sensory systems to specify the number of responses sought, and carry out a qualitative study that addresses clinical reasoning of school-based therapists and why different modalities and activities are chosen.

Conclusion

A survey study was conducted to describe the current use of a multisensory approach to handwriting remediation by school-based occupational therapists. Results revealed a large number of multisensory modalities and activities being used by occupational therapists. However, only a few of them were used often or very often by at least half of the respondents. The number of different modalities and activities identified in this study as being used in a multisensory approach to handwriting remediation is greater than previously expected and indicates room for creativity when designing individual treatment. Consensus among respondents about the primary sensory systems targeted by the modalities and activities is inconclusive. On the basis of the broad and varied results obtained in this study, further quantitative and qualitative research is needed in this area to examine further therapists' clinical reasoning related to a multisensory treatment approach to handwriting problems. A clearer understanding of the reasoning leading to the different modalities and activities identified may help with the efficiency and effectiveness of school-based occupational therapy focused on handwriting.

This understanding, in turn, may improve students' occupational performance in handwriting.

Acknowledgments

We thank the survey respondents who participated in this study; Susie Amundson, MS, OTR/L; Sandi Koch, OTR/L; Juli McGruder, PhD, OTR/L; Zadie Rogers, OTR/L; and Katherine Stewart, MS, OTR/L, for their participation in this study's pilot study; and Martins Linauts, PhD, PT, for his knowledge and guidance. We also thank the University of Puget Sound Enrichment Committee for its research grant.

This article is based on the first author's thesis completed in partial fulfillment of the requirements for a master's degree in occupational therapy at the University of Puget Sound in Tacoma, WA.

Appendix 3.1.
Multisensory Modalities and Activities Used in Handwriting Remediation Found in the Literature

- Bags of hair gel for finger tracing
- Bead stringing
- Black construction paper covered with salt
- Block design
- Carpet squares and chalk
- Chalk and chalkboard
- Colored or embossed lined paper
- Colored writing lines that represent the sky, grass, and dirt
- Copying and tracing letters on regular lined paper
- Design copying on paper strips and masking tape on the floor
- Dried glue for writing lines
- Forming letters in a tray of rice or sand with a finger

(continued)

- Grease pencils on a plastic template over letters
- Letter forming with a finger or dowel in clay
- Magic markers or felt pens
- Paper folding
- Parquetry
- "Rainbow writing" using different colors to copy the same letter
- Shape tracing behind a masking box with vision occluded
- "Sky writing" letters in the air
- Tracing letters with a magic marker over cellophane
- Tracing or copying letters over a rough surface
- Verbal descriptions of letter shapes while student writes
- Viscous substances, such as shaving cream, for finger writing
- Wrist weights

Note. Compiled from Amundson, 1998; Harris & Livesey, 1992; Lockhart & Law, 1994; Oliver, 1990; Weiser, 1986.

References

Amundson, S. J. (1992). Handwriting: Evaluation and intervention in school settings. In J. Case-Smith & C. Pehoski (Eds.), *Development of hand skills in the child* (pp. 63–78). Rockville, MD: American Occupational Therapy Association.

Amundson, S. J. (1998). *TRICS for written communication: Techniques for rebuilding and improving children's school skills.* Homer, AK: O.T. Kids.

Amundson, S. J., & Weil, M. (1996). Prewriting and handwriting skills. In J. Case-Smith, A. S. Allen, & P. N. Pratt (Eds.), *Occupational therapy for children* (pp. 524–544). St. Louis, MO: Mosby.

Bergman, K. E., & McLaughlin, T. F. (1988). Remediating handwriting difficulties with learning disabled students: A review. *B.C. Journal of Special Education, 12,* 101–120.

Clark-Wentz, J. (1997). Improving students' handwriting. *OT Practice, 2*(9), 29–33.

Cornhill, H., & Case-Smith, J. (1996). Factors that relate to good and poor handwriting. *American Journal of Occupational Therapy, 50,* 732–739.

Dennis, J. L., & Swinth, Y. (2001). Pencil grasp and children's handwriting legibility during different-length writing tasks. *American Journal of Occupational Therapy, 55,* 175–183.

Halpin, G., & Halpin, G. (1976). Special paper for beginning handwriting: An unjustified practice? *Journal of Educational Research, 69,* 267–269.

Harris, S. J., & Livesey, D. J. (1992). Improving handwriting through kinaesthetic sensitivity practice. *Australian Occupational Therapy Journal, 39,* 23–27.

Humphries, T., Wright, M., Snider, L., & McDougall, B. (1992). A comparison of the effectiveness of sensory integrative therapy and perceptual-motor training in treating children with learning disabilities. *Journal of Developmental and Behavioral Pediatrics, 13*(1), 31–40.

Krzesni, J. S. (1971). Effect of different writing tools and paper on performance of the third grader. *Elementary English, 7,* 821–824.

Lamme, L. L., & Ayris, B. M. (1983). Is the handwriting of beginning writers influenced by writing tools? *Journal of Research and Development in Education, 17,* 32–38.

Laszlo, J. I., & Bairstow, P. J. (1984). Handwriting: Difficulties and possible solutions. *School Psychology International, 5,* 207–213.

Lindsay, G. A., & McLennan, D. (1983). Lined paper: Its effects on the legibility and creativity of young children's writing. *British Journal of Educational Psychology, 53,* 364–368.

Lockhart, J., & Law, M. (1994). The effectiveness of a multisensory writing programme for improving cursive writing ability in children with sensorimotor difficulties. *Canadian Journal of Occupational Therapy, 61,* 206–214.

Oliver, C. E. (1990). A sensorimotor program for improving writing readiness skills in elementary-age children. *American Journal of Occupational Therapy, 44,* 111–116.

Parham, L. D., & Mailloux, Z. (1996). Sensory integration. In J. Case-Smith, A. S. Allen, & P. N. Pratt (Eds.), *Occupational therapy for children* (pp. 307–356). St. Louis, MO: Mosby.

Reis, E. M. (1990). Multisensory approaches for teaching handwriting to learning-disabled children. *Journal of Instructional Psychology, 17*(4), 190–193.

Reisman, J. E. (1991). Poor handwriting: Who is referred? *American Journal of Occupational Therapy, 45*, 849–852.

Rutherford, L. H. (1991, November/December). For sweet success, use multisensory approaches to teach writing. *Social Studies*, pp. 243–244.

Salant, P., & Dillman, D. (1994). *How to conduct your own survey*. New York: Wiley.

Statistical Package for the Social Sciences, release 6.1 [Computer program]. (1995). Chicago: SPSS, Inc.

Tseng, M. H., & Cermak, S. A. (1993). The influence of ergonomic factors and perceptual-motor abilities on handwriting performance. *American Journal of Occupational Therapy, 47*, 919–926.

Vickery, K. S., & Cochran, S. W. (1987). Multisensory teaching approach for reading, spelling and handwriting, Orton-Gillingham based curriculum, in a public school setting. *Annals of Dyslexia, 37*, 189–200.

Weil, M. J., & Amundson, S. J. (1994). Relationship between visuomotor and handwriting skills of children in kindergarten. *American Journal of Occupational Therapy, 48*, 982–988.

Weiser, D. (1986). Handwriting: Assessment and remediation. *Developmental Disabilities Special Interest Section Newsletter, 9*(3), 4–5.

II
Scholarship of Integration

CHAPTER 4

Eliciting Children's Voices in Qualitative Research

Clare Curtin

Clare Curtin, PhD, OTR, *is school-based occupational therapist, Jefferson County Public Schools, Golden, CO, and private practitioner, Children and Youth First Services, 1524 19th Avenue, Longmont, CO 80501.*

Children can be reliable informants and provide accurate accounts of their experiences (Lamb, Sternberg, Orbach, Hershkowitz, & Esplin, 1999; Zwiers & Morrissette, 1999). However, engaging children in qualitative research and eliciting their voices involve different challenges and research methods than research with adults. The purpose of this chapter is to identify these challenges and provide practical suggestions for talking with and obtaining the perspectives of preschool- and elementary-school-age children. Implications for clinical practice also are presented.

Qualitative researchers can reap benefits from involving children as informants, especially when examining childhood occupations (e.g., play) or pediatric occupational therapy practice. This involvement provides an opportunity for the researcher to learn about the children's worlds and perspectives, including the personal meanings children attribute to events and actions. The researcher can learn from the children's own knowledge and experience and gain a better understanding of the phenomena being studied. In addition, children can benefit from being active participants in the research process. The experience of having a voice may give children practice in making life decisions and may help develop perceptions of control and the view of being altruistic (Weithorn & Scherer, 1994). Children's participation in decision making may also promote a sense of being responsible for their own lives versus being "powerless victims of the whims of adults" (Weithorn, 1983, p. 241).

Yet, at least three major impediments to incorporating children as research participants can exist. The first is that the researcher may assume that children are less competent participants and maintain a conscious or unconscious belief of his or her superior knowledge. Acting on these beliefs, the researcher may not even think to include children as active contributors in the research, may focus only on what children cannot do, or may not value the children's perspectives. Second, in the typical adult–child relationship, an inequality in the

Originally published 2001 in *American Journal of Occupational Therapy,* 55, 295–302.

power relations exists because the adult is considered the authority (Alldred, 1998). This difference in power may affect the children's comfort in expressing their thoughts and feelings and the adult's evaluation of the children's ideas. Third, children and adults have different communication styles. For example, children more than adults often rely on nonverbal language and silence as primary methods of communication (Curtin, 1995). Consequently, the researcher may find it more difficult and challenging to communicate with children than with adults to elicit information of depth and richness.

Therefore, to involve children as research participants, the researcher is challenged to (a) examine his or her own beliefs regarding children's competencies, (b) define a different adult–child relationship that minimizes the power differential (Fine, 1987), and (c) learn the children's communication styles in order to elicit the children's perspectives and develop a common language (Curtin, 1995). In addition, the researcher needs to use research techniques that do not rely only on verbal language.

Methodological Challenges

Examining Beliefs Regarding Children's Competence

In past studies of children, researchers tended to focus more on children as "objects of inquiry" (Graue & Walsh, 1995, p. 136) than as informants. These studies typically examined developmental processes instead of children's perspectives of their own world (Alldred, 1998). Oakley (1994) argued that in the theoretical frameworks underlying many studies of children, "the emphasis is not on what children are, but on what they are not" (p. 22). She proposed that this stance is prevalent in theories of development.

Graue and Walsh (1995) maintained that a lack of studies with children as informants exists because researchers have assumed that "children are too developmentally immature to be able to think conceptually or to have the language necessary to be able to express their ideas" (p. 146). Similarly, Waksler (1986) argued that there are two prevalent beliefs regarding children's competencies. The first is that adults tend to think of children as being not grown up, immature, and thus "not something" (p. 74). She maintained that adults tend to view children as knowing less, being less serious, and being less important than themselves. The second belief is that "children are routinely wrong, in error, and don't understand" (p. 76). Thus, Waksler contended that adults tend to assume that they are superior to children because of their maturity and experience. She advocated the viewpoint that children are different from adults, not inferior. Qvortrup (1994) also stressed the importance of viewing children as "human beings, not only 'human becomings'" (p. 18).

Tammivaara and Enright (1986) argued that "adultcentrism" has led researchers to underestimate children's abilities (p. 227). This stance is seen when researchers assume that they know all about children because they once were children. When adultcentrism occurs, researchers tend to stay with their own frames of reference versus being open to learning from the different perspectives of children (Fine, 1987).

Another problem in past research is that when children had difficulty responding or completing a task, they were often considered incompetent in that area. Yet researchers have not always examined their own roles in the research, such as checking whether the children understood what the researcher was really asking. For instance, when researchers presented Piaget's research questions in a manner that was more related to the children's life experience and clarified what concept was being tested, the children knew more than what Piaget had proposed (Donaldson, 1978). In a study of how occupational therapists collaborated with children in treatment planning (Curtin, 1995), I found one 9-year-old child losing interest in drawing and talking about his experience in therapy. At first, I started to doubt his competence to express himself. However, when I changed my approach and created a guessing game that still involved questions about his experience, he eagerly directed the game and began talking again.

In studies in which children have been informants, researchers have gained a better understanding of children's competencies and their perspectives. The researchers also had some unexpected findings. For example, in a 9-month ethnography of an oncology unit, Bluebond-Langner (1978) interviewed and observed children 3 to 9 years of age who were dying. She discovered that the children's understanding of death progressed through stages that depended on individual experiences (e.g., knowing a child who died), not on their ages. Children knew that they had cancer and would die even when adults did not tell them this was the case. They came to this conclusion by talking with peers on the unit, interpreting the serious expressions of everyone around them, and making sense of unusual behaviors in others (e.g., getting numerous gifts). The children perceived what the adults could handle and responded in a way to match this. For example, some parents would maintain a pretense that the children would recover. Even though the children knew they would die, they engaged in this mutual pretense with their parents. Bluebond-Langner found that the children viewed supporting others as their life task. She was also surprised by the staff members' unawareness or denial of the depth of the children's knowledge.

Chalhub de Oliveira (1997) conducted an ethnography of homeless children in Rio de Janeiro. She found that even though the children encountered violence and hunger, some actually preferred living on the street instead of being with their families. A number of the children liked the freedom and independence they had on the street. Maria, a 10-year-old, described how she liked to be "free to go and stay anywhere" (p. 170). She also told the researcher,

> I don't know what I'm going to eat tomorrow. I don't care. Somehow I will have something. Somebody will feel sorry to see a cute, dirty, and hungry little girl on the sidewalk crying, begging for food . . . I don't need to know about tomorrow. I don't have anything to worry about . . . at home I had everything, but my mother wanted to control everything I did. (p. 170)

Therefore, the first challenge is for the researcher to examine his or her beliefs regarding children's competencies. This examination requires ongoing reflection and being prepared to learn from children. The researcher needs to recognize children as experts about their own lives and to be open to the idea that children may have competencies of which adults may not know. The researcher also needs to recognize that if children are having difficulty answering a question or participating in the research, it does not automatically mean that the children are incompetent. Instead, the researcher needs to examine the entire situation, including the context, the child's age, and especially his or her own role (e.g., reflecting on how the questions are worded).

Overcoming Inequality in the Typical Adult–Child Relationship

Adults often tell children what they should or should not do, and children are socialized to conform to adult's wishes (Koocher & Keith-

Spiegel, 1994). For example, children are taught to follow their teacher's instructions and the school rules. Children also learn that when a teacher asks questions, they need to try to determine what the teacher wants to hear and guess at the right answer (Tammivaara & Enright, 1986). Thus, when an adult asks children questions, the children may think there is a right answer that the adult, as the authority, already knows. As a result, children may try to guess at an answer instead of expressing their own thoughts.

In the typical adult–child relationship, Waksler (1986) also argued that if children challenge what an adult says, the children's views are "routinely discounted" (p. 77); therefore, "children have learned to keep their thoughts from adults" (Fine & Glassner, 1979, p. 170). Additionally, children are careful about how they act in the presence of adults, and, consequently, a "'hidden world' of childhood" exists that adults do not see (Fine & Sandstrom, 1988, p. 43). Unless the researcher conveys to the children the desire to hear their perspectives and learn about their worlds, the researcher risks that children may not express their thoughts or act naturally while he or she is present.

The second challenge then is to develop a relationship and clarify a role (e.g., define rules for interaction) that decrease the differences in power between the researcher and children and convey the researcher's desire to learn. The researcher would need to convey to the children the importance of hearing the children's perspectives and to employ specific strategies to reduce authoritarian, judgmental, or interfering behavior. In addition, the researcher would assume a responsive versus a dominating stance to the children's actions and words. This relationship could be considered that of an "out-of-the-ordinary" adult (Tammivaara & Enright, 1986, p. 229) or the assumption of the "least adult role"

(Mandell, 1988, p. 435). When this type of relationship is clear to the children, it is reflected in their descriptions of the researcher. For example, the children called Fine (1987) an "honorary kid" (p. 238).

Establishing a different type of relationship can be difficult at times for the researcher because children often react with bewilderment and then test the limits of the relationship. The children may find a nondirective and nonauthoritarian adult–child relationship puzzling if it is a new experience for them. For instance, when one researcher observed children getting into trouble and did nothing, a child yelled, "What's wrong with you, mister, aren't you going to report us?" (Fine & Sandstrom, 1988, p. 53). In Mandell's (1988) study, whenever she acted differently from other adults, the children often asked, "Who are you?" Mandell maintained, "The main reason children have difficulty in accepting an adult as nondirective stems from their lack of experience of adults as participatory, enjoyable, and nonjudgmental" (p. 442). However, she found that when the children were viewed seriously, they responded with joy.

Children may also challenge the researcher to see whether this is truly a different adult–child relationship. For example, children will watch the researcher's reactions in situations not tolerated by most adults. The children also will check to see whether they can trust the researcher. Bluebond-Langner's (1978) relationship was tested by a child named Benjamin. Benjamin asked her what happened to Maria, a girl on the unit. Bluebond-Langner replied, "She was very sick, much sicker than you are, and she died" (p. 188). Later, she found out that Benjamin asked everyone he saw what happened to Maria. When she asked him why he did that, he said, "The ones who tell me are my friends. I knew Maria died. I saw the cart come for her. They told everyone to go in their rooms. I wanted to see if you were really my friend" (p. 188).

The researcher also can encounter difficulties in assuming a nondirective and nonauthoritarian role because as an adult, he or she is morally and legally responsible for protecting children from harm (Fine, 1987), especially if the researcher is the only adult present. If any possibility exists that the children may get hurt, the researcher needs to take action. At the same time, the researcher has to be careful not to get into a policing role (Fine, 1987). This dual role requires a delicate balance. The researcher seeks an understanding of the children's worlds (including deviant behavior), but if he or she intervenes as an authority, the children may limit what they say.

Bridging Different Styles of Communication

Children often communicate differently from adults (Baumann, 1997). Preschoolers may use babble or nonstandard English in a way that other children, but not always adults, can understand the meaning (Mandell, 1988). Children also display a greater reliance on nonverbal language and silence for communication. For example, in my study (Curtin, 1995), Lisa (pseudonym) spoke in short sentences but varied the pitch, tone, and loudness of her voice to clarify the meaning. Once the therapist learned Lisa's facial and voice cues, she said, "She really was very communicative, even though it wasn't always verbal. Even her facial expression, you can just see when she's sad or see when she's angry. I mean her whole mannerism changes" (p. 81).

Children also tend to use fewer words to encapsulate the meaning of their message (Curtin, 1995). When asked, "What is important for therapists to know when they work with chil-

dren," Lisa responded, "How to talk to them." After a few probing questions, she added, "That they understand what you are saying" (p. 69). Her message is poignant because of her hospital experience. Until the occupational therapist began treatment, Lisa did not know why she was hospitalized or why she was getting medical tests. She told the therapist, "They don't tell me nothin' " (p. 64).

When asked general or vague questions, children may give minimal information. Pipe, Gee, and Wilson (1993) described an interview of a 6-year-old child:

> *Interviewer:* A couple of weeks ago you came and saw a magic show. Well, I'd like you to tell me all about it. Let's start at the beginning . . . someone came to get you out of your class. What happened then?
>
> *JR:* We did a magic show. (p. 25)

However, when young children are asked more specific questions about their present experience, more information can be elicited. The statements young children make may appear meaningless or shallow because of the lack of verbal detail, but when examined, they are often rich with meaning (Zwiers & Morrissette, 1999).

Thus, communicating with children can take more time and effort if the researcher wants to learn about the children's perspectives. Tammivaara and Enright (1986) contended that difficulties in communicating have kept researchers "from examining the world of the child from the vantage point of the child for many years" (p. 226). Often, researchers rely only on the parents or other adults to speak for the children. Yet parents do not always know what their children are thinking (Biklen & Moseley, 1988).

Therefore, the researcher's third challenge is to learn and use ways of communicating that bridge the different styles. The researcher needs to look for the meaning conveyed in short phrases. It is important for the researcher to learn "kid's language," including the nonstandard use of words, to allow the children enough time to answer, and to ask questions in more than one way. The researcher also needs to learn which words children understand and try not to use "big words" or complex language. When I worked in an oncology clinic, one child made this point in his story for the group newspaper:

> When I was in the hospital I felt really bad at the time because I didn't know what was going on at the time. I didn't know what kind of medicine that was going in my body and when I was going to radiation they was trying to explain to me. But I didn't understand because the kind of words that they was using.

Lastly, the researcher needs to be willing to adapt and use a variety of nonverbal techniques (e.g., drawing) to elicit the children's perspectives.

Considerations and Adaptations

A number of adaptations can be made to successfully include children as valuable research participants. Because all children have competencies, the researcher is responsible for using techniques that will elicit the competencies needed to participate in the research. If the researcher considers different ways of getting children's perspectives, successful participation becomes more feasible.

Developmental Considerations

When working with children, it is helpful for the researcher to be aware of development norms and that development varies with experience. However, the researcher also needs to be open to the idea that children may be able to do

and understand more than has been stated in previous research and theories of development. Reexamination of Piaget's work provides a good example (Donaldson, 1978).

The following developmental patterns affect children's abilities to describe their experiences. By 3 years of age, children tend to be able to recall and tell about events that they have experienced, often in an outline format with few details (Saywitz, 1990). Their memories are more accurate with meaningful and familiar events than hypothetical stories, but children tend to lose detail as time passes (Lamb et al., 1999; Steward, Bussey, Goodman, & Saywitz, 1993). A 3-year-old may find it difficult to remember "peripheral details" (e.g., location) and events they consider unimportant (Saywitz, 1990, p. 333). Although preschool children are more easily misled and affected by suggestion than adults, they are less suggestible when recounting life experiences (Zwiers & Morrissette, 1999).

Preschoolers tend to have the vocabulary needed to talk about the present but are still learning concepts regarding time and the use of words involving past tense (Steward et al., 1993). In first grade, children can talk concretely about events in the past and are better able to answer questions starting with "how," "why," or "when" (Steward et al., 1993). However, children under 7 years of age tend to have difficulty answering questions involving abstractions with a variety of dimensions (Hatch, 1990).

At 7 years of age, children can discriminate the different feelings and actions that occur in various situations, such as recognizing that they are more competent in one subject (e.g., art) than another (Zwiers & Morrissette, 1999). They also appear to distinguish between external and internal events at the same level as adults (Lamb et al., 1999). By 8 years of age, children describe more details in their accounts of their experience, and by 10 years of age, they are similar to adults in their recall of historical events (Zwiers & Morrissette, 1999).

Ethical Considerations

Researchers have found that most elementary-school-age children have the capacity to provide assent as defined by federal regulations (Weithorn & Scherer, 1994). The children need to be given an explanation of the research in words that they can understand and be told with whom the information will be shared. Children also need to be told that they have a right to dissent, that a decision not to participate will be respected, and that they can stop at any time with no consequences.

As in all research, the researcher is ethically responsible for being sensitive to signs of distress or anxiety so as to not harm the children (Crowley, 1996). Throughout the research, children should have opportunities to ask questions and express concerns (Kendall, 1997).

Children may want their real names to be used in the study. When I told a child in my study that I needed to change his name, he replied, "That's dumb." I explained that it was necessary and had him pick the name to use. Some of the children in Fine's (1987) study also wanted their names used, but he used pseudonyms because he had documented the children's deviant behaviors and was concerned about ramifications in the future.

The Setting

When eliciting children's perspectives, it is best to be in a place that is quiet and private. The location needs to be a neutral place where the children feel comfortable and free to talk. If possible, the researcher should let the children choose the location (Faux, Walsh, & Deatrick, 1988). If this is not possible and a strange setting is used, the researcher needs to allow time for the children to get familiar with the setting (Yarrow, 1960). It also is helpful if child-sized chairs are available and the researcher sits at the same level as the children. Younger children usually are more comfortable with their parents or other children present (Koocher & Keith-Spiegel, 1994).

Adaptations for Preschoolers

The use of drawing or play materials is especially useful for eliciting the perspectives of preschoolers (Deatrick & Faux, 1991). Therefore, one way to adapt an interview is to ask a question and have the preschooler respond with pictures (Garbarino & Stott, 1989). Otherwise, preschoolers do best when questions come from the immediate situation or are embedded in an activity that is familiar (Deatrick & Faux, 1991; Tammivaara & Enright, 1986). Also helpful is if the researcher develops questions that use words introduced by the child or that respond to the child's actions or drawings (Garbarino & Stott, 1989) and keeps in mind that preschoolers are better at describing events, persons, or objects than reflecting or clarifying (Garbarino & Stott, 1989; Yarrow, 1960). Preschoolers also will do better if names are used instead of pronouns (Garbarino & Stott, 1989). Lastly, because preschoolers can be suggestible, opening up the range of possible answers is important (Parker, 1984); otherwise, the researcher's questions may directly influence the children's responses.

Adaptations for Elementary-School-Age Children

Because an interview highly depends on the relationship established between the interviewer and the person being interviewed, the researcher in an interview with a child can decrease the differences in power by being flexible and informal (Deatrick & Faux, 1991). The opening question "sets the tone of the relationship" and conveys what is expected (Yarrow, 1960, p. 580). To help the interview flow, a few key questions prepared ahead of time can be helpful, especially because children do better with some structure in the interview (Yarrow, 1960). However, if the interview is too highly structured, the children may think it is a classroom lesson with predetermined answers (Tammivaara & Enright, 1986). Asking the children to tell the researcher when they want a break or when they do not understand a question is a helpful strategy (Zwiers & Morrissette, 1999).

One way a researcher can start an interview is to have the children bring a picture or something they made (Yarrow, 1960). By encouraging children to talk about their work, they are put into the role of an expert and given the message that their thoughts are valued (Yarrow, 1960). Another strategy for beginning an interview and decreasing anxiety is to ask the children to either share three wishes or describe who they would like to become (Faux et al., 1988).

Methods of Eliciting the Children's Perspectives

Children's perspectives can be elicited through a variety of ways. The child can draw pictures, make a videotaped story, talk to a pretend friend, or act out different roles or scenes. Other ideas include drawing and writing in a diary (Sorensen, 1989), completing sentences (Kendall, 1997), explaining a videotape the researcher shows (Graue & Walsh, 1998), or participating in a focus group (Shaw, 1996). The use of props (e.g., talking through a doll or toy phone) can be especially effective with preschoolers (Yarrow, 1960).

The Art of Questioning

When asking children questions, it is helpful to inform the children (a) that there are no right or wrong answers and (b) that it is all right if they do not have an answer (Faux et al., 1988). It is best to avoid the use of double negatives and vague references to time (e.g., "a few months ago") (Zwiers & Morrissette, 1999). The researcher also needs to monitor his or her responses, being careful not to use judgmental phrases like "that's right" or "that's good." Faux et al. (1988) also recommended that questions gradually shift from least to most sensitive, general to detailed, concrete to abstract. Children find it easier to answer questions about the present and events they have just experienced than about the past (Amato & Ochiltree, 1987; Hatch, 1990). The researcher also needs to keep in mind that questions starting with "why" are the most difficult because they require knowledge about causality (Saywitz, 1990). The researcher should word questions with only three to five more words than the children's average number of words in a sentence (Garbarino & Stott, 1989). To learn about the children's level of vocabulary, the researcher can read storybooks that children typically read at that age (Zwiers & Morrissette, 1999).

In the interview, the researcher should try to avoid initiating all conversation, controlling the children's behavior, interrupting with many questions, and responding with an additional question (Faux et al., 1988; Garbarino & Stott, 1989; Tammivaara & Enright, 1986). Instead, the interview needs to be more similar to a casual conversation and stopped if it becomes more like an interrogation. If the interview is too formal, children may think it is a test (Hatch, 1990).

A researcher can encourage children to talk more by using props (e.g., photographs, videotapes, toys, or objects) related to the phenomena being studied (Pipe et al., 1993). Hatch (1990) gave the example of how a researcher studying children's perspectives in sharing would elicit more information if the children carry an object (e.g., a toy) that they have had to share. The children can then look and touch the object as they talk about their thoughts and feelings about sharing it.

Group interviewing is a format that can elicit more information (Graue & Walsh, 1995). Children tend to be more comfortable talking with other children than with an adult and will be more likely to direct the conversation (Graue & Walsh, 1995). When children guide the conversation, the researcher learns what the children consider important.

To get more information from children, the researcher can ask for examples for clarification. Another strategy is "playing dumb," in which the researcher asks the children to help him or her to understand (Tammivaara & Enright, 1986, p. 231). A third suggestion is for the researcher to repeat the same question in a different way or restate the children's words or feelings in a questioning manner (Faux et al., 1988; Garbarino & Stott, 1989). Biklen and Moseley (1988) recommended asking about persons, things, and activities separately or dividing requests for information into parts and ask questions about each part. If the researcher asks children about a difficult topic, Yarrow (1960) suggested giving the children a chance to say something positive before asking questions that might entail a negative response. He also suggested mentioning that other children may feel the same way. Faux et al. (1988) recommended asking children about what they would do in a certain situation as a way to elicit their feelings.

Sensitivity to Signs of Fatigue, Disinterest, or Lack of Understanding

Elementary-school-age children often can tolerate 30-minute interviews (Faux et al., 1988).

However, the researcher needs to watch for nonverbal signs of fatigue or decreased attention and allow for diversions (Faux et al., 1988; Garbarino & Stott, 1989). If children are using the same phrase repeatedly, it may be an indication that they do not know the answer, may not understand the question, or may think the question is unimportant (Biklen & Moseley, 1988). Additionally, quick or easy answers may mean that they are bored or tired (Faux et al., 1988). The researcher needs to realize that until 10 or 11 years of age, children may not be able to say what they do not know, understand, or remember (Garbarino & Stott, 1989). If a child does not understand a question, the researcher can help by rewording the question instead of repeating it (Garbarino & Stott, 1989). When checking for understanding, the researcher should ask children to repeat what they have heard rather than asking "Do you understand?" (Garbarino & Stott, 1989, p. 190).

Occupational Therapists as Qualitative Researchers With Children

Pediatric occupational therapists who become researchers bring with them a wealth of knowledge regarding children. They have experience interpreting children's nonverbal language, talking at the children's level, and involving children as active participants in the therapy process. These skills are valuable assets for doing research with children. Occupational therapists also have a history of being problem solvers who discover creative solutions to various difficulties. This skill can be applied to discovering inventive ways of eliciting children's voices. For example, when the 9-year-old child in my study (Curtin, 1995) stopped talking, I used my skills as a therapist to analyze the situation. I realized that he may have been bored, felt pressured to talk, or did not like talking in front of an audience (i.e., his mother, younger brother, and myself). So I created two games and wrapped them up like presents. In the next session, he was intrigued. He smiled as he opened the packages. I told him that he had a choice of a matching game (matching his experiences in therapy with pictures of children with different feelings) or a guessing game. He chose the guessing game in which each card had a question about his experience in therapy and the four of us had to guess at the answer. The child was pleased to tell us the right answer (which also meant that he told us about his experience). By being creative and playful, I discovered a way to elicit this child's perspective.

Implications for Clinical Practice

Therapists can use the ideas presented in this article to help them collaborate with children. Although occupational therapists tend to be skilled at giving children a voice in treatment activities, involving children in defining the purpose of therapy is more challenging. Yet if therapists want children to learn to speak and act for themselves, they can start by eliciting and strengthening the children's voices in defining the focus of therapy. By engaging the children in dialogue combined with other methods (e.g., drawing, using props), the therapist may increase the likelihood of participation and in the process gain an understanding of the children's perspectives.

It has been my experience that children are often more comfortable talking while engaged in an activity. Consequently, if children know that the therapist is interested in their thoughts and will listen to them, they often share their concerns in the midst of an activity. Because it is their choice whether or not to focus on the

activity or to talk, the children do not feel pressured to talk as in a formal interview. Therefore, occupational therapists often can be in a position of listening and helping children.

Children appreciate having an opportunity to talk with a therapist who cares and values what they have to say. When two children in my study were asked about their time in occupational therapy, Tony (pseudonym) said, "We had fun while she was asking me the questions and I was telling her the answers. It was like fun doing that." Lisa said that she liked "the stitching and the talking." When asked what she liked about her therapist, she replied, "She's fun, she's got a lot of neat things to do, and we talk" (Curtin, 1995, pp. 68–69).

Conclusion

Occupational therapy researchers will gain a better understanding of childhood occupations and pediatric practice by eliciting children's voices in research. For example, researchers may learn how children's hidden worlds affect their functioning and about children's experiences in therapy. This information can assist therapists in providing treatment that is more meaningful to children's lives. In addition, when children are given the opportunity to be informants, they may also benefit from the research experience. For instance, in my study Tony reviewed the videotape of his interview where he talked about his experiences in therapy. He said that he liked the tape because of the way he was talking and sitting: It was "like I'm a real professional."

Although it may be more difficult for a researcher to engage children in research than to work with adults, the impediments are not insurmountable. The researcher can make a number of adaptations and adjustments to elicit children's perspectives and explore children's worlds. By doing so, the researcher will find that children can be active research participants who will help expand the knowledge base of occupational therapy. In addition, the researcher will be giving children an opportunity to have a voice like "real professionals."

Acknowledgment

I thank Rebecca Burns, who reviewed this manuscript.

References

Alldred, P. (1998). Ethnography and discourse analysis: Dilemmas in representing the voices of children. In J. Ribbens & R. Edwards (Eds.), *Feminist dilemmas in qualitative research: Public knowledge and private lives* (pp. 147–170). London: Sage.

Amato, P. R., & Ochiltree, G. (1987). Interviewing children about their families: A note on data quality. *Journal of Marriage and the Family, 49,* 669–675.

Baumann, S. L. (1997). Qualitative research with children as participants. *Nursing Science Quarterly, 10,* 68–69.

Biklen, S. K., & Moseley, C. R. (1988). "Are you retarded?" "No, I'm Catholic": Qualitative methods in the study of people with severe handicaps. *Journal of the Association for Persons With Severe Handicaps, 13,* 155–162.

Bluebond-Langner, M. (1978). *The private worlds of dying children.* Trenton, NJ: Princeton University.

Chalhub de Oliveira, T. (1997). Homeless children in Rio de Janeiro: Exploring the meaning of street life. *Child and Youth Care Forum, 26,* 163–174.

Crowley, A. (1996). Whose life is it anyway? In I. Butler & I. Shaw (Eds.), *A case of neglect? Children's experiences and the sociology of childhood* (pp. 107–124). Brookfield, VT: Ashgate.

Curtin, C. (1995). *Collaborative treatment planning with children.* Unpublished doctoral dissertation, University of Illinois at Chicago.

Deatrick, J. A., & Faux, S. A. (1991). Conducting qualitative research with children and adolescents. In J. M. Morse (Ed.), *Qualitative nursing research: A contemporary dialogue* (pp. 203–223). Newbury Park, CA: Sage.

Donaldson, M. (1978). *Children's minds.* New York: Norton.

Faux, S. A., Walsh, M., & Deatrick, J. A. (1988). Intensive interviewing with children and adolescents. *Western Journal of Nursing Research, 10,* 180–194.

Fine, G. A. (1987). *With the boys: Little League baseball and preadolescent culture.* Chicago: University of Chicago Press.

Fine, G. A., & Glassner, B. (1979). Participant observation with children: Promise and problems. *Urban Life, 8,* 153–174.

Fine, G. A., & Sandstrom, K. L. (1988). *Knowing children: Participant observation with minors* (Vol. 15). Newbury Park, CA: Sage.

Garbarino, J., & Stott, F. M. (1989). *What children can tell us.* San Francisco: Jossey-Bass.

Graue, M. E., & Walsh, D. J. (1995). Children in context: Interpreting the here and now of children's lives. In J. A. Hatch (Ed.), *Qualitative research in early childhood settings* (pp. 135–154). Westport, CT: Praeger.

Graue, M. E., & Walsh, D. J. (1998). *Studying children in context: Theories, methods, and ethics.* Thousand Oaks, CA: Sage.

Hatch, J. A. (1990). Young children as informants in classroom studies. *Early Childhood Research Quarterly, 5,* 251–264.

Kendall, J. (1997). The use of qualitative methods in the study of wellness in children with attention deficit hyperactivity disorder. *Journal of Child and Adolescent Psychiatric Nursing, 10,* 27–38.

Koocher, G. P., & Keith-Spiegel, P. (1994). Scientific issues in psychosocial and educational research with children. In M. A. Grodin & L. H. Glantz (Eds.), *Children as research subjects: Science, ethics, and law* (pp. 47–80). New York: Oxford University Press.

Lamb, M. E., Sternberg, K. J., Orbach, Y., Hershkowitz, I., & Esplin, P. W. (1999). Forensic interviews of children. In A. Memon & R. Bull (Eds.), *Handbook of the psychology of interviewing* (pp. 253–277). New York: Wiley.

Mandell, N. (1988). The least-adult role in studying children. *Journal of Contemporary Ethnography, 16,* 433–467.

Oakley, A. (1994). Women and children first and last: Parallels and differences between children's and women's studies. In B. Mayall (Ed.), *Children's childhoods: Observed and experienced* (pp. 13–32). London: Falmer.

Parker, W. C. (1984). Interviewing children: Problems and promise. *Journal of Negro Education, 53*(1), 18–28.

Pipe, M., Gee, S., & Wilson, C. (1993). Cues, props, and context: Do they facilitate children's event reports? In S. Goodman & B. L. Bottoms (Eds.), *Child victims, child witnesses: Understanding and improving testimony* (pp. 25–45). New York: Guilford.

Qvortrup, J. (1994). Childhood matters: An introduction. In J. Qvortrup, M. Brady, G. Sgritta, & H. Wintersberger (Eds.), *Childhood matters: Social theory, practice and politics* (pp. 1–23). Brookfield, VT: Ashgate.

Saywitz, K. (1990). The child as witness: Experimental and clinical considerations. In A. La Greca (Ed.), *Through the eyes of the child: Obtaining self-reports from children and adolescents* (pp. 329–367). Boston: Allyn & Bacon.

Shaw, I. (1996). Unbroken voices: Children, young people and qualitative methods. In I. Butler & I. Shaw (Eds.), *A case of neglect? Children's experiences and the sociology of childhood* (pp. 19–36). Brookfield, VT: Ashgate.

Sorensen, E. (1989). Using children's diaries as a research instrument. *Journal of Pediatric Nursing, 4,* 427–431.

Steward, M. S., Bussey, K., Goodman, G. S., & Saywitz, K. J. (1993). Implications of developmental research for interviewing children. *Child Abuse and Neglect, 17,* 25–37.

Tammivaara, J., & Enright, D. S. (1986). On eliciting information: Dialogues with child informants. *Anthropology and Education Quarterly, 17,* 218–238.

Waksler, F. C. (1986). Studying children: Phenomenological insights. *Human Studies, 9,* 71–82.

Weithorn, L. A. (1983). Involving children in decisions affecting their own welfare. In G. B. Melton, G. P. Koocher, & M. J. Saks (Eds.), *Children's competence to consent* (pp. 235–260). New York: Plenum.

Weithorn, L. A., & Scherer, D. G. (1994). Children's involvement in research participation decisions: Psychological considerations. In M. A. Grodin & L. H. Glantz (Eds.), *Children as research subjects: Science, ethics, and law* (pp. 133–179). New York: Oxford University Press.

Yarrow, L. J. (1960). Interviewing children. In P. H. Mussen (Ed.), *Handbook of research methods in child development* (pp. 561–602). New York: Wiley.

Zwiers, M. L., & Morrissette, P. J. (1999). *Effective interviewing of children: A comprehensive guide for counselors and human service workers.* Philadelphia: Taylor & Francis.

CHAPTER 5

Traumatic Brain Injury in Children

Issues in Community Function

Anne Frances Cronin

Anne Frances Cronin, PhD, OTR, BCP, *is assistant professor, West Virginia University, Morgantown, WV 26505; acronin@hsc.wvu.edu.*

Lazar and Menaldino (1995) identified traumatic brain injury (TBI) as the leading cause of acquired disability in childhood, estimating that 5 million children sustain TBI yearly. No typical clinical picture of TBI exists because differences in the original brain insult can result in widely disparate outcomes. Early in the recovery process, most children with TBI are classified by degree of impaired consciousness based on the Glasgow Coma Scale (GCS; Teasdale & Jennett, 1974). The GCS is used to predict rehabilitation outcomes (Jennett & Bond, 1975) on the basis of four categories: mild (good recovery), moderate (independence in activities of daily living [ADL] with disability), severe (dependency), and vegetative state (see Table 5.1). More than 90% of children with TBI fall within the mild or moderate range (Lowenthal, 1998; Shurtleff, Massagli, Hays, Ross, & Sprunk-Greenfield, 1995). Most are discharged to their home communities, often with little follow-up or support services (DiScala, Osberg, Gans, Chin, & Grant, 1991).

Children with motor limitations are often referred for physical therapy and occupational therapy during the recovery period after TBI. Although research indicates that even children with mild or moderate TBI without motor impairments demonstrate reduced functional performance, children without obvious motor or medical limitations seldom receive specialized therapy or support (Coster, Haley, & Baryza, 1994; Kinsella et al., 1997). Psychosocial and behavioral sequelae of pediatric head injury are less likely to receive medical attention, although they are consistently reported to be present and problematic (Lazar & Menaldino, 1995; Serio, Kreutzer, & Gervasio, 1995).

Asarnow, Satz, Light, and Neumann (1991) reported a high incidence of behavior problems in children with TBI. Researchers agree with this finding regarding children with severe head injuries but have contested it for the mild and moderate groups (Massagli et al., 1996). Some of the discrepancy between results may stem from the types of assessments typically used with children.

Originally published 2001 in *American Journal of Occupational Therapy, 55,* 377–384.

Table 5.1. Glasgow Coma Scale: Outcomes

Category and Score	Description
Vegetative state (< 5)	A persistent state of impaired consciousness.
Severe (5–8)	Child is conscious but requires 24-hour care and supervision because of cognitive, behavioral, or physical disabilities. Slow response time and difficulties with short-term memory predominate.
Moderate (9–12)	Child is expected to achieve eventual independence in activities of daily living and home and community activities with persistent disability. Children in this group may have memory impairments, hemiparesis, dysphagia, ataxia, and other neuromotor problems.
Mild (13–15)	Good recovery is expected. Child is able to reintegrate into normal social life. There may be mild persisting sequelae.

Note. From "Head Injury," by P. Winkler, 1995, in *Neurological Rehabilitation* (3rd ed., p. 429), by D. Umphred (Ed.), St. Louis, MO: Mosby. Copyright © by W. B. Saunders Company. Adapted with permission from Elsevier.

Tests of cognitive performance do not assess function in natural environments. Current research indicates that cognitive status does not accurately predict level of behavioral functioning or adaptive skills (Lazar & Menaldino, 1995).

Children recovering from TBI are seldom referred for rehabilitation services of any kind. DiScala, Osberg, and Savage (1997) followed 24,021 children and adolescents hospitalized for TBI. They found that 27% left the hospital "with apparent functional limitation" (p. 5), as defined by these researchers. Functional limitations considered were those in the areas of vision, hearing, speech, self-feeding, bathing, dressing, walking, cognition, or behavior. Of this group, 75% were discharged to home. According to the researchers, "[A]mong school-age children with limitations who returned to their homes, only 1.8% were referred for special education services" (p. 8). They expressed concern regarding the apparent discrepancy between numbers of children with TBI eligible for and those receiving special education and related services under the Individuals With Disabilities Education Act of 1990 (IDEA; P.L. 101–476).

In this chapter, I review the literature on motor, communication, cognitive, behavioral, and psychosocial sequelae of pediatric TBI. Issues in family adjustment, community function, and implications for school-based occupational therapists are considered.

TBI: Pathology and Complications

Traumatic head injuries usually occur as part of a multitrauma event, such as an automobile accident or a fall. At the time of the incident, the child often presents with contusions, cranial fractures, extraparenchymal or intracranial hematomas, cranial nerve injuries, and edema (Blaskey & Jennings, 1999). Cerebral damage after head injury may be primary to the trauma or secondary to complications of the injury. Secondary damage includes insults that immediately follow the impact and insults that occur during the emergency medical intervention process. Primary cerebral damage is usually permanent (Bruce, 1990). Both types of damage can lead to limitations in functional outcomes.

In children, most primary focal injuries are frontal and temporal (Blaskey & Jennings, 1999). Computed tomography scan after an injury helps the clinician predict the types and degree of functional limitation likely to follow. Diffuse axonal injuries (DAI) are the result of shearing forces at the time of impact. DAI are usually identified through the use of magnetic resonance imaging and involve the brainstem and corpus callosum (Berker, 1996). DAI often result in edema, increased intracranial pressure, and diffuse axonal deafferentation accompanied by denervation hypersensitivity (Povlishock & Christman, 1995).

Children's brain tissue is developmentally different from that of adults, and very young children are particularly vulnerable to damage from secondary trauma (Johnston, 1995). Secondary trauma complications include vasospasm, cerebral swelling, cerebral edema, and hematomas (Pang, 1985), which typically result in increased intracranial pressure, hypoxia, ischemia, and hypotension. Infarction, brain herniation, and pressure necrosis may occur in the immediate posttrauma period. In children, damage from these secondary complications is more likely to be diffuse than in adults and more likely to resolve during the child's recovery and rehabilitation period. About 59% of pediatric TBI cases are classified as mild, 8% as moderate, and 11.5% as severe (DiScala et al., 1997).

In DiScala et al.'s (1997) sample, the mean length of hospital stay of children with TBI was 6 days, and 90% of the children were hospitalized for less than 15 days. The children were screened for functional limitations before discharge, although the methodology associated with this screening was not presented. More than 68% of the children discharged were described as having no functional limitations, and 16% were described as having one to three limitations. Within these groups, all of the children with no functional limitations and more than 90% of those with one to three limitations were discharged to home. Less than one-third of the children discharged to home were recommended for outpatient rehabilitation services. Epidemiological evidence suggests that only children with severe impairments following TBI are referred to rehabilitation hospitals (DiScala et al., 1997). According to DiScala et al.,

> A large gap exists between percentages of children discharged to home with specific types of limitations and those receiving post-acute referrals. Over half of the children were discharged with limitations in walking, bathing, and/or

dressing, while only 13.2% were referred to occupational therapy, and only 23.7% to physical therapy…. A total of 18.7% of these children were discharged with cognitive limitation, but only 1.8% were referred to special education. (p. 6)

The authors also reported low referrals for children with TBI to community-based services. Even fewer children actually received the services because of limitations in financial, social, and emotional resources. Families may lack an understanding of the potential problems, or some cultural influences may exist that lead the family to avoid "medical" support (Humphry & Case-Smith, 1996; Vessey, 1997).

Prognostic Indicators

The functional impact of head injury includes physical, mental, information-processing, language, socioemotional, and medical impairments (Blaskey & Jennings, 1999). Rehabilitation of persons with TBI focuses on nonphysiologic interventions directed at these impairments. Traditionally, length of coma, changes in the GCS score in the first 24 hours, age, and the availability of rehabilitation services are considered prognostic indicators (Blaskey & Jennings, 1999). Gilchrist and Wilkinson (1979) questioned the predictive validity of the GCS for functional outcomes and suggested that a better predictor of outcome is the rate and quality of return of intellectual and memory functions.

Pediatric TBI and Rehabilitation

The benefit of rehabilitation services at any stage of recovery is poorly documented (Hall & Cope, 1995; High, Boake, & Lehmkuhl, 1995). Although they did not use control groups, several studies have demonstrated positive relationships between improved functional outcome and rehabilitation. Decreased length of coma (Mackay, Berstein, Chapman, Morgan, & Milazzo, 1992), improved functional outcomes (Heinemann et al., 1990), and decreased hospital stays (Hall & Cope, 1995) are attributed to early rehabilitation services. Because of the lack of uniformity within these studies and difficulties with instrumentation, researchers still debate whether rehabilitation actually optimizes functional outcomes or "simply expedite[s] the time to reaching a functional plateau" (Hall & Cope, 1995, p. 11). Hall and Cope responded to this argument with the following statement:

> There is substantial evidence that plateaus do not represent maximum functional improvement, based on the positive changes reported by numerous studies in "stable" populations. If rehabilitation only expedited time to maximum function for an individual, then improvement might not be evidenced in many cases for years after injury. (p. 11)

The occupational therapy literature tends to deal with TBI in terms of specific impairments. The rehabilitation approach varies by individual limitations, point of service delivery, and length of time after trauma. Occupational therapy interventions in acute stage head trauma recovery include positioning, range of motion, and sensory stimulation (Scott & Dow, 1995; Winkler, 1995). In intermediate care, interventions broaden, including improving motor control and training in ADL, cognitive–perceptual remediation, and community reentry skills. Cognitive disability can greatly limit recovery because voluntary control and independent function rely on cognition (Blaskey & Jennings, 1999). In their study of children with multisystem trauma discharged to home, Wesson et al. (1992) reported a substantial incidence of physical and psychosocial morbidity as much as 1 year after discharge. Their study compared children with TBI to children experiencing other types of severe multisystem trauma

and reported that many injured children in both groups are left with behavioral disturbances and lower academic scores after discharge.

The IDEA legislation requires states and schools to provide eligible children with special services, including occupational therapy, physical therapy, and speech therapy, to assure academic access. TBI is a disability category under IDEA, and children exhibiting functional problems are eligible for referral and screening for early intervention or school services. The public schools and school-based therapists are well placed to identify and recognize the special needs of children recovering from TBI (Blosser & Pearson, 1997). According to D'Amato and Rothlisberg (1996), any child having a history of TBI should be considered at risk for academic problems, so ideally, schools will be informed if a student incurs, or has incurred, a TBI. Not every child returning to school after TBI will need special services, but classroom monitoring of these children is recommended.

Brain Injury From a Developmental Perspective

The medical and physical needs that result from childhood trauma are the focus of emergency room and acute hospital caregivers. After the child is medically stable, the developmental issues become more prominent. According to Lazar and Menaldino (1995),

> In the context of a child recovering from TBI, taking a developmental perspective refers to recognizing that the dynamic process of recovery from TBI is superimposed in time over maturational/developmental changes in neural structures, as well as developmental changes in cognitive, behavioral, emotional, and social functioning. (p. 56)

This recovery approach underlies the recent interest in longitudinal studies of pediatric TBI.

The effects of TBI grow more complex as the child matures and faces new challenges. Although neuroplasticity allows young children to develop alternative neural pathways, these pathways may be less efficient and may compromise the original function of the compensating structures (Lazar & Menaldino, 1995). Through alternative pathways, the child may develop compensatory or atypical strategies to achieve desired skill levels. These strategies will improve function at the child's current developmental level but may interfere with the overall developmental process and cause delays at some future point in development. The child's compensatory "swapping" of functions allows the overriding of a system or a function that the young child does not yet need, resulting in other impairments that appear much later. The very young child is considered particularly vulnerable to impairment, as studies have shown that developmental skill areas undergoing rapid change are more vulnerable to damage secondary to TBI (Ewing-Cobb et al., 1997). Preschool children are believed to fare less well than older children and adults after TBI (Lazar & Menaldino, 1995).

Impairments Associated With Brain Injury in Children

Children with severe brain injuries are most likely to exhibit motoric impairment. Children with motor impairments after TBI are reported to have a good prognosis (Blaskey & Jennings, 1999; Winkler, 1995). Children with mild and moderate TBI have fewer limitations but often experience a number of transient impairments that may affect school performance (Kinsella et al., 1997; Shurtleff et al., 1995).

Decreased Motor Control

Common motoric problems seen in children with TBI include velocity-dependent muscle stiffness (i.e., spasticity), velocity of movement problems (i.e., ataxia), changes in muscle elastic properties (i.e., contractures), paralysis, and speech impairments. The incidence and severity of these motor disorders increase with the length of coma following the head trauma (Blaskey & Jennings, 1999). Between 5% and 30% of children with TBI manifest some motor control sequelae and may show improvements for up to 7 years after the injury (Klonoff, Clark, & Klonoff, 1993). Some long-term musculoskeletal problems are muscle contracture, altered joint mobility or stability, muscle disuse resulting in atrophy or muscle weakness, and decreased muscular endurance (Winkler, 1995). The clinical intervention literature clearly describes interventions for both the immediate and long-term problems associated with motor impairment secondary to TBI (Blaskey & Jennings, 1999; Scott & Dow, 1995; Winkler, 1995).

Orthopedic Impairments

Spasticity and prolonged posturing during the recovery period may lead to limitations in joint range of motion. Blasier and Letts (1989) documented the common orthopedic problems associated with severe brain injuries and the average time of deformity onset. Contractures can be prevented through ongoing skilled positioning and motor interventions (Moseley, 1997; Nuismer, Ekes, & Holm, 1997; Prosser, 1996). In addition to occupational therapy and physical therapy, several surgical and pharmacological treatments are available to address motor problems.

Somatosensory System Impairments

Sensory perception may be impaired following TBI. Commonly reported difficulties are impaired postural awareness and orientation, sensation impairments (e.g., impaired proprioception, tactile hypersensitivity), difficulty grading muscle force, and increased latency before muscle firing (Blaskey & Jennings, 1999). In addition, children may demonstrate impaired motor planning, tactile sensory dysfunction, and spatial disorientation (Carney & Gerring, 1990). These problems sometimes lead to specific problems with swallowing and eating (Porr, 1999).

Sensory System Impairments

Audiological and visual system impairments may develop as a result of brain injury (DiScala et al., 1997). Common visual problems include diploplia, hemianopsia, and changes in visual acuity (Massagli et al., 1996). Visual perceptual problems are described for the adult TBI populations and are assumed to be equally common in children, although little literature exists to support this assumption (Farmer, Clippard, Luehr-Wiemann, Wright, & Owings, 1996; Massagli et al., 1996).

Cardiopulmonary Impairments

Hypertension and decreased heart rate variability are common aftereffects of TBI (Blaskey & Jennings, 1999). Although the bulk of the problems are expected to resolve with neurological recovery, in some cases, continued cardiopulmonary inefficiencies persist. These persistent inefficiencies are attributed to brainstem disturbances and secondary deconditioning. Cardiopulmonary limitations of this type could exaggerate the functional impairment associated with other limitations the child may have in motor performance or cognitive organization.

Cognitive Impairments

Deficits in cognition cause some of the most severe sequelae of TBI. The motor problems described previously are interrelated with cognitive and behavioral problems (Warren, 1991). The most common persistent cognitive deficit areas in children with TBI are attention, concentration, judgment, and impulse control

(Anderson, Fenwick, Manly, & Robertson, 1998). Functional limitations associated with these cognitive deficits can include poor initiation of tasks and poor task orientation. Difficulties with memory and decreased information processing speed often are lasting changes following TBI (Porr, 1999).

Psychosocial and Behavioral Impairments

Postconcussion syndrome may be seen after any type of head injury, including mild injuries. This syndrome involves personality changes, mood lability, loss of self-confidence, impaired short-term memory, headaches, and other subtle cognitive impairments (Walleck & Mooney, 1994). Functional problems described as part of postconcussion syndrome are lack of goal direction and initiative, social withdrawal, depression, denial of disabilities, immature behavior, apathy, self-centeredness, disinhibition, and aggression (Carney & Gerring, 1990; Miller, 1991). Brown, Chadwick, Shaffer, Rutter, and Traub (1981) found an increased rate of psychiatric disorders in children with TBI.

Coster et al. (1994) reported that the functional performance of young children from 1 month to 5.6 years of age (M = 2.97 years) with head injuries did not differ from their uninjured peers at 1 month or 6 months after discharge, but there was evidence of increased caregiver assistance in self-care and social functioning required by the group with head injuries. The children with head injuries were performing the same activities as their age peers but needed more supervision and direction to complete the task. Similarly, Mazaux et al. (1997) reported a loss of social autonomy in adults with TBI. Behavioral adjustment and adaptive functioning impairments are more severe in children with more severe injuries but can be found to a lesser degree throughout the post-TBI population (Lazar & Menaldino, 1995).

Most studies find no relationship between cognitive outcome and behavioral adjustment (Lazar & Menaldino, 1995; Perrot, Taylor, & Montes, 1991). Based on the absence of premorbid behavior data on the children in these studies, whether the child's behavioral difficulties predated the head injury is unclear. Some authors accept this "premorbid problem" approach; others have suggested "a cumulative negative effect of the interactions of the child's early cognitive deficits; loss of self-esteem; the impact of the head injury on family, friends, teachers; and their responses" (Lazar & Menaldino, 1995, p. 59). It is believed that the cumulative impact of these pressures on the child starts a downward spiral, resulting in a pattern of maladaptive behavior (Shurtleff et al., 1995).

Communication Impairments

Impairments in both expressive and receptive language are common in children with TBI (Ewing-Cobb et al., 1997). In children with mild to moderate TBI, expressive language tends to be more impaired than receptive. Commonly noted are deficits of memory, word retrieval, labeling, verbal organization, efficient verbal learning, and effective use of spoken language (Porr, 1999). Improvements in speech (expressive language) correlate with improvements in motor function. Receptive language improvements correlate with gains in cognitive and perceptual function (Ewing-Cobb et al., 1997).

Long-Term Developmental Impairments

Of the few studies describing long-term recovery from pediatric head injury, most indicate that children have far fewer residual deficits than adults (Bruce, 1990). Recent studies suggest, however, that children demonstrate less damage early in recovery, but deficits can emerge later as

the child matures (Lazar & Menaldino, 1995). All of the children in Ewing-Cobb et al.'s (1997) study showed improvement on neuropsychological testing throughout the first 6 months after the trauma; during the subsequent 18 months, a combination of persistent deficits impaired the children's ability to acquire new skills. As in the 6-month trends of Coster et al.'s (1994) study, 5% (n = 79) of the adult participants in Mazaux et al.'s (1997) 5-year study continued to need supervision in one or more areas of daily function. Common problems included need for supervision in administrative tasks and financial management, writing letters and calculating numbers, driving, planning the week, and using public transportation. These problems can be subtle and difficult to identify in children because during childhood, autonomous function gradually develops.

School and Community Reentry Needs

There is extensive documentation of academic difficulties in children with TBI (Lazar & Menaldino, 1995). Educators indicate a need for support and additional education in managing students with TBI (Clark, 1996; Kehle, Clark, & Jenson, 1996). The child with TBI must be supported in the transition to school and provided continuing support "beyond the point of apparent cognitive recovery" (Lazar & Menaldino, 1995, p. 59). Recommended transition services are (a) establishing communication among all persons involved in caring for the child, (b) initiating the evaluation process, (c) integrating assessment information in an interdisciplinary forum, (d) planning and adapting education programs to meet the student's needs, (e) preparing the student for transitions, and (f) providing ongoing monitoring for late-emerging functional deficits (Blosser & Pearson, 1997; DiScala et al., 1997; Shurtleff et al., 1995).

Some children with head injuries exhibit chronic neurobehavioral and psychosocial impairments, necessitating ongoing monitoring and intervention in community settings. Families may need support well beyond the time of hospital discharge (Lazar & Menaldino, 1995; Serio et al., 1995). Community-based access to rehabilitation services in either outpatient settings or the public schools is limited by low referral rates, poor interagency communication, inadequate family resources, and incomplete understanding of long-term sequelae by families and community service providers. Protocols for school reentry abound in the literature (DiScala et al., 1997; Kinsella et al., 1997; Parkin, Maas, & Rodger, 1996), but they rely on the family reporting the TBI to school personnel. According to Shurtleff et al. (1995), "Because of their often excellent physical recovery, the cognitive and behavior effects of TBI may go unrecognized or be minimized" (p. 65). Mild cognitive problems often result in vague signs that families may not link to the injury (Savage, 1991). Researchers argue that school and primary care personnel need education on the signs of "late" problems that are likely to appear only after an extended period.

Occupational Therapy Intervention in the Community and Implications From the Literature

TBI in Infants: Early Intervention Services

Children who sustain a TBI before 3 years of age are an at-risk population and eligible for early intervention services. Because there is usually excellent physical recovery in this population, it is easy to overlook functional problems associated with cognition (Coster et al., 1994). Occupational therapists in early intervention programs may need to carefully assess the amount of caregiver support a child needs to perform age-appropriate activities. Children with TBI may pass the items on a developmental scale yet function in a manner atypical for their developmental level in terms of the external support needed. Increased need for caregiver assistance may reflect problems in cognitive functioning that emerges as greater developmental demands are placed on the child. Interventions for these problems are parent support, education, and training to create an environment that maximizes the child's ability to work independently. The occupational therapist following the young child with TBI can consult with the family about transition planning. One of the common cognitive impairments associated with TBI is difficulty processing new information and acquiring new skills. As the child matures, impairments may become more apparent as the child is expected to learn in new and different ways.

TBI in Preschoolers: School-Based Services

IDEA mandates preschool (3–5 years) services, including occupational therapy, for children qualifying for special education. TBI is one of the diagnostic categories that will qualify a child for services under IDEA if the resulting impairments affect his or her ability to benefit from special education. Children in this age group with impairments from TBI may be seen by an occupational therapist. Occupational therapists in preschool settings play a crucial role in planning the child's transition to elementary school and are well placed to advocate continued monitoring for late-emerging deficits. As with the younger children, patterns to look for are the need for more adult or environmental support in routine activities than is typical and difficulty in acquiring new skills.

TBI in School-Age Children: School-Based Services

Children not qualifying for special education in the preschool period may qualify during their later school years. As academic and developmental demands increase, late-emerging problems may surface. Problems with postural awareness and orientation, visual perception, tactile hypersensitivity, and spatial disorientation are seen in children with TBI. In a classroom setting, the occupational therapist may see difficulties with handwriting and atypical classroom behavior. All children with TBI should be reviewed periodically for the need for special services (Blosser & Pearson, 1997; DiScala et al., 1997; Lazar & Menaldino, 1995; Shurtleff et al., 1995). As with younger children, a concern in the school-age population is the amount of caregiver assistance required for ordinary function. The occupational therapy evaluation provides needed information for the educational team. The therapist collaborates with the team to obtain this information and to alert other team members to the potential for late-emerging deficits. Table 5.2 lists common problems that children with mild brain injury experience. These indicators of possible TBI-related impairments should be made available to the child and to all persons involved in the child's care.

Conclusion

Because TBI is the leading cause of acquired disability in childhood, clinicians and educators need to be aware of the potential immediate and late-emerging sequelae of pediatric TBI. Education is needed for specialists and families about the potential challenges that even children with mild and moderate injuries may face. Providing information on the common psychosocial and physical problems reported in children with TBI and offering therapeutic support

Table 5.2. Common Problems After Mild Brain Injury in Children

Problem	Description
Physical	• Dizziness (rare after 8 weeks) • Fatigue • Headaches • Visual complaints • Sleep disturbance
Thinking	• Difficulty concentrating • Memory problems • Poor reasoning and judgment • Difficulty in school • Acting on impulse • Slow to complete tasks • Difficulty putting thoughts into words
Behavior and emotions	• Depression • Anger outbursts • Irritability • Personality changes • Difficulty getting along with friends

Note. From "Screening Children and Adolescents With Mild or Moderate Traumatic Brain Injury to Assist School Reentry," by H. Shurtleff, T. Massagli, R. Hays, B. Ross, & H. Sprunk-Greenfield, 1995, *Journal of Head Trauma Rehabilitation, 10,* 76. Copyright © 1995 by Aspen Publishers. Adapted with permission.

in the classroom setting may maximize these children's opportunities for success.

References

Anderson, V., Fenwick, T., Manly, T., & Robertson, I. (1998). Attentional skills following traumatic brain injury in childhood: A componential analysis. *Brain Injury, 12,* 937–949.

Asarnow, R., Satz, P., Light, R., & Neumann, E. (1991). Behavior problems and adaptive functioning in children with mild and severe closed head injury. *Journal of Pediatric Psychology, 16,* 543–555.

Berker, E. (1996). Diagnosis, physiology, pathology and rehabilitation of traumatic brain injuries. *International Journal of Neuroscience, 85,* 195–220.

Blasier, D., & Letts, R. (1989). Pediatric update 7: The orthopedic manifestations of head injury in children. *Orthopedics Review, 18,* 350–358.

Blaskey, J., & Jennings, M. (1999). Traumatic brain injury. In S. Campbell (Ed.), *Decision making in pediatric neurologic physical therapy* (pp. 84–140). New York: Churchill Livingstone.

Blosser, J., & Pearson, S. (1997). Transition coordination for students with brain injury: A challenge schools can meet. *Journal of Head Trauma Rehabilitation, 12,* 21–31.

Brown, G., Chadwick, O., Shaffer, D., Rutter, M., & Traub, M. (1981). A prospective study of children with head injuries: III. Psychiatric sequelae. *Psychological Medicine, 11,* 63–78.

Bruce, D. (1990). Head injuries in the pediatric population. *Current Problems in Pediatrics, 20,* 61–107.

Carney, J., & Gerring, J. (1990). Return to school following severe closed head injury: A critical phase in pediatric rehabilitation. *Pediatrician, 17,* 222–229.

Clark, E. (1996). Children and adolescents with traumatic brain injury: Reintegration challenges in educational settings. *Journal of Learning Disabilities, 29,* 549–560.

Coster, W. J., Haley, S., & Baryza, M. J. (1994). Functional performance of young children after traumatic brain injury: A 6-month follow-up study. *American Journal of Occupational Therapy, 48,* 211–218.

D'Amato, R., & Rothlisberg, B. (1996). How education should respond to students with traumatic brain injury. *Journal of Learning Disabilities, 29,* 670–683.

DiScala, C., Osberg, J., Gans, B., Chin, L., & Grant, C. (1991). Children with traumatic head injury: Morbidity and post acute treatment. *Archives of Physical Medicine and Rehabilitation, 72,* 662–666.

DiScala, C., Osberg, J., & Savage, R. (1997). Children hospitalized for traumatic brain injury: Transition to postacute care. *Journal of Head Trauma Rehabilitation, 12,* 1–10.

Ewing-Cobb, L., Fletcher, J., Levin, H., Francis, D., Davidson, K., & Miner, M. (1997). Longitudinal neuropsychological outcome in infants and preschoolers with traumatic brain injury. *Journal of the International Neuropsychological Society, 3,* 581–591.

Farmer, J., Clippard, D., Luehr-Wiemann, Y., Wright, E., & Owings, S. (1996). Assessing children with traumatic brain injury during rehabilitation: Promoting school and community reentry. *Journal of Learning Disabilities, 29,* 532–548.

Gilchrist, E., & Wilkinson, M. (1979). Some factors determining prognosis in young people with severe head injuries. *Archives of Neurology, 36,* 355–359.

Hall, K., & Cope, D. (1995). The benefit of rehabilitation in traumatic brain injury: A literature review. *Journal of Head Trauma Rehabilitation, 10,* 1–13.

Heinemann, A., Saghal, V., Cichowski, K., Ginsburg, K., Tuel, S., & Betts, H. (1990). Functional outcome following traumatic brain injury rehabilitation. *Journal of Neurologic Rehabilitation, 4,* 27–37.

High, W. M., Jr., Boake, C., & Lehmkuhl, L. D. (1995). Critical analysis of studies evaluating the effectiveness of rehabilitation after traumatic brain injury. *Journal of Head Trauma Rehabilitation, 10,* 14–26.

Humphry, R., & Case-Smith, J. (1996). Working with families. In J. Case-Smith, A. Allen, & P. Pratt (Eds.), *Occupational therapy for children* (3rd ed., pp. 67–94). St. Louis, MO: Mosby.

Individuals With Disabilities Education Act. (1990). Pub. L. 101–476, 20 U.S.C., Ch. 33.

Jennett, B., & Bond, M. (1975). Assessment of outcome after severe brain damage: A practical scale. *Lancet, 1,* 480–484.

Johnston, M. (1995). Neurotransmitters and vulnerability of the developing brain. *Brain Development, 17,* 301–306.

Kehle, T., Clark, E., & Jenson, W. (1996). Interventions for students with traumatic brain injury: Managing behavioral disturbances. *Journal of Learning Disabilities, 29,* 633–642.

Kinsella, G., Prior, M., Sawyer, M., Ong, B., Murtagh, D., Eisenmajer, R., et al. (1997). Predictors and indicators of academic outcome in children 2 years following traumatic brain injury. *Journal of the International Neuropsychological Society, 3,* 608–616.

Klonoff, H., Clark, C., & Klonoff, P. (1993). Long-term outcome of head injuries: A 23-year follow-up study of children with head injuries. *Journal of Neurology and Neuroscience in Psychiatry, 56,* 410–425.

Lazar, M. R., & Menaldino, S. (1995). Cognitive outcome and behavioral adjustment in children following traumatic brain injury: A developmental perspective. *Journal of Head Trauma Rehabilitation, 10,* 55–63.

Lowenthal, B. (1998). Traumatic brain injury in early childhood: Developmental effects and interventions. *Infant–Toddler Intervention: The Transdisciplinary Journal, 8,* 377–388.

Mackay, L., Berstein, B., Chapman, P., Morgan, A., & Milazzo, L. (1992). Early intervention in severe head injury: Long-term benefits of a formalized program. *Archives of Physical Medicine and Rehabilitation, 73,* 635–641.

Massagli, T., Jaffe, K., Fay, G., Polissar, N., Liao, S., & Rivara, J. (1996). Neurobehavioral sequelae of severe pediatric traumatic brain injury: A cohort study. *Archives of Physical Medicine and Rehabilitation, 77,* 223–231.

Mazaux, J., Masson, F., Levin, H., Alaoui, P., Maurette, P., & Barat, M. (1997). Long-term neuropsychological outcome and loss of social autonomy after traumatic brain injury. *Archives of Physical Medicine and Rehabilitation, 78,* 1316–1320.

Miller, L. (1991). Significant others: Treating brain injury in the family context. *Journal of Cognitive Rehabilitation, 9,* 16–25.

Moseley, A. (1997). The effect of casting combined with stretching on passive ankle dorsiflexion in adults with traumatic head injuries. *Physical Therapy, 77,* 240–247.

Nuismer, B. A., Ekes, A. M., & Holm, M. B. (1997). The use of low-load prolonged stretch devices in rehabilitation programs in the Pacific Northwest. *American Journal of Occupational Therapy, 51,* 538–543.

Pang, D. (1985). Pathophysiologic correlates of neurobehavioral syndromes following closed head injury. In M. Ylvisaker (Ed.), *Head injury rehabilitation: Children and adolescents* (pp. 3–70). San Diego, CA: College Hill Press.

Parkin, A., Maas, F., & Rodger, S. (1996). Factors contributing to successful return to school for students with acquired brain injury: Parent perspectives. *Australian Journal of Occupational Therapy, 43,* 133–141.

Perrot, S., Taylor, H., & Montes, J. (1991). Neuropsychological sequelae, familial stress, and environmental adaptation following pediatric head injury. *Developmental Neuropsychology, 7,* 69–86.

Porr, S. (1999). Children with traumatic brain injury. In S. Porr & E. Rainville (Eds.), *Pediatric therapy: A systems approach* (pp. 525–544). Philadelphia: F. A. Davis.

Povlishock, J., & Christman, C. (1995). The pathobiology of traumatically induced axonal injury in animals and humans: A review of current thoughts. *Journal of Neurotrauma, 12,* 555–564.

Prosser, R. (1996). Splinting in the management of proximal interphalangeal joint flexion contracture. *Journal of Hand Therapy, 9,* 378–386.

Savage, R. (1991). Identification, classification, and placement issues for students with traumatic brain injuries. *Journal of Head Trauma Rehabilitation, 6,* 1–9.

Scott, A., & Dow, P. (1995). Traumatic brain injury. In C. Trombly (Ed.), *Occupational therapy for physical dysfunction* (4th ed., pp. 705–733). Baltimore: Williams & Wilkins.

Serio, C., Kreutzer, J., & Gervasio, A. (1995). Predicting family needs after brain injury: Implications for intervention. *Journal of Head Trauma Rehabilitation, 10,* 32–45.

Shurtleff, H., Massagli, T., Hays, R., Ross, B., & Sprunk-Greenfield, H. (1995). Screening children and adolescents with mild or moderate traumatic brain injury to assist school reentry. *Journal of Head Trauma Rehabilitation, 10,* 64–79.

Teasdale, G., & Jennett, B. (1974). Assessment of coma and impaired consciousness: A practical scale. *Lancet, 2,* 81–84.

Vessey, J. (1997). School services for children with chronic conditions. *Pediatric Nursing, 23,* 507–510.

Walleck, C., & Mooney, K. (1994). Neurotrauma: Head injury. In E. Barker (Ed.), *Neuroscience nursing* (pp. 324–351). St. Louis, MO: Mosby.

Warren, M. (1991). Strategies for sensory and neuromotor remediation. In C. Christiansen & C. Baum (Eds.), *Occupational therapy: Overcoming human performance deficits* (pp. 634–662). Thorofare, NJ: Slack.

Wesson, D., Scorpio, R., Spence, L., Kenney, B., Chipman, M., Netley, C., et al. (1992). The physical, psychological and socioeconomic costs of pediatric trauma. *Journal of Trauma, 33,* 252–257.

Winkler, P. (1995). Head injury. In D. Umphred (Ed.), *Neurological rehabilitation* (3rd ed., pp. 421–453). St. Louis, MO: Mosby.

CHAPTER 6

Young Children's Occupations
Explicating the Dynamics of Developmental Processes

Ruth Humphry

Ruth Humphry, PhD, OTR/L, *is professor, Division of Occupational Science, University of North Carolina at Chapel Hill, CB 7120, Chapel Hill, NC 27599-7120; rhumphry@med.unc.edu.*

Originally published 2002 in *American Journal of Occupational Therapy,* 56, 171–179.

Our profession believes that children's occupational engagement is both the process for and the outcome of development (Coster, 1998), but occupational therapists need to articulate further their view of young children as developing occupational beings. Leaders within occupational therapy stress the importance of placing occupation at the core of our knowledge and practice (Fisher, 1998; Wood, 1998). Conceptual models of occupation do not elaborate on processes underlying age-related changes in children, and developmental models of practice focus either on sensory integration and motor impairments or on stages of change in other performance components (Law, Missiuna, Pollock, & Stewart, 2001). In addition, clarity is needed to respond to expectations that professionals serving young children work from a theoretical foundation and develop evidence regarding *which* group of children under *what* conditions benefit from their services (Guralnick, 1998; McWilliam, 1999). As a first step in meeting these pressures to understand child development as it relates to occupation, this chapter examines assumptions made in pediatric practice and proposes a conceptual model of dynamic processes underlying the development of young children as occupational beings.

One difficulty in articulating occupational therapy's unique body of knowledge and our related role in early intervention is our overreliance on another academic field, psychology, as our primary source of knowledge about young children. Psychologists' traditional way of viewing behavior appears to have shaped occupational therapists' beliefs regarding development of daily activities. Illustrating this approach to development, Zelazo and Zelazo (1998) started with a complex behavior, functional object play, and explained changes in play as arising from developmental shifts in memory and mental representation, thus implying that intrinsic changes are prerequisites to new behaviors. Assuming that daily activities have a prerequisite foundation in performance components, occupational therapists might adapt activities or create special environments to stimulate growth of selected components, anticipating that occupational performance subsequently will improve. Intervention models that explain acquisition of skills in daily activities in terms of changing a performance component, such as sensory integration or fine motor abilities, are of concern because evidence suggests that cognition, motor, sensory systems, and emotion develop and operate simultaneously, so meaningful separation is questionable (Diamond, 2000; Magnusson, 2000; Thelen, 1995). Furthermore, suggesting internal change as the causal factor underlying development of occupation is not consistent with the conceptualization of occupation as emerging from person–environment interactions (Law et al., 2001).

Compounding the problem of overreliance on psychology, occupational therapy builds on historic, grand theories (e.g., those of Erikson, Gesell, and Piaget) for understanding children's behaviors (Coster, 1995; Law et al., 2001). The classic theorists generated descriptions of succeeding stages of development that were assumed to apply to all children. Overreliance on descriptions of average changes in groups of children who are typically developing is reflected by therapists' use of developmental norms as a "gold standard" in practice (Dunn, 2000, p. 34). To assume a universal sequence of stages is questionable, because growing consensus is that development is not predetermined and multiple developmental pathways exist (Horowitz, 2000).

Finally, by building practice around classic psychological theories, therapists have not been informed about occupation and development (Coster, 1995). Although psychology's contemporary theories recognize a reciprocity between the child and environment, psychology's description of experience is not well articulated (Horowitz, 2000). Without clarity in the forms of experience under consideration, psychological theories of development offer little evidence regarding what types or patterns of daily activities are most relevant and the mechanisms through which occupations affect children's lives.

One step in building our own body of knowledge is to consider available research, asking how it informs our understanding of the developing occupational human and how to arrange these ideas into a developmental model with occupation at the core. Such a conceptual model will serve as a metaphor to help organize ideas. Consequently, this type of model in itself is not evidence to guide practice but suggests relevant aspects of children's development for future study and can help to generate occupation-centered models of practice for young children with developmental delays.

Definitions

Humans, as multifaceted, living systems, grow and develop at several levels. Transformations within each level represent complex phenomena influenced by all other levels; therefore, no one level is a foundation for another, but all share reciprocal relationships (Gottlieb, 1996; Kelso, 2000). The study of age-related change in humans is an interdisciplinary effort. Although appreciating the transformations at every level contributes to a holistic picture, a discipline's philosophy determines the most relevant area for special study (Magnusson & Cairns, 1996). As pointed out earlier, occupational therapists have focused on changes within the child. Here, body structures (e.g., the limbic or musculoskeletal systems) and body functions (e.g., sensory processing, memory, motor control) are seen to have bidirectional influence with each other and are defined as a young child's intrinsic capacities for interactions with the environment. Based on our profession's philosophy, the model proposed here addresses change at a different level—children's occupation. *Occupation,* then, is defined as culturally valued, coherent patterns of actions that emerge through transactions between the child and environment and as activities the child either wants to do or is expected to perform.

This definition highlights some aspects of children's occupations that warrant comment. First, although culturally valued, not every childhood occupation is modeled for a child. Rather, an activity might be a child-generated pattern of intentional acts that meets the child's own needs (e.g., dipping a hand into applesauce and rubbing it on the high chair tray to explore the texture). These occupations reflect a cultural nature, as certain forms of child-directed activities are tolerated in one group but not in others (Humphry & Thigpen-Beck, 1997; Valsiner, 1997). At the same time, someone besides the child selects and orchestrates many other childhood occupations, assuming the child will participate. For instance, a parent feeding a 7-month-old determines the food, time, and place, expecting the child to share in the activity. Finally, children's occupations can be composed of actions, but not all of a child's acts are occupational. Children's universal, functional acts (e.g., scratching an itch) and acts without meaning to the child (e.g., gazing blankly at a television screen) are not occupational. Rather, actions become occupational in nature when they reflect the unique aspect of the physical and social environment and, when viewed in context, appear intentional (Wood, Towers, & Malchow, 2000).

The nature of young children's intent is crucial to understanding development. If young children started with the goal of sensorimotor imitation of others' actions without some appreciation of the outcome, their first efforts would mirror functional activities of caregivers (e.g., trying to spoon-feed another person). Rather, children initially organize their behaviors to experience an effect or achieve an outcome relative to themselves and create novel solutions in trying to reach desired outcomes, suggesting a consciousness of

what they intend to do. For example, young children in Japan who try to use chopsticks for self-feeding before they are able to control both sticks in one hand will hold one stick in each hand and stab at the food, something they never observe adults doing (J. Kurosawa, Minami Osaka Ryouikuen Hospital for Children, personal communication, July 20, 2000). The developmental processes enabling occupational behaviors in children and the acquisition and refinement of occu-pations are the focus of the remainder of this article.

Young Children's Occupational Behaviors

To communicate how young children can produce occupational behaviors and how occupational engagement serves as a change mechanism, I turn to concepts from a dynamic system approach. Originating in the physical sciences, dynamic system models are often used to explicate how patterns of organization form from interactive component parts and how change occurs. Concepts from this approach have been applied to organization of the nervous system, motor control, attachment behaviors, and adolescent development (Gottlieb, 1996; Kelso, 2000; Lewis, Lamey, & Douglas, 1999; Magnusson & Cairns, 1996). Occupational therapists have used a dynamic system perspective in their work (Case-Smith, 2000; Gray, Kennedy, & Zemke, 1996; Kielhofner, 1995). Here, a dynamic system perspective is integrated with research to suggest a conceptual model of developmental processes in early childhood.

Wilcock (1998) argued that evolutionary pressures created the occupational nature of humans; therefore, I assume that the same pressures shaped developmental processes. In proposing this model, four issues are considered. First, what leads infants to experience actions as intentional and to appreciate subjective feelings associated with activities? The second and third issues relate to mechanisms that enable very young children to generate occupational behaviors and to do so in a manner consistent with the sociocultural group in which the child is a member. The fourth issue addresses how engaging in occupation is the condition that leads to developmental changes, the acquisition of new skills, and performance refinement.

Experiences With Intention and Occupation

We assume that a young child's goal or expected outcome of his or her occupation determines behavior, which raises the question of how infants come to be aware of actions as purposeful and to associate emotional reactions with activities. Rather than genetically encoded characteristics of occupation, evolution favored conditions in which very young children bring a developmental readiness that is complemented by learning opportunities. Thus, both children's innate characteristics and the context in which they are raised enable very young children to perceive that sequences of action have an outcome and hold meaning to the actor.

Readiness to learn about intention is reflected by observations that infants and toddlers track adults' visual attention and strive to join with others in communication about objects and events (Carpenter, Nagell, & Tomasello, 1998). Infants' inherent traits also extend to interests in what others do with their hands, and they attend better to hand actions that are functional and look less at random, nonfunctional movements (Woodward, 1999). By the end of their first year, infants appear to perceive units in the flow of adults' actions that are marked by an outcome, such as picking up a towel after it has fallen to the floor (Baldwin, Baird, Saylor, & Clark, 2001).

The child's inherent interest in the intentional behaviors of others would have evolved only if the young were exposed to experiences that support learning about occupation. The discussion turns, then, to what provides optimal learning opportunities. Dewey (1939/1958) noted that experience is a continuous interaction between an organism and the environment, but a sense of *completion* of that interaction is prerequisite to *perceiving* the experience. Although exploration and play are universal behaviors of infants and toddlers (Bornstein, Haynes, Pascual, Painter, & Galperin, 1999; Gibson, 1988), in some cultures these may be solitary activi-ties and without marked points of conclusion. Receiving care, sharing in activities of others, and observing household routines offer more universal opportunities for young children to experience a sequence of actions with recognized points of completion. Hence, in their daily routines, others, especially caregivers, create temporal patterns of action punctuated by outcomes as the context for infants to learn about occupation. Enhancing this process, their gestures, words, and facial expressions focus children's attention on relevant features of tasks and the intended outcome (Perinant & Sadurni, 1999; Vygotsky, 1978).

An example of a routine that exposes a young child to occupation as a unit of sequenced actions marked by points of completion is seen when a mother feeds her infant. The mother who tells her 5-month-old son, "Time for your dinner; let's try squash," frames the occupation. The mealtime experiences include being placed in an infant seat, donning a bib, having the mother repeatedly bring a spoon with food to his mouth, and having his face wiped. Throughout this process, animated interaction occurs where the mother expresses affective reactions marking the end of various activities and comments as the baby anticipates or reacts to these different events.

Children's subjective interpretation of the purpose and meaning of activities they observe or share in has not been studied explicitly. Because of developmental differences in intrinsic capacities and more limited ranges of experiences with activities, young children's perspectives are expected to be different from those of an adult. For example, when given objects they have seen adults use, infants persist at reproducing simple functional acts, and although they enjoy adults' attention, infants do not respond to cues to complete the task (Barrett & Morgan, 1995). Thus, a 1-year-old girl could define bringing the spoon to the rim of the bowl and up to her mouth as her intended outcome of spoon use. Her sense of purpose and meaning is further suggested by the fact that she is untroubled by the lack of food on the spoon.

Producing Occupational Behaviors

In interactions with caregivers, and through exploration and play, children optimize their own development. Evolution, then, would not have yielded a developmental process that brought intrinsic capacities to a level of maturity *before* they were applied occupations. Rather, species survival favored efficiently using intrinsic capacities (at any level of maturity) to maximize an individual's ability to solve everyday challenges (Cosmides & Tooby, 1987). Thus, the second issue explored here is how very young children are able to generate occupational behaviors, despite immature capacities.

Three interrelated dynamic system constructs help with understanding production of occupational behaviors. *Self-organization* describes a living system's pattern formation drawing on subsystems to generate ordered actions (Kelso, 2000; Lewis et al., 1999). Subsystems, or intrinsic capacities, may be at any level of maturity and are brought together in a pattern organized to achieve the intended outcome of the occupational behav-

ior. Intrinsic capacities interact, influencing each other as they are used in the action. The second construct, *complex, nonlinear relationships*, states that with this interrelationship, more than an additive effect exists in how intrinsic capacities affect the characteristics of occupational behavior. Rather, the behavior is determined by a synergistic interaction of the more and less mature capacities brought together to achieve an outcome. With a nonlinear relationship, isolating a single element's effect on performance is not meaningful (Kelso, 2000). As the child combines intrinsic capacities into a pattern that meets a need or responds to expectations of others, his or her behavior can be said to emerge, the final construct. The idea of *emergent behaviors* implies no predetermined patterns, as actions are put together as needed in response to a particular task and situation (Thelen, 1995).

Observations of two young girls learning to use a spoon demonstrate these constructs (self-organization, nonlinear complexity, emergent behaviors). The first toddler, confronted with her inability to master the spatial task of scooping food with a spoon, solves the problem by using another person as an agent of action. That is, she hands the utensil to her mother to have the spoon's bowl filled before grabbing the handle and transporting the spoon to her mouth. The other toddler integrates her intrinsic capacities to find a different solution to the same spatial problem. She holds the spoon in one hand and uses the other hand to place pieces of food onto the utensil before transporting it to her mouth. In both situations, the toddler's occupation is eating a meal, and self-feeding with a spoon is the intended outcome or occupational behavior. Self-organization processes generated solutions that fit the intended outcome. The presence of nonlinear complexity is reflected by how each toddler combined her more and less mature intrinsic capacities so that her solution could not have been predicted.

Rather, the emergent behavior results from a unique pattern of organization brought out by each girl engaging in her occupation.

Fitting Into a Sociocultural Niche

Being occupational is more than acquiring universal acts or survival skills. Parallel to *Homo sapiens's* evolving abilities in functional activities was the evolution of culture (Tomasello, Kruger, & Ratner, 1993; Wilcock, 1998). Therefore, evolution would select for developmental processes where mastering culturally determined elements of behavior would be inseparable from learning to do an activity. The issue, then, is what characteristics within children combine synergistically with contextual factors to ensure that infants' and toddlers' emerging occupational behaviors incorporate the cultural features of the group.

The first trait within the infant is an inclination to reproduce observed behavior. Proclivity to imitate is part of early infancy and becomes a social, purposeful activity before the end of the first year (Uzgiris, 1999). Reflecting the occupational nature of imitation, young children are more inclined to imitate activities that seem to have purpose (Bellagamba & Tomasello, 1999), and they do not have to actually see successfully completed actions. Instead, they seem to "fill in" what adults meant to do and organize their efforts to imitate intended actions (Meltzoff, 1995). In this way, imitation brings the child into a situation that supports a social, cultural learning process where the child, in generating occupational behaviors with an anticipated outcome in mind, has opportunity for feedback regarding both the outcome and how it was achieved.

Besides being oriented toward people and imitating their occupations, children are open systems and conform their behaviors to the unique features of the environment (Dunn, 2000; Horowitz, 2000). The power of external factors to determine or modify actions is illustrated by

research where environmental conditions seem to govern what type of grasp an infant uses. Newell, Scully, Tenenbaum, and Hadiman (1989) reported that when blocks were scaled to the size of infants' hands, precision grip emerged at a much younger age than typically expected. This finding exemplifies how a range of actions might be within the child's repertoire and how external forces determine which behavior emerges as part of an occupation.

As children's behaviors are influenced by their social and physical environments, caregiving becomes a mechanism in the cultural learning process. Universal adult practices, such as proximity with the young child, an interactive speaking style, and scaffolding activities, suggest that evolutionary pressures shaped adult behaviors to capitalize on the child's interest in people and their occupations (Papousek & Papousek, 1995; Rogoff, Mosier, Mistry, & Goncu, 1993). Furthermore, by deciding what objects and people a child can access, in promoting some and limiting other activities, and through organization of daily routines, caregivers create their own sociocultural niches for children (Bornstein et al., 1999; Pierce, 2000; Rogoff et al., 1993; Valsiner, 1997). In this way, caregiving creates a unique ecology for each child and ensures that childhood occupations reflect the cultural characteristics of the group.

Developmental Changes

The final issue explores mechanisms underlying the appearance of new forms of occupational behavior and how performance is refined. The proposed model considers three general types of observable change. Some behaviors surface as completely new abilities, transforming the overall nature of the child's occupation. Appearance of dramatically new behavior reflects what has been thought of as a developmental milestone. Sometimes, instead of entirely new forms of occupation, some changes reflect finding alternative behavioral strategies to achieve the desired outcome. These more subtle modifications in how occupations are enacted reflect a second type of developmental change. Finally, children's occupational behaviors might retain the same observable characteristics, and development leads to skill refinement and generalization of the activity to new contexts.

Because developmental milestones seem to show up in children at approximately predictable ages, the nervous system's maturation has been a long-favored explanation. A dynamic system approach offers an alternative way to address the issue (Thelen, 1995). Recognizing the complex, nonlinear organization that assembles intrinsic capacities into behavior suggests that maturation of a variety of components plays a role. Capacities mature secondarily to age-related growth and as a result of general use in other occupations. For a period, a cluster of essential capacities can be too immature, so the self-organization process cannot circumvent these limits. When maturation of these performance-limiting capacities is sufficient, the self-organization process is brought into play as opportunities for the activity are created by the caregiver.

Eating pureed food illustrates a dynamic system perspective of dramatic transformations in an occupation. A variety of factors limit the infant's ability to eat from a spoon (Carruth, Skinner, & Nevling, 1993). These factors can include persistence of the extrusion reflex that pushes food out of the mouth, poor postural control in supported sitting, inability to orient the head, intolerance of some oral sensory experiences, structure of the oral cavity, and lack of organization needed to communicate interest and satiety. Just as the synergistic combination of capacities shape emerging behaviors, no one of these factors acts alone to determine readiness to eat from a spoon. Over the first 6 months, the capacities mature so that

when given the opportunity, infants use the self-organization process to generate a completely new form of eating—taking food from a spoon. Performance is not perfect, and there is a learning period while the child masters what needs to occur and how to do it (Gentile, 1998). Learning how to achieve an intended outcome brings intrinsic capacities to an even greater level of maturity.

Development of occupational behavior can be subtler than a sequence of major transformations in children's occupations. To understand the mechanism behind these more subtle changes, what occurs as the child masters an age-appropriate occupation must be considered. In a dynamic system, variability while learning is expected and reflects experimentation with alternative organizational patterns (Case-Smith, 2000; Lockman, 2000). An inclination to repeat a pattern occurs when the emergent behavior achieves the intended outcome. When a child uses a familiar pattern of organization, he or she is thought to approach an *attractor state* for that behavior (Lewis et al., 1999). Settling into a repeatable pattern for an occupation eases the energy burden imposed by having to organize intrinsic capacities each time the child engages in that activity. An attractor state is not a set, inflexible pattern but a dynamic one, and either internal or external factors can disrupt it. The two types of developmental change discussed here are the consequences of a recurring sequence of organization stability, instability, and reorganization to achieve an intended outcome.

In the first type of developmental change, factors such as changes in mood, intrinsic capacities, or altered interpretation of experiences with the occupation can destabilize an attractor state. When the disruptive force is sufficient, a child might not return to the familiar occupational behavior, and a new organization of intrinsic capacities leads to an alternative behavior to reach the intended outcome. For example, Gibson (1988) argued that perceptual development is a process of acquiring ever greater understanding of the opportunities for action that objects afford. Thus, a toddler initially may use a fork by scooping with it like a spoon (application of an existing attractor state). Observations of others and experience with utensils alters the perceptual understanding of the fork so that the child recognizes the opportunities for stabbing offered by the tines. This shift in intrinsic capacity produces instability in the existing attractor state, and the child enters a period of transition. Utensil use becomes messier (more variable) as a new pattern of self-feeding (stabbing food with the fork) emerges and application becomes differentiated from the original attractor state for spoon use. This process of having repeatable behavior, destabilization because one or more internal forces disrupt the attractor state, and then emergence of a new strategy illustrates how children's behavioral repertoire for an occupation can become more complex.

Contextual changes may also interrupt an attractor state so that an alternative behavior is needed to achieve an intended outcome. If the parent decides it is time for baby to try a new type of food, for example, a cracker that breaks into crumbs that do not dissolve easily with saliva, coughing confirms that the mouthing and sucking strategies used on pureed foods do not effectively manage solid pieces. The new food texture forces the baby to bring attention to feelings in the mouth to a more mature level and to reorganize oral-motor actions to generate new eating strategies (e.g., tongue lateralization and munching). Food texture acts as a *control parameter,* an external condition triggering a shift to a different pattern of behavior (Thelen, 1995). With experience in an activity, the child perceives the characteristics of control parameters and switches between the alternative forms of behavior.

Settling into a repeatable pattern does not suggest adultlike functioning, and the third type of change addresses how reorganization of intrinsic capacities results in performance refinement and alternative patterns of organization so that the occupation is generalized to new situations. In selecting a process whereby occupational behaviors emerge, evolution favored a mechanism that could accommodate changes in intrinsic capacities and the child's changing interpretation of an occupation. For example, arm length, in-hand manipulation, emotional regulation, and awareness of how others act all change at different rates during childhood. Thus, a preschooler who has mastered occupational behaviors for eating a meal at one age still undergoes changes. Through reorganization, new combinations of intrinsic capacities enable the child to adjust to changing body structures and functions as well as to new insights about "proper" mealtime behaviors. By reorganizing intrinsic capacities into new patterns to sustain occupational engagement, no major behavioral changes in self-feeding occur, but skill refinement and more socially desirable elements emerge (e.g., less spilling, not pushing food onto the spoon with the other hand).

Children also face environments where unanticipated events and new expectations produce ever-shifting occupational contexts. Because emergent behaviors are task and context specific, novel conditions that challenge existing attractor states can lead to reorganization to continue the activity. Thus, effort at maintaining occupational engagement in a variety of situations leads to generalization of existing behaviors as the child uses different patterns of intrinsic capacities. For example, a toddler having mastered self-feeding with a short-handled infant spoon in her own home might temporarily lose an attractor state for spoon use when eating in a restaurant. She retains the idea of her intended outcome, so reorganization occurs as she brings her capacities into a different pattern to generate the same behavior. With this new blend of intrinsic capacities, she uses a teaspoon in a distracting setting.

Discussion

Our profession's need to understand occupation brings the issue of how children develop as occupational beings to the foreground of our discussion. In putting forth the model of developmental processes, a key concept was that young children organize their behaviors around their ideas about the outcome of their occupational efforts. Infants appear sensitive to cues about intent and emotional reactions of others, so experiences of receiving care and watching significant others provide an introduction to the intentional nature of activities. A self-organization process allows infants to synthesize intrinsic capacities into a pattern of occupational behavior and to engage in their own intentional behaviors. Innate traits that lead to cultural learning include an inclination to imitate occupations of others and the open nature of emerging behavior. In combination with the sociocultural niche created by caregivers, the culturally determined characteristics of occupation are not added on but are part of the child's learning to do the activity.

After describing how very early occupational engagement is possible, discussion turns to using the construct of self-organization to understand how occupation serves as the medium for change. The proposed model suggests that some completely new occupations appear when the combined readiness of intrinsic capacities and a caregiver's expectations for new occupations converge. But the model of developmental processes introduces other forms of change where the instability of self-organized patterns, or attractor state for an occupational behavior, is the basis for further development. Destabilization of patterns can be from a single factor or a confluence of several internal or external factors. Within the

child, maturation of intrinsic capacities or altered subjective interpretation about an occupation can be sufficient to disrupt an attractor state. Control parameters can include any event, person, or object that alters the occupational context sufficiently to challenge emerging behavior. The iterative flow of having an intended outcome, organization for action, destabilization of the attractor state, and reorganization to produce occupational behaviors under new conditions generates alternative behavioral strategies or refined, more flexible performance. By highlighting the child's intention in occupation as part of the self-organization process, the model clarifies how occupational engagement, not use of performance components in actions, serves as the medium for development.

Use of dynamic system concepts and this synthesis of research to propose a conceptual model of developmental processes is in its early stages. The existing framework provides a way to speak of multifaceted processes, but limitations exist. The paradigm shift to a dynamic system view of development is compatible with understanding individual differences and developmental mechanisms. But the shift away from framing development in terms of normative behaviors of children results in the need for new research methods (Lewis et al., 1999; Magnusson & Cairns, 1996). Many of the studies cited here used traditional methodology and were conducted to understand development of young children's intrinsic capacities rather than occupation. Therefore, in an effort to start a dialogue about occupation and child development, I have extrapolated from available literature to propose this model. Furthermore, illustrative application was made to a socially negotiated occupation—eating a meal. Understanding how the model applies to behavioral changes in more child-directed occupations and development at different ages across the life span will be illuminating.

Clearly, there are many ramifications for further study, so only initial questions about early intervention issues are proposed here. One concern is the implications of a dynamic systems view of occupation for traditional pediatric models of practice that focus on impairments. If several intrinsic capacities are combined, having a synergistic effect on an emergent occupation, the dominance of one capacity in the developmental process is difficult to argue. Although these practice models illuminate impairments, can services focused on remediation of sensory or motor deficits continue to be justified for children with delays, as they are based on models that suggest that one capacity serves as a unique foundation for development of occupations?

The model of developmental processes suggests that through use and reorganization efforts to sustain occupational engagement, intrinsic capacities are brought to a more mature level. These changed capacities, in turn, bring about further reorganization so that more efficient performance occurs. The reciprocity between development of occupation and maturing performance components is not new. The model of developmental processes, in highlighting intention, suggests that the bidirectional influence between occupation and intrinsic capacities is more specific to an activity as carried out in a particular context than previously recognized. In light of this specificity, an issue becomes this: What activities are the most effective therapeutic media? Would therapist-generated, remedial activities using special toys or therapeutic equipment that do not appear in the child's daily environments be as effective as enabling occupations embedded in family life, child care programs, and educational settings?

Finally, this conceptual model suggests that development of the occupational being is not something that happens exclusively within the child and argues that participation in family life and sharing activities with significant others are

crucial developmental mechanisms. If subjective experiences with an activity and mastering cultural aspects of performance are inseparable from learning to do it, involving family members, significant others, and peers in intervention is probably crucial. In light of the importance of contexts in development, it would be difficult to justify serving a child with delays if significant others are not an integrated part of the process of the child learning an occupation. The proposed model is consistent with a family-centered practice and occupational therapy delivered in inclusive settings.

Conclusion

This chapter is an effort to move toward clarity regarding the body of knowledge needed to understand development of young children as occupational beings. In putting forward the model of developmental processes, the complexity of learning to do and refining occupations is described. Practice issues will be resolved through research that explicitly addresses children's occupations in naturally occurring environments, and with knowledge based on understanding children's developing occupations, therapists will be ready to determine which childhood activities in what settings promote optimal development for what particular group of young children.

Acknowledgments

I thank my colleagues in the Division of Occupational Science at the University of North Carolina at Chapel Hill for sharing in constructive dialogues about occupation, especially Wendy Wood, PhD, OTR/L, FAOTA, for our conversations about behavior and occupation. A study leave through the division gave me essential time to reflect on the implications of occupational engagement and human development. I also thank Grace Baranek, PhD; Sally Bober, MS; and Wendy Wood for their feedback on earlier versions of this manuscript.

Several of the examples illustrating the concepts came from raw data collected through collaborative student projects. I particularly thank Sally Bober, Heather Casewell, Amanda Core, Paula Knowlton, Kristin Rogers, and Dona Swahlan for their work.

References

Baldwin, D. A., Baird, J. A., Saylor, M. M., & Clark, M. A. (2001). Infants parse dynamic action. *Child Development, 72,* 708–717.

Barrett, K. C., & Morgan, G. A. (1995). Continuities and discontinuities in mastery motivation during infancy and toddlerhood: A conceptualization and review. In R. H. MacTurk & G. A. Morgan (Eds.), *Mastery motivation: Origins, conceptualizations, and applications* (pp. 57–93). Norwood, NJ: Ablex.

Bellagamba, F., & Tomasello, M. (1999). Re-enacting intended acts: Comparing 12 and 18 month olds. *Infant Behavior and Development, 22,* 277–282.

Bornstein, M. H., Haynes, O. M., Pascual, L., Painter, K. M., & Galperin, C. (1999). Play in two societies: Pervasiveness of process, specificity of structure. *Child Development, 70,* 317–331.

Carpenter, M., Nagell, K., & Tomasello, M. (1998). Social cognition, joint attention and communicative competence from 9 to 15 months of age. *Monograph of the Society for Research in Child Development, 63.*

Carruth, B. R., Skinner, J. D., & Nevling, W. L. (1993). Eating readiness: Reading the cues. *Pediatric Basics, 63,* 2–8.

Case-Smith, J. (2000). Development of childhood occupations. In J. Case-Smith (Ed.), *Occupational therapy for children* (4th ed., pp. 71–94). St. Louis, MO: Mosby.

Cosmides, L., & Tooby, J. (1987). From evolution to behavior: Evolutionary psychology as the missing link. In J. Dupre (Ed.), *The latest on the best essays on evolution and optimality* (pp. 277–306). Cambridge, MA: MIT Press.

Coster, W. (1995). Developmental aspects of human occupation. In C. B. Royeen (Ed.), *Curriculum for the practice of the future: Putting occupation back into therapy.* Bethesda, MD: American Occupational Therapy Association.

Coster, W. (1998). Occupation-centered assessment of children. *American Journal of Occupational Therapy, 52,* 337–344.

Dewey, J. (1958). Having an experience. In *Art as experience* (pp. 35–57). New York: Capricorn Books. (Original work published 1939)

Diamond, A. (2000). Close interrelation of motor development and cognitive development and of the cerebellum and prefrontal cortex. *Child Development, 71,* 44–56.

Dunn, W. (2000). *Best practice occupational therapy: In community service with children and families.* Thorofare, NJ: Slack.

Fisher, A. G. (1998). Uniting practice and theory in an occupational therapy framework [1998 Eleanor Clarke Slagle Lecture]. *American Journal of Occupational Therapy, 52,* 509–522.

Gentile, A. M. (1998). Implicit and explicit processes during acquisition of functional skills. *Scandinavian Journal of Occupational Therapy, 5,* 7–16.

Gibson, E. J. (1988). Exploratory behavior in the development of perceiving, acting, and the acquiring of knowledge. *Annals of Reviews in Psychology, 39,* 1–41.

Gottlieb, G. (1996). Developmental psychobiological theory. In R. B. Cairns, G. H. Elder, & E. J. Costello (Eds.), *Developmental science* (pp. 63–77). New York: Cambridge University Press.

Gray, J. M., Kennedy, B. L., & Zemke, R. (1996). Application of dynamic systems theory to occupation. In R. Zemke & F. Clark (Eds.), *Occupational science: The evolving discipline* (pp. 309–324). Philadelphia: F. A. Davis.

Guralnick, M. (1998). Effectiveness of early intervention for vulnerable children: A developmental perspective. *American Journal of Mental Retardation, 102,* 319–345.

Horowitz, F. D. (2000). Child development and the PITS: Simple questions, complex answers, and developmental theory. *Child Development, 71,* 1–10.

Humphry, R., & Thigpen-Beck, B. (1997). Caregiver role: Ideas about feeding infants and toddlers.

Occupational Therapy Journal of Research, 17, 237–264.

Kelso, J. A. S. (2000). Principles of dynamic pattern formation and change for a science of human behavior. In L. R. Bergman, R. B. Cairns, L. Nilsson, & L. Nystedt (Eds.), *Developmental science and the holistic approach* (pp. 63–83). Mahwah, NJ: Erlbaum.

Kielhofner, G. (1995). Human system. In G. Kielhofner (Ed.), *A model of human occupation: Theory and application* (pp. 9–25). Baltimore: Williams & Wilkins.

Law, M., Missiuna, C., Pollock, N., & Stewart, D. (2001). Foundations for occupational therapy practice with children. In J. Case-Smith (Ed.), *Occupational therapy for children* (4th ed., pp. 39–70). St. Louis, MO: Mosby.

Lewis, M. D., Lamey, A. V., & Douglas, L. (1999). A new dynamic systems method for the analysis of early socioemotional development. *Developmental Science, 2,* 457–475.

Lockman, J. J. (2000). A perception–action perspective on tool use development. *Child Development, 71,* 137–144.

Magnusson, D. (2000). The individual as the organizing principle. In L. R. Bergman, R. B. Cairns, L. Nilsson, & L. Nystedt (Eds.), *Developmental science and the holistic approach* (pp. 33–47). Mahwah, NJ: Erlbaum.

Magnusson, D., & Cairns, R. B. (1996). Developmental science: Toward a unified framework. In R. B. Cairns, G. H. Elder, & E. J. Casello (Eds.), *Developmental science* (pp. 7–30). New York: Cambridge University Press.

McWilliam, R. A. (1999). Controversial practices: The need for a reacculturation of early intervention fields. *Topics in Early Childhood Special Education, 19,* 1777–1788.

Meltzoff, A. (1995). Understanding the intentions of others: Re-enactment of intended acts by 18-month-old children. *Developmental Psychology, 31,* 838–850.

Newell, K. M., Scully, D. M., Tenenbaum, F., & Hadiman, S. (1989). Body scale and the development of prehension. *Developmental Psychobiology, 22,* 1–13.

Papousek, H., & Papousek, M. (1995). Intuitive parenting. In M. H. Bornstein (Ed.), *Handbook of parenting: Biology and ecology of parenting* (Vol. 2, pp. 117–136). Mahwah, NJ: Erlbaum.

Perinant, A., & Sadurni, M. (1999). The ontogenesis of meaning: An interactional approach. *Mind, Culture, and Activity, 6,* 53–76.

Pierce, D. (2000). Maternal management of the home as a developmental play space for infants and toddlers. *American Journal of Occupational Therapy, 54,* 290–299.

Rogoff, B., Mosier, C., Mistry, J., & Goncu, A. (1993). Toddlers' guided participation with their caregivers in cultural activity. In E. A. N. Minick & C. A. Stan (Eds.), *Context for learning: Sociocultural dynamics in children's development* (pp. 230–235). New York: Oxford University Press.

Thelen, E. (1995). Motor development: A new synthesis. *American Psychologist, 50*(2), 79–95.

Tomasello, M., Kruger, A. C., & Ratner, H. H. (1993). Cultural learning. *Behavioral and Brain Sciences, 16,* 495–511.

Uzgiris, I. C. (1999). Imitation as activity: Its developmental aspects. In J. Nadel & G. Butterworth (Eds.), *Imitation in infancy* (pp. 186–206). Cambridge, UK: Cambridge University Press.

Valsiner, J. (1997). *Culture and the development of children's action: A theory of human development* (2nd ed.). New York: Wiley.

Vygotsky, L. S. (1978). *Mind in society: The development of higher psychological processes.* Cambridge, MA: Harvard University Press.

Wilcock, A. A. (1998). *An occupational perspective of health.* Thorofare, NJ: Slack.

Wood, W. (1998). Nationally speaking—It is jump time for occupational therapy. *American Journal of Occupational Therapy, 52,* 403–411.

Wood, W., Towers, L., & Malchow, J. (2000). Environment, time-use, and adaptedness in prosimians: Implications for discerning behavior that is occupational in nature. *Journal of Occupational Science, 7,* 5–18.

Woodward, A. L. (1999). Infants' ability to distinguish between purposeful and non-purposeful behaviors. *Infant Behavior and Development, 22,* 145–160.

Zelazo, P. R., & Zelazo, P. D. (1998). The emergence of consciousness. In H. H. Jasper, L. Descarries, V. F. Casellucci, & S. Rossignol (Eds.), *Consciousness: At the frontiers of neuroscience: Advances in neurology.* Philadelphia: Lippincott-Raven.

III
Scholarship of Assessment

CHAPTER 7

Grip Form and Graphomotor Control in Preschool Children

Allen W. Burton and Michael J. Dancisak

Allen W. Burton, PhD, *is associate professor, Division of Kinesiology, 1900 University Avenue, SE, University of Minnesota, Minneapolis, MN 55455-0155; awb@tc.umn.edu.*

Michael J. Dancisak, MA, *was doctoral student, Division of Kinesiology, University of Minnesota, at the time of this study, and is now director of graduate studies for the College of Education, Concordia University, St. Paul.*

Difficulty with graphomotor skills—handwriting or drawing—is often why children in public schools are referred for occupational therapy services (Diekema, Deitz, & Amundson, 1998; Reisman, 1991; Tseng & Cermak, 1993). To address these types of problems, occupational therapists need to be able to assess graphomotor performance, identify the grip on the writing or drawing implement, and understand the variables that may affect the performance or the grip. Focusing on three issues subsumed under the last two categories, this study was designed to examine (a) the utility of the grip scale presented by Schneck and Henderson (1990), (b) the effect of grip form on drawing accuracy, and (c) the effect of implement diameter on grip form and drawing accuracy.

First, Schneck and Henderson's (1990) developmental grip scale has often been cited and recommended for use by occupational therapists (e.g., Amundson, 1992; Amundson & Weil, 1996; Tseng & Cermak, 1993; Ziviani, 1995), but there has been no published confirmation of the utility of the scale for categorizing all variations of grips and the generalizability of the relative occurrence of each grip for children 3 to 5 years of age. Second, grip is often mentioned as a possible source of graphomotor problems, but the extent to which an atypical grip can contribute to poor writing or drawing has not been clearly established (Benbow, 1995; Graham & Weintraub, 1996; Tseng & Cermak, 1993). Third, manipulating the size of the writing or drawing tool has been suggested as an ergonomic therapeutic strategy to facilitate a better grip or improve graphomotor performance (Amundson, 1992; Amundson & Weil, 1996; Tseng & Cermak, 1993), but little empirical evidence supports this recommendation.

Researchers have reported two general types of grip assessment systems: component and whole configuration. In component systems, separate components of the grip—the position of each finger and the thumb, position of the grip along the length of the implement, or the forearm position relative to

Originally published 2000 in *American Journal of Occupational Therapy,* 54, 9–17.

the table—are evaluated. Researchers using a component assessment system include Blote and colleagues (Blote & van Gool, 1989; Blote & Van Haasteren, 1989; Blote, Zielstra, & Zoetewey, 1987); Sassoon, Nimmo-Smith, and Wing (1986); and Martlew (1992). In whole-configuration systems, all of the components of an observed grip are described together, and the grip, considered as a discrete behavior, is given an appropriate label. A good example of a whole-component assessment system is Schneck and Henderson's (1990) scale. The main advantage of a component system is that the many combinations of possible features allow just about any grip, even unusual configurations, to be coded.

Conversely, the primary advantage of a whole-configuration system is that a single judgment from a limited set of choices is made, rather than from a series of judgments. A key assumption in whole-configuration systems is that the identified grips represent the most common component combinations and account for most grip possibilities.

Schneck and Henderson's (1990) developmental grip scale describes 10 pencil and crayon grips (see Table 7.1 and Figure 7.1). To test their developmental grip progression, they had 320 children who were 3, 4, 5, and 6 years of age perform two trials of a drawing task and two trials of a coloring task. Based on their results,

Table 7.1. Descriptions of 10 Grips and 5 Grip Levels According to Schneck and Henderson (1990) and Schneck (1991)

Grip No.[a]	Level No.[b]	Description
1	1	*Radial cross palmar grasp:* implement positioned across palm radially (thumb down); implement held with fisted hand; forearm fully pronated; full arm movement
2	2	*Palmar supinate grasp:* implement positioned across palm projecting ulnarly (thumb up); implement held with fisted hand; wrist slightly flexed and supinated away from midposition; full arm movement
3	2	*Digital pronate grasp, only index finger extended:* implement held in palmar grasp; index finger extended along pencil toward tip; arm not supported on table; full arm movement
4	3	*Brush grasp:* implement held with fingers; eraser end positioned against palm; hand pronated with wrist movement present; whole arm movement; forearm positioned in air
5	3	*Grasp with extended fingers:* implement held with fingers; wrist straight and pronated with slight ulnar deviation; forearm moves as a unit
6	4	*Cross thumb grasp:* fingers fisted loosely into palm; implement held against index finger; thumb crossed over pencil toward index finger; finger and wrist movement; forearm positioned on table
7	4	*Static tripod grasp:* implement stabilized against radial side of third digit by thumb pulp; index pulp on top of shaft; thumb stabilized in full opposition; wrist slightly extended; hand moves as a unit; implement rests in open web space; forearm resting on table
8	4	*Four fingers grasp:* implement held with four fingers in opposition; wrist and finger movement; forearm positioned on table
9	5	*Lateral tripod grasp:* implement stabilized against radial side of third digit by thumb pulp; index pulp on top of shaft of implement; thumb adducted and braced over or under anywhere along lateral border of index finger; wrist slightly extended; fourth and fifth digits flexed to stabilize the metacarpophalangeal arch and third digit; localized movements of digits of tripod and wrist movements on tall and horizontal strokes; forearm resting on table
10	5	*Dynamic tripod grasp:* implement stabilized against radial side of third digit by thumb pulp; index pulp on top of shaft of implement; thumb stabilized in full opposition; wrist slightly extended; fourth and fifth digits flexed to stabilize the metacarpophalangeal arch and third digit; localized movements of digits of tripod and wrist movements on tall and horizontal strokes; forearm resting on table

[a] From Schneck and Henderson (1990).
[b] From Schneck (1991).

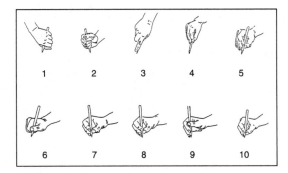

Figure 7.1. Illustrations of the 10 grip forms from Schneck and Henderson (1990). From "Descriptive Analysis of the Developmental Progression of Grip Position for Pencil and Crayon Control in Nondysfunctional Children" by C. M. Schneck & A. Henderson, 1990, *American Journal of Occupational Therapy, 44*, p. 895. Copyright 1993 by The American Occupational Therapy Association, Inc.

Schneck and Henderson labeled the first five grips "primitive," because they were rarely observed after 4 years of age; the next three grips "transitional," because their use decreased with age but still continued into the 6th year; and the last two grips "mature," because their use increased with age. However, Schneck and Henderson acknowledged that a developmental progression from immature to transitional to mature grips for individual children was not a reasonable expectation. The authors reported a reliability of .90 but did not specify the type of reliability coefficient used. Their 10-grip assessment system offers the simplicity needed by clinicians, but does it account for all grip possibilities? The first purpose of the present study was to examine this question.

After the 1990 study, Schneck (1991) considered whether first-grade children with difficulties in forming letters show less mature grips than do their peers without handwriting difficulties. For this research, she collapsed the 10 grips in the original scale into five levels by grouping together grips that were found to have mean ages within 2 months of each other (see Table 7.1).

With this five-point scale, she found that the children with writing difficulties obtained a significantly lower mean grip score (4.70) than the other children (4.93), and those with poor proprioceptive–kinesthetic finger awareness obtained a significantly lower mean grip score (4.33) than the others (4.94).

However, other researchers have found limited evidence of a relationship between writing performance and the grip used. In their study of writing skill among 8- to 14-year-olds, Ziviani and Elkins (1984) found that the way their 8- to 14-year-old participants held their pencils did not necessarily affect their speed or legibility of writing. Similarly, Blote et al. (1987) reported only low correlations between 5- to 6-year-olds' written products and different indices of body movement and grip. The tripod posture has been traditionally viewed as the most effective grip, but Sassoon et al. (1986) found no advantage in terms of writing speed with a tripod grip compared with other grips, and Martlew (1992) found only slight indications that 4- to 5-year-olds using a tripod grip could produce more accurate letter and word forms. In their review of handwriting research from 1980 to 1994, Graham and Weintraub (1996) concluded that "although the studies reviewed here suggest that variations in handwriting grip do not influence how fast or clearly children write, the generality of this conclusion requires further testing" (p. 24). Given the contrasting findings, the second purpose of the study was to investigate the effect of grip on drawing accuracy.

The third purpose of this study was to examine the effect of implement diameter on both grip form and performance. Large-diameter pencils became available from school supply houses in the 1920s and were recommended for young children to encourage correct finger position, discourage finger movement, improve control, and reduce cramping (Carlson & Cunningham,

1990; Graham & Weintraub, 1996). However, the advantages of larger diameter implements over standard-sized implements have not been demonstrated in the few studies carried out in this area. Wiles (1942–43), who had first graders exclusively use pencils of one of three diameters—7.4, 8.6, or 9.8 mm—over an entire school year, reported little correspondence between the quality of handwriting and pencil size at any of the three assessment intervals. Lamme and Ayris (1983) randomly assigned five different writing tools (large primary pencils, small primary pencils, standard #2 pencils, #2 pencils with triangular grip, fine-line felt-tip pens) to 35 first-grade classes to be used for one semester. They found no significant differences in writing legibility across the five tool groups and concluded that "teacher and/or student differences within each tool group were greater than tool differences, and that both teachers and students varied in their reactions to the different writing tools" (p. 37). More recently, Carlson and Cunningham (1990) examined the effect of pencil diameter (7.5 mm, 10.0 mm) on drawing and writing performance and grip used by 4- and 5-year-olds. Ten grips were identified in a whole-configuration system, but they were reduced to three ordinal grip levels for the analyses. They found no differences in performance or grips related to pencil diameter, but their results and those reported by Wiles (1942–43) and Lamme and Ayris (1983) must be interpreted cautiously because the range of pencil diameters was quite limited in all three studies.

Accordingly, three sets of hypotheses were established, corresponding to the three purposes of the study. First, in regard to the utility of Schneck and Henderson's (1990) whole-configuration grip scale, (a) all observed grips were expected to fit into one of Schneck and Henderson's 10 categories, and (b) the relative frequency of each of the five grip levels (using Schneck's [1991] sim-

plified system) for 3-, 4-, and 5-year-olds was expected to be within 5% of the values reported by Schneck and Henderson for the same age groups. Second, level of grip was not expected to significantly affect drawing accuracy. Third, contrary to current knowledge, increasing implement diameter was expected to significantly decrease the frequency of higher level grips and significantly decrease drawing accuracy.

Method

Participants

Sixty 3-, 4-, and 5-year-old boys and girls recruited from a public preschool program in metropolitan Minneapolis–St. Paul, Minnesota, participated in this study, with 10 in each of the 6 age–gender groups. None of the participants had prior formal instruction in writing or drawing grips. Most participants wrote only with their right hand (82%), but 13% wrote only with their left hand, and 5% wrote with both hands. The mean ages of the participants in each group, along with handedness information, are presented in Table 7.2. A parent or guardian of all participants signed an informed consent form.

Table 7.2. Age, Handedness, and Finger Length of the Participants According to Age–Gender Group

| | Age | | Hands | | | |
| | | | No. Using Right Only | No. Using Left Only | No. Using Both | Finger Length (mm) |
Group	M (Year-Month)	SD (Year-Month)				
3 years						
Boys	3-8	0-2	8	1	1	42–52
Girls	3-8	0-3	9	0	1	40–52
4 years						
Boys	4-5	0-3	7	2	1	43–54
Girls	4-5	0-3	7	3	0	40–52
5 years						
Boys	5-5	0-2	10	0	0	47–55
Girls	5-4	0-1	8	2	0	43–55

Apparatus

The participants were seated in a plastic-and-metal chair (with the seat 29.2 cm high) at a matching desk with a wood-grain laminate top (66.0 cm square, 50.8 cm high). Each participant was given a booklet composed of 20 half-sheet, standard white pages (21.6 cm x 14.0 cm). At the center of each sheet, a square shape with only three sides was drawn. A 3.2-mm-wide writing path was created by drawing the same three-sided pattern just to the outside of the first. The two open ends of the path terminated in 9.5 mm x 6.4 mm rectangles, with an ant drawn in one and a star in the other (see Figure 7.2). Finally, the background around the pattern was colored gray to highlight the white writing path. The inside lengths of the three sides were scaled to be approximately 40% of the participant's index finger length (measured from the web of skin between the index and middle fingers to the tip of the index finger) by using three different-sized squares. A small square (15.9 mm long) was used for finger lengths between 40 mm and 43 mm (37%–40%), a medium square (19.1 mm long) for finger lengths between 44 mm and 51 mm (37%–43%), and a large square (22.2 mm long) for finger lengths between 52 mm and 55 mm (40%–43%). If the writing paths were not scaled to finger length, then children with shorter fingers would face relatively longer paths and might

need to adjust their hand position or grip more often, which could affect drawing performance (Newell, McDonald, & Baillargeon, 1993; Newell, Scully, McDonald, & Baillargeon, 1989; Newell, Scully, Tenebaum, & Hardiman, 1989).

The drawing task was designed to require the fine motor skill needed in handwriting and precise drawing, but to minimize nonmotor factors that could affect movement behavior, such as perception and knowledge and understanding of the alphabet, language, and specific types of manuscript or cursive handwriting formats. Additionally, the task was designed for the degree of movement control to be easily and objectively quantified. Amundson and Weil (1996) asserted that fine motor control is an important component of handwriting readiness and that occupational therapists must determine when it is appropriate for a child to work on prerequisite handwriting skills, the functional skill of handwriting, or both.

Each participant performed the drawing task with implements of five different diameters: 4.7 mm (3/16 in.), 7.9 mm (5/16 in.), 11.1 mm (7/16 in.), 14.3 mm (9/16 in.), and 17.5 mm (11/16 in.). The 7.9-mm diameter matched that of a standard pencil or pen, the 11.1-mm and 14.3-mm diameters matched that of a small marker, and the 17.5-mm diameter matched that of a large marker. The implement barrels were made from Plexiglas™[1] rods, painted flat black, and fitted with a .5-mm ultra-fine Uni-ball™[2] metal-point pen refill (#UBR-5P). All implements were 13.8 cm long. A pen was used instead of a pencil, as reported by Schneck and Henderson (1990), because the special barrels could not easily accommodate pencil inserts, either sharpened or mechanical pencils. The use

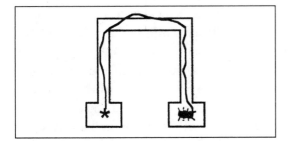

Figure 7.2. One page from the testing booklet, presenting a medium-sized drawing path (19.1 mm long), with the open end oriented up.

[1]Rohm & Haas Company, 222 West Washington Square, Philadelphia, PA 19106.
[2]Faber-Castell USA, PO Box 7013, Bedminster, NJ 07921.

of a pen rather than a pencil was assumed to have little effect on drawing grips, although some participants were observed to move the implement up to a steeper angle when they discovered that the pen would not write at a shallow angle like a pencil. As the participants performed the drawing task, the palmar aspect of the writing hand was videotaped with a VHS camcorder.

Procedure

Before testing, each participant's index finger length was measured to determine which of the three pattern sizes would be needed. Once seated at the table, participants were instructed to "draw a line from the ant to the star, staying only in the white path." They were given no practice trials and no demonstration by the experimenter. The participants performed 20 trials, four with each of the five implements. On the four consecutive trials with a particular implement, the open end of the square pattern was placed up, down, left, and right. Additionally, before each trial, the writing end of the implement was oriented toward the open end of the pattern. This systematic variation of the implement orientation was designed to prevent any bias of grip forms from the implement orientation. In a pilot study, some 3- and 4-year-olds were observed to not adjust their grip after initially picking it up, consistent with research on in-hand manipulation skills (Pehoski, 1995). The order of the five implements was varied using a Latin-square design, with each order repeated twice within each group of 10 participants.

Design and Analysis

This study involved three primary independent variables—age (3), gender (2), and implement diameter (5)—and two dependent variables—grip form and drawing accuracy. Grip form was coded according to the 10 developmentally ordered patterns presented by Schneck and Henderson (1990). In a later paper, Schneck (1991) reduced the scale to five levels, grouping together grips that were achieved within 2 months of each other (see Table 7.1). One rater coded all 1,200 trials according to Schneck and Henderson's levels, noting all deviations from the specified levels. The rater recoded the trials of two participants from each of the six age–gender groups, yielding a .75 proportion of perfect agreement. When the 10 levels were converted to Schneck's (1991) five-point system, the intrarater proportion of perfect agreement was .87, with a kappa of .75. Similarly, a second rater coded the trials of two participants from each of the six age groups, yielding a .67 proportion of perfect agreement between raters. When the 10 levels were converted to the five-point system, the interrater proportion of perfect agreement was .80, with a kappa of .64.

Drawing accuracy was measured by a six-point ordinal scale developed for the study and designed to discriminate between levels of drawing deviations from the specified path (see Table 7.3). For example, the sample presented in Figure 7.2 would be scored as a 4. All 1,200 trials by all participants were judged by two independent raters, yielding an interrater proportion of perfect agreement of .80 and a kappa value of .73. One of the raters also reevaluated the performance of 12 participants (2 randomly chosen from each age–gender group), yielding an intrarater proportion of perfect agreement of .90 and a kappa value of .87.

Because of the ordinal nature of the grip and accuracy scores, chi-square analyses were used to address the experimental hypotheses related to the effects of age, gender, and implement diameter. An alpha of .01 was chosen rather than the traditional .05 to minimize the degree of error potentially created by conducting repeated chi-square analyses.

Table 7.3. Descriptions of Accuracy Levels

Level No.	Level Description
1	*Task not completed:* lines not within 6.4 mm of starting boxes or ending boxes and/or gaps > 6.4 mm in the middle.
2	*One or more large deviations over inside or outside edge of the pattern:* (a) the perpendicular distance of deviations to edge or corner > 3.2 mm or (b) the perpendicular distance of deviations to edge or corner > 1.6 mm and < 3.2 mm, and length > 12.8 mm.
3	*One or more medium deviations over inside or outside edge of the pattern:* (a) the perpendicular distance of deviations to edge or corner > 1.6 mm and < 3.2 mm, and length < 12.8 mm, or (b) the perpendicular distance of deviations to edge or corner < 1.6 mm and length > 12.8 mm, but less than length of side.
4	*One or more small deviations over inside or outside edge of the pattern:* the perpendicular distance of deviations to edge or corner < 1.6 mm and length < 12.8 mm.
5	*All lines within the pattern, with some touching the edge.*
6	*All lines within the pattern.*

Results

Grip Form

The predominant grips used by all three age groups were Levels 4 and 5, accounting for 79.5% (3-year-olds), 92.3% (4-year-olds), and 98.8% (5-year-olds) of all trials (see Figure 7.3). No participants showed a Level 1 grip, and no 5-year-olds showed a Level 2 grip. The chi-square analysis of the effect of age on the frequency of all four observed grip levels (2–5) was significant, $\chi^2(6, N = 1,200) = 125.7, p < .001$. In addition, the chi squares for each grip level (2–5) were significant, $\chi^2(2, n = 71) = 73.4, \chi^2(2, n = 47) =$

14.6, $\chi^2(2, n = 450) = 22.6, \chi^2(2, n = 632) = 15.2, ps < .001$, with 5-year-olds by far showing the most Level 5s, 4-year-olds showing the most Level 4s, and 3-year-olds showing the most Levels 2s and 3s.

The chi square analyzing the effect of gender on the frequency of the four grip levels also was significant, $\chi^2(3, n = 1,200) = 64.3, p < .001$. Subsequent chi squares on the individual grip levels showed that boys demonstrated significantly more Level 4 grips, $\chi^2(1, n = 450) = 6.6, p < .01$, but the girls demonstrated significantly more Level 5 grips, $\chi^2(1, n = 632) = 10.8, p < .001$. Thus, the overall grip levels were higher for girls than boys.

Figure 7.4 shows that Level 4 steadily increased over the four largest diameters and Level 5 decreased over the three largest diameters. The effect of implement diameter on the frequency of the four grip levels was significant, $\chi^2(12, n = 1,200) = 27.5, p < .01$, but only the individual chi square for Level 3 was significant, $\chi^2(4, n = 47) = 15.0, p < .01$. The significant decrease of Level 3 and general increase of Level 2 as the implement became wider, coupled with the general decrease in Level 5 and increase in Level 4, indicated that lower level grips were used as diameter increased. The average percentage difference across the five grips was 4.3% for 3-year-olds, 5.7% for 4-year-olds, and

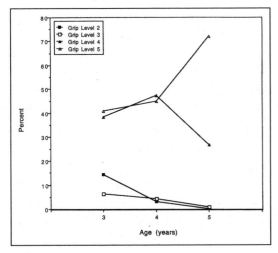

Figure 7.3. Percentage of grip levels by age group.

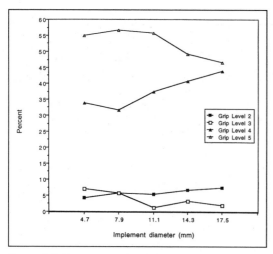

Figure 7.4. Percentage of grip levels by implement diameter.

Drawing Accuracy

3.3% for 5-year-olds (10 of the 15 differences were less than 5%).

Drawing Accuracy

The two highest drawing accuracy scores (5 and 6) increased with age, and the three lowest scores (1, 2, and 3) decreased with age (see Figure 7.5). The chi-square analysis of the effect of age on the frequency of all six accuracy scores was signifi-

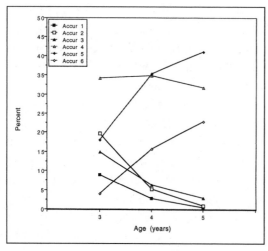

Figure 7.5. Percentage of accuracy scores by age group.

cant, $\chi^2(10, N = 1,200) = 252.6$, $p < .001$. In addition, the chi squares for scores of 1, 2, 3, 5, and 6 were significant, $\chi^2(2, n = 49) = 37.6$, $\chi^2(2, n = 104) = 89.1$, $\chi^2(2, n = 97) = 38.2$, $\chi^2(2, n = 377) = 36.5$, $\chi^2(2, n = 170) = 50.7$, $ps < .001$. Clearly, the older children demonstrated more accurate drawings than did the younger children.

More girls showed the three highest accuracy scores (4, 5, and 6), and more boys showed two of the lowest accuracy scores (2 and 3), but the chi square analyzing the effect of gender on the frequency of the six accuracy scores was not significant ($p > .05$).

The percentages of the poorest accuracy scores (1, 2, and 3) were low and consistent across the five implement diameters, all less than 10.0% and varying by 3.3% or less. The most common scores—4 and 5—averaged 32.4% across the first four diameters, with the difference between the two always 6.7% or less, but at the 17.5-mm diameter, the percentage of 4s increased to a high of 39.2% and the percentage of 5s decreased to a low of 27.1%. The chi square analyzing the effect of diameter on the frequency of the six accuracy scores was not significant ($p > .05$).

The question of whether certain grips allowed for more accurate drawing was answered by examining the relative occurrence of the four grips (2–5) for each accuracy score (1–6). The chi-square analysis of the effect of accuracy score on grip percentages was significant, $\chi^2(15, n = 400) = 61.1$, $p < .001$ (see Figure 7.6). Subsequent chi-square analyses of individual accuracy scores were significant only for the most accurate score (6), $\chi^2(3, n = 38.9) = 16.2$, $p < .01$, and the least accurate score (1), $\chi^2(3, n = 20.3) = 23.3$, $p < .001$. For an accuracy score of 6, the highest level grip (5) was used almost as often (19.0%) as the other three grip levels combined (19.9%), and for an accuracy score of 1, the lowest level grip observed (2) was used more than one-and-a-half times as often (19.7%) as the

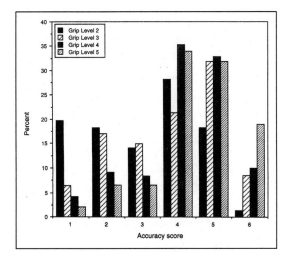

Figure 7.6. Percentage of grip levels by accuracy score. For each grip level separately, the frequency of each accuracy score was divided by the total frequency of the grip level and then multiplied by 100.

other three grip levels combined (12.7%). Additionally, Spearman's rho, quantifying the relationship between grip level and accuracy score, yielded a value of −.305.

Discussion

Utility of Schneck and Henderson's Grip Scale

As hypothesized, all observed grips in the 1,200 trials fit into one of Schneck and Henderson's (1990) 10 categories. However, individual participants often showed idiosyncratic finger positions that did not match any of the grips described by Schneck and Henderson, but the general characteristics of the grip allowed it to be classified according to the 10-level system. For Grip 8—four fingers grasp—13 participants held the implement with three instead of four fingers on 74 trials, and 3 participants pronated their wrist as in Grip 1 on 10 trials. For Grips 7 to 10, 10 participants did not place their forearm on the table on 54 trials.

The interrater reliability on the 10 categories, as measured by proportion of perfect agreement, was considerably lower (.67) than expected and likely was accounted for by these variations from the specified grip descriptions. The interrater reliability coefficient reported by Schneck and Henderson (1990) was .90, but they did not indicate exactly what type of measure was used.

Schneck and Henderson (1990) reported the relative occurrence of 10 grips for 3-, 4-, 5-, and 6-year-olds using a #2 pencil in a drawing task and a crayon in a coloring task. Their percentages of the 10 grips for the drawing task only, considered according to Schneck's (1991) five-level system, were found to be very close to those found in the present study for 3-, 4-, and 5-year olds. Across all implement diameters, the percentage differences between the two studies were not less than 5% as predicted for all grip levels by age, but 10 of the 15 differences were less than 5% and the average percentage difference for each age group was less than 6%. For the standard pencil diameter only (7.9 cm), 11 of the 15 differences were less than 5% and the average percentage difference for each age group also was less than 6%.

Based on the results of this study, use of Schneck and Henderson's (1990) 10-grip scale is recommended only for documenting the grips of individual persons and changes in their grips. If comparisons between persons are desired, then Schneck's (1991) five-level scale should be used. In addition, two important limitations in the 10-grip scale were identified. First, the description for Grip 8 indicates that the implement is held with four fingers in opposition, but 21.7% of our participants showed a three-finger opposition grip (and were coded as an 8). Second, forearm position relative to the table is mentioned in Grips 3 and 4 and 6 to 10, but this aspect of the grip did not always match the rest of the descriptions. Consistent with this second recommendation, Blote et al. (1987), in their work with 5- and 6-year-olds, reported that "in most cases the children started writing with their forearm and elbow resting on the table, but only in about half of the cases is their forearm and elbow still on the table at the end of the line" (p. 333). Thus, forearm position appears to be related to the extent of the writing rather than to a specific grip form.

A major limitation of the present study is the use of a ballpoint pen rather than a pencil or marker. Preschool children usually use pencils or colored markers, which can be held at steeper angles than ballpoint pens to make even marks or lines. Some participants were observed trying to write at steeper angles than possible with the pens and then adjusting the angle but not their grip when they saw that they were not making even marks. However, some of the grips reported in this study might not be the same if the children had used pencils or markers of the same diameter. A .5-mm metal-point pen refill was used because, after some exploration of other alternatives, it was found to best accommodate the Plexiglas implement barrels of varying diameters. Additionally, two other advantages of using a pen rather than a pencil were that the point was always the same and never had to be sharpened.

Effect of Grip on Drawing Accuracy

The second hypothesis predicted that the level of grip would not significantly affect drawing accuracy. However, when the relative distribution of accuracy scores for each grip level was calculated and then the grip percentages compared for each accuracy score, the relative occurrence of the grips was not equitably distributed for the most accurate and least accurate scores. Indeed, the highest grip level was used most often with the highest accuracy score (6), and the lowest observed grip level was used most often with the lowest accuracy scores (1–3), but the grips were fairly evenly distributed at accuracy scores of 4 and 5. This nonlinear effect of grip level on accuracy scores—significant only at the two extremes of the accuracy scale—helps explain the fairly low Spearman's rho value of −.305 between grip level and accuracy score. This nonlinear effect may have been masked in previous studies that showed only a minimal relationship between grip and graphomotor performance because most of these studies relied on mean performance measures across all levels of skill.

Children who perform at the low end of the accuracy scale are the ones most likely to be treated by occupational therapists and may be able to improve their writing or drawing accuracy by modifying their grip. Teaching or eliciting a different grip by manipulating the writing implement or other variables may be a fruitful strategy when working with persons with poor graphomotor skill, but persons should not be referred to occupational therapists just because of an unusual or "immature" grip (Amundson, 1992; Sassoon et al., 1986; Tseng & Cermak, 1993; Ziviani, 1995).

The highest level grip (5) was observed in more than half of the 1,200 trials (52.7%), with 35.3% dynamic tripods (Schneck & Henderson, 1990; Grip 10) and 17.4% lateral tripods (Grip 9). About the same ratio between the two tripod grips was reported by Schneck and Henderson (1990) for the 3- to 5-year-olds (42.5% vs. 15.9%) and 6-year-olds (67.5% vs. 25.0%). Bergmann (1990) reported that 88% of a broad sample of adults used the dynamic tripod grip to write but that about 9% used the lateral tripod grip. Interpreting their own and Bergmann's results, Schneck and Henderson concluded that "until further studies are conducted, the lateral tripod grasp should be considered an acceptable alternative to the dynamic tripod grasp" (p. 898).

This conclusion can be tested in the present study by comparing accuracy scores on the two types of tripod grips. Compared with the lateral tripod, the dynamic tripod yielded a higher percentage of the two highest accuracy scores (56.8% vs. 43.5%) and a lower percentage of the two lowest scores (4.9% vs. 12.0%). However, a chi-square analysis showed that the effect of these two grips on accuracy scores was not significant ($p > .05$). This result based on 632 observations provides further evidence that the lateral tripod should be considered an acceptable alternative to the dynamic tripod. What remains to be investigated, however, is the relative effectiveness of the lateral tripod over long bouts of writing or drawing and its resistance to fatigue (Tseng & Cermak, 1993).

Effect of Implement Diameter on Grip and Drawing Accuracy

The third hypothesis, predicting that increasing implement diameter would significantly decrease the frequency of higher level grips and significantly decrease drawing accuracy, was supported for grip form but not accuracy. Lower level grips, particularly Level 5 instead of Level 4, were used as diameter increased over the four largest implements. One explanation of why these results were different than the null effect reported earlier by Wiles (1942–43), Lamme and Ayris (1983), and Carlson and Cunningham (1990) relates to the wider range of diameters experienced by the participants in the present study—4.7 mm to 17.5 mm—as opposed to a range of 7.5 mm to 10.0 mm in the other studies. Thus, the use of implements commonly available to preschool children, such as color markers ranging in diameter from 10 mm to 18 mm, may elicit lower level grips.

Even across a diameter range of 12.8 mm, accuracy scores did not significantly change. The most marked change was a decrease in over-

all scores from the 14.3-mm to the 17.5-mm diameter, but the overall effect was not significant. The grip and accuracy results together indicate that, although larger diameter implements may often lead to lower level grips, accuracy changes very little, even on the precision drawing task used in this study. Hence, teachers and therapists should not be concerned about possible grip changes that may occur as children choose larger writing implements. However, they may encourage children who demonstrate very poor graphomotor skills to use smaller diameter implements, which may elicit higher level grips.

Conclusion

The first issue addressed in this study was the usefulness of Schneck and Henderson's (1990) grip scale for occupational therapy and other professionals working with children on graphomotor skills. The results showed that all grips used by the 3- to 5-year-olds could be categorized according to Schneck and Henderson's system and that the relative usage of the five grip levels (Schneck, 1991) was very close to that reported by Schneck and Henderson. Therapists are recommended to use the 10-grip scale only for documenting the grips of individual persons and changes in their grips, but if comparisons between persons are desired, then Schneck's (1991) five-level scale, which affords greater generalizability, should be used.

The second and third issues addressed in this study were the effect of grip on drawing performance and the effect of implement diameter on grip level and drawing performance. These issues are important for occupational therapists because of the potential implications for helping children with graphomotor deficits. Amundson and Weil (1996) recommend five approaches to handwriting intervention: neurodevelopmental, acquisitional, sensory integration, biomechanical, and behavioral. The strategies of manipulating grip level or implement size relate to the bio-mechanical approach or Tseng and Cermak's (1993) "ergonomic" approach.

The key question is whether changing grips can improve graphomotor performance. Our results indicate an equivocal "maybe." Although the lowest observed grip level (2) was used most often with the lowest accuracy scores (1–3), the grip levels were fairly evenly distributed at accuracy scores of 4 and 5. Only at the highest accuracy score (6) did the highest grip level (5) make a difference. Thus, children with graphomotor performance deficits are not likely to benefit from grip manipulations, because such strategies were shown to improve only performance that was already good. Moreover, this conclusion also emphasizes the point that persons should not be referred to occupational therapists just because of an unusual or "immature" grip (Amundson, 1992; Sassoon et al., 1986; Tseng & Cermak, 1993; Ziviani, 1995).

A final point on the issue of grip intervention is that "any grip, efficient or inefficient, that has been used over time becomes kinesthetically locked in" (Benbow, 1995, p. 267) and that "by the beginning of the second grade, changing a child's grasp pattern may be so stressful that the effort should be abandoned" (Amundson & Weil, 1996, p. 537). If a child is using an oversized implement (i.e., 11.1-cm diameter or larger), reducing the diameter—a "bypass strategy" within an ergonomic approach (Tseng & Cermak, 1993)—may help improve the grip form, but decreasing implement diameter from the standard 7.9 cm is likely to change grip form very little.

References

Amundson, S. J. (1992). Handwriting: Evaluation and intervention in school settings. In J. Case-Smith & C. Pehoski (Eds.), *Development of hand skills in the child* (pp. 63–78). Rockville, MD: American Occupational Therapy Association.

Amundson, S. J., & Weil, M. (1996). Prewriting and handwriting skills. In J. Case-Smith, A. S. Allen, & P. N. Pratt (Eds.), *Occupational therapy for children* (3rd ed., pp. 524–541). St. Louis, MO: Mosby.

Benbow, M. (1995). Principles and practices of teaching handwriting. In A. Henderson & C. Pehoski (Eds.), *Hand function in the child: Foundations for remediation* (pp. 255–281). St. Louis, MO: Mosby.

Bergmann, K. (1990). Incidence of atypical pencil grasps among nondysfunctional adults. *American Journal of Occupational Therapy, 44,* 736–740.

Blote, A. W., & van Gool, H. (1989). Writing behaviour of children aged four to five and half years. *Journal of Human Movement Studies, 17,* 133–152.

Blote, A. W., & Van Haasteren, R. (1989). Developmental dimensions in the drawing behaviour of pre-school children. *Journal of Human Movement Studies, 17,* 187–205.

Blote, A. W., Zielstra, E. M., & Zoetewey, M. W. (1987). Writing posture and writing movement of children in kindergarten. *Journal of Human Movement Studies, 13,* 323–341.

Carlson, K., & Cunningham, J. L. (1990). Effect of pencil diameter on the graphomotor skill of preschoolers. *Early Childhood Research Quarterly, 5,* 279–293.

Diekema, S. M., Deitz, J., & Amundson, S. J. (1998). Test–retest of the Evaluation Tool of Children's Handwriting–Manuscript. *American Journal of Occupational Therapy, 52,* 248–255.

Graham, S., & Weintraub, N. (1996). A review of handwriting research: Progress and prospects from 1980 to 1994. *Educational Psychology Review, 8,* 7–87.

Lamme, L. L., & Ayris, B. M. (1983). Is the handwriting of beginning writers influenced by writing tools? *Journal of Research and Development in Education, 17*(1), 32–38.

Martlew, M. (1992). Pen grips: Their relationships to letter/word formation and literacy knowledge in children starting school. *Journal of Human Movement Studies, 24,* 165–185.

Newell, K. M., McDonald, P. V., & Baillargeon, R. (1993). Body scale and infant grip configurations. *Developmental Psychobiology, 26,* 195–205.

Newell, K. M., Scully, D. M., McDonald, P. V., & Baillargeon, R. (1989). Task constraints and infant grip configurations. *Developmental Psychobiology, 22,* 817–832.

Newell, K. M., Scully, D. M., Tenebaum, F., & Hardiman, S. (1989). Body scale and the development of prehension. *Developmental Psychobiology, 22,* 1–13.

Pehoski, C. (1995). Object manipulation in infants and children. In A. Henderson & C. Pehoski (Eds.), *Hand function in the child: Foundations for remediation* (pp. 136–153). St. Louis, MO: Mosby.

Reisman, J. E. (1991). Poor handwriting: Who is referred? *American Journal of Occupational Therapy, 45,* 849–852.

Sassoon, R., Nimmo-Smith, I., & Wing, A. M. (1986). An analysis of children's penholds. In H. Kao, G. van Galen, & R. Hoosain (Eds.), *Graphonomics: Contemporary research in handwriting* (pp. 93–106). Amsterdam: North-Holland.

Schneck, C. M. (1991). Comparison of pencil-grip patterns in first graders with good and poor writing skills. *American Journal of Occupational Therapy, 45,* 701–706.

Schneck, C. M., & Henderson, A. (1990). Descriptive analysis of the developmental progression of grip position for pencil and crayon control in nondysfunctional children. *American Journal of Occupational Therapy, 44,* 893–900.

Tseng, M. H., & Cermak, S. A. (1993). The influence of ergonomic factors and perceptual-motor abilities on handwriting performance. *American Journal of Occupational Therapy, 47,* 919–926.

Wiles, M. E. (1942–43). Effect of different sizes of tools on the handwriting of beginners. *Elementary School Journal, 43,* 412–414.

Ziviani, J. (1995). The development of graphomotor skills. In A. Henderson & C. Pehoski (Eds.), *Hand function in the child: Foundations for remediation* (pp. 184–193). St. Louis, MO: Mosby.

Ziviani, J., & Elkins, J. (1984). An evaluation of handwriting performance. *Education Review, 36,* 249–261.

CHAPTER 8

Classroom-Based Assessment
Validation for the School AMPS

Pat Fingerhut, Helen Madill, Johanna Darrah,
Megan Hodge, and Sharon Warren

Pat Fingerhut, MSc, OTR,
is occupational therapist in private practice, Pediatric Therapy Center, 8323 Southwest Freeway, Suite 101, Houston, TX 77074.

Helen Madill, PhD,
is professor, Department of Occupational Therapy, University of Alberta, Edmonton, Alberta, Canada.

Johanna Darrah, PhD,
is assistant professor, Department of Physical Therapy, University of Alberta, Edmonton, Alberta, Canada.

Megan Hodge, PhD,
is associate professor, Department of Speech and Language Pathology, University of Alberta, Edmonton, Alberta, Canada.

Sharon Warren, PhD,
is professor, Faculty of Rehabilitation Medicine, University of Alberta, Edmonton, Alberta, Canada.

Originally published 2002 in *American Journal of Occupational Therapy, 56,* 210–213.

"Occupational therapists working in school systems are concerned with a student's functional performance [and] in the activities or occupational tasks of self-care, leisure and productivity required to participate in the school setting" (Graham, Kennedy, Phibbs, & Stewart, 1990, p. 5). The role of the school-based occupational therapist is to facilitate a student's task performance or ability to do purposeful and meaningful activities so that the student can benefit from the educational experience.

To practice effectively in a school setting, occupational therapists need to develop methods of evaluation and intervention that address functional performance from an occupational therapy perspective. Their focus needs to be on the person–environment interactions, with evaluation at the level of occupational performance (Law, Baum, & Dunn, 2001). Occupational therapy models of practice are moving toward a top–down approach, where occupational performance is the basis for evaluation and measurement of performance components added to clarify deficit areas (Fisher & Short-DeGraff, 1993). For the school-age child, occupational performance occurs in the classroom (the naturalistic setting), with the child doing the activities required of him or her in the student role (Magalhaes, 1995). For effective model-based practice, clinicians must understand the theory and model underlying the assessments they use and what constructs the assessment addresses.

Unfortunately, many assessments either involve removing the child from the classroom for evaluation or use a series of clinical observations that have not been tested for validity and reliability (Atchison, Fisher, & Bryze, 1998). However, assessments are being developed that measure children's occupational performance within a naturalistic setting. For example, the School Function Assessment (Coster, Deeney, Haltiwanger, & Haley, 1998) measures the student's participation, task supports, and activity performance with a rating scale completed by a person familiar with the child's classroom performance (e.g., teacher, teaching assistant). The School Version of the Assessment of Motor and Process Skills (School AMPS; Fisher & Bryze, 1998) is a psychometrically sound tool that focuses on functional school-related skills in the classroom. Motor and process elements of schoolwork performance (i.e., school motor skills, school process skills) are evaluated by an occupational therapist through observation in the classroom setting. School motor skills include quality of performance in areas of posture, mobility, coordination, strength and effort, and energy. School process skills include quality of performance in areas of attention, using knowledge, temporal organization, using space and objects, and adaptation. The School AMPS was originally developed by Magalhaes (1995) and revised by Fisher and Bryze (1998).

The purpose of this study was to validate the School AMPS further. No gold standard has been established to measure the constructs of school motor and school process performance. Hypotheses regarding correlations to other instruments where the constructs are better established are needed to build a composite picture of how well the School AMPS is measuring what it intends. Within the school system in Alberta, Canada, where this study was conducted, occupational therapists frequently use the Peabody Developmental Motor Scale–Fine Motor (PDMS–FM; Folio & Fewell, 1983) to evaluate children of kindergarten age who are referred for productivity problems in the classroom. This assessment measures the performance component of fine motor development. It is a standardized, product-based assessment conducted in a one-to-one testing format outside of the classroom.

The School AMPS measurement of the construct of school motor skills was compared to the PDMS–FM. A moderate correlation was expected because of the similarity in tasks measured

(e.g., cutting, drawing, manipulating small objects) and common elements of fine motor performance. A higher correlation was not expected because of dissimilarities between the two assessments. The School AMPS (motor) tests the quality of all motor performance (e.g., fine motor, gross motor, locomotion, strength, endurance), whereas the PDMS–FM is restricted to fine motor skills only. The School AMPS is focused on occupational performance in a naturalistic setting, whereas the PDMS–FM is functionally based and evaluates the performance component of fine motor development in a controlled clinical environment.

The School AMPS process scale was compared to the PDMS–FM on the assumption that the two scales would measure different constructs. Deficits in process skills (e.g., attention, organization, use of knowledge) can severely affect a child's occupational performance but be unrelated to motor deficits; hence, a lower correlation would be expected between the assessments. Some correlation would be expected, however, because children with motor problems frequently have process problems as well.

The research questions for this study were the following:

- What is the relationship between the PDMS–FM and the School AMPS motor ability measure (correlation of PDMS–FM and School AMPS motor ability measure)?
- What is the relationship between the PDMS–FM and the School AMPS process ability measure (correlation of PDMS–FM and School AMPS process ability measure)?

Method

Sample

Forty-two children from five public school kindergarten classes were included in the study.

This sample of convenience included all children in the kindergarten classes between 5 and 7 years of age for whom a signed consent from the parents was received. Children with neuromuscular conditions (e.g., cerebral palsy, spina bifida), autism, severe sensory disability (e.g., severe vision or hearing impairment), or severe behavior problems cannot be assessed with the PDMS–FM using standardized testing procedures, so they were excluded from the study.

The kindergarten classes comprised children with a range of academic and motor abilities. Fourteen children had been identified as having special needs and were integrated into the regular kindergarten program. The children with special needs had a variety of delays, including speech, motor, perceptual, and cognitive. A mix of lower-income and middle-income families reside in the catchment area.

Procedure

Each child was assessed with the School AMPS and the PDMS–FM on the same day (morning or afternoon, depending on the kindergarten placement of the child). Children were randomly assigned to groups where either the School AMPS or PDMS–FM was given first. To administer the PDMS–FM, the child was taken to a quiet room away from the classroom. All items were administered with the child seated at a child-sized table. Because the School AMPS is an observational tool, it was administered in the classroom. A number of typical classroom activities, such as copying text or cutting and pasting, fit the School AMPS criteria for assessment tasks. To administer the School AMPS, each child was observed doing two of these tasks. A short interview with the teacher was conducted before the evaluation to clarify such issues as what product was in keeping with the teacher's expectations for a child who is typically developing and what level of independence and cleanup was expected as rec-

ommended by Atchison et al. (1998) and Magalhaes (1995).

The first author (rater) assessed all children. She has extensive experience in using the PDMS–FM and had attended courses in the administration of both the AMPS (Fisher, 1997) and the School AMPS to qualify in administration of the School AMPS. The rater was not informed of the children's classroom performance or the nature of their special needs before evaluation.

Results

Each child was scored on the three different tests. For the PDMS-FM, z scores were calculated from the test manual (Folio & Fewell, 1983). For the School AMPS motor scale and process scale, logits (log-odds probability units) were derived from the many-faceted Rasch measurement computer program, FACETS (Linacre, 1987–1994). The PDMS–FM had a mean z score of –.17 (SD = 1.19, range = –2.33–1.64). The School AMPS motor scale had a mean of 2.03 logits (SD = .63, range = .69–3.60). The School AMPS process scale had a mean of .73 logits (SD = .67, range = –1.13–3.01).

Pearson product-moment correlation coefficients were calculated to examine the relationship between the scores of each child on the two instruments. The results were as expected with the School AMPS motor scale, correlating higher with the PDMS–FM ($r = .45$) than the School AMPS process scale with the PDMS–FM ($r = .35$). Figures 8.1 and 8.2 show the scatter of individual students' scores on these instruments. The scores shown in Figure 8.1 have more of a linear relationship than those in Figure 8.2.

Discussion

As expected, the construct of fine motor development is more closely related to school motor

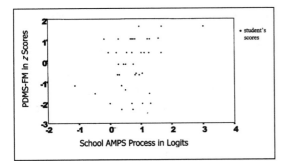

Figure 8.1. The scores of the kindergarten children on the Peabody Developmental Motor Scale–Fine Motor (PDMS–FM) and the School Version of the Assessment of Motor and Process Skills (School AMPS) motor scale.
Note. z scores = standard scores; logits = log-odds probability units.

task performance than school process task performance. This finding supports the assertion that the School AMPS motor and process scales measure different constructs. The fact that the correlation between the PDMS–FM and School AMPS motor scale was only moderate supports the assertion that the School AMPS motor scale assesses more than just fine motor skills, although similar tasks are used in the two assess-

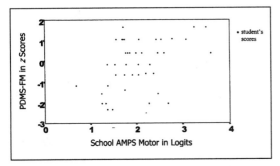

Figure 8.2. The scores of the kindergarten children on the Peabody Developmental Motor Scale–Fine Motor (PDMS–FM) and the School Version of the Assessment of Motor and Process Skills (School AMPS) process scale.
Note. z scores = standard scores; logits = log-odds probability units.

ments. These results also may support the assertion that occupational performance in the naturalistic setting may not necessarily correlate highly with functional assessment of performance components in the laboratory or clinical setting.

The assessment results show the unique patterns of performance by individual students. Some performed poorly or well on all three scales; others had significant areas of strengths and weaknesses. The fact that the School AMPS can identify the effect of deficits in process skills on performance and contributions of deficits in motor skill is valuable in planning effective intervention. Different intervention strategies would be implemented for a child experiencing difficulty with organizing his or her space and task approach than for a child struggling with motor control.

The School AMPS continues to be developed through ongoing research of validity, reliability, and clinical use (Atchison et al., 1998; Fisher, Bryze, & Atchison, 2000). The results of this study support the assertions that the School AMPS is not measuring the same constructs as the PDMS–FM and that it measures two different aspects of occupational performance labeled school motor skills and school process skills.

Limitations and Directions for Future Research

This study used a convenience sample of kindergarten children from regular and special education settings in one school system in Alberta, Canada. Replication of results with children of other ages and other socioeconomic and ethnic backgrounds is needed before these findings can be generalized. As well, the high prevalence of children with identified special needs in this sample may have resulted in higher correlations than would have been obtained had children been randomly drawn from the general school population, as the identified children would increase the variability of the group. However, the assessments used in this study are designed to be used with children with special needs and would not be used clinically with children who are not experiencing productivity problems in the classroom.

As cautioned by Magalhaes (1995), Atchison et al. (1998), and Fisher and Bryze (1998), it is important to choose an assessment task that challenges the child to maximize observations. For the purposes of this study, no prior knowledge beyond eligibility for participation was obtained about the children before evaluation. Tasks, therefore, were chosen to accommodate the setting and time. In clinical use, prior discussion with the classroom teacher would reveal referral concerns about the child, which would allow the occupational therapist to choose "the just-right challenge." It is likely that this choice would result in increased reliability of the assessment results.

Continued validation studies contribute to the clinical use of an instrument. The usual method of referral for occupational therapy services in school-based practice is through teacher identification. In clinical practice then, only those children who are determined to be having difficulty in the classroom would actually be assessed with the School AMPS. Once cut-off scores have been determined for the School AMPS, a study using discriminant analysis to determine how well the School AMPS (motor and process scales) scores and classroom teachers agree in identifying children who need services would be valuable both for School AMPS validation and evaluation of current referral practices.

Continued reliability and validity studies of the School AMPS will contribute to its clinical use. It appears that the School AMPS would be a desirable tool for evaluation of outcomes in the clinical setting because its observational format allows multiple data collections over time. As an observational assessment, no bias is created by the participant's learning of test items, which would facilitate its use for measurement of change. Clinical trials using this assessment would provide feedback to guide clinicians in its possibilities for clinical use.

Implications for Occupational Therapy Practice

This study contributes to the validation of the School AMPS as an instrument to measure the occupational constructs of school motor skills and school process skills in a naturalistic setting. Occupational therapists in school-based practice need assessments that evaluate occupational performance so that they can provide service from an occupational perspective. Ideally, these tools need to have adequate validity, reliability, and sensitivity in identifying children in need of occupational therapy services and in measuring change.

References

Atchison, B. T., Fisher, A. G., & Bryze, K., (1998). Rater reliability and internal scale and person response validity of the School Assessment of Motor and Process Skills. *American Journal of Occupational Therapy, 52,* 843–850.

Coster, W. J., Deeney, T., Haltiwanger, J., & Haley, S. M. (1998). *School Function Assessment.* San Antonio, TX: Psychological Corporation.

Fisher, A. G. (1997). *Assessment of motor and process skills* (2nd ed.). Fort Collins, CO: Three Star Press.

Fisher, A. G., & Bryze, K. (1998). *School AMPS: School Version of the Assessment of Motor and Process Skills* (2nd research ed.) Fort Collins, CO: Three Star Press.

Fisher, A. G., Bryze, K., & Atchison, B. T. (2000). Naturalistic assessment of functional performance in school settings: Reliability and validity of the

School AMPS scales. *Journal of Outcome Measures, 4,* 491–512.

Fisher, A. G., & Short-DeGraff, M. (1993). Nationally speaking—Improving functional assessment in occupational therapy: Recommendations and philosophy for change. *American Journal of Occupational Therapy, 47,* 199–201.

Folio, M. R., & Fewell, R. (1983). *Peabody Developmental Motor Scales and Activity Cards.* Chicago: Riverside.

Graham, D. R., Kennedy, D., Phibbs, C., & Stewart, D. (1990). *Position paper on occupational therapy in schools.* Ottawa, ON: Canadian Association of Occupational Therapists.

Law, M., Baum, C., & Dunn, W. (2001). *Measuring occupational performance.* Thorofare, NJ: Slack.

Linacre, J. A. (1987–1994). *FACETS: Many-faceted Rasch measurement computer program.* Chicago: MESA.

Magalhaes, L. C. (1995). *Assessing motor and process skills during naturalistic classroom observation: Pilot study.* Unpublished doctoral dissertation, University of Illinois at Chicago.

CHAPTER 9

The Evaluation of Sensory Processing
A Validity Study Using Contrasting Groups

Cheryl L. Johnson-Ecker and L. Diane Parham

Cheryl L. Johnson-Ecker, MA, OTR/L, BCP, *is occupational therapist, Therapy in Action, 18522 Oxnard Street, Tarzana, CA 91356.*

L. Diane Parham, PhD, OTR, FAOTA, *is associate professor, Department of Occupational Science and Occupational Therapy, University of Southern California, Los Angeles.*

Sensory history questionnaires are clinical assessment tools that are traditionally used in occupational therapy to assess children with known or suspected sensory integration problems. These instruments usually are parent questionnaires consisting of items that inquire about a child's responses to sensory experiences in the context of everyday life. In one exhaustive search of the sensory history questionnaire literature (LaCroix, 1993), 15 different instruments by different authors, all printed in the 1970s and 1980s, were found. Thus, for over 20 years, sensory history questionnaires have been used by occupational therapists to supplement formal testing, observation, and interviewing (Parham & Mailloux, 1996). These instruments are thought to be useful for the identification of children who would benefit from occupational therapy designed to enhance participation in childhood occupations by reducing the impact of sensory processing problems. Before such instruments can be used with confidence, however, qualities such as reliability and validity must be examined.

The purpose of this study was to examine the criterion-related validity of a sensory history questionnaire, the Evaluation of Sensory Processing (ESP), using contrasting groups. The term "sensory processing" in the name of the instrument refers to the brain's handling of sensory information for the purpose of enabling a person's engagement in occupations. This is synonymous with what Ayres (1979) called "sensory integration": the brain's coordination of various forms of sensory information in order to support participation in daily life activities. The present study was designed to identify ESP items that differentiate between responses of parents whose children have sensory integrative dysfunction, and responses of parents whose children are typically developing.

Literature Review

Several studies have been conducted to estimate the validity of a variety of sensory history parent questionnaires. The earliest published validity study, by

Originally published 2000 in *American Journal of Occupational Therapy,* 54, 494–503.

Larson (1982), examined whether sensory history items discriminated between developmentally delayed children with and without tactile defensiveness. Although her questionnaire consisted of items that were judged by a panel of experts to be representative of tactile defensive behaviors, only 16% of the items differentiated statistically between the tactile defensive and nondefensive groups.

Royeen later developed a questionnaire to measure tactile defensiveness in elementary-school-aged children entitled Touch Inventory for Elementary-School-Aged Children (Royeen, 1986; Royeen & Fortune, 1990) and a parent or teacher questionnaire for preschoolers entitled the Touch Inventory for Preschoolers (Royeen, 1985, 1987). The content validity of the questionnaires was supported by expert reviewers (Royeen, 1985), and the Touch Inventory for Elementary-School-Aged Children was shown to distinguish between groups of children with and without tactile defensiveness (Royeen, 1986).

Spyropulos (1991) examined content and construct validity of a sensory history survey constructed by Clark and Parham (1984) that used items from older unvalidated instruments that measured a variety of aspects of sensory processing. Of the 39 items, 37 were considered to have good content validity with a criterion of at least 80% agreement among a panel of experts. However, only 11 items were found to differentiate between responses of parents of children with and without sensory integrative dysfunction.

The Sensory Rating Scale (SRS) is a parent questionnaire developed specifically to identify sensory defensiveness in infants and young children from birth to 3 years (Provost, 1991; Provost & Oetter, 1993). Content validity of the SRS was assessed informally by three experts and their suggestions were used to improve the clarity of items. Provost (1991) administered the SRS to parents of 120 typically developing children

and an equal number of parents of children at risk for or with developmental delays. The at-risk/delayed children had considerably higher SRS scores, indicating a higher occurrence of reported behaviors associated with sensory defensiveness. In addition, the children with multiple developmental problems or more severe developmental delays were found to have a higher incidence of sensory defensive behaviors, as indicated by parent ratings, than children who had less severe delays.

Dunn and her colleagues have conducted the most extensive validity research on a sensory history questionnaire. In the initial study of Dunn's instrument, the Sensory Profile (Dunn, 1994), 67 of 99 items met a criterion for uncommon behaviors ("rarely" or "never" response ratings for at least 80% of children who were typically developing). Dunn and Westman (1997) then collected data on 1,115 typically developing children using a revised version of the Sensory Profile on which 26 items were added. Ninety-one of 125 items met the above criterion for uncommon behaviors in typical children. A factor analysis of Sensory Profile ratings for these typically developing children identified item loadings into nine patterns of behavior related to sensory modulation and responsiveness (Dunn & Brown, 1997). Kientz and Dunn (1997) identified 84 of the 99 items on the original Sensory Profile that distinguished between children with and without autism. Ermer and Dunn (1998) administered the Sensory Profile to parents of children with autism or pervasive developmental disorder, children with attention deficit hyperactivity disorder, and typically developing children. Using factor scores on the Sensory Profile, and discriminant analysis, they found that 89% of the children were classified into the correct diagnostic group.

LaCroix (1993) initiated the development of the ESP, the instrument that is used in the study reported here. Following rigorous procedures for instrument development outlined by Benson and Clark (1982), LaCroix gathered questionnaire items from published and unpublished questionnaires and generated items on sensory integrative dysfunction from literature and from personal contacts with therapists and parents, creating a collection of 679 items. A panel of experts in sensory integration then were asked to rate items for their representativeness of each of seven sensory systems and to identify which items were thought to be "good items" for clinical use. The index of item–objective congruence (Rovinelli & Hambleton, 1977) was calculated for each of the items to evaluate content validity. The 200 items selected for inclusion in the ESP had good content validity, defined as an index of item–objective congruence of .70 or higher, and were designated as a "good item" by raters. Content validity results were used to group the 200 items into seven sensory systems: auditory, gustatory, olfactory, proprioception, tactile, vestibular, and visual. Items then were formatted into a Likert scale (Likert, 1932) with response choices of always, often, sometimes, rarely, never, and not applicable.

LaCroix and Mailloux (1995) conducted a validity study on the ESP involving parent ratings of typically developing preschoolers ($n = 37$). Results identified 116 items on which 75% or more of the parents responded with ratings of "rarely" or "never." These findings suggested that these items describe behaviors that are not typical of preschoolers. To examine the meaningfulness of ESP items to parents, LaCroix and Mailloux additionally conducted interviews of mothers who completed the ESP, two of whom had children with sensory integrative problems. LaCroix and Mailloux found that the mothers of children with sensory integrative dysfunction felt a need to discuss items more expansively than the mothers of children without sensory integrative dysfunction. Because ESP items are designed to detect unusual behaviors, many items seemed to have greater relevance and meaning to the mothers of children with sensory integrative dysfunction.

The ESP is similar to other sensory history questionnaires, yet it has certain unique characteristics. The instruments developed by Larson (1982) and Royeen (1985, 1987) address only tactile defensiveness rather than a variety of aspects of sensory processing across multiple sensory systems. Provost (1991) addressed multiple sensory systems but focused specifically on sensory defensiveness. Moreover, her instrument is designed for infants and toddlers, not older preschoolers or school-aged children. The questionnaire studied by Spyropulos (1991) addressed multiple aspects of sensory integration, but its items overall did not differentiate between parent ratings for children with and without dysfunction.

Of the published instruments, the Sensory Profile (Dunn, in press) is most similar to the ESP. Both the Sensory Profile and the ESP assess a variety of aspects of sensory processing in multiple sensory systems. In addition, they are intended for assessment of children from preschool through elementary school. The ESP, however, is distinctive in containing only items that are specific to particular sensory systems. This feature is related to the extensive content validity procedures used to develop the ESP. In contrast, the Sensory Profile contains many items that are not related to a particular sensory system and may not in themselves be indicative of sensory processing problems. Because of this distinction, both the Sensory Profile and the ESP are likely to be clinically useful, but for somewhat different purposes. Of the two instruments, the Sensory Profile may be better suited for assessing a broad range of clinically significant problem behaviors, including behaviors that are not necessarily related to sensory processing. The ESP is designed to identify behaviors that are specifically indicative of sensory processing problems.

Method

Participants

Parents of 89 children participated in this study by completing the ESP. Written informed consent was required of all participants prior to participation. Of the parents in the study, 30 had children ranging in age from 3 years to 6 years 11 months who were identified as having sensory integrative dysfunction by occupational therapists with training and clinical experience in sensory integration. These children had not yet participated in any intervention involving sensory integration treatment techniques. This criterion was deemed important because the ESP is intended to be used primarily as an initial evaluation tool, and child behavior related to sensory processing is thought to change intervention. In addition, parents whose children have been involved in therapy may have a more sophisticated understanding of sensory processing issues and a heightened sensitivity to the behaviors identified in the ESP compared with parents who have not had this exposure. Thus, exposure to sensory integration-based intervention may affect parental ratings. Another criterion for inclusion in the sensory integrative dysfunction group was that the child was not medicated for or diagnosed with a developmental disability such as cerebral palsy, mental retardation, autism, or seizures.

Information about the procedures and criteria for participation in the study was provided to therapists who recruited parents of eligible children with sensory integrative dysfunction into the study. Following completion of data collection, the questionnaire for each child identified as having sensory integrative dysfunction was matched with a questionnaire for a child from the typically developing group.

Parents of children in the typically developing group ($n = 59$) were contacted through daycare programs, preschools, and an adult education center offering parenting classes. Questionnaires for a subgroup of 30 typically developing children were used in the statistical analysis of the study. These 30 typically developing children were matched as closely as possible to the children in the sensory integrative dysfunction group for age, gender, geographic location, ethnicity, and socioeconomic status. Age was the primary criterion for matching because sensory integrative functioning is known to be age dependent (Ayres, 1979, 1989). Children in the two groups whose data were statistically analyzed were matched for age within 6 months. Table 9.1 summarizes additional demographic characteristics of all the children whose parents participated in the study.

Instrument

The ESP was used in the current study. Prior to data collection, five parents completed the questionnaire and were interviewed to ensure that items were accurately understood. Several changes to items were made after the interviews: Examples of behaviors were added to 14 questions, 27 others were reworded for greater clarity, and 8 were eliminated because they contained professional jargon that was not understood by the parents. A total of 192 items were used in subsequent data collection and analysis.

Procedures

Of 520 questionnaires distributed to day care programs, preschools, and the adult education center for recruitment of participants, 84 were returned for children in the typically developing group. Twenty-five were excluded because the children's ages were not within the parameters of the inclusionary criteria or the children had a medical diagnosis related to learning or developmental disability. Of 160 questionnaires distrib-

Table 9.1. Characteristics of the Children

Demographic	Total in Typically Developing Group ($n = 59$)	Typically Developing Group in Matched Sample ($n = 30$)	Group With Sensory Integrative Disorders ($n = 30$)	Total ($N = 89$)
Children				
Gender				
Male	23	16	21	44
Female	36	14	9	45
Geographic area				
Southern California	43	24	24	67
Eastern Washington	5	1	1	6
Phoenix, Arizona, vicinity	2	1	1	3
Boston, Massachusetts, vicinity	2	2	2	4
Miami, Florida, vicinity	6	1	1	7
Minneapolis, Minnesota, vicinity	1	1	1	2
Ethnicity				
White	52	28	27	79
Asian	2	1	2	4
Other or Mixed Race	5	1	1	6
Socioeconomic status				
Class 1 (highest)	5	1	7	12
Class 2	26	14	6	32
Class 3	24	13	11	35
Class 4	4	2	4	8
Class 5	0	0	0	0
Class unknown	0	0	2	2

Note. Socioeconomic status was rated using the Hollingshead (1957) Two-Factor Index of Social Position.

uted to therapists for recruitment of parents of children with sensory integrative dysfunction, 59 were returned. Twenty-nine of these were excluded from the study either because of age or diagnosis that was not within the parameters of the inclusionary criteria, because there were missing data that could not be retrieved, or because a match from the typically developing group could not be identified.

If any questionnaire had more than six "not applicable" responses, the investigator contacted the parent by telephone to discuss the items in question to ensure that the parent was not confusing "not applicable" with "never." Care was taken not to bias responses of parents during these discussions. The questionnaire responses were then recoded, if appropriate. Additionally, three parents for whom English was a second language were contacted by phone, and the entire questionnaire was reviewed carefully to ensure that the questionnaire ratings accurately reflected their perceptions of their children.

Data Analysis

Frequency distributions and measures of central tendency of item ratings were calculated on all questionnaires included in the study. Separate calculations were made for the total group of children without sensory integration disorders ($n = 59$), the matched sample of children without sensory integration disorders ($n = 30$), and the group of children with sensory integration disorders ($n = 30$). The questionnaires for the matched groups were analyzed further using the Wilcoxon signed rank test for nonparametric comparison of the medians of the paired samples (Pagano & Gauvreau, 1993). A nonparametric test was indicated because of the ordinal data and lack of normal distributions of scores for most items. All analyses were conducted using the Statistical Analysis System (SAS) computer software package.

Results

Examination of frequency distributions indicated that data for nearly all items were highly skewed. This was particularly so for typically developing children. In this group (*n* = 59), 127 items had distributions in which 75% or more children were rated at the extreme ranges of the scale (*rarely* and *never*, or *always* and *often*).

The Wilcoxon signed rank test was computed for each item, and a statistically significant difference (*p* ≤ .05) between matched groups was found for 84 of the 192 items on the ESP. Of the significant items, 16 were in the auditory section, 0 in the gustatory section, 2 in the olfactory section, 10 in the proprioceptive section, 24 in the tactile section, 19 in the vestibular section, and 13 in the visual section. Table 9.2 summarizes results for these 84 items.

Score distributions were examined for each of the items that significantly differentiated between the matched groups. For most items, scores of all groups of children were highly skewed, and the scores of children with sensory integrative disorders tended to be more variable than those of children without dysfunction.

Of the 84 items that significantly differentiated between the groups, 48 were characterized by clearly skewed score distributions in the same direction for both groups. An example is shown in Figure 9.1. In this example, as in all items that fit this pattern, the score distribution for the children with dysfunction is flatter than that of the comparison group, because scores are spread more evenly across the response categories. This pattern indicates that ratings at the extreme end of the response continuum (*always* and *often*, or *rarely* and *never*) were unusual in both groups, but appeared more frequently in the group with sensory integrative problems.

The next most common pattern of item score distributions, seen for 14 of the significant items, shows ratings for the dysfunctional group approximating a bimodal distribution, whereas the ratings for the typically developing group are skewed, either positively or negatively. Figure 9.2 illustrates this score distribution pattern.

This pattern indicates that, for the typically developing group, ratings tend to fall at one end of the response continuum. For the example in Figure 9.2, these are ratings of "rarely" or "never." In contrast, for the children with sensory integrative problems, ratings suggest the existence of two subgroups: one whose ratings indicate that behavior is biased toward one end of the response continuum and another whose ratings tend to fall toward the opposite end of the continuum. For the item shown in Figure 9.2, one subgroup of children with sensory integration disorders is characterized by the "often" response, and the other subgroup is characterized by the "never" response.

On 10 items, scores for the children with dysfunction approximated a normal distribution, whereas the comparison children's scores were skewed. This indicates that, for these items, typically developing children were usually given ratings at one end of the response continuum, in contrast to the children with sensory integration problems, who most commonly were rated at the middle of the continuum, with some scores falling at either side.

Various combinations of bimodal, flat, normal, and skewed curves were identified among the remaining items. These items were less frequently observed, and in some cases, less easily defined than the patterns discussed above.

(*text continues on page 105*)

Table 9.2. Item Analysis and Frequency Distributions for the Evaluation of Sensory Processing

Question	p	Group	A	O	S	R	N
Auditory System							
3. Does your child have trouble understanding what other people mean when they say something?	.001	1	0.0	0.0	18.6	49.2	32.2
		2	0.0	0.0	20.0	46.7	33.
		3	0.0	16.7	36.7	36.7	10.0
4. Does your child seem to hear sounds that other people tend to not notice?	.039	1	1.7	0.0	16.9	32.2	49.2
		2	3.3	0.0	23.3	23.3	50.0
		3	0.0	23.3	26.7	23.3	26.7
5. Do you notice your child being bothered by any sounds which occur during daily life tasks such as tasks of personal hygiene, dressing, eating, home making, schoolwork, play/leisure?	.012	1	0.0	0.0	8.5	10.2	81.4
		2	0.0	0.0	10.0	6.7	83.3
		3	3.3	6.7	13.3	33.3	43.3
7. Does your child seem to have trouble remembering what is said to him or her?	.012	1	0.0	0.0	30.5	45.8	23.7
		2	0.0	0.0	20.0	46.7	33.3
		3	0.0	6.7	53.3	20.0	20.0
8. Is your child bothered by the sounds of any household or ordinary items, such as squeaky shoes, the vacuum, the blowdryer, dog barking, etc.?	.016	1	0.0	8.5	18.6	20.3	52.5
		2	0.0	6.7	20.0	16.7	56.7
		3	6.7	13.3	36.7	16.7	26.7
9. Does your child seem to understand oral directions?	<.001	1	55.9	40.7	3.4	0.0	0.0
		2	63.3	33.3	3.3	0.0	0.0
		3	23.3	53.3	23.3	0.0	0.0
10. Does your child fail to follow through to act upon a request to do something or to understand directions?	.001	1	0.0	3.4	40.7	45.8	10.2
		2	0.0	3.3	36.7	50.0	10.0
		3	0.0	30.0	53.3	10.0	6.7
16. Is your child distracted by sounds not normally noticed by average persons?	<.001	1	0.0	0.0	0.0	25.4	74.6
		2	0.0	0.0	0.0	26.7	73.3
		3	0.0	13.3	30.0	20.0	36.7
19. Is your child frightened of sounds which would not normally convey alarm for other children the same age?	.005	1	0.0	0.0	3.4	13.6	83.1
		2	0.0	0.0	3.3	16.7	80.0
		3	6.7	10.0	16.7	20.0	46.7
20. Does your child hear sounds other people don't notice, or have trouble tuning out certain sounds, such as a clock or watch ticking?	.011	1	0.0	0.0	3.4	13.6	83.1
		2	0.0	0.0	6.7	10.0	83.3
		3	0.0	13.3	16.7	16.7	53.3
21. Does your child ask others not to talk or sing or make noise?	.015	1	0.0	1.7	44.1	32.2	22.0
		2	0.0	0.0	43.3	36.7	20.0
		3	3.3	13.3	53.3	20.0	10.0
24. Does your child have trouble interpreting the meaning of simple or common words?	.002	1	0.0	0.0	3.4	15.3	81.4
		2	0.0	0.0	0.0	20.0	80.0
		3	0.0	3.3	20.0	33.3	43.3
26. Does your child seem confused as to the direction of sounds or where sound is coming from?	.026	1	0.0	0.0	5.1	30.5	64.4
		2	0.0	0.0	0.0	30.0	70.0
		3	0.0	0.0	20.0	30.0	50.0
27. Does your child have difficulty paying attention when there are other noises nearby?	.002	1	0.0	0.0	39.0	30.5	30.5
		2	0.0	0.0	40.0	36.7	23.3
		3	3.3	23.3	50.0	13.3	10.0
28. Is your child easily distracted by irrelevant or background noises such as a lawn mower outside, children talking in the back of the room, crinkling paper, air conditioners, refrigerators, fluorescent lights?	<.001	1	0.0	0.0	13.6	33.9	52.5
		2	0.0	0.0	13.3	36.7	50.0
		3	3.3	16.7	33.3	30.0	16.7
29. Does your child seem too sensitive to sounds?	.002	1	0.0	0.0	11.9	23.7	64.4
		2	0.0	0.0	10.0	26.7	63.3
		3	3.3	23.3	20.0	26.7	26.7

(continued)

Question	*p*	Group	A	O	S	R	N
Olfactory System							
5. Is your child able to identify smells of scratch-n-sniff stickers?	.008	1	34.8	54.3	10.9	0.0	0.0
		2	41.7	58.3	0.0	0.0	0.0
		3	11.8	41.2	41.2	5.9	0.0
12. Does your child interact with objects by smelling?	.022	1	0.0	6.8	30.5	39.0	23.7
		2	0.0	10.0	33.3	36.7	20.0
		3	0.0	6.7	16.7	23.3	53.3
Proprioception System							
1. Does your child grasp objects so tightly that it is difficult to use the object?	.020	1	0.0	0.0	5.1	30.5	69.5
		2	0.0	0.0	10.0	10.0	80.0
		3	3.3	10.0	13.3	26.7	46.7
2. Does your child tire easily after sitting or lying in the same position for a while?	.009	1	1.7	1.7	22.0	37.3	37.3
		2	3.3	0.0	13.3	43.5	40.0
		3	3.3	16.7	40.0	13.3	26.7
6. Does your child like giving bear hugs?	.006	1	20.3	39.0	32.2	6.8	1.7
		2	26.7	40.0	26.7	6.7	0.0
		3	10.0	20.0	43.3	20.0	6.7
7. Does your child seem unsure of how far to raise or lower the body during movement such as sitting down or stepping over an object?	<.001	1	0.0	0.0	8.5	32.2	59.3
		2	0.0	0.0	10.0	26.7	63.3
		3	0.0	16.7	33.3	23.3	26.7
12. Does your child grasp objects so loosely that it is difficult to use the object?	.002	1	0.0	0.0	3.4	25.4	71.2
		2	0.0	0.0	3.3	30.0	66.7
		3	3.3	23.3	10.0	20.0	43.3
17. Does your child have difficulty positioning himself or herself in a chair?	<.001	1	0.0	1.7	8.5	27.1	62.7
		2	0.0	0.0	6.7	26.7	66.7
		3	3.3	13.3	16.7	43.3	23.3
19. Does your child seem generally weak?	<.001	1	1.7	1.7	0.0	11.9	84.7
		2	3.3	0.0	0.0	10.0	86.7
		3	6.7	13.3	13.3	13.3	53.3
21. Does your child like getting bear hugs?	.011	1	30.5	39.0	27.1	1.7	1.7
		2	40.0	36.7	23.3	0.0	0.0
		3	10.0	40.0	40.0	6.7	3.3
22. Does your child taste or chew on toys, clothes, or other objects more than other children?	.002	1	0.0	3.4	8.6	25.9	62.1
		2	0.0	0.0	6.7	26.7	66.7
		3	6.7	3.3	20.0	36.7	33.3
25. Does your child have difficulty sitting erect, or choose to lie down instead of sitting up?	.002	1	0.0	1.7	8.5	23.7	66.1
		2	0.0	3.3	10.0	23.3	63.3
		3	3.3	10.0	30.0	36.7	20.0
Tactile System							
4. Does your child pull away from light touch?	.006	1	0.0	0.0	5.1	16.9	78.0
		2	0.0	0.0	3.3	13.3	83.3
		3	3.3	0.0	20.0	33.3	43.3
5. Does your child seem to lack the normal awareness of being touched?	.009	1	0.0	0.0	0.0	8.5	91.5
		2	0.0	0.0	0.0	10.0	90.0
		3	0.0	0.0	10.3	27.6	62.1
8. Does your child tend to prefer to wear long sleeved shirts and long pants regardless of the weather, for instance prefers to wear long sleeves even when it is warm outside?	.005	1	1.7	1.7	3.4	11.9	81.4
		2	0.0	0.0	0.0	10.0	90.0
		3	0.0	6.7	13.3	20.0	60.0
10. Does your child like to cuddle up with a blanket or stuffed animal or special pillow?	.030	1	23.7	27.1	32.2	11.9	5.1
		2	33.3	26.7	23.3	16.7	0.0
		3	16.7	30.0	16.7	16.7	20.0

(*continued*)

Table 9.2. Item Analysis and Frequency Distributions for the Evaluation of Sensory Processing (*Continued*)

Question	p	Group	A	O	S	R	N
12. Does your child avoid playing with "messy" things (e.g., finger paint, mud, sand, glue, glitter, clay)?	.029	1	0.0	5.1	18.6	18.6	57.6
		2	0.0	6.7	20.0	20.0	53.3
		3	10.0	13.3	20.0	30.0	26.7
13. Does your child show an unusual dislike for having his or her hair combed, brushed, or styled?	.049	1	1.7	10.2	18.6	39.0	30.5
		2	0.0	6.7	26.7	33.3	33.3
		3	6.7	30.0	16.7	16.7	30.0
16. Does your child prefer to touch rather than be touched?	.025	1	1.7	0.0	16.9	16.9	64.4
		2	0.0	0.0	16.7	16.7	66.7
		3	3.3	13.3	20.0	26.7	36.7
22. Does your child tend to wear coats or sweaters when they are not needed?	.012	1	0.0	1.7	5.1	13.6	79.7
		2	0.0	0.0	3.3	10.0	86.7
		3	0.0	3.4	17.2	17.2	62.1
23. Does your child appear to lack the normal awareness of being touched?	.047	1	0.0	0.0	1.7	8.5	89.8
		2	0.0	0.0	3.3	6.7	90.0
		3	0.0	3.3	10.0	20.0	66.7
28. Does your child struggle against being held?	.003	1	0.0	0.0	6.8	45.8	47.5
		2	0.0	0.0	3.3	43.3	53.3
		3	3.3	3.3	33.3	30.0	30.0
34. Does your child demonstrate an aversion to any form of clothing?	.019	1	0.0	3.4	23.7	27.1	45.8
		2	0.0	0.0	16.7	26.7	56.7
		3	3.3	13.3	23.3	20.0	40.0
36. Does it bother your child to have his or her face touched?	<.001	1	0.0	0.0	8.5	37.3	62.7
		2	0.0	0.0	10.0	20.0	70.0
		3	3.3	16.7	30.0	20.0	30.0
37. Does it bother your child to have his or her face washed?	.035	1	1.7	8.5	20.3	40.7	28.8
		2	0.0	6.7	16.7	46.7	30.0
		3	3.3	26.7	33.3	13.3	23.3
38. Does your child object to being touched by familiar people?	.013	1	0.0	0.0	8.5	27.1	64.4
		2	0.0	0.0	10.0	20.0	70.0
		3	3.3	0.0	26.7	30.0	40.0
39. Does it bother your child if he or she cannot see who is touching him or her when among familiar people at home or school?	.024	1	0.0	5.1	5.1	32.2	57.6
		2	0.0	6.7	0.0	33.3	60.0
		3	6.7	6.7	33.3	10.0	43.3
41. Does your child resist or dislike wearing short sleeved shirts or short pants?	.001	1	0.0	0.0	5.1	15.3	79.7
		2	0.0	0.0	0.0	10.0	90.0
		3	0.0	6.7	3.3	33.3	56.7
47. Does your child have an unusually high tolerance for pain?	.005	1	0.0	6.8	11.9	27.1	54.2
		2	0.0	6.7	13.3	23.3	56.7
		3	10.3	10.3	24.1	34.5	20.7
48. Does your child demonstrate an excessive need to touch?	.013	1	0.0	0.0	15.3	23.7	61.0
		2	0.0	0.0	13.3	26.7	60.0
		3	10.0	3.3	16.7	30.0	40.0
50. Does your child startle easily when being touched unexpectedly?	.008	1	0.0	3.4	8.5	44.1	44.1
		2	0.0	0.0	14.0	46.7	46.7
		3	6.7	13.3	16.7	26.7	36.7
53. Does your child tend to feel pain less than others?	.006	1	0.0	1.7	6.8	23.7	67.8
		2	0.0	0.0	10.0	23.3	66.7
		3	10.3	10.3	13.8	20.7	44.8
55. Does your child avoid touching different textures?	.001	1	0.0	0.0	1.7	16.9	81.4
		2	0.0	0.0	0.0	20.0	80.0
		3	0.0	0.0	26.7	23.3	50.0
58. Does your child avoid foods of certain textures?	.046	1	1.7	5.1	23.7	16.9	52.5
		2	0.0	6.7	26.7	13.3	53.3
		3	3.3	16.7	20.0	36.7	23.3

(continued)

Table 9.2. Item Analysis and Frequency Distributions for the Evaluation of Sensory Processing (*Continued*)

Question	p	Group	A	O	S	R	N
59. Does your child avoid getting his or her hands in finger-paint, paste, sand, clay, mud, glue, etc.?	.032	1	0.0	1.7	13.6	20.3	64.4
		2	0.0	3.3	10.0	23.3	63.3
		3	3.3	13.3	13.3	40.0	30.0
61. Does it bother your child to have his or her hair cut?	<.001	1	1.7	1.7	17.2	19.0	60.3
		2	0.0	3.3	10.0	23.3	63.3
		3	13.3	10.0	26.7	20.0	30.0

Vestibular System

Question	p	Group	A	O	S	R	N
2. Does your child seem excessively fearful of movement (e.g. going up and down stairs, riding swings, teeter totters, slides, or other playground equipment)?	.002	1	0.0	0.0	0.0	18.6	81.4
		2	0.0	0.0	0.0	20.0	80.0
		3	0.0	13.3	23.3	13.3	50.0
4. Does your child like to swing?	.002	1	50.8	35.6	13.6	0.0	0.0
		2	63.3	26.7	10.0	0.0	0.0
		3	20.0	43.3	26.7	6.7	3.3
5. Does your child demonstrate distress when he or she is moved or on moving equipment?	<.001	1	0.0	0.0	5.1	27.1	67.8
		2	0.0	0.0	6.7	23.3	70.0
		3	0.0	13.3	30.0	23.3	33.3
8. Does your child have good balance?	<.001	1	52.5	42.4	5.1	0.0	0.0
		2	63.3	33.3	3.3	0.0	0.0
		3	10.0	26.7	36.7	20.0	6.7
9. Does your child have to exert more effort to move than others, tire easily from exertion, and/or require more sleep than others?	<.001	1	0.0	0.0	3.4	22.0	74.6
		2	0.0	0.0	0.0	23.3	76.7
		3	10.0	10.0	16.7	40.0	23.3
10. Does your child avoid balance activities such as walking on curbs or uneven ground?	<.001	1	0.0	0.0	3.4	8.5	88.1
		2	0.0	0.0	3.3	10.0	86.7
		3	3.3	13.3	20.0	30.0	33.3
14. Does your child like fast-spinning carnival rides such as merry-go-rounds?	.002	1	29.3	34.5	24.1	8.6	3.4
		2	44.8	27.6	20.7	6.9	0.0
		3	16.7	30.0	23.3	16.7	13.3
15. Is your child fearful of activities which require good balance?	<.001	1	0.0	0.0	8.5	22.0	69.5
		2	0.0	0.0	6.7	16.7	76.7
		3	3.3	13.3	23.3	43.3	16.7
16. When your child shifts his or her body, does he or she sometimes fall out of the chair?	.020	1	0.0	1.7	8.5	39.0	50.8
		2	0.0	3.3	3.3	40.0	53.3
		3	0.0	16.7	6.7	46.7	30.0
17. Is your child sometimes unable to catch himself or herself when falling?	.018	1	0.0	6.8	16.9	49.2	27.1
		2	0.0	6.7	16.7	50.0	26.7
		3	0.0	26.7	13.3	46.7	13.3
20. Does your child seem generally weak?	.005	1	1.7	0.0	1.7	5.1	91.5
		2	3.3	0.0	0.0	3.3	93.3
		3	3.3	16.7	10.0	16.7	53.3
22. Does your child rock himself or herself when stressed?	.028	1	0.0	0.0	1.7	5.1	93.2
		2	0.0	0.0	0.0	6.7	93.3
		3	0.0	0.0	13.3	16.7	70.0
23. Does your child like to be inverted or tipped upside down or enjoy doing things like hanging upside down, somersaults, etc.?	.034	1	22.0	37.3	35.6	1.7	3.4
		2	30.0	33.3	33.3	3.3	0.0
		3	17.2	24.1	48.3	0.0	10.3
24. Is your child fearful of swinging or bouncing, or was as an infant?	<.001	1	0.0	0.0	0.0	13.6	86.4
		2	0.0	0.0	0.0	10.0	90.0
		3	0.0	16.7	13.3	26.7	43.3
29. Does your child avoid rapid or spinning movement?	.013	1	0.0	3.4	8.5	37.3	50.8
		2	0.0	3.3	3.3	30.0	63.3
		3	0.0	16.7	20.0	30.0	33.3
30. Is your child fearful of activities in which he or she moves through space?	<.001	1	0.0	0.0	10.2	35.6	54.2
		2	0.0	0.0	6.7	30.0	63.3
		3	0.0	10.0	36.7	30.0	23.3

(*continued*)

Table 9.2. Item Analysis and Frequency Distributions for the Evaluation of Sensory Processing (*Continued*)

Question	*p*	Group	A	O	S	R	N
31. Does your child demonstrate distress when his or her head is in any other position than upright or vertical, such as having the head tilted backward or upside down?	<.001	1	0.0	0.0	5.1	23.7	71.2
		2	0.0	0.0	3.3	23.3	73.3
		3	3.3	6.7	20.0	40.0	30.0
32. Does your child react negatively to, dislike, appear threatened by, or exhibit a fear reaction to movement?	<.001	1	0.0	0.0	1.7	22.0	76.3
		2	0.0	0.0	0.0	13.3	86.7
		3	0.0	3.3	40.0	23.3	33.3
33. Does your child enjoy excessive spinning and whirling?	.020	1	8.5	11.9	28.8	22.0	28.8
		2	10.0	13.3	33.3	20.0	23.3
		3	6.7	6.7	10.0	36.7	40.0

Visual System

Question	*p*	Group	A	O	S	R	N
1. Does your child have trouble telling the difference between different printed figures that appear similar, for example, confusing b with p, or + with x?	.043	1	1.8	8.8	19.3	31.6	38.6
		2	3.4	10.3	6.9	44.8	34.5
		3	7.4	22.2	29.6	22.2	18.5
4. Is your child able to look at something far away?	.004	1	66.1	28.8	5.1	0.0	0.0
		2	70.0	23.3	6.7	0.0	0.0
		3	33.3	46.7	13.3	0.0	6.7
5. Does your child have difficulty keeping his or her eyes on the task or activity at hand?	<.001	1	0.0	1.7	25.4	40.7	32.2
		2	0.0	0.0	33.3	43.3	23.3
		3	6.7	36.7	40.0	10.0	6.7
6. Does your child have trouble maintaining his or her visual focus on one task or object very long?	.002	1	1.7	1.7	35.6	30.5	30.5
		2	3.3	0.0	40.0	33.3	23.3
		3	6.7	40.0	26.7	16.7	10.0
8. Does your child have difficulty with visually focusing on things far away?	.026	1	0.0	0.0	1.7	15.3	83.1
		2	0.0	0.0	3.3	16.7	80.0
		3	0.0	0.0	24.1	24.1	51.7
9. Does your child become easily distracted by visual stimuli?	<.001	1	3.4	3.4	20.3	42.4	30.5
		2	6.7	3.3	20.0	43.3	26.7
		3	10.0	30.0	36.7	16.7	6.7
11. Does your child close one eye and/or tip his or her head back when looking at something or someone?	.007	1	0.0	0.0	0.0	8.5	91.5
		2	0.0	0.0	0.0	3.3	96.7
		3	0.0	0.0	16.7	16.7	66.7
12. Does your child have difficulty with unusual visual environments such as a bright colorful room or a dimly lit room?	.018	1	0.0	0.0	3.4	16.9	79.7
		2	0.0	0.0	3.3	10.0	86.7
		3	0.0	3.3	6.7	36.7	53.3
13. Does your child have difficulty with visually focusing on things close?	.036	1	0.0	0.0	0.0	8.5	91.5
		2	0.0	0.0	0.0	6.7	93.3
		3	0.0	0.0	3.4	6.9	21.0	69.0
14. Does your child have difficulty controlling eye movements during activities such as following objects with eyes, keeping place while reading, or copying from blackboard to desk?	<.001	1	0.0	0.0	1.7	18.6	79.7
		2	0.0	0.0	0.0	20.0	80.0
		3	0.0	10.7	21.4	28.6	39.3
15. Compared to other children the same age, does your child seem to be easily distracted by visual stimuli?	<.001	1	0.0	5.1	10.2	30.5	54.2
		2	0.0	6.7	0.0	33.3	60.0
		3	6.7	26.7	36.7	13.3	16.7
16. Does your child have trouble following objects with his or her eyes?	<.001	1	0.0	0.0	0.0	20.3	79.7
		2	0.0	0.0	0.0	13.3	86.7
		3	0.0	6.7	26.7	23.3	43.3
17. Does your child have difficulty naming, discriminating, or matching colors, shapes, sizes?	.007	1	0.0	1.7	6.8	27.1	64.4
		2	0.0	3.3	3.3	26.7	66.7
		3	0.0	6.7	26.7	30.0	36.7

Note. A = always; O = often; S = sometimes; R = rarely; N = never. Numbers in the A, O, S, R, and N columns indicate percentages of responses in the respective group. Group 1 = parents of children without disorders, *n* = 59; Group 2 = parents of children without disorders included in the matched study, *n* = 30; Group 3 = parents of children with sensory integrative disorders, *n* = 30. *p* values are from the Wilcoxon signed rank test performed with Group 2 and Group 3.

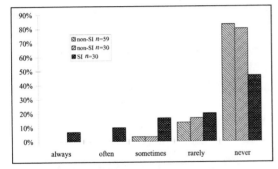

Figure 9.1. Score distributions of Item 19, Auditory section: Is your child frightened by sounds which would not normally convey alarm for other children the same age?
Note. SI = sensory integration.

Discussion

This study demonstrated that parent ratings for 84 of the 192 ESP items differentiated significantly between groups with and without sensory integrative dysfunction. In general, these results are encouraging in that nearly half of the items can be considered to provide information that is clinically meaningful. The effort made to ensure that the clinical group had not received sensory integration–based intervention strengthens the conclusion that these items are likely to be useful in clinical assessment.

However, it is clear that some aspects of the ESP are problematic. Some items are re-

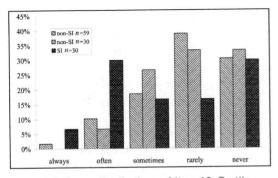

Figure 9.2. Score distributions of Item 13, Tactile section: Does your child show unusual dislike for having his or her hair combed, brushed, or styled?
Note. SI = sensory integration.

dundant and could be revised or eliminated to make the instrument more concise. No gustatory items and only two olfactory items differentiated between the groups, so these items cannot be assumed to have clinical relevance given these data. On the other hand, it is fortunate that the sensory systems with the highest number of significant items, tactile and vestibular, are key areas of concern in sensory integration theory.

As noted earlier, past studies of sensory history questionnaires have evaluated item validity through analysis of frequency distributions of ratings for children without any known dysfunction (Dunn, 1994; LaCroix & Mailloux, 1995). Items in these studies were accepted as "good items" if more than 75% or 80% of participant responses were in the extreme ranges of the scale, such as "rarely" and "never," or "always" and "often," depending on the wording of the question. In the LaCroix and Mailloux (1995) study using an early version of the ESP, 116 of the items met their criterion of 75%. In the present study using a revised ESP, 127 items met this same criterion. However, if frequency distribution of the typically developing group was the only criterion for item elimination on the ESP, 27% of the items identified as discriminating in the Wilcoxon signed rank analysis would have been missed. One item that would have been missed is shown in Figure 9.2, where scores of the group without dysfunction are skewed yet are distributed across all response choices. The scores of this group were significantly different from those of the group with sensory integrative dysfunction, whose distribution was bimodal. The use of contrasting groups additionally made it possible to identify items that were not good discriminators of sensory integrative dysfunction even though the score distribution of the typically developing group was concentrated at the extreme end of the response continuum.

The high degree of variability in scores of children with sensory integrative dysfunction is consistent with sensory integration theory (Ayres, 1972, 1979, 1989). Sensory integrative dysfunction is a heterogeneous category. Children with sensory integrative dysfunction do not all manifest it in the same way or in the same sensory systems. For example, it is possible for a child to demonstrate proprioception-seeking behaviors, while also having aversive responses to tactile stimuli and perceptual problems in the visual system. On the ESP, this child might have parent ratings similar to typically developing children on the auditory, olfactory, gustatory, and vestibular items, while ratings are atypical for some proprioceptive, tactile, and visual items. Another child with sensory integrative dysfunction may have a completely different pattern of ESP ratings.

Further study of the effects of age, gender, and ethnicity on ESP ratings is warranted, as these issues could influence clinical interpretation (Benson & Clark, 1982; Gwyer, 1989). It is possible that gender and ethnicity of the child may influence ESP scores, but this could not be ascertained in the current study due to sample limitations (i.e., the limited degree to which gender was matched, the limited variation in ethnic diversity of the children rated). Parent characteristics such as gender, ethnicity, and number of children may also affect ratings that are assigned to a child.

Although not all of the questionnaires for the large group of typically developing children ($n = 59$) were used in the statistical analysis, Table 9.2 includes frequency distributions of item ratings for this group to provide clinicians with expanded data on typically developing children. Distributions for this larger group and for the subset of 30 matched typically developing children are, not surprisingly, similar to each other. It is recommended that clinicians examine distributions for the larger group to gain insight into the range and frequency of ratings typically reported for children without disability on particular items and thus to increase confidence in clinical interpretation of ESP ratings.

Acknowledgments

This chapter is based on a master's thesis completed by the first author at the University of Southern California, under the guidance of the second author. We appreciate the comments of the other thesis committee members, Ann Neville-Jan and Florence Clark. We are also grateful for the assistance of John Morrison and Mike Carlson. The work of the second author was partially supported by the U.S. Department of Health and Human Services, Public Health Service, Health Resources and Services Administration, Maternal and Child Health Bureau, Grant MCJ 009048-11. This study could not have been completed without the commitment of the individuals and facilities across the United States who assisted with data collection. These data collection efforts are greatly appreciated.

References

Ayres, A. J. (1972). *Sensory integration and learning disorders.* Los Angeles: Western Psychological Services.

Ayres, A. J. (1979). *Sensory integration and the child.* Los Angeles: Western Psychological Services.

Ayres, A. J. (1989). *Sensory integration and praxis tests.* Los Angeles: Western Psychological Services.

Benson, J., & Clark, F. (1982). A guide for instrument development and validation. *American Journal of Occupational Therapy, 36,* 789–800.

Clark, F., & Parham, L. D. (1984). *USC sensory history survey.* Unpublished instrument, University of Southern California.

Dunn, W. W. (1994). Performance of typical children on the sensory profile: An item analysis. *American Journal of Occupational Therapy, 48,* 967–974.

Dunn, W. W. (in press). *Sensory profile*. San Antonio, TX: Therapy Skill Builders.

Dunn, W., & Brown, C. (1997). Factor analysis on the sensory profile from a national sample of children without disabilities. *American Journal of Occupational Therapy, 51*, 490–495.

Dunn, W., & Westman, K. (1997). The sensory profile: The performance of a national sample of children without disabilities. *American Journal of Occupational Therapy, 51*, 25–34.

Ermer, J., & Dunn, W. W. (1998). The sensory profile: A discriminant analysis of children with and without disabilities. *American Journal of Occupational Therapy, 52*, 283–290.

Gwyer, J. (1989). Designing and implementing research on the development editions of the test. In L. J. Miller (Ed.), *Developing norm-referenced standardized tests* (pp. 43–62). New York: Haworth Press.

Hollingshead, A. B. (1957). *Two-Factor Index of Social Position*. Unpublished manuscript, Yale University, New Haven, CT.

Kientz, M., & Dunn, W. (1997). Comparison of the performance of children with and without autism on the sensory profile. *American Journal of Occupational Therapy, 51*, 530–537.

LaCroix, J. E. (1993). *A study of content validity using the sensory history questionnaire*. Unpublished master's thesis, University of Southern California, Los Angeles.

LaCroix, J. E., & Mailloux, Z. (1995, April). *Evaluation of sensory processing*. Paper presented at the American Occupational Therapy Association National Conference, Denver, CO.

Larson, K. A. (1982). The sensory history of developmentally delayed children with and without tactile defensiveness. *American Journal of Occupational Therapy, 36*, 590–596.

Likert, R. A. (1932). A technique for the measurement of attitudes. *Archives of Psychology, 52*, 140.

Pagano, M., & Gauvreau, K. (1993). *Principles of biostatistics*. Belmont, CA: Wadsworth.

Parham, L. D., & Mailloux, Z. (1996). Sensory integration. In J. Case-Smith, A. S. Allen, & P. N. Pratt (Eds.), *Occupational therapy for children* (3rd ed., pp. 307–356). St. Louis: Mosby.

Provost, E. (1991). *Measurement of sensory behaviors in infants and young children*. Unpublished dissertation, University of New Mexico.

Provost, B., & Oetter, P. (1993). The Sensory Rating Scale for infants and young children: Development and reliability. *Physical and Occupational Therapy in Pediatrics, 13*(4), 15–35.

Rovinelli, F. J., & Hambleton, R. K. (1977). On the use of content specialists in the assessment of criterion-referenced test item validity. *Dutch Journal for Educational Research, 2*, 49–60.

Royeen, C. B. (1985). Domain specifications of the construct tactile defensiveness. *American Journal of Occupational Therapy, 39*, 596–599.

Royeen, C. B. (1986). The development of a touch scale for measuring tactile defensiveness. *American Journal of Occupational Therapy, 40*, 414–419.

Royeen, C. B. (1987). TIP—Touch Inventory for Preschoolers: A pilot. *Physical and Occupational Therapy in Pediatrics, 7*, 29–40.

Royeen, C. B., & Fortune, J. C. (1990). Touch Inventory for Elementary-School-Aged Children. *American Journal of Occupational Therapy, 44*, 155–159.

Spyropulos, P. (1991). *Sensory history survey: The relationship between sensory responsiveness, sensory integration, and learning handicaps*. Unpublished master's thesis, University of Southern California, Los Angeles.

CHAPTER 10

Construct-Related Validity of the Toglia Category Assessment and the Deductive Reasoning Test With Children Who Are Typically Developing

Naomi Josman and Tal Jarus

Naomi Josman, PhD,
is lecturer, Department of Occupational Therapy, a joint program of the Faculty of Welfare and Health Studies, University of Haifa, and Technion, Mount Carmel, Haifa, Israel; naomij@construct.haifa.ac.il.

Tal Jarus, PhD, OTR,
is lecturer, Department of Occupational Therapy, School of Allied Health, Medical Faculty of Tel Aviv University, Tel Aviv, Israel.

Originally published 2001 in *American Journal of Occupational Therapy*, 55, 524–530.

Both classification and deductive reasoning are essential cognitive components underlying any learning process (Rosser, 1994). Children with developmental or learning disabilities frequently demonstrate cognitive disabilities that limit their occupational performance at school and home. Those children who demonstrate decreased performance are typically referred to occupational therapy for intervention (Polatajko et al., 1995). Notwithstanding the importance of cognitive skills in children, none of the standardized assessments developed and used by occupational therapists specifically assess or measure children's classification and deductive reasoning abilities. Occupational therapists need appropriate cognitive assessments to evaluate these abilities in children.

The Toglia Category Assessment (TCA) and the Deductive Reasoning test are standardized assessments used with adults to evaluate their ability to establish categories, switch conceptual sets, and carry out deductive reasoning. Both tools are potentially suitable for evaluating children insofar as they use functional rather than abstract objects that are familiar to children. Both tools emphasize the qualitative aspects of performance and are based on dynamic interactional principles of testing. Hence, they examine the ability to profit from cues and task modifications (Toglia, 1994).

A dynamic assessment aims to establish the degree to which individual performance may be modified or changed. This concept is based on Vygotsky's (1978) principle of the Zone of Proximal Development (ZPD), which is defined as the difference between unaided performance and performance achieved by guidance or cuing. Thus, the ZPD is an index of the difference between the child's level of performance when functioning independently and the level of performance when interacting with a more knowledgeable partner. Vygotsky hypothesized that the ZPD reveals the child's potential for learning and characterizes differences in ability not identified by static tests.

Dynamic assessment strategies have been applied successfully to standardized tools that measure school achievement and children's learning potential (Campione & Brown, 1990). Both the TCA and the Deductive Reasoning test entail methods of dynamic assessment by which the evaluator intervenes to provide cues to the participant whenever needed. The information obtained from this approach can then be used to construct individualized treatment plans (Josman, 1999). The purpose of this study was to establish construct-related validity of the TCA and the Deductive Reasoning test for children who are typically developing.

Constructs Assessed in the TCA and Deductive Reasoning Test

Categorization

Categorization is defined as a method of creating concepts about the world by organizing stimuli and classifying them into groups possessing similar characteristics (Rosser, 1994). *Categorization* is the predominant term used in the neuropsychology literature, whereas *classification* is the term most commonly used in developmental psychology (e.g., Inhelder & Piaget, 1964). The two terms are often used interchangeably. Categorization is essentially a way of simplifying the world around us. The ability to assign a new object to an existing category makes it possible to change the unknown into the known insofar as we attribute to the new object all the information previously acquired about its category. Furthermore, this ability to organize the world influences the prediction and anticipation of similar events in the future (Rosser, 1994). These basic cognitive processes are involved in every thinking activity, such as identifying details, making comparisons, solving problems, and acquiring new knowledge. Categorization also requires the

ability to perform a shift in a conceptual set. This ability to shift ideas and actions and to adopt different perspectives of a concept is termed *cognitive flexibility* (McCarthy & Warrington, 1990). The ability to create categories and store information in an organized manner reduces the load on memory and facilitates efficient processing of information (Markman, 1989).

Difficulty in executing categorization affects functional performance in daily life as well as learning processes. Through a series of studies, Scott and Greenfield (1991) were able to support their hypothesis that children with learning disabilities have a specific difficulty in categorical ability. Moreover, the evaluation of categorization ability in groups of children at high risk for learning disabilities was deemed to be both important and critical because it may provide a predictive tool for expected difficulties in school.

Deductive Reasoning

The two main types of inferences that exist in everyday life are called *inductive* and *deductive*. In inductive reasoning, the main interest is in prediction based on partial data. Thus, an element of uncertainty and probability is involved. In deductive reasoning, one of the subjects of this chapter, a new conclusion is based on the primary data at one's disposal. This ability to make inferences and draw conclusions is critical for evaluating information, solving problems, and making decisions.

In the process of deductive reasoning, the person draws conclusions on the basis of available information, perceptual observations, memory, beliefs, and imagination. Conclusions may be based on each individual component or on all of them (Johnson-Laird & Byrne, 1991). Reasoning is a deliberate process of thought that enables a person to derive new information from old on the basis of a set of systematic principles establishing specific relations between premises and conclusions (Rosser, 1994). The correct conclusion is reached if one has rationally followed the initial hints provided and has confirmed or disproved assumptions formed in the process. Thus, at the end of the process, an option that seems to be correct is singled out.

The use of deductive reasoning processes can already be discerned in young children. In the early stages, deductions arrived at by the child may appear to be somewhat amusing to the adult observer, but an analysis of the child's deductive reasoning will show that a correct logical process has transpired and that the eventual deduction is quite logical and sound. In recent years, didactic games requiring this type of reasoning, such as "Guess Who,"[1] have been developed. Because deductive reasoning is central to the thinking processes of judgment, problem solving, and decision making, it is central to a child's stages of development and influences the child's learning ability in kindergarten and school. As such, it should be a prime area for evaluation and, when necessary, treatment.

Metacognition

Metacognition refers to a person's knowledge of his or her own cognitive processes, the tasks to be accomplished, and the strategies to be used (Flavell, 1985). The term *metacognition* includes awareness and executive functions. Awareness refers to one's consciousness of the existence of a problem and the capacity to analyze his or her ability (or inability) to solve it. Executive functions are the activities that govern the person's performance (Brown, 1987). The ability to initiate, set a goal, and plan and carry out behaviors directed toward that goal through the use of effective strategies and self-regulation are all con-

sidered to be executive functions (Katz & Hartman-Maier, 1998). Metacognition mediates cognitive abilities and provides the basis for generalization and the transfer of acquired abilities to daily functioning.

Many aspects of awareness can be observed either preceding, during, or immediately succeeding the completion of a certain activity (Toglia, 1998). The issue of awareness is of central importance in the treatment of children because the awareness of their own strengths and weaknesses influences learning and its generalization (Belmont, Butterfield, & Ferretti, 1982). None of the tests commonly used include an evaluation of self-awareness. The assessments used in the present study combine a metacognitive component with the cognitive examination. Awareness of one's own capacities is assessed with each of the tools both before and after the performance of the test itself.

The purpose of this study is to examine the construct-related validity of both the TCA and the Deductive Reasoning test for a population of children who are typically developing. Two research questions were addressed:

1. Is there a difference in performance on each test among children of various age groups?
2. Is there a relationship between the children's self-awareness of their competence in each test and their actual abilities?

Because cognitive abilities are typically expected to increase with age during childhood, a corresponding increase in test scores would be expected if the tests are indeed valid. Therefore, it was expected in the current study that differences in performance in both the TCA and Deductive Reasoning test would be found among children in various age groups, meaning that younger children would score lowest and that the scores would increase with age.

---

[1]Milton Bradley, Toy World, Newton Square, Philadelphia, PA.

Method

Sample

The study population consisted of 235 children, 5 to 11 years of age (112 [47.7%] boys, 123 [52.3%] girls) who were typically developed, attending public schools in northern Israel, and receiving no form of treatment. The children were recruited from several schools, with a convenience sample used for data collection. The Ministry of Education granted approval for conducting the study, and the parents gave written permission to include their children in the study. The sample was divided into six age groups of varying sizes (see Table 10.1). The number of boys and girls in each age group differed; however, no significant differences in test scores between boys and girls were found in the *t* test analysis.

Instruments

TCA. The TCA (Toglia, 1994) employs every-day objects to evaluate categorization abilities in persons who have experienced brain injury. Participants are asked to sort plastic food utensils into three groups: kinds of utensils (fork, spoon, knife), size (big, small), and color (green, yellow, red). The evaluation is dynamic–interactive, and the evaluator supplies cues as necessary. These cues are arranged in a hierarchical order, starting

Table 10.1. Mean Scores and Standard Deviations of the Different Age Groups in Categorization and Deductive Reasoning

Age Group (Years)	Categorization[a]			Deductive Reasoning[b]		
	n	*M*	*SD*	*n*	*M*	*SD*
5	22	7.485	.389	21	4.87	.211
6	71	8.319	.216	66	5.61	.119
7	46	8.514	.269	38	5.561	.157
8	37	9.396	.300	35	6.20	.163
9	30	10.089	.333	30	6.422	.177
10–11	29	10.345	.339	29	6.609	.180

[a]Possible score range is 1–1.
[b]Possible score range is 1–7.

from (a) repeating the instructions to (b) general feedback to (c) specific feedback to (d) demonstration and finally to (e) reducing the number of objects. The range of scores for each categorization is 1 to 11, with each intervention used resulting in a lowering of the score. In addition, an overall score (3–33) is obtained from the sum of the scores attained on all three subtests (Toglia, 1994).

To test participants' awareness of their own abilities, two awareness questions are posed before the assessment (prediction questions), and two additional awareness questions are asked after test completion (estimation questions). The participants are asked for their opinions regarding how they will perform or have performed on the assessment. In the second estimation question (after completion of test), participants are asked whether their performance had improved from the first categorization to second and from second to third. Information obtained from the awareness questions is then correlated with the assessment score itself. For the purpose of this study, another part was added to the test. After completion of the assessment, the evaluator noted whether performance improved on the second or third categorization compared with the first. This score is called "eval" and ranges from 1 = *not improved* to 4 = *improved.*

The findings of a previous study with adults (Josman, 1999) indicated that the TCA has an interrater reliability of *r* = .87, internal consistency ranging from .74 to .80 (*p* < .001), and a concurrent validity with the Riska Object Classification (Williams & Allen, 1985) of *r* = .52 (*p* < .001). No discriminant validity was obtained.

Deductive reasoning. The Deductive Reasoning test is essentially an extension of the categorization assessment, is administered after the TCA, and incorporates a game of questions using the food utensil set (Toglia, 1994). The evaluator informs the participant that he or she is thinking about an item from the set, and the participant is asked to discover which item is being thought about by asking questions to which the evaluator can answer only "yes" or "no." The participant is instructed to use a minimum of questions and may not ask specific questions, such as, "Did you select the small red fork?"

The Deductive Reasoning test also is dynamic–interactive and includes cues that are hierarchically arranged (Toglia, 1994). The scores range from 1 to 7 (1 = *unable to guess the chosen item,* 7 = *able to guess the chosen item with five questions or fewer*); every needed incident of cuing lowers the score. The test involves three trials; after the participant correctly guesses the first item, the evaluator says "Let's try it again" for a second and third trial. The final score is a sum of the scores obtained in the three trials. If the participant has obtained the highest mark of 7 twice, there is no need to continue, and the final score is 21. As in the TCA, awareness questions in this assessment are divided into prediction questions asked before starting the test and estimation questions asked on completion of the test. For the purpose of this study, another part was added to the test to compare objective progress in the test as observed by the evaluator with progress in the test as estimated by the participant. After completion of the assessment, the evaluator noted whether performance improved from the second to the third trial. This score is calculated by subtracting the score of the second trial (DR2) from the score of the third trial (DR3). Information obtained from the awareness questions is compared with the score obtained in the assessment itself. The Deductive Reasoning test is in use by clinicians treating persons experiencing head injuries, but no research has yet been carried out regarding its validity or reliability.

The questions and the cues included in both tests were translated into Hebrew and adapted to the participants' language level before beginning the study. Demographic data about age, gender, locality of residence, and parents' education (expressed as years of schooling) were obtained from the parents.

Data Collection

The first author collected data at each participating school with each child individually and without the presence of other persons. Administration of the TCA and Deductive Reasoning test lasted approximately 30 min for each child. Both tests were administered according to standard protocol (Toglia, 1994).

Data Analysis

Categorization. Following administration of the TCA, three scores were recorded for each participant, one each for color, type, and size. The possible scores for each parameter ranged from 1 to 11, and the positive overall score, which is the sum of the three parameters, ranged from 3 to 33.

For the statistical analysis, a three-way analysis of variance (ANOVA) with repeated measures was performed, using a 6 (age group) 3 3 (parameter of categorization) design. Post hoc tests were then performed using Scheffé multiple comparison and simple contrast procedures to test for significant differences between the age groups and categorization parameters (Kirk, 1982; Rohlf & Sokal, 1981).

Deductive reasoning. Three scores, one for each of the three interventions, ranged from 1 to 7. The overall (final) score, which is the sum of the three interventions (i.e., three trials for guessing), ranged from 3 to 21.

For the statistical analysis, a three-way ANOVA with repeated measures was performed, using a 6 (age group) 3 3 (intervention) design. To investigate the correlation between categorization and deductive reasoning, a Pearson product-moment correlation was conducted on the final scores of TCA and Deductive Reasoning test.

Awareness. The awareness questions in both the TCA and Deductive Reasoning test were divided into two components: (a) prediction questions before test performance and (b) estimation questions after test performance. To investigate self-awareness ratings, Pearson product-moment correlations between self-prediction and estimation to actual performance (final score) were conducted for both assessments. In addition, the improvement scores (eval, DR3 – DR2) were correlated with the second estimation question on how the participants judged their improvement during the assessment. The level of significance was set at .05 for all statistical tests.

Results

Categorization

The results of the ANOVA indicated a significant main effect for the parameter of categorization, $F(2,458) = 28.038$, $p < .001$. The children performed more accurate categorizations according to color ($M = 9.39$, $SD = 2.6$) and type ($M = 9.51$, $SD = 2.49$) than according to size ($M = 7.88$, $SD = 3.09$) (see Figure 10.1).

A significant main effect for age was obtained for performance, $F(5, 229) = 11.234$, $p < .001$. Performance of the three older age groups (8–11-

year-olds) was more accurate than that of the youngest age group (5-year-olds), and the two older age groups (9–11-year-olds) performed more accurately than the 6-year-olds and 7-year-olds (see Table 10.1). All differences in performance between the group ages were significant.

No significant interaction between the parameter of categorization and age group was obtained, $F(10, 458) > 1$, implying that the same pattern of performance was evident in the three kinds of categorization in several age groups.

Deductive Reasoning

The results of the ANOVA indicated a significant main effect for trials of deductive reasoning, $F(2, 426) = 59.24$, $p < .001$. The children improved significantly from the first trial to the second and then to the third (see Table 10.2).

A significant main effect for age was obtained from the performance, $F(5, 213) = 12.35$, $p < .001$. Performance of the three older age groups (8–11-year-olds) was more accurate than performance of the youngest age group (5-year-olds), and the two older age groups (9–11-year-olds) performed more accurately than the 6-year-olds and 7-year-olds (see Table 10.1).

The interaction between trial of deductive reasoning and age group was significant, $F(10, 426) = 2.00$, $p < .05$. Post hoc analyses indicated that the significant interaction is due to the

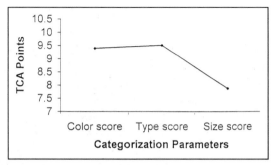

Figure 10.1. Main effect for parameters of categorization for all participants.
Note. TCA = Toglia Category Assessment.

Table 10.2. Means and Standard Deviations in the Three Trials of Deductive Reasoning According to Age Groups

Age Group (Years)	n	Trial 1 M	Trial 1 SD	Trial 2 M	Trial 2 SD	Trial 3 M	Trial 3 SD
5	21	4.3333	1.3166	5.2381	1.3002	5.0476	1.7169
6	66	4.9848	1.2949	5.6667	1.2930	6.1818	1.1490
7	38	4.8947	1.3313	5.6579	1.4003	6.1316	1.3591
8	35	5.8857	1.3009	6.2000	1.1581	6.5143	0.8869
9	30	6.0000	0.8305	6.5333	0.5713	6.7333	0.7397
10–11	29	6.3103	0.8906	6.6897	0.6603	6.8276	0.6017
Total	219	5.3653	1.3491	5.9635	1.2298	6.2785	1.2040

difference among the age groups in their improvement from the first and second trials to the third (see Table 10.2). The 5-year-olds did not improve from the second trial to the third compared with the other age groups (see Figure 10.2). In addition, on the first trial, the three youngest age groups performed less accurately than the three older age groups. On the second trial, the two youngest age groups performed less accurately than the two older age groups, and the 7-year-olds performed less accurately than the oldest age group. On the last trial, all the children performed better than the 5-year-olds. A significant positive correlation between the overall TCA score and the overall Deductive Reasoning test score ($r = .46$, $p = .0001$) implied that high child performance on the TCA is concomitant with high performance on the Deductive Reasoning test, and alternately, poor performance on the TCA is coupled with similar poor performance on the Deductive Reasoning test.

Awareness

With regard to awareness, the following relationships were analyzed: (a) the relationship between participants' levels of awareness of their performances before the assessment and outcome score, (b) correlation between TCA overall final scores and estimation scores, and (c) correlation between the actual improvement in performance and the child's estimation of improvement.

Categorization. No significant correlation between the actual performance and the child's prediction was obtained for any of the age groups. On the other hand, the results showed a significant correlation between the TCA final score and the children's (except for the 7-year-olds') estimation of their performance. These correlations are stronger for 8 years of age and up (see Table 10.3).

The correlation between the actual improvement in performance and the child's estimation of improvement was significant only for the 10-year-olds to 11-year-olds but in the wrong direction ($r = -.377$, $p < .05$). The better the child performed as measured on the TCA, the lower the accuracy of the child's estimation of performance.

To sum up the relationship between awareness and performance of categorization, none of the children in the assessed age groups were capable of accurately predicting their categorization ability. From 8 years of age, however, children were moderately capable of estimating their performance on the classification tasks.

Deductive reasoning. The results showed that there was a significant correlation between the deductive reasoning final score and the children's

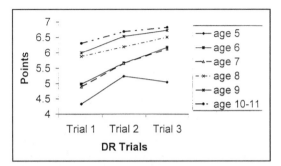

Figure 10.2. Interaction effects between the three deductive reasoning trials and age.
Note. DR = Deductive Reasoning test.

Table 10.3. Spearman Rank Order Correlations of Toglia Category Assessment Final Scores and Awareness Questions

Age Group (Years)	n	Prediction 1	Prediction 2	Estimation 1
All	221	−.122	−.088	−.368***
5	17	−.287	−.386	−.523*
6	71	−.22	.197	−.241*
7	46	−.184	−.188	−.121
8	36	−.009	−.214	−.597***
9	30	.068	.341	−.589***
10–11	29	.051	−.197	−.715***

*$p < .05$. **$p < .01$. ***$p < .001$.

estimation of their performance only for the 5-year-olds ($r = -.669$, $p < .01$) and 7-year-olds ($r = -.325$, $p < .05$) and for all participants as a group ($r = -.241$, $p < .001$). No significant correlation was found between the actual performance of deductive reasoning and the child's prediction in any of the age groups. The correlation between the actual improvement in performance and the child's estimation of improvement was significant only for the 5-year-olds ($r = -.565$, $p < .05$).

To sum up the relationship between awareness and performance of deductive reasoning, none of children in the assessed age groups were capable of predicting their deductive reasoning ability. Only the 5-year-olds and 7-year-olds adequately estimated their performance on deductive reasoning.

Discussion

The findings of this study support the suitability of the TCA and the Deductive Reasoning test with children. The TCA evaluates categorization ability, which is fundamental and central to children's everyday functioning. In every area of life, ranging from getting up in the morning and selecting suitable clothes to engaging in school activities, children must implement their classification skills. The Deductive Reasoning test evaluates deductive reasoning ability, which is also central to children's everyday functioning, such as solving problems and, especially, strengthening learning abilities. Therefore, it is essential that occupational therapists evaluate and, if necessary, treat these cognitive components.

The tools in these assessments consist of plastic utensils of various colors and sizes. These are everyday objects that are familiar to children of all ages and from different cultures. In the course of the study, the children's reactions to these objects were positive. No child refused to participate in the evaluation; indeed, most seemed to enjoy the classification test and even more so the deductive reasoning test. Some children requested to change roles with the evaluator, underlining the general belief that the tool neither poses a threat nor arouses anxiety. This conclusion is an important starting point for adapting a new tool for the evaluation of children.

Both instruments used in this study employed a dynamic assessment approach. In recent years, the field of dynamic assessment in general and in occupational therapy in particular has made great strides (Hadas-Lidor & Katz, 1998). One advantage to this approach is that in addition to the child's final score, it is possible to point to the cues or evaluator interventions that mediated the child to succeed at the task. Although this type of mediation may reduce the child's overall score, it enables him or her to uncover a new classification criterion and to demonstrate flexibility in thinking. In addition, the information thus obtained augments the evaluator's information about the kinds of cues likely to help the participant.

The first research question addressed whether differences in performance on the TCA and Deductive Reasoning test would be found between children of different age groups. This question was only partially answered. Although differences emerged in the average scores, significant differences were found mainly between the youngest and the oldest age groups, not among all age groups. This finding strengthens the construct-related validity of the TCA and Deductive Reasoning test and provides the foundation for applying and implementing these assessments with children.

The fact that no significant differences were observed between age groups by year is not surprising. Theory pertaining to the development of categorization and deductive reasoning skills does not address single-year differences, and stages of cognitive development, as described by Piaget

(1970), are not manifested in 1-year segments. Notably, in a previous study concurrent validity for the TCA compared with the Riska Object Classification was supported for adults with head injuries and schizophrenia (Josman, 1999). To date, no systematic study has determined the validity and reliability of the Deductive Reasoning test. It is recommended that both assessments be studied further to amplify their validity. In addition, studies should investigate whether the tools discriminate between children with and without disabilities. Although a sample of convenience was used for data collection in the present study, we recommend that a random sample be sought to represent the child population more reliably. Additionally, large-scale studies are needed to establish scale norms on the basis of age.

The second research question addressed the nature of the relationship between children's awareness of their capabilities and their actual performances, as assessed by correlating the prediction estimation questions and actual performance. Similar results were obtained for the TCA and the Deductive Reasoning test, showing no relationship between the children's *predictions* of their abilities to categorize and their actual performances. However, a significant relationship was found between children's *estimations* of their performances and their actual performances, except for the 7-year-olds, on the TCA (see Table 10.3); the same significant relationship was found for only the 5-year-olds and 7-year-olds on the Deductive Reasoning test.

Children's predictive abilities are based on their capacities to focus on and recall situations similar to that in which they are now being asked to perform and, on the basis of that knowledge, to predict how they will succeed on the test about to be tackled. The ability to estimate, on the other hand, is based on the activity just completed. Thus, it is feasible to hypothesize that estimation ability would be somewhat easier for children

insofar as their awareness is enhanced once an activity is performed. Children who are aware of their strengths and weaknesses may be able to devote more effort to activities with which they have difficulty. Accordingly, they might more readily seek or accept strategies to assist in their attempts at overcoming their difficulties. In any case, it may be important for occupational therapists to aim to bolster children's awareness of both pretest and posttest performance. In addition, if therapists have knowledge of children's awareness already in the evaluation stage, then they will be better able to plan the course of treatment and appropriate interventions.

Conclusion

The results of this study contribute to the validity of the TCA and Deductive Reasoning test as used with a sample of children who are typically developing. We recommend that research with large-scale studies be conducted to establish score norms on the basis of age. We also recommend the establishment of discriminative validity for both assessments by conducting a comparative study with a clinical population, such as children with learning disabilities and controls, to investigate manifestations of significant performance differences. Once discriminative validity as well as test norms are established, the TCA and the Deductive Reasoning test may be recommended for use in evaluating children in occupational therapy.

Acknowledgments

We thank all the children and their parents for participation in this study.

References

Belmont, J. M., Butterfield, E. C., & Ferretti, R. P. (1982). To secure transfer of training: Instruct self-management skills. In D. K. Detterman & R. J. Stemberg (Eds.), *How and how much can intelligence be increased.* Norwood, NJ: Ablex.

Brown, A. L. (1987). Metacognition, executive control, self-regulation, and other more mysterious mechanisms. In F. E. Weinert & R. H. Kluwe (Eds.), *Metacognition, motivation and understanding* (pp. 88–127). Hillsdale, NJ: Erlbaum.

Campione, J. C., & Brown, A. L. (1990). Guided-learning and transfer: Implications for approaches to assessment. In J. R. Frederiksen (Ed.), *Diagnostic monitoring of skill and knowledge acquisition* (pp. 141–172). Hillsdale, NJ: Erlbaum.

Flavell, J. H. (1985). *Cognitive development.* Englewood Cliffs, NJ: Prentice Hall.

Hadas-Lidor, N., & Katz, N. (1998). A dynamic model for cognitive modifiability: Application in occupational therapy. In N. Katz (Ed.), *Cognition and occupation in rehabilitation: Cognitive models for intervention in occupational therapy* (pp. 281–304). Bethesda, MD: American Occupational Therapy Association.

Inhelder, B., & Piaget, J. (1964). *The early growth of logic in the child.* London: Routledge & Kegan Paul.

Johnson-Laird, P. N., & Byrne, M. J. (1991). *Deduction.* Hillsdale, NJ: Erlbaum.

Josman, N. (1999). Assessment of categorization skills in brain-injured and schizophrenic persons: Validation of the Toglia Category Assessment (TCA). *Canadian Journal of Occupational Therapy, 2,* 33–42.

Katz, N., & Hartman-Maier A. (1998). Metacognition: The relationships of awareness and executive functions to occupational performance. In N. Katz (Ed.), *Cognition and occupation in rehabilitation: Cognitive models for intervention in occupational therapy* (pp. 323–342). Bethesda, MD: American Occupational Therapy Association.

Kirk, R. E. (1982). *Experimental design: Procedures for the behavioral science* (2nd ed.). Pacific Grove, CA: Brooks/Cole.

Markman, E. M. (1989). *Categorization and naming in children.* Cambridge, MA: MIT Press.

McCarthy, R. A., & Warrington, E. K. (1990). *Cognitive neuropsychology: A clinical introduction.* New York: Academic Press.

Piaget, J. (1970). Piaget theory. In P. H. Mussen (Ed.), *Carmichael's manual of child psychology* (3rd ed., pp. 703–732). New York: Wiley.

Polatajko, H. J., Macnab, J. J., Anstett, B., Malloy-Miller, T., Murphy, K., & Noh, S. (1995). A clinical trial of process-oriented treatment approach for children with developmental coordination disorder. *Developmental Medicine and Child Neurology, 37,* 310–319.

Rohlf, F. J., & Sokal, R. R. (1981). *Statistical tables* (2nd ed.). New York: Freeman.

Rosser, R. (1994). *Cognitive development: Psychological and biological perspectives.* Newton, MA: Allyn & Bacon.

Scott, M. S., & Greenfield, D. B. (1991). The screening potential of taxonomic information task for the detection of learning disabled and mildly retarded children. *Journal of Applied Development Psychology, 12,* 429–446.

Toglia, J. P. (1994). *Dynamic assessment of categorization. TCA: The Toglia Category Assessment.* New York: Maddak.

Toglia, J. P. (1998). A dynamic interactional model to cognitive rehabilitation. In N. Katz (Ed.), *Cognition and occupation in rehabilitation: Cognitive models for intervention in occupational therapy* (pp. 1–50). Bethesda, MD: American Occupational Therapy Association.

Vygotsky, L. S. (1978). *Mind in society: The development of higher psychological processes.* Cambridge, MA: Harvard University Press.

Williams, L. R., & Allen, C. K. (1985). Research with nondisabled population. In C. K. Allen (Ed.), *Occupational therapy for the psychiatric diseases: Measurement and management of cognitive disabilities* (pp. 315–338). Boston: Little, Brown.

CHAPTER 11

Prediction of School Performance Using the Miller Assessment for Preschoolers (MAP)
A Validity Study

Shula Parush, Monica Winokur, Sarina Goldstand, and Lucy Jane Miller

Shula Parush, PhD, OTR, *is lecturer and assistant director, School of Occupational Therapy, Hebrew University, PO Box 24026, Mount Scopus, Jerusalem, Israel; msshulap@pluto.huji.ac.il.*

Monica Winokur, MSc, OTR, *is national counselor for special needs populations, Ministry of Education, Israel, Preschool Education Division, Tel Aviv.*

Sarina Goldstand, OTR/L, *is pediatric clinician and graduate student, School of Occupational Therapy, Hebrew University, Jerusalem, Israel.*

Lucy Jane Miller, PhD, OTR, *is assistant professor, University of Colorado, Health Sciences Center, Department of Pediatrics, Denver.*

Originally published 2002 in *American Journal of Occupational Therapy, 56,* 547–555.

Evaluation of the young child and his or her family is one of the most basic aspects of occupational therapy services in pediatrics and includes both screening and diagnostic instruments (Dunn, 2000a). The goal of screening is to identify children who may be candidates for in-depth testing of whether they could benefit from preventive or remedial intervention programs (Carran & Scott, 1992; Dunn, 2000a; Gredler, 1997; May & Kundert, 1997; Miller, 1988a, 1988c). As such, screening is an example of occupational therapy service delivery within the context of the current health care paradigm that emphasizes preventive services (Dunn, 2000a), maintenance and enhancement of the individual's functional status (Baum, 2000), and consideration of cost–benefit ratios in care (Wenner, 1995).

Screening is especially relevant for the families of young children because research supports that early intervention enhances long-term functioning in all occupational areas (Gallagher, 1993; Henderson & Hall, 1982; McLaughlin & Wehman, 1992). Effective screening can facilitate family-centered therapy (Dunn, 2000a) in that parents' knowledge of their child's condition leads to parent involvement in evaluation and therapy and, as a result, to enhanced functional outcomes (Calnan et al., 1994; King, King, & Rosenbaum, 1996; Rosenbaum, King, Law, King, & Evans, 1998).

Evidence-based practice demands the selection of the current best tools (Tickle-Degnen, 1999). Pragmatic characteristics, such as ease of administration and appropriate content domains, are crucial (Gredler, 1997; Meisels & Wasik, 1990). Another feature of an effective screening tool is that it should have at least one cut-point below which children are considered "at risk" and in need of referral for further assessment (Crossland, 1994).

Another critical issue in selecting an evidenced-based screening tool is the determination of appropriate levels of sensitivity and specificity. These data are essential to evaluating the accuracy with which the test detects the target population. Sensitivity indicates the extent to which the test detects dysfunction when it is actually present; specificity indicates the extent to which the test accurately rules out dysfunction. False negatives result in a lack of special services to children who could benefit from the services; false positives result in identifying children who are actually typically developing as at risk. Both types of mislabeling can have serious consequences.

A primary concern in the selection of a screening instrument is predictive validity, which refers to the tool's ability to predict accurately persons who will develop future problems versus those who will not (Barnes, 1982; Lichtenstein & Ireton, 1991). Predictive validity requires that longitudinal analysis be accomplished through the use of follow-up studies (Carran & Scott, 1992). Follow-up studies that compare screening test scores with later target performance abilities of similar subjects evaluate the screening prediction relative to the later measured outcome (Miller, Lemerand, & Schouten, 1990). A screening instrument that demonstrates a high level of accuracy after a long interval is the most useful (Barnes, 1982).

The literature on preschool screening is replete with calls for longitudinal research; however, the predictive validity of only a few preschool screening tests is available (Badian, 1988; Gredler, 1997). Simner (1996) found that kindergarten children with lower scores on the Caregiver's School Readiness Inventory (Simner, 1989), a nontraditional preschool screening for school failure, were likely to exhibit poor academic performance at the end of second grade. Kelly and Peverly (1992) demonstrated that the Kindergarten Screening Battery (Belkin & Sugar, 1985) was an effective predictor of academic achievement in reading, mathematics, and listening comprehension in first and second graders. The Brigance K and 1 Screen (Brigance, 1982) and the Merrill Language Screening Test (Mumm, Secord, & Dykstra, 1980) were predictive of kindergarten teachers' recommendations for referral to remedial programs and for retention (Wenner, 1995). The Early Screening Inventory (Meisels, Henderson, Liaw, Browning, & Have, 1993) and the Early Prevention of School Failure (Roth, McCaul, & Barnes, 1993) also have shown predictive utility, particularly in fine motor and auditory modalities. The Revised Denver Developmental Screening Test (Frankenburg, Fandel, Sciarillo, & Burgess, 1981) was found to be an efficient prognostic tool of formal assessment results for 3- to 4-year-old preschool children at risk for language impairments over a 6-month test interval (Feeney & Bernthal, 1996).

The Miller Assessment for Preschoolers (MAP; Miller, 1988c) is a widely used preschool screening test. The MAP taps into sensory, motor, perceptual, cognitive, and verbal performance components in children and contains activities that are easily administered in an appealing game format.

Several longitudinal studies have been performed in the United States with the purpose of establishing the predictive validity of the MAP. Cohn (1986) performed a follow-up study after an interval of 2 years from screen testing with the MAP. In Cohn's study, the MAP's prediction of at risk versus not at risk was evaluated in relation to teachers' ratings of overall academic performance and assignment to special services in first grade. Results indicated that the means of the MAP scores distinguished between groups of at-risk and not-at-risk children in their first school year in accordance with teachers' ratings. In another study, Lemerand (1988) found that the classification analysis of the MAP's 25% cut-point, after a 1-year interval, indicates sound sensitivity and specificity rates (≥ 0.70) in predicting children who later had difficulty in kindergarten.

Miller (1988a, 1988b) conducted a follow-up study of the MAP standardization sample and examined the results of intelligence and achievement tests conducted on the participants 4 years after screening (Miller, 1988b). She found that the highest correlation was between the MAP total score and the Wechsler Intelligence Scale for Children (WISC; Wechsler, 1991) criteria ($r =$ .45–.50) (Miller, 1988c). Strong relationships also were found between the MAP and achievement tests, such as the Woodcock measures (Woodcock & Johnson, 1977) ($r = $.35–.38). These studies demonstrate that the MAP, when given to preschoolers, adequately predicted intelligence and academic performance 4 years later (Miller, Lemerand, & Cohn, 1987).

The purpose of the present study was to cross-validate the previous findings that the MAP is a screening tool capable of predicting performance of school-age children over a substantial period (7 years). Therefore, the assessments selected for the follow-up testing were designed to tap into a wide range of performance components that spanned the areas of motor, perception, cognition, and functional academic performance, such as reading and writing. Because the normative data for the MAP were obtained in 1980, this study attempts to provide evidence to update and substantiate previous claims of predictive validity.

Moreover, comparing screening results with relevant aspects of future functional status gives us insight into the relationship between performance components and functional outcomes, a concept about which many have theorized (Case-Smith, 2000; Coster, 1998) yet for which almost no empirical data can be found. It is noteworthy that this study was conducted on Israeli children and used the Hebrew version of the MAP, which was standardized on a sample of Israeli preschool children (Schneider, Parush, Katz, & Miller, 1995). The Israeli standardization study found no significant differences with respect to MAP total scores between the norms established by Miller on American preschoolers and Israeli preschoolers. Therefore, this follow-up study that examines functional outcomes and occupational performance of school children from another culture affords us additional insight about the functioning of school-age children irrespective of the cultural context.

Method

Design

Establishing predictive validity of a screening tool is a process that is tested over time. This research is a follow-up study examining academic outcome and performance components of school children who had been previously classified (5–7 years before) through the MAP as being at risk or not at risk for pre-academic problems.

Sample

A convenience sample of 30 children (14 girls, 16 boys) in grades 4 through 7 from two cities in central Israel participated in the present study. They were selected from a total of 128 MAP test protocols that had been administered to all the children registered in four Mother and Child Health Care centers. The original screening was administered as part of an early screening project carried out between the years 1989 and 1992, with follow-up occurring 5 to 7 years later.

The 30 children were divided into two groups according to the risk criteria devised by MAP total scores. The children in the not-at-risk group ($n = 15$; 9 girls, 6 boys) were within normal limits on the MAP on the original screening (i.e., scores between 25% and 99%). The children in the at-risk group ($n = 15$; 5 girls, 10 boys) had MAP scores between 1% and 25%. The mean age for the sample was 3 years, 10 months, at the time of the original screening. At follow-up, the mean age was 11 years, 11 months, for the at-risk group and 11 years, 4 months, for the not-at-risk group (a nonsignificant group difference). All children in both groups were living with their two-parent families (biological or legal) at the time the research took place.

Socioeconomic status (SES) was established through Hartman's (1975) formula and grading, which takes into consideration both parents' educational background and the father's present occupation. No significant differences between groups were found in these demographic variables (see Table 11.1).

Instrument

The MAP score (Miller, 1988c) was the independent variable. The MAP is an individually administered test that identifies children between the ages of 2 years, 9 months, and 5 years, 8 months, who may be at risk for mild to moderate pre-academic problems. It examines performance components that may affect school function and includes 27 subtests in 5 domains: neurological foundations, motor coordination, language, nonverbal cognition, and complex tasks (combined domains). The total MAP score is expressed in percentiles, and the cutpoints are 0% to 5% (Red; likely problem, refer for evaluation), 6% to 25% (Yellow; possible problem, watch carefully and use clinical judgment about the need to refer for evaluation), and 26% to 99% (Green; unlikely to have problems, do not refer for evaluation).

The MAP has excellent internal reliability ($r = .79–.82$) and interrater reliability ($r = .98$) (Daniels & Bressler, 1990; Miller, 1988c). Test–retest reliability for total score is $r = .81$ (Miller, 1988c). Content validity for the MAP is supported in the literature as MAP total score correlates significantly with the WISC–R IQ scale ($r = .50–.45$) and with the Woodcock–Johnson Math, Reading and Language subtests ($r = .38–.35$) (Miller, 1988c). In the present study, the translated version of the MAP was used, for which test–retest reliability for the total score is $r = .74$, and interrater reliability is $r = .91$ (Schneider et al., 1995). The follow-up dependent measures were as follows.

Motor performance components. The Bruininks–Oseretsky Test of Motor Proficiency (BOTMP), Short Form (Bruininks, 1978) is an individually administered test that assesses the gross and fine motor performance components of children from 4 1/2 to 14 1/2 years of age. The Short Form consists of 14 items from the complete battery. It contains a brief survey of general motor proficiency: running speed and agility, balance, bilateral coordination, strength, upper-limb coordination, response speed, visual–motor control, and upper-limb speed and dexterity. Interrater reliability ranges from $r = .80$ to .97, and test–retest reliability ranges from $r = .86$ to .97 (Bruininks, 1978).

Visual–motor performance components. The Developmental Test of Visual–Motor Integration (VMI; Beery, 1989) is a developmental

Table 11.1. Demographic Characteristics of Children in the At-Risk and Not-At-Risk Groups

Characteristic	At Risk		Not At Risk			
	M	*SD*	*M*	*SD*	*Z*[a]	*p*
School grade	5.47	0.99	5.33	0.98	−.433	NS
Number of siblings	2.67	0.90	2.67	1.05	−.116	NS
Siblings with learning problems	0.33	0.49	0.33	0.49	0	NS
Birth order	2.07	0.96	2.00	0.93	−.131	NS
Socioeconomic status	2.95	0.92	3.08	1.16	−.438	NS

Note: NS = not significant.
[a]Mann–Whitney *U* test.

sequence of 24 geometric forms to be copied with paper and pencil. The age range includes preschool children through adults. This scale correlates significantly with academic achievement (correlations ~ .50). Interrater reliability is $r = .93$, and test–retest reliability ranges from $r = .75$ to .92 (Beery, 1989).

Cognitive performance components. The Pictorial Sequence subtest of the Loewenstein Occupational Therapy Cognitive Assessment (LOTCA; Itzkovich, Elazar, & Averbuch, 1993) comprises two series of pictorial sequences that assess the sequential thinking performance of children. The children are asked to arrange picture cards according to what they consider to be a logical sequence and to describe the resulting story. Each subtest is scored on a scale from 1 (*unable to perform*) to 4 (*good performance*). Interrater reliability ranges from $r = .82$ to .97, and the alpha coefficient for internal consistency is .85. Construct validity has been demonstrated (Averbuch & Katz, 1991).

The Visual Aural Digit Span Test (VADS; Koppitz, 1977) measures both cross-modal sensory integration and short-term memory performance components. This test detects learning problems in children from 5 years, 6 months to 12 years of age. It consists of four subtests: Aural–Oral, Visual–Oral, Aural–Written, and Visual–Written. Reliability for subtest scores ranges from $r = .72$ to .90. The VADS score for kindergarten children has concurrent validity for second- through fifth-grade children's reading achievement scores (Koppitz, 1977).

The Conners Abbreviated Symptom Questionnaire (ASQ; Goyette, Conners, & Ulrich, 1978), a parent rating scale, was completed by the parents to detect attention deficits and hyperactivity. This 10-item index reflects the most frequently endorsed items in Conners's more extensive Teacher and Parent Rating Scales

(Conners, 1985). Scaling for each item ranges from 0 to 3, and total scores above 15 are considered to suggest hyperactive behavior. The appropriate ages for administration of this questionnaire range from 3 years to 17 years. Interrater reliability is not reported; however, interparent agreement is $r = .55$ to .71, and parent–teacher agreement is $r = .49$ (Goyette et al., 1978).

Academic performance area. The Hebrew Handwriting Evaluation (HHE; Erez & Parush, 1999) was administered to assess handwriting proficiency, handwriting speed, self-comprehension, and subjective legibility and spelling in copying and dictation conditions. A total score is calculated for Handwriting–Copying and Handwriting–Dictation by summing the scores of the different relevant subtests. Good interrater ($r = .75–.79$) and internal ($r = .81$) reliability correlations have been established for this scale, and construct validity has been demonstrated (Devash, Levi, Traub, & Shapiro, 1995).

Reading ability was tested by the diagnostic–didactic tests developed and used at Nizan, the Israeli Center for Learning Disabled Children. The tests measure a child's level of proficiency in silent reading and in recitation (Kidron, 1990) in the Hebrew language. A total score was calculated for reading proficiency by summing the scores of the different reading subtests (silent, recitation). Although these tests are widely used in Israel, no reliability or validity data have been reported.

Child placement and intervention information. A parent questionnaire requiring yes and no responses was used to gather data about the following dependent variables: (a) rate of special education attendance currently or during kindergarten, (b) rate of kindergarten retention, and (c) number of special services interventions (e.g., speech therapy, occupational therapy, psychology) the children received.

Procedure

The original MAP screening was administered by two qualified occupational therapists who were trained by an expert examiner in a special workshop for MAP administration. The current sample for the follow-up testing was selected in three stages: (a) examining MAP protocols, (b) tracing the potential participants, and (c) procuring agreement (informed consent). MAP scores were obtained by retrospective analysis of test protocols from the centers' archives. Children who had incomplete MAP protocols were excluded. One hundred twenty-eight children met entrance criteria, of which 69 families were located. Of the 69 families, 26 had children who were identified as at risk according to MAP criteria, and 15 agreed to participate in the study. From the not-at-risk children (43), a control sample of 15 was matched for age and SES to the at-risk children.

Each follow-up test session lasted approximately 2 hours. All testing was done by the second author at the child's home during the afternoon hours. She also administered the reading tests under the supervision of two didactic testing professionals. It is noteworthy that the second author did not participate in the original MAP screening, eliminating a possible source of experimenter bias.

Data Analysis

All data were expressed as raw scores because the standard scores and percentiles of the different measures were not standardized on Israeli children. It is noteworthy that raw scores are considered a more reliable indication of change over time (Wilson, Polatajko, Kaplan, & Faris, 1995); therefore, use of the raw score may facilitate further research with these children.

Depending on the level of the measurement scale, the variable Mann–Whitney U and t tests were used to compare the demographic and test performance data of the two groups across time. To determine the extent to which our results might depend on our sample size, post hoc power estimates were calculated according to the observed sample mean difference, the sample standard deviations, and the sample sizes. Results are interpreted as the probability that this effect size will be detected; the higher the obtained number, the higher the probability of detection of a given effect.

Results

The MAP total scores (in percentiles) ranged from 3 to 25 for the at-risk group and from 47 to 92 for the not-at-risk group. The mean total scores were 16.13% ($SD = 7.77$) for the at-risk group and 73.33% ($SD = 18.57$) for the not-at-risk group. Meaningful differences were seen between both groups with regard to child placement and intervention services. In the not-at-risk group, all the children attended regular kindergartens, and none were retained for a second year. Moreover, none of the children in this group required special education services, and only 4 received developmental special services interventions. In contrast, 4 children in the at-risk group were placed in special education kindergartens. Three of these children continued on in special education frameworks, with 2 in special education classes within regular schools and 1 attending a segregated special education school. This child had the lowest MAP score from within the follow-up research sample. In addition to the 4 children in special education, 10 children in the at-risk group received special services intervention in one developmental area (e.g., speech therapy), and 7 children were receiving two types of treatment simultaneously (e.g., occupational therapy and physical therapy).

Many of the outcomes for the tests administered in this study—BOTMP, VADS, VMI, Conners ASQ, LOTCA, and handwriting and reading scales—demonstrated significant group differences, with the not-at-risk group performing better on these measures than the at-risk group. Raw scores in the not-at-risk group indicated better performance than those of the at-risk group on all tests. To correct for the number of t tests, we adjusted the alpha level to .01. Group differences were significant at the .01 level or less in 13 of the 26 subtests. Tables 11.2 and 11.3 compare the groups' performances on all the follow-up tests. They indicate that significant differences exist, especially in cognitive and visual–motor performance components (i.e., LOTCA, VMI) and academic performance area (handwriting, three of five subtests in reading) (see Table 11.3).

To determine the extent to which these results might depend on the size of the sample, post hoc calculations of power estimates were done (Cohen, 1992). These estimates yielded the following results: BOTMP, .14; Conners ASQ, .30; VADS, .50; VMI, .87, LOTCA, .98; HHE (copy), .98; HHE (dictation), .87; and reading proficiency, .87. These data indicate that had a larger sample size been used, greater group differences would have resulted on the VMI, LOTCA, HHE (copy and dictation), and reading proficiency. In contrast, a larger sample size would not have changed the differences between the scores

of the groups on the BOTMP, the Conners ASQ, and the VADS.

Sensitivity and specificity were calculated only for those tests that were found to be significantly different between groups. Table 11.4 displays the sensitivity and specificity values of the tests that were found to be significant in predicting children's future performance (i.e., VMI, reading proficiency, HHE [copy and dictation]).

Discussion

The findings from this study are consistent with those from the longitudinal studies undertaken in the United States to establish the predictive validity of the MAP with American children (Humphry & King-Thomas, 1993; Miller, 1988a). The longitudinal studies found consistent group differences between children at risk and not at risk in class retention, assignment to special services, and assignment to special education classes (Cohn, 1986; Lemerand, 1988; Miller, 1988a; Miller et al., 1987). As Miller (1988a) stated, "The MAP Total Score effectively differentiated problem and no-problem children" (p. 13).

In addition to cross-validating previous U.S. results, the current findings indicate that the not-

Table 11.2. Comparison of Results—BOTMP Short Form, VADS, and VMI

| Test | At-Risk Group | | Not-At-Risk Group | | | | |
	M	SD	M	SD	t	df	p
BOTMP							
Raw score	64.40	10.03	67.40	7.63	−1.004	28	.324
Standard score	51.13	17.09	58.20	13.61	−1.252	28	.221
VADS							
Aural–Oral	5.53	0.99	6.20	0.86	−1.967	28	.059
Visual–Oral	6.20	0.94	6.47	0.64	−0.907	28	.372
Aural–Written	5.13	1.19	5.93	1.10	−1.915	28	.066
Visual–Written	5.53	0.74	6.33	0.82	−2.806	28	.009
Total scores	22.40	3.64	24.93	2.87	−2.118	28	.043
VMI							
Total score	31.07	6.64	38.87	6.41	−3.273	28	.003

Note. BOTMP = Bruininks–Oseretsky Test of Motor Proficiency; VADS = Visual Aural Digit Span Test; VMI = Developmental Test of Visual–Motor Integration.

Table 11.3. Comparison of Scores—Conners ASQ, LOTCA, and Handwriting and Reading Proficiency

Test	At-Risk Group		Not-At-Risk Group		Z^a	p
	M	SD	M	SD		
Conners ASQ						
Total point score	10.81	5.71	7.27	4.40	−1.657	.098
LOTCA						
Total point score	5.73	1.49	7.53	0.74	−3.487	.000
HHE						
Copy						
Speed	2.73	0.70	3.53	0.52	−3.102	.002
Self-comprehension	3.40	0.63	3.87	0.35	−2.318	.200
Subjective legibility	2.67	0.62	3.53	0.52	−3.510	.000
Spelling	2.80	0.94	3.87	0.37	−3.405	.001
Dictation						
Speed	2.67	0.82	3.47	0.74	−2.573	.100
Self-comprehension	3.13	0.74	3.73	0.59	−2.645	.008
Subjective legibility	2.47	0.74	3.33	0.72	−2.849	.004
Spelling	2.47	0.74	3.53	0.64	−3.518	.000
Reading proficiency (Nizan)						
Recitation						
Speed	3.27	0.70	3.73	0.46	−1.963	.050
Comprehension	2.80	0.77	3.67	0.62	−3.121	.002
Accuracy	3.00	0.85	3.67	0.49	−2.408	.016
Silent reading						
Speed	3.40	0.83	3.87	0.35	−1.998	.046
Comprehension	2.87	0.83	3.73	0.59	−3.084	.002

Note. Conners ASQ = Conners Abbreviated Symptom Questionnaire; LOTCA = Loewenstein Occupational Therapy Cognitive Assessment (the Pictorial Sequence subtest); HHE = Hebrew Handwriting Evaluation.
[a]Mann–Whitney *U* test.

at-risk group performed significantly better than the at-risk group in the perceptual, cognitive, and functional academic performance areas that were tested. Specifically, the not-at-risk group had higher scores than the at-risk group on the visual–motor integration, pictorial sequencing and narrative, the auditory and visual short-term memory, and the handwriting and reading proficiency tests.

Table 11.4. Sensitivity and Specificity of the Miller Assessment for Preschoolers

Criterion Test	Sensitivity (%)	Specificity (%)	x^2	p
VMI	85.71	60.87	4.64	.01
Reading	87.50	63.64	6.14	.01
Writing–copy	80.00	65.00	5.40	.02
Writing–dictation	76.92	70.59	6.65	.01

Note. VMI = Developmental Test of Visual–Motor Integration.

No significant differences were detected in motor proficiency between the study groups on the BOTMP at follow-up. Motor proficiency, however, is reported to be an important indicator of future school success (Ellwein, Walsh, Eads, & Miller, 1991; Roussounis, Gaussen, & Stratton, 1987). We believe that methodological factors related to instrumentation might account for this finding. The BOTMP Short Form, used to avoid overtiring the children during testing sessions, has some limitations compared with the longer BOTMP. Because the short form contains fewer items, it might not be sensitive enough to detect a problem in a specific motor area. Additionally, the overall score of the BOTMP Short Form provides only one composite result without subtest results. Therefore, it can only indicate the existence of general problems.

Further, because many of the children in the at-risk group received occupational therapy or physical therapy in the intervening years, their motor performance might have improved as a result of treatment effects over time.

The results of our study indicate that no significant differences existed in the Conners ASQ between the groups at follow-up. Because the Conners ASQ taps into parental perceptions of the attention and hyperactive behaviors of their children, the results suggest that the MAP is not sensitive to these areas. These findings may be explained by noting that the MAP is a "child-friendly" assessment. The different items are presented in a playful fashion and are devised to be executed in short periods of time, up to a few minutes each, so that even children with short attention spans can demonstrate their optimal abilities. Given the importance of the behavioral issues in academic achievement, the results of this study might indicate that the MAP should be reinforced with a complementary test (e.g., an index of hyperactivity) that refers specifically to this variable.

Another limitation of this study is sample size. Power estimates indicated that had a larger sample size been used, the VMI, LOTCA, HHE (copy and dictation), and reading proficiency scores would have discriminated between the groups even more. In contrast, the results of those tests for which group scores did not reach significant differences (BOTMP, Conners ASQ, VADS) would not have been affected by increasing the number of participants. These findings support the reliability of our current study results despite the small sample size.

To achieve optimal predictability, tests that intend to screen for developmental risk during a presymptomatic period must be sensitive to participants who demonstrate later developmental difficulties (Meisels & Wasik, 1990). Sensitivity and specificity indexes were calculated for the MAP with respect to each one of the outcome criteria variables that demonstrated statistical differences between the groups. The highest coherence was between the MAP and the VMI and the reading and writing proficiency tests. These findings are congruent with the MAP objectives of predicting academic performance (Miller, 1988a, 1988b, 1988c; Miller et al., 1987).

The use of a long prediction interval (5–7 years) is an important new issue addressed by this study. Although literature on young children's screening tools frequently calls for long-term longitudinal research, few scales actually demonstrate this attribute (Badian, 1988; Gredler, 1997). The heterogeneous nature of learning disabilities makes their long-term prediction more challenging; shorter periods for prediction increase the likelihood that predictive statistics will appear high. A critical problem with short-term follow-up is that the cognitive levels of proficiency demonstrated by young children are discontinuous when compared with later academic tasks. Different cognitive tasks represent relevant markers for academic success at later ages. Thus, the weaknesses that appear in earlier ages may be expressed in cognitive processes at a later age. In addition, no academic difficulties may be evidenced until children are required to address more complex or abstract subjects in their curriculum (Lavin, 1995). A relatively long time lapse, such as that seen in this study, increases the chance of uncontrolled-for effects of history; intervening experiences may weaken the association between screening outcomes and follow-up criteria (Miller, 1988a, 1988b). Perhaps the inclusion of verbal and nonverbal cognitive items in the MAP that demand memory and problem-solving skills has given it the predictive power to relate to aspects of future cognitive, perceptual–motor, and academic performance, such as reading and handwriting proficiency.

Conclusion

The results of this study strengthen the assertion that the use of the MAP can be very beneficial in clarifying potential sources of observed deficits in important daily tasks (Coster, 1998; Dunn, 2000b). Significant differences were demonstrated in school performance between the two groups of children (at risk, not at risk) as designated by the original MAP results across a substantial period of time (5–7 years). These results provide evidence of the strong predictive capability of the MAP in accurate prediction of academic performance. In addition, the examination of academic and varied performance components in another cultural context allows for better insight into the aspects of performance that impinge on the occupational performance of school-age children irrespective of cultural context.

Acknowledgments

We thank Beit Issie Shapiro for its cooperation in providing access to the original MAP screening data that formed the basis for our follow-up findings. We especially acknowledge the assistance of Dana Roth, PhD, Director of Research and Development at Beit Issie Shapiro, Raanana, Israel, and Michele Shapiro, MSc, OT, who initiated and conducted the difficult yet important task of screening the preschool children of Raanana.

This study was done in partial fulfillment of the second author's requirement for a master's degree in occupational therapy from the School of Occupational Therapy, The Hebrew University–Hadassa Medical School.

References

Averbuch, S., & Katz, N. (1991). Age level standards of the Loewenstein Occupational Therapy Cognitive Assessment (LOTCA). *Israel Journal of Occupational Therapy, 1,* E1–E2.

Badian, N. A. (1988). The prediction of good and poor reading before kindergarten entry: A nine-year follow-up. *Journal of Learning Disabilities, 21,* 98–103.

Barnes, K. E. (1982). *The measurement and prediction of children at-risk.* Springfield, IL: Charles C Thomas.

Baum, C. (2000, January 3). Occupation-based practice: Reinventing ourselves for the new millennium. *OT Practice,* pp. 12–15.

Beery, K. E. (1989). *VMI—Developmental Test of Visual–Motor Integration. Administration, scoring and teaching manual.* New York: Modern Curriculum Press.

Belkin, A. S., & Sugar, F. (1985). *The Kindergarten Screening Battery.* Unpublished manuscript.

Brigance, A. H. (1982). *Brigance K & 1 Screen for Kindergarten and First Grade.* Billerica, MA: Curriculum Associates.

Bruininks, R. H. (1978). *The Bruininks–Oseretsky Test of Motor Proficiency.* Circle Pines, MN: American Guidance Service.

Calnan, M., Katsouyiannopoulos, V., Ovcharov, V. K., Prokhoskas, R., Pramic, H., & Williams, S. (1994). Major determinants of consumer satisfaction with primary care in different health systems. *Family Practice, 11,* 468–478.

Carran, D. T., & Scott, K. G. (1992). Risk assessment in preschool children: Research implications for the early detection of educational handicaps. *Topics in Early Childhood Education, 12,* 196–211.

Case-Smith, J. (2000). Effects of occupational therapy services on fine motor and functional performance in preschool children. *American Journal of Occupational Therapy, 54,* 372–380.

Cohen, J. (1992). A power primer. *Psychological Bulletin, 112*(1), 155–159.

Cohn, S. H. (1986). *An analysis of the predictive validity of the Miller Assessment for Preschoolers in a suburban public school district.* Unpublished doctoral dissertation, University of Denver, Denver, CO.

Conners, C. K. (1985). *The Conners Rating Scales: Instruments for the assessment of childhood psychopathology.* Unpublished manuscript, Children's Hospital National Medical Center, Washington, DC.

Coster, W. (1998). Occupation-centered assessment of children. *American Journal of Occupational Therapy, 52,* 337–344.

Crossland, H. (1994). Screening early literacy: Ideology, illusion, and intervention. *Educational Review, 46,* 47–62.

Daniels, L. E., & Bressler, S. (1990). The Miller Assessment for Preschoolers: Clinical use with children with developmental delays. *American Journal of Occupational Therapy, 44,* 48–53.

Devash, L., Levi, M., Traub, R., & Shapiro, M. (1995). *Reliability and validity of the Hebrew Handwriting Evaluation.* Jerusalem: School of Occupational Therapy, Faculty of Medicine, Hebrew University.

Dunn, W. (2000a). The screening, pre-assessment, and referral process. In W. Dunn (Ed.), *Best practice occupational therapy: In community service with children and families* (pp. 55–78). Thorofare, NJ: Slack.

Dunn, W. (2000b). Using frames of reference and models of practice to guide practice. In W. Dunn (Ed.), *Best practice occupational therapy: In community service with children and families* (pp. 27–54). Thorofare, NJ: Slack.

Ellwein, M. C., Walsh, D. J., Eads, G. M., & Miller, A. (1991). Using readiness tests to route kindergarten students: The snarled intersection of psychometrics, policy, and practice. *Educational Evaluation and Policy Analysis, 13,* 159–175.

Erez, N., & Parush, S. (1999). *The Hebrew Handwriting Evaluation* (2nd ed.). Jerusalem: School of Occupational Therapy, Faculty of Medicine, Hebrew University.

Feeney, J., & Bernthal, J. (1996). The efficiency of the Revised Denver Developmental Screening Test as a language screening tool. *Language Speech and Hearing Services in Schools, 27,* 330–332.

Frankenburg, W. K., Fandel, A., Sciarillo, W., & Burgess, D. (1981). The newly abbreviated and revised Denver Developmental Screening Test. *Journal of Pediatrics, 99,* 995–999.

Gallagher, G. G. (1993). Preventive intervention. *Pediatric Clinics of North America, 20,* 3.

Goyette, C. H., Conners, C. K., & Ulrich, R. F. (1978). Normative data on the revised Conners Parent and Teacher Rating Scales. *Journal of Abnormal Child Psychology, 6,* 221–236.

Gredler, G. R. (1997). Issues in early childhood screening and assessment. *Psychology in the Schools, 34,* 99–106.

Hartman, M. (1975). *Prestige grading of occupations with sociologists as judges.* Paper presented at the 70th meeting of the American Sociological Association, Chicago.

Henderson, S. E., & Hall, D. M. B. (1982). Concomitants of clumsiness in young school children. *Developmental Medicine and Child Neurology, 24,* 448–460.

Humphry, R., & King-Thomas, L. (1993). A response and some facts about the Miller Assessment for Preschoolers. *Occupational Therapy Journal of Research, 13,* 34–49.

Itzkovich, M., Elazar, B., & Averbuch, S. (1993). *LOTCA: Loewenstein Occupational Therapy Cognitive Assessment: Manual.* Pequannock, NJ: Maddak.

Kelly, M. S., & Peverly, S. T. (1992). Identifying bright kindergartners for learning difficulties: Predictive validity of a kindergarten screening tool. *Journal of School Psychology, 30,* 245–258.

Kidron, R. (1990). *Reading proficiency: Diagnostic didactic tests.* Jerusalem: Nitzan, The Israeli Center for Learning Disabled Children and the Division of Special Education, Ministry of Education.

King, G., King, S., & Rosenbaum, P. (1996). Interpersonal aspects of care-giving and client outcomes: A review of the literature. *Ambulatory Child Health, 2,* 151–160.

Koppitz, E. M. (1977). *Visual Aural Digit Span Test (VADS) manual.* New York: Grune & Stratton.

Lavin, C. (1995). Clinical applications of the Stanford–Binet Intelligence Scale: Fourth edition to reading instruction of children with learning disabilities. *Psychology in the Schools, 32,* 255–263.

Lemerand, P. A. (1988). Predictive validity of the Miller Assessment for Preschoolers (MAP). *Sensory Integration News, 16*(1), 1–8.

Lichtenstein, R., & Ireton, H. (1991). Preschool screening for developmental and educational problems. In B. A. Bracken (Ed.). *Psychoeducational assessment of preschool children* (pp. 486–513). Boston: Allyn & Bacon.

May, D. C., & Kundert, D. K. (1997). School readiness practices and children at risk: Examining the issues. *Psychology in the Schools, 34,* 73–84.

McLaughlin, P. J., & Wehman, P. (1992). Preface. In P. J. McLaughlin & P. Wehman (Eds.), *Developmental disabilities: A handbook for best practices* (pp. xiii–xvi). Stoneham, MA: Butterworth-Heinemann.

Meisels, S. J., Henderson, L. W., Liaw, F., Browning, K., & Have, T. T. (1993). New evidence for the effectiveness of the Early Screening Inventory. *Early Child Research Quarterly, 8,* 327–346.

Meisels, S. J., & Wasik, B. A. (1990). Who should be served? Identifying children in need of early intervention. In S. J. Meisels & J. P. Shonkoff (Eds.), *Handbook of early intervention* (pp. 605–632). New York: Cambridge University Press.

Miller, L. J. (1988a). Differentiating children with school-related problems after four years using the Miller Assessment for Preschoolers. *Psychology in the Schools, 25,* 10–15.

Miller, L. J. (1988b). Longitudinal validity of the Miller Assessment for Preschoolers: Study II. *Perceptual and Motor Skills, 66,* 811–814.

Miller, L. J. (1988c). *Miller Assessment for Preschoolers: MAP manual* (rev. ed.). San Antonio, TX: Psychological Corporation.

Miller, L. J., Lemerand, P. A., & Cohn, S. H. (1987). A summary of three predictive studies with the MAP. *Occupational Therapy Journal of Research, 7,* 378–381.

Miller, L. J., Lemerand, P. A., & Schouten, P. G. W. (1990). Interpreting evidence of predictive validity for developmental screening tests. *Occupational Therapy Journal of Research, 10,* 74–86.

Mumm, M., Secord, W., & Dykstra, K. (1980). *Merrill Language Screening Test: Examiner's manual.* Columbus, OH: Merrill.

Rosenbaum, P., King, S., Law, M., King, G., & Evans, J. (1998). Family-centered service: A conceptual framework and research review. *Physical and Occupational Therapy in Pediatrics, 18*(1), 1–20.

Roth, M., McCaul, E., & Barnes, K. (1993). Who becomes an "at-risk" student? The predictive value of a kindergarten screening battery. *Exceptional Children, 59,* 348–358.

Roussounis, S. H., Gaussen, T. H., & Stratton, P. (1987). A 2-year follow-up study of children with motor coordination problems identified at school entry age. *Child: Care, Health, and Development, 13,* 377–391.

Schneider, E., Parush, S., Katz, N., & Miller, L. J. (1995). Performance of Israeli versus U.S. preschool children on the Miller Assessment for Preschoolers. *American Journal of Occupational Therapy, 49,* 19–23.

Simner, M. L. (1989). *Caregiver's School Readiness Inventory.* London: Phylmar Association.

Simner, M. L. (1996). Predictive validity of the Caregiver's School Readiness Inventory. In M. Luther, E. Cole, & P. Gamlin (Eds.), *Dynamic assessment for instruction: From theory to application* (pp. 56–62). New York: Captus Press.

Tickle-Degnen, L. (1999). Evidence-Based Practice Forum—Organizing, evaluating, and using evidence in occupational therapy practice. *American Journal of Occupational Therapy, 53,* 537–539.

Wechsler, D. (1991). *Wechsler Intelligence Scale for Children.* San Antonio, TX: Harcourt.

Wenner, G. (1995). Kindergarten screens as tools for the early identification of children at risk for remediation or grade retention. *Psychology in the Schools, 32,* 249–254.

Wilson, B. N., Polatajko, H. J., Kaplan, B. J., & Faris, P. (1995). Use of the Bruininks–Oseretsky Test of Motor Proficiency in occupational therapy. *American Journal of Occupational Therapy, 49,* 8–17.

Woodcock, R. W., & Johnson, M. B. (1977). *Woodcock–Johnson Psycho–Educational Battery.* Hingham, PA: Teaching Resources.

CHAPTER 12

Comparison of Sensory Profile Scores of Young Children With and Without Autism Spectrum Disorders

Renee L. Watling, Jean Deitz, and Owen White

Renee L. Watling, MS, OTR, *is doctoral student, Division of Occupational Therapy, Department of Rehabilitation Medicine, University of Washington, Box 356490, Seattle, WA 98195; rwatling@u.washington.edu.*

Jean Deitz, PhD, OTR, FAOTA, *is professor, Division of Occupational Therapy, University of Washington, Seattle.*

Owen White, PhD, *is professor, College of Education, University of Washington, Seattle.*

Originally published 2001 in *American Journal of Occupational Therapy, 55,* 416–423.

The ability to respond to sensation with appropriate physical and emotional responses depends on effective integration of perceptual and sensorimotor information. Piaget (1952) described perceptual development in early childhood as a series of stages, each of which creates a foundation for the next. Ayres (1972) described the process of *sensory integration* as "the organization of sensation for use" (p. 1), stating that integration of sensory information was necessary for a child to interact effectively with his or her world. Children who do not acquire developmentally mature perceptual and sensory integrative abilities often display maladaptive emotional and physical responses to environmental stimuli (Ayres, 1979; DeGangi, 1991; Murray & Anzalone, 1991; Williamson & Anzalone, 1997).

Sensory and perceptual abnormalities are common in persons with autism. Based on reviews of research, firsthand reports, and clinical accounts, between 30% and 100% of children with autism spectrum disorders are believed to have sensory–perceptual abnormalities of some kind (Dawson & Watling, 2000). Among these are tactile defensiveness (Grandin, 1995; McKean, 1994), auditory hypersensitivity (Grandin, 1992; Williams, 1994), olfactory hypersensitivity (Stehli, 1991), and sensory overload (Williams, 1994). Hyporeactivity and hyperreactivity to sensory stimuli (Wing & Wing, 1971), inappropriate responses to multiple sensory stimuli (Goldfarb, 1961; Hermelin & O'Connor, 1970; Lovaas, Schreibman, Koegel, & Rehm, 1971), and faulty modulation of sensory input (Ornitz, 1974) are also described.

Abnormal responses to sensory stimulation may differentiate young children with autism from children with typical development and children with mental retardation. For example, Dahlgren and Gillberg (1989) found that sensitivity to auditory stimuli in infancy was a powerful discriminator between children with and without autism ($N = 26$). Mayes and Calhoun (1999) examined diagnostic criteria for autism and found that 100% of their sample ($N = 24$)

exhibited somatosensory characteristics and suggested that this element should be included as part of the diagnostic criteria. More recently, Baranek (1999) found significant differences in the sensorimotor behaviors of infants 9 months to 12 months of age in her group comparison study of children with autism, children with mental retardation, and children with typical development. These studies provide evidence that sensory–perceptual abnormalities are prevalent among young children with autism. Much of the research in this area, however, is methodologically weak, and more data are needed to determine the prevalence, nature, and characteristics of the sensory–perceptual deficits that persons with autism spectrum disorders experience.

Occupational therapists frequently measure sensory processing in their comprehensive assessments because faulty processing can have a negative impact on the performance of daily life activities (DeGangi, 1991; Dunn, 1997; Murray & Anzalone, 1991; Williamson & Anzalone, 1997). Current methods of assessment typically consist of clinical observations, informal questionnaires, and parent interviews. These approaches lack standardization and the normative data necessary for establishing consistent interpretation of sensory–processing abilities. The Sensory Profile (Dunn, 1999), a 125-item parent-report questionnaire, is the first available sensory–processing assessment for which normative data have been reported.

To date, two studies using the Sensory Profile with children with autism have been reported in the literature. In a preliminary study (N = 32) using a pilot version of the Sensory Profile, Kientz and Dunn (1997) found that 3-year-old to 13-year-old children with autism performed differently ($p < .000$) from 3-year-old to 10-year-old children with typical development. A univariate analysis revealed that 84 of the 99 items on the pilot version accounted for the differences between

the groups in this study; however, no specific items on the Sensory Profile were considered common for children with autism. In a subsequent study, Ermer and Dunn (1998) identified 46 items and 4 factors from the Sensory Profile that discriminated among children with autism spectrum disorders (n = 38), children with attention deficit hyperactivity disorder (ADHD; n = 61), and children without disabilities (n = 1,075). The 4 factors were Sensory Seeking, Oral–Motor, Inattention/Distractibility, and Fine Motor/ Perceptual. The authors concluded that the Sensory Profile was an effective tool for discriminating between children in these three groups and that children with autism displayed a specific pattern of sensory responses that was identified by the Sensory Profile.

The studies by Kientz and Dunn (1997) and Ermer and Dunn (1998) provide an excellent beginning in examining the sensory–processing differences between children with and without autism. Additional research is necessary to continue developing knowledge in this area. Given the possibility that sensory–processing abilities may vary at different ages or stages of development, the next step in this line of inquiry is to examine the sensory–processing abilities of children with and without autism within distinct age groups. The present study sought to describe the Sensory Profile factor scores of 3-year-old through 6-year-old children with and without autism and to compare the factor score patterns of the two groups. The following research questions were addressed:

1. Do significant differences exist between the scores of children with autism or pervasive developmental delay and children who are typically developing on those Sensory Profile factors representing areas of sensory processing described in the literature as frequently deficient in persons with autism (i.e., Sensory Seeking,

Emotionally Reactive, Oral Sensitivity, Inattention/Distractibility, Poor Registration, Sensory Sensitivity)?

2. Can patterns of sensory-based behaviors be identified in the Sensory Profile factor scores of young children with autism?

Method

Sample

A group comparison design was used to describe sensory-based behaviors of 40 children with autism spectrum disorders and 40 children without any known disabilities. (The sample included children with autism or pervasive developmental delay. To minimize cumbersome sentences, the text refers to "children with autism.") Parents of two groups of children between 36 months and 83 months of age (3 years, 0 months and 6 years, 11 months) participated. Each child with autism was matched to a child without disabilities on the variables of age and gender. The study design also sought to match children on ethnicity; however, all children in the study were Caucasian. Three children with autism who initially were recruited for the study were eliminated during the screening process because of an inability to find appropriately matched children without disabilities. The parents of two children without disabilities who began the study did not complete all steps (i.e., did not return consent form or complete the demographic interview), and the children were replaced in the final sample. Age categories were established in 6-month increments from 3 years through 6 years, 11 months. The mean age differences between the two groups were less than 1 month for all age categories under 6.5 years. For the 6.6 year to 6.11 year category, the mean age difference was 1.4 months. Compared with prevalence data identifying a gender ratio for autism of 4 boys to 1 girl (Bryson, 1996), the gender distribution of participants in the present study was 7 boys to 1 girl. Inclusion criteria for children with autism were (a) age within the specified range and (b) diagnosis of an autism spectrum disorder (e.g., autism, pervasive developmental delay). Inclusion criteria for the comparison group were (a) age within the specified range, (b) absence of a diagnosed medical condition that might compromise development (e.g., ADHD, Down syndrome, cerebral palsy), and (c) no siblings with an autism spectrum disorder.

Parents of children with and without autism spectrum disorders were recruited from three sites representing both urban and suburban communities: a diagnostic center, a hospital-based therapy clinic, and a public preschool. At the diagnostic center, the occupational therapist who had participated on the diagnostic team contacted parents by telephone. The therapist explained the study and then mailed a cover letter and consent form to those parents interested in participating. The study questionnaire was mailed to the parent when the researchers received the completed consent form. At the therapy clinic, therapists working with children with autism described the study to parents and distributed the cover letter and consent form. On receipt of the completed consent form, the therapist distributed the study questionnaire. At the school, teachers distributed the cover letter and consent forms to parents by placing a packet in each child's backpack. The study questionnaire was distributed via the child's backpack after the parent returned a completed consent form to the school. All forms were coded numerically to allow for tracking while maintaining confidentiality.

Instrument

The research version of the Sensory Profile (Dunn & Westman, 1995) was used in this study. The 125 items and 10 factors included in this version are identical to the published questionnaire (Dunn,

1999), except for grammatical changes in item wording. The 10 Sensory Profile factors are Sensory Seeking, Emotionally Reactive, Low Endurance/Tone, Oral Sensitivity, Inattention/Distractibility, Poor Registration, Sensory Sensitivity, Sedentary, Fine Motor/Perceptual, and Other. To complete the Sensory Profile, parents used a 5-point Likert scale ranging from *always* to *never* to record the frequency with which their child displayed each behavior. Each parent completed the questionnaire independently. The primary investigator was available by telephone to answer questions. The primary investigator contacted each parent by telephone 1 week after the parent received the Sensory Profile to answer questions related to the questionnaire or study procedures and to gather demographic data.

Data Analysis

The completed Sensory Profile questionnaires were scored according to guidelines presented at the 1996 American Occupational Therapy Association Annual Conference (Ermer & Dunn, 1996) and later published in the *Sensory Profile User's Manual* (Dunn, 1999). Each parental response was converted to a numerical value corresponding to the frequency of each behavior (i.e., 1 = *always*, 5 = *never*). Using this conversion, behaviors that occur frequently receive low scores. The Sensory Profile items are written such that frequent behaviors are undesirable. For example, a child who received a 1 for "twirls/spins self frequently throughout the day" would, according to parent report, always demonstrate this behavior, whereas a child who received a 5 on this item would never display the behavior. Thus, low scores are undesirable because they suggest that a child has sensory–processing difficulties, and high scores are desirable because they suggest appropriate responses to sensory stimuli.

Factor scores were calculated by converting parent responses to numerical values, entering item scores onto the factor grid (Dunn, 1996), and calculating the sum for each factor. The data were analyzed with Microsoft Excel 97 (Microsoft Corporation, 1997), Data Desk 6.0 (Data Description, 1997), and the Statistical Package for the Social Sciences, 9.0.0 for Windows (SPSS, 1998). Because the primary research question involved multiple comparisons, 1 for each of the 10 factors, the probability of making a Type I error was increased. Therefore, the alpha level was set at $p \leq .005$ (two-tailed), using Bonferroni's adjustment whereby the desired alpha level (in this case, $p = .05$) is divided by the number of comparisons (Godfrey, 1985).

Results

Of the 40 children with autism in this study, 39 attended public preschool or kindergarten programs, and 1 did not attend school. Of the 39, 30 were in inclusive classrooms and 9 in self-contained classrooms. Thirty-six of the children without autism attended school (27 public, 9 private), and 4 did not attend school. Twelve children with autism received speech–language therapy at school, 4 received private services, and 18 received both. Nine children with autism received school-based occupational therapy services, 7 received private services, and 18 received both. Ten children with autism were taking medication at the time of the study. Although three of the children without autism had received speech–language therapy before the time of the study, none of them were receiving special services or taking medication at the time of the study.

Parents of children in both groups reported a similar occurrence of family history of disability. Family history was considered positive if (a) the child's parent, aunt, uncle, cousin, or grandparent had autism, learning disability, or attention deficit disorder or (b) a sibling of the child had attention deficit disorder, learning disability, or developmental delay. Twelve children with autism and 10 without autism met the criteria for a positive family history of disability. Three families in each group reported that they did not know their family histories.

Developmental information was gathered from parent report to determine group differences in achievement of general milestones. Children in both groups achieved motor milestones at similar ages, with a mean difference of .4 months for age of sitting and a mean difference of .2 months for walking. However, substantial group differences occurred in toilet training. At the time of data collection, only 20 (50%) of the children with autism had achieved independent toileting. By contrast, 36 (90%) of the children without autism had mastered the skill.

The Sensory Profile scores between the groups were compared by examining the performance of each group on each factor. Figure 12.1 presents bar graphs for each group's factor scores. The graphs indicate the lowest and highest scores received as well as the number of children from each group receiving a score in the designated range. On the Emotionally Reactive factor, 67.5% of the children with autism displayed more frequent sensory behaviors than any of the children without autism. On the Low Endurance/Tone factor, children with autism received scores across a broad range, whereas 77.5% of the children without autism clustered at the highest end of the scale. On the Poor Registration factor, 62.5% of the children without autism scored higher than any of the children with autism. On the Other factor, 65% of the children with autism had scores lower than any of the children without autism.

Table 12.1 displays the descriptive statistics and findings related to the first research question: Do significant differences exist between children with and without autism in Sensory Profile factor scores? As a group, young children with autism

tended to have lower scores than children without autism. In addition, the scores of children with autism were more widely distributed across the possible range of scores. Score differences between the groups were significant on 8 of the 10 factors, with no significant differences found for the Sensory Sensitivity and Sedentary factors.

Further analyses were conducted to answer the second research question, Can patterns be identified in the Sensory Profile factor scores of children with autism? Twenty-seven children with autism received lower scores than the children without autism on the Emotionally Reactive factor, and 26 received lower scores on the Other factor. Many children with autism ($n = 16$) had scores lower than the children with typical development on the Poor Registration factor. In most cases, these children also had lower scores on either the Emotionally Reactive factor or the other factor, or both. Further, we determined the number of factors on which each child with autism had scores lower than those of the children without autism. For children with autism, this number ranged from 0 to 6 factors, with 34 (85%) children receiving scores lower than any of the children without autism on at least 1 factor. Of those 34, 6 had scores lower than any child without autism on 1 factor, 11 on 2 factors, 5 on 3 factors, 6 on 4 factors, 4 on 5 factors, and 2 on 6 factors.

Discussion

The major finding from this study is that the scores of children with autism were significantly different from those of children without autism on eight Sensory Profile factors: Sensory Seeking, Emotionally Reactive, Low Endurance/Tone, Oral Sensitivity, Inattention/Distractibility, Poor Registration, Fine Motor/Perceptual, and Other. This finding is consistent with the literature that describes hyposensitivities and hypersensitivities to sensory stimuli (Poor Registration factor),

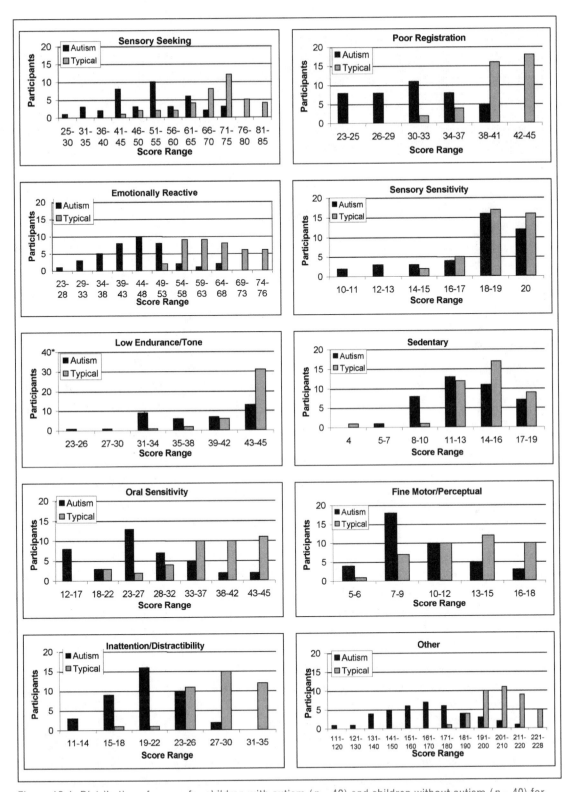

Figure 12.1. Distribution of scores for children with autism (*n* = 40) and children without autism (*n* = 40) for each Sensory Profile factor. Low scores are undesirable and represent more frequent demonstration of the behaviors; high scores are desirable and represent infrequent demonstration of the behaviors.

Note. * = scale of *y* axis is 40 on the Low Endurance/Tone graph.

Table 12.1. Factor Scores for Children With and Without Autism

Factor	Floor[a]	Ceiling[b]	M	Median	SD	Low/High	Mann–Whitney U
Sensory Seeking	17	85					p < .0001
Autism			52.6	51.5	11.9	25/73	
Typical development			68.7	70.5	9.8	41/82	
Emotionally Reactive	16	80					p < .0001
Autism			45.6	46.0	8.7	23/65	
Typical development			63.7	63.5	7.9	49/76	
Low Endurance/Tone	9	45					p < .0001
Autism			37.0	36.5	6.4	23/45	
Typical development			43.1	44.0	2.9	31/45	
Oral Sensitivity	9	45					p < .0001
Autism			26.3	27.0	8.6	12/44	
Typical development			36.1	37.5	6.9	18/45	
Inattention/Distractibility	7	35					p < .0001
Autism			20.4	21.0	4.2	11/28	
Typical development			28.2	29.0	3.8	17/35	
Poor Registration	9	45					p < .0001
Autism			30.6	30.0	4.8	23/39	
Typical development			40.2	41.0	3.4	30/45	
Sensory Sensitivity	4	20					p = .1962
Autism			17.7	19.0	2.8	10/20	
Typical development			18.7	19.0	1.4	14/20	
Sedentary	4	20					p = .0490
Autism			13.0	13.0	3.2	5/19	
Typical development			14.3	15.0	2.8	4/9	
Fine Motor/Perceptual	4	20					p < .0001
Autism			9.7	9.0	3.0	5/16	
Typical development			12.8	13.0	3.4	5/18	
Other	46	230					p < .0001
Autism			165.7	166.5	22.2	111/213	
Typical development			204.2	203.0	12.5	173/228	

[a]Lowest score possible on subscale.
[b]Highest score possible on subscale.

sensitivities to auditory and visual stimuli (Sensory Sensitivity factor), picky eating habits (Oral Sensitivity factor), poor attention and play skills (Inattention/Distractibility factor), poor coping and variability in emotional responses (Emotional Reactivity factor), hyperactivity (Sensory Seeking factor), and a variety of other abnormal perceptual responses (Other factor) among children with autism or pervasive developmental delays (see Baranek, Foster, & Berkson, 1997; O'Neill & Jones, 1997; Wing & Wing, 1971). The significant differences in Sensory Profile factor scores of 3-year-old through 6-year-old children with and without autism strengthen the argument that sensory–processing is an important area of differ-

ence between these groups. This finding also supports using the Sensory Profile to identify the sensory–processing tendencies of these age groups.

As a group, the children with autism also had scores that tended to spread further across the possible score ranges than the scores of the children without autism, suggesting that this group may not be homogenous. This wide spread of scores is evident in the distributions on the Low Endurance/Tone, Oral Sensitivity, Sensory Sensitivity, and Fine Motor/Perceptual factors (see Figure 12.1). This finding suggests that, although many children with autism may have compromised sensory processing, the sensory processing of some children with autism may be similar to that of children without autism. This inconsistency highlights the individuality of each child and reminds therapists that a specific child may or may not exhibit differences from the group to which he or she belongs. Therefore, clinicians must remain objective when assessing a young child with autism and conduct a thorough evaluation of sensory–processing abilities to determine whether that child's sensory processing is compromised.

Another important finding was the way in which patterns of low scores for the group of children with autism were distributed across the Sensory Profile factors. A majority of these children scored lower than any child without autism on the Emotionally Reactive ($n = 27$) and Other ($n = 26$) factors. A large number of children with autism ($n = 16$) also had scores lower than any child without autism on the Poor Registration factor. This cluster of low scores for a majority of children with autism suggests the possibility that, taken together, these 3 factors may be helpful in discriminating between children with and without autism in the 3-year-old through 6-year-old age range.

The finding that children with autism scored lower (more frequent behaviors) than children without autism on the Sensory Seeking and Emotionally Reactive factors is interesting, although not unexpected, given that these 2 factors have good face validity for being sensory-based measures and that the items included on these factors are similar to the sensory-based behaviors frequently described in the literature. However, this finding contrasts with that of Ermer and Dunn (1998), who reported a lower incidence of the behaviors on the Sensory Seeking factor for children with autism. This difference in the data gathered from two different samples highlights the importance of conducting multiple studies in an effort to replicate the findings of an initial study. Further, clinicians must exercise cau-

tion when interpreting scores on the Sensory Profile only on the basis of preliminary findings. Further research is needed to determine whether any of the Sensory Profile factors will be helpful in discriminating between young children with and without autism on the basis of sensory–processing abilities. Even so, the finding that 85% of the children with autism scored lower than any of the children without autism on at least 1 factor suggests that clinicians should conduct further assessments of any child from 3 through 6 years of age who obtains 1 or more Sensory Profile factor scores that are lower than those of the children without autism in this study. (See Table 12.1 for the low and high factor scores of each group.)

The low score patterns of children with autism were investigated in an effort to identify potential subgroups. Eight children with autism had scores lower than the children without autism on the Oral Sensitivity, Emotionally Reactive, and Other factors. In a similar pattern, 7 children with autism had scores lower than the children without autism on the Inattention/Distractibility, Emotionally Reactive, and Other factors. Two children with autism had low scores on the Oral Sensitivity and Inattention/Distractibility factors. Further, children with autism who had lower scores than children without autism on Low Endurance ($n = 5$), Sensory Seeking ($n = 5$), and Sensory Sensitivity ($n = 5$) also always had lower scores on either the Emotionally Reactive or the Other factors. These findings suggest that there may be subgroups of children with autism who display distinct profiles of sensory processing. Because of our small sample size, however, these findings could not be examined thoroughly. Further investigation using larger samples to determine whether such subgroups can be identified on the basis of sensory–processing behaviors is necessary.

Of the 40 children with autism in this study, 6 did not have any factor scores lower than the children without autism. We conducted exploratory analyses to determine whether these children were truly different from the group. Analysis of the raw data showed that some parents of these 6 children did not provide responses at the extreme high or low ends of the Likert scale. Two possibilities explain this occurrence. First, the parents accurately reported their children's behavior, and their children's scores fell in the range of scores demonstrated by the children without autism. However, clinical observations of 2 of these 6 children suggest that the parent report did not reflect the behaviors exhibited in the clinical setting. Although the possibility exists that some children with autism do not demonstrate extreme sensory behaviors, it also is possible that the intensity of some behaviors exhibited by the children in this study were moderated by parent report. The second possible explanation for the difference in scores is that some of the parents of children with autism may have reported extreme behaviors because they expected that their children were different. These questions regarding the accuracy of parent report underscore the importance of incorporating clinical observations and professional judgment with results from parent report questionnaires, such as the Sensory Profile.

Implications for Occupational Therapy Practice

The results of this study support the need to measure sensory–processing abilities in young children with autism during occupational therapy evaluations. The Sensory Profile may be a valuable tool in accomplishing this goal. As with all parent-report measures, however, information provided on the Sensory Profile may be inconsistent with clinical observations of sensory processing. Therefore, clinicians should consistently supplement parent report with clinical observations and structured situations in which sensory–processing abilities may be assessed. Clinical observations,

behavior during standardized assessment, and structured play observations may be helpful.

The Sensory Profile does not provide diagnostic information, and this study did not contrast the Sensory Profile score patterns of children with autism with those of children in other diagnostic groups who frequently demonstrate sensory–processing deficits. Further, this study did not examine the ability of the Sensory Profile to discriminate between children with and without autism. Therefore, clinicians should use caution not to assume a diagnosis when a child demonstrates a pattern of sensory behaviors similar to those identified for the children with autism in this study. Further research is necessary to determine whether the pattern of behaviors identified in this study is unique to children with autism and to determine whether Sensory Profile scores discriminate between children with and without autism spectrum disorders.

Limitations

The small sample size in this study and the fact that the sample represented only one region of the country are the primary limitations of this study. Although these may limit the generalizability of the findings, the careful matching of children in the two groups strengthened the design and increased confidence that results are relevant when using the Sensory Profile with young children with autism. Future studies could be strengthened by including mental age testing and a control group of children with developmental delays.

Conclusion

Findings from this study provide clear support for the presence of sensory–processing differences between 3-year-old through 6-year-old children with and without autism. Differences were significant in behaviors related to sensory registration, sensory sensitivity, sensory seeking, emotional reactivity, oral sensitivity, distractibility, and other sensory-based behaviors. Exactly 50% of the children with autism had scores that were lower than any of the children without autism on both the Emotionally Reactive and Other factors, suggesting that these Sensory Profile factors may be especially useful in identifying sensory–processing deficits in children with autism. Clinicians are cautioned, however, to use the Sensory Profile in combination with clinical observations and other measures of sensory–processing abilities to ensure that a child's full range of behaviors are assessed. Additional research with larger groups is needed to fully understand the nature and prevalence of sensory–processing dysfunction in children with autism.

Acknowledgments

We thank Good Samaritan Hospital Children's Therapy Unit, Puyallup, Washington; Center on Human Development and Disability, University of Washington, Seattle; and Experimental Education Unit, University of Washington, Seattle, for their assistance in recruiting participants for this study. We also thank Sue Wendel, MS, OTR, for her assistance in data collection.

This study was funded in part by the Maternal and Child Health Bureau, Division of Health and Human Services ("Leadership Education in Neurodevelopmental Disorders," MCJ 539159-08-0) and the U.S. Department of Education ("Preparing Leaders for Careers in Transdisciplinary Professional Development, Research, and Administration in the Education of Children with Disabilities," H029D70035).

References

Ayres, A. J. (1972). *Sensory integration and learning disorders.* Los Angeles: Western Psychological Services.

Ayres, A. J. (1979). *Sensory integration and the child.* Los Angeles: Western Psychological Services.

Baranek, G. (1999). Autism during infancy: A retrospective video analysis of sensory–motor and social behaviors at 9–12 months of age. *Journal of Autism and Developmental Disorders, 29,* 213–224.

Baranek, G. T., Foster, L. G., & Berkson, G. (1997). Tactile defensive and stereotyped behaviors. *American Journal of Occupational Therapy, 51,* 91–95.

Bryson, S. E. (1996). Brief report: Epidemiology of autism. *Journal of Autism and Developmental Disorders, 26,* 165–168.

Dahlgren, S. O., & Gillberg, C. (1989). Symptoms in the first two years of life: A preliminary population study of infantile autism. *European Archives of Psychiatry and Neurological Sciences, 238,* 33–52.

Data Description. (1997). Data Desk 6.0 [Computer software]. Ithaca, NY: Author.

Dawson, G., & Watling, R. (2000). Interventions to facilitate auditory, visual, and motor integration: A review of the evidence. *Journal of Autism and Developmental Disorders, 30,* 415–421.

DeGangi, G. (1991). Assessment of sensory, emotional, and attentional problems in regulatory disordered infants: Part 1. *Infants and Young Children, 3*(3), 1–8.

Dunn, W. (1996). *Sensory Profile factor grid.* Kansas City: University of Kansas.

Dunn, W. (1997, March). The Sensory Profile: A discriminating measure of sensory processing in daily life. *Sensory Integration Special Interest Section Newsletter, 20,* pp. 1–3.

Dunn, W. (1999). *Sensory Profile user's manual.* San Antonio, TX: Psychological Corporation.

Dunn, W., & Westman, K. (1995). *Sensory Profile (1995 version).* Unpublished manuscript, University of Kansas Medical Center, Kansas City.

Ermer, J., & Dunn, W. (1996, April). *Interpretation of Sensory Profile scores: Preliminary data.* Poster session presented at the American Occupational Therapy Association Annual Conference and Exposition, Chicago.

Ermer, J., & Dunn, W. (1998). The Sensory Profile: A discriminant analysis of children with and without disabilities. *American Journal of Occupational Therapy, 52,* 283–290.

Godfrey, K. (1985). Statistics in practice: Comparing the means of several groups. *New England Journal of Medicine, 313,* 1450–1456.

Goldfarb, W. (1961). *Childhood schizophrenia.* Cambridge, MA: Harvard University Press.

Grandin, T. (1995). *Thinking in pictures.* New York: Doubleday.

Hermelin, B., & O'Connor, N. (1970). Perception and perceptual deficits. In B. Hermelin & N. O'Connor (Eds.), *Psychological experiments with autistic children* (pp. 24–60). Oxford, UK: Pergamon.

Kientz, M. A., & Dunn, W. (1997). The performance of children with and without autism on the Sensory Profile. *American Journal of Occupational Therapy, 51,* 530–537.

Lovaas, O., Schreibman, L., Koegel, R., & Rehm, R. (1971). Selective responding by autistic children to multiple sensory input. *Journal of Abnormal Psychology, 77,* 211–222.

Mayes, S. D., & Calhoun, S. L. (1999). Symptoms of autism in young children and correspondence with the DSM. *Infants and Young Children, 12*(2), 90–97.

McKean, T. (1994). *Soon will come the light.* Arlington, TX: Future Horizons.

Microsoft Corporation. (1997). Microsoft Excel 97 [Computer software]. Redmond, WA: Author.

Murray, E. A., & Anzalone, M. (1991). Integrating sensory integration theory and practice with other intervention approaches. In A. G. Fisher, E. A. Murray, & A. C. Bundy (Eds.), *Sensory integration theory and practice* (pp. 354–384). Philadelphia: F. A. Davis.

O'Neill, M., & Jones, R. S. P. (1997). Sensory–perceptual abnormalities in autism: A case for more research? *Journal of Autism and Developmental Disorders, 27,* 283–293.

Ornitz, E. (1974). The modulation of sensory input and motor output in autistic children. *Journal of Autism and Childhood Schizophrenia, 4,* 197–215.

Piaget, J. (1952). *The origins of intelligence in children.* New York: Norton.

SPSS Inc. (1998). Statistical Package for the Social Sciences for Windows, release 9.0.0, standard version [Computer software]. Chicago: Author.

Stehli, A. (1991). *The sound of a miracle: A child's triumph over autism.* New York: Doubleday.

Williams, D. (1994). *Somebody somewhere.* London: Doubleday.

Williamson, G. G., & Anzalone, M. (1997). Sensory integration: A key component of the evaluation and treatment of young children with severe difficulties in relating and communicating. *Zero to Three, 17,* 29–36.

Wing, L., & Wing, J. K. (1971). Multiple impairments in early childhood autism. *Journal of Autism and Childhood Schizophrenia, 1,* 256–266.

CHAPTER 13

Reliability and Validity of a Parent Questionnaire on Childhood Motor Skills

Brenda N. Wilson, MS, OT(C), *is researcher, Behavioural Research Unit, Alberta Children's Hospital Research Centre, 1820 Richmond Road, SW, Calgary, Alberta T2T 5C7 Canada; brenda.wilson@crha-health.ab.ca.*

Bonnie J. Kaplan, PhD, *is professor of pediatrics, University of Calgary, and director, Behavioural Research Unit, Alberta Children's Hospital Research Centre, Calgary, Alberta, Canada.*

Susan G. Crawford, MSc, *is study coordinator, Behavioural Research Unit, Alberta Children's Hospital Research Centre, Calgary, Alberta, Canada.*

Anne Campbell, BSc, OT(C), *is occupational therapist, Renfrew Educational Services, Calgary, Alberta, Canada.*

Deborah Dewey, PhD, *is associate professor of pediatrics, University of Calgary, and psychologist, Behavioural Research Unit, Alberta Children's Hospital Research Centre, Calgary, Alberta, Canada.*

Originally published 2000 in *American Journal of Occupational Therapy,* 54, 484–493.

Brenda N. Wilson, Bonnie J. Kaplan, Susan G. Crawford, Anne Campbell, and Deborah Dewey

Occupational therapy has long been involved in the treatment of children with developmental and mild motor problems. The prevalence is estimated to be at least 6% (American Psychiatric Association, 1994) and higher in children with other developmental or learning problems (Fox & Lent, 1996). It is now recognized that most children are not likely to outgrow their clumsiness (Losse et al., 1991). The academic, social, and emotional impact of this chronic condition affects the occupational performance of school-age children, resulting in frequent referrals to occupational therapy (Cantell, Smyth, & Ahonen, 1994; Missiuna, 1996; Schoemaker & Kalverboer, 1994). While the condition has many names (Missiuna & Polatajko, 1995), the DSM-IV defines *developmental coordination disorder* (DCD) as "a marked impairment in the development of motor coordination....[which] significantly interferes with academic achievement or activities of daily living"(American Psychiatric Association, 1994).

The need for valid and reliable assessment tools in identifying children who have motor coordination problems has been advocated by occupational therapists (McConnell, 1995; Missiuna & Pollock, 1995). Burton and Miller (1998) reviewed 45 tests of motor skills and abilities, but many are not appropriate for use with school-age children. Of the tests most commonly used in North America with this age group, the Bruininks–Oseretsky Test of Motor Proficiency (BOTMP; Bruininks, 1978) is among the most appropriate. The Movement Assessment Battery for Children (Movement ABC; Henderson & Sugden, 1992) is a relatively new test used extensively in Europe and Asia but is not well known in North America. The Test of Gross Motor Development (Ulrich, 1985) is a useful assessment of the *process* used to perform skilled movement but requires exceptional observational skills and is best suited to children 5 to 7 years of age. The Sensory Integration and Praxis Tests (Ayres, 1989) is a well designed and validated set of tests but is lengthy and expensive to administer, and the economic cutbacks in the health care and educational systems often preclude its use. Methodologically strong but succinct measurements are needed.

Parent report of childrens' current skills and deficits has consistently been shown to be a sensitive, reliable, and valid source of information (Faraone, Biederman, & Milberger, 1995; Glascoe & Dworkin, 1995). In addition to being time-effective and possibly more accurate than some standardized tests (Fox & Lent, 1996), parental perceptions used as part of a client-centered approach are advocated by occupational therapists (Townsend et al., 1997). In addition, they may help overcome the difficulty in assessing skills relevant to children's daily living when using objective measures (Miyahara & Mobs, 1995). Judgment-based assessments have many advantages and offer a balance between objective standardized tests and the subjective nature of clinical observations (Burton & Miller, 1998). Parent questionnaires can provide qualitative, accurate assessment of their children's skills in a naturalistic environment.

The Movement ABC (Henderson & Sugden, 1992) and the Teacher Identification of Children With Movement Skill Problems (Missiuna & Pollock, 1995) were both developed for use by teachers to augment standardized tests in the identification of children with movement disorders. In considering the use of either of these scales with parents, we found that many questions were difficult for parents to answer; however, no other questionnaire that specifically assessed parent perceptions of their children's motor abilities had been reported in the literature. As the practice of occupational therapy encompasses family-centered care (Pollock & Stewart, 1998), our aim was to develop a measure of motor skills for parents.

We also wanted to make the questionnaire applicable across all school ages by asking parents to compare their child with other children his or her own age. This objective was made possible when we conducted a series of studies with

360 children, who underwent several days of assessment, including 3 hours of testing of motor, visual motor, and visual perceptual skills (Kaplan, Wilson, Dewey, & Crawford, 1998). Parents spent several hours being interviewed and completing questionnaires about their children. These families agreed to participate in the first and third studies.

This chapter describes the procedures involved in the development of the Developmental Coordination Disorder Questionnaire (DCDQ), a parent questionnaire used to identify children with motor problems. We also report the evaluation of the questionnaire's reliability and validity and two additional studies that investigate the use of the DCDQ.

Study 1
Method
Procedure

We developed a scale with 35 items based on our review of three commonly used questionnaires: Parent Rating Scale of Everyday Cognitive and Academic Abilities (Williams, Ochs, Williams, & Mulhern, 1991), the Movement ABC (Henderson & Sugden, 1992), and the Teacher Identification of Children With Movement Skill Problems (Teacher Identification Checklist) (Missiuna & Pollock, 1995). After reviewing this version ith researchers and clinicians and having four families evaluate it for clarity and ease, the questionnaire was reduced to 22 items. For each item, parents were asked to compare the degree of coordination of their child with that of other children of the same age, and to rate this on a 5-point Likert scale ranging from *not at all like this child* to *extremely like this child*. Examples of items are (a) throws a ball in a controlled and accurate fashion, compared with other children this age, and (b) learned to ride a bike later than his or her friends.

The questionnaire was not forced choice; parents had the option of answering "Don't know" to each question. Most items were written so that a high score on the scale reflected good coordination, but eight were written so that the same high score reflected poor coordination; these items, worded in a negative direction, were interspersed with positively worded items to reduce response set.

The questionnaire was mailed to a sample of 345 families who participated in the series of studies, with a cover letter inviting them to complete it and return by mail or to call and complete it through a phone interview. A large proportion (two-thirds) of the sample had reading disorders in the family, which might have affected the parent's ability to respond to a questionnaire, so offering to complete the questionnaire through a phone interview should have improved both the response rate and the validity of the answers. Of the 345 questionnaires mailed, 96% were returned: 252 by mail and 80 by telephone interview.

Four items in the DCDQ were answered "Don't know" over 5% of the time; therefore, they were dropped from the questionnaire. Two of these items required the parents to remember when their child first learned a motor skill (e.g., skipping, using a knife), and the other two involved assessing how well their child "dribbled" or kicked a ball, which many parents reported not observing directly. One other item involving the parent's description of their child's pencil grasp was excluded because parents seemed unable to define a grasp beyond "typical" or "atypical," which did not provide the range of comparison that other items gave us. The final 17-item version of the questionnaire was used in the analyses reported here. The values of items worded in the negative direction were reversed (e.g., 5 became 1), and the scores for each item were added to give a total DCDQ score.

Measurement Tools

No single test has been accepted as a gold standard for DCD (Henderson, 1987; Kaplan, Wilson, et al., 1998; Polatajko, 1999). Maeland (1992) used two standardized tests and one questionnaire to assess over 300 children for the presence of DCD. Each of the three tests tended to identify 5% of the population-based sample; however, each test tended to identify a slightly different 5% group of children. Studies like this have led to a common practice of "triangulation" to determine a diagnostic when no gold standard exists (Levine, Busch, & Aufseeser, 1982; Missiuna & Pollock, 1995; Wright & Sugden, 1996). This approach was used in our studies, where two measures commonly used to assess motor competence in school-aged children were administered to define DCD and to examine the concurrent validity of the DCDQ. The BOTMP (Bruininks, 1978) is a 46-item test that assesses the motor functioning of children from 4.5 to 14.5 years of age. The Movement ABC (Henderson & Sugden, 1992) also assesses motor difficulties in children. It contains eight tasks for each of four different age groups: 4 to 6 years, 7 to 8 years, 9 to 10 years, and 11 to 12 years. The total impairment score is interpreted in terms of age-related percentile norms.

Participants

Between 1992 and 1997, a study conducted at the Alberta Children's Hospital Research Center examined physiological, behavioral, and genetic correlates of learning and attention problems (Kaplan, Dewey, Crawford, & Fisher, 1998). Three hundred seventy-nine children and their families participated: 224 index children with learning or attention disorders referred by agencies and private schools, and 155 control participants with no apparent learning or attention problems. The control group consisted of 112 children, individually matched to every second index child with regard to age, sex, and socioeconomic status, and 43 control participants from another study concerning children with a history of family health problems (e.g., a parent with a physical disability) on whom we had identical data. All children were between the ages of 8 and 18 years. Of the 379 children, 73 were above the age limit of the BOTMP (14 years, 6 months) and were not included. Although none of the children was referred to this study specifically because of motor or coordination problems, a substantial number displayed such difficulties. Table 13.1 describes the remaining sample of 306 participants in terms of age, gender, socioeconomic status (determined by parental occupation), and the presence or absence of a learning, attention, or motor problem using the following criteria.

Reading Disability. To be categorized as having a reading disability, child participants could have any of three different types of reading difficulties: (a) deficits in basic reading skills (scoring at or below the 16th percentile on the Basic Reading cluster of the Woodcock–Johnson Psychoeducational Battery–Revised (WJ–R; Woodcock & Johnson, 1989); (b) deficits in reading comprehension (scoring at or below the 16th percentile on the WJ–R Reading Comprehension cluster); or (c) deficits in phonological awareness (scoring below the 24th percentile on the WJ–R Word Attack subtest, and scoring at or below the 16th percentile on the Wide Range Achievement Test–Revised [WRAT–R; Jastak & Wilkinson, 1984) spelling subtest or the WJ–R spelling subtest, and scoring less than or equal to 16 on the Auditory Analysis Test (Rosner & Simon, 1971]).

Attention-Deficit Hyperactivity Disorder (ADHD). To be categorized as ADHD, child participants had to (a) meet diagnostic criteria for ADHD, determined by the Diagnostic Interview Schedule for Children (DISC) (Costello, Edelbrock, & Costello, 1985) through the DSM in 1992 (DSM-III-R) (current at the time the study began); or (b) be diagnosed as ADHD by a physician and be currently taking Ritalin; or (c) obtain a *T* score greater than or equal to 70 (the conventional clinical cutoff is 67) on the Attention Scale of the Child Behavior Check List (CBCL; Achenbach, 1991) and score greater than or equal to one standard deviation above the mean for age and sex on the Abbreviated Symptom Questionnaire (ASQ; Conners, 1991).

Table 13.1. Subject Characteristics (Study 1)

Category	Age M (SD)	Sample Size	SES % Low % Middle % High	% Meeting Criteria for RD	% Meeting Criteria for ADHD	% Meeting Criteria for ADHD and RD
DCD	11.01 (1.3)	n = 38 22 boys 16 girls	20.6 55.9 23.5	13	29	29
Suspect	11.20 (1.48)	n = 45 28 boys 17 girls	20.0 48.8 30.2	6	22	20
Non-DCD	11.02 (1.72)	n = 223 174 boys 49 girls	20.3 52.6 27.1	11	14	15
Total	11.05 (1.64)	N = 306 224 boys 82 girls	20.4 52.4 27.1	11	17	17

Note. ADHD = attention deficit hyperactivitiy disorder; DCD = developmental coordination disorder; RD = reading disability.

Levine (Levine et al., 1982; Levine & Satz, 1984) defined important principles about the detection and selection of children with ADHD, advocating that diagnosis be made only after a review of information from multiple observation sources, as information from a variety of sources may differ due to inadequacy of the testing instruments, personal biases, political or funding agendas, or the fact that the child may manifest the problem variably in different settings. For these reasons, several sources of data were used in our evaluation of ADHD. The majority of children meeting the criteria for ADHD (91%) met the criteria on the DISC, with the remaining children meeting other criteria based on the CBCL, ASQ, and physician diagnosis.

Developmental Coordination Disorder. To evaluate the validity of the DCDQ in identifying children with motor problems, it was necessary to categorize each child participant in our study as DCD or non-DCD. For this task, the BOTMP and the Movement ABC were used, yielding a total of five scores. The BOTMP provided Fine Motor, Gross Motor, Battery Composite, and Short Form scores. The Short Form was used only if the Battery, Fine Motor, or Gross Motor Composites were unavailable for a child, which was the case for 17 participants. The Movement ABC provided one score and was used with about half of the children; it had not been published when our research began in 1992. One hundred twenty children had all five scores, and 183 had four scores (missing the Movement ABC). Three children had only two scores, but both scores were below the 10th percentile, which indicated that they met the criteria for DCD.

Because of the difficulty in establishing cutoff scores on standardized tests for the identification of DCD, we felt it appropriate to assign participants to one of three categories: DCD, Suspect, and non-DCD. The criteria used for each category were as follows: (1) DCD, $\leq$ 10th percentile on at least 2 of the 5 possible scores obtained; (2) Suspect, (a) $\geq$ 11th percentile and $\leq$ 25th percentile score on at least 2 of the 5 tests or (b) $\leq$ 10th percentile score on 1 of the 5 tests plus $\geq$ 11th percentile score and $\leq$ 25th percentile score on 1 of the 5 tests; and (3) non-DCD, $\geq$ 25th percentile score on at least 4 of the 5 tests.

The inclusion of a Suspect category is useful in identifying those children who do not exhibit serious motor delays but whose skills are not clearly within the average range. Other standardized measures, such as the Bayley Scales of Infant Development (Bayley, 1983), have used similar categories to define risk groups.

Three considerations led to a decision to define DCD on at least two measures. First, this definition avoided categorizing the child who had only an occasional problem with motor skills (poor performance on a single measure) as DCD. Second, it had been observed that it was not uncommon for children to score within the average range on one test or part of a test, but below average on another test or part of it. Defining DCD by low performance on at least two measures took into account this type of variability. Last, the practice of triangulation, or using more than one score from a single data base to identify learning and developmental problems, is recommended by many professionals (Levine et al., 1982; Missiuna & Pollock, 1995; Wright & Sugden, 1996).

Results

Sample Characteristics

In classifying the subjects as DCD, Suspect DCD, or non-DCD, there were no group differences on age ($F(2, 305)$ = .23, n.s.) or SES ($\chi^2(4)$ = .51, n.s.). There were significantly more boys in the non-DCD group than in the Suspect or the DCD groups ($\chi^2(2)$ = 9.95, $p < .01$).

Reliability

Internal Consistency

Cronbach's coefficient alpha was used to examine how well all items measured the same construct and contributed to the total assessment, with .70 specified as an acceptable level (see Table 13.2). The alpha coefficient for the total test was .88. The alpha of each item, if that item was deleted, measured greater than .87 (range, .87–.88). The deletion of any item did not increase the alpha coefficient of other items.

The total score of the DCDQ was significantly correlated with each of the items of the test, another measure of internal consistency. These item total correlations ranged from $r = .40$ to $r = .76$, with all significant at the probability level of .0001.

Concurrent Validity

The total score of the DCDQ was significantly correlated with the four composite scores of the BOTMP ($r = .46–.54$, $p < .0001$). The DCDQ

Table 13.2. Internal Consistency as Measured by Cronbach's Alpha Coefficient (Study 1)

Item	Correlation Between Item and Total Test Score	Correlation Alpha If Item Was Deleted
Bull in china shop	.4248	.8790
Catch ball	.6317	.8716
Hit ball or birdie	.6233	.8714
Throw ball	.7164	.8681
Cutting	.5847	.8728
Avoids sports	.5090	.8756
Rides bicycle	.3037	.8838
Fatigues easily	.4402	.8784
Jump over	.5890	.8730
Run and stop	.6634	.8700
Team sports	.3117	.8839
Writing legibly	.5503	.8740
Writing speed	.4936	.8767
Pencil pressure	.5206	.8752
Awkward	.4509	.8780
Learns skills	.6008	.8719
Plan activity	.5550	.8753

Note. N = 204.

was also significantly correlated with the total impairment score of the Movement ABC ($r = –.59$, $p < .0001$). The correlations between the DCDQ and the BOTMP are positive values, as high scores reflect better performance on both of these tests. The correlation with the Movement ABC, however, is negative as the two scores are scaled in opposite directions: High Movement ABC Impairment Scores reflect poor performance. These correlations indicate an acceptable level of concurrent validity of the DCDQ.

Construct Validity

The groups differed significantly on the total DCDQ score ($F (2, 203) = 29.43$, $p < .001$), demonstrating that the DCDQ measures a motor construct (see Table 13.3). Using the Scheffe test for post hoc group comparisons, it was found that the DCD group scored significantly lower than the Suspect DCD group and the non-DCD group. The Suspect group also scored significantly below the non-DCD group. Boys and girls did not differ ($F (1, 203) = .32$, n.s.), and age and total score did not correlate significantly ($r = –.075$, n.s.), indicating that the scale is valid for use with both genders and between the ages of 8 and 14 1/2 years.

Discriminant Function Analysis

A discriminant function analysis was performed using the 17 items of the DCDQ as predictors of

Table 13.3. Total Scores on the DCDQ by Group (Study 1)

Group	DCD Group M (SD)	Suspect DCD Group M (SD)	Non-DCD Group M (SD)
Boys	47.83 (10.90)	63.09 (11.74)	68.78 (10.37)
Girls	52.20 (12.21)	60.83 (13.18)	70.39 (12.15)
Total	49.82 (11.45)	62.29 (12.11)	69.11 (10.74)

Note. DCD = developmental coordination disorder; DCDQ = Developmental Coordination Disorder Questionnaire.

membership in three groups: DCD, Suspect DCD, and non-DCD. Of the entire sample of 306 children, 102 had at least one item score (a variable) missing and were therefore excluded from this analysis, resulting in a sample size of 204. Two discriminant functions were identified, with a combined χ^2 (34) = 99.14, p < .00001. These two discriminant functions accounted for 87.4% of the between-group variability. After removal of the first function, no association was found between groups and predictors. The first discriminant function separated children with DCD and those suspect for DCD from the children in the non-DCD group. The best predictors for distinguishing between non-DCD children and the other two groups were the following items: catching a ball, running and stopping, throwing a ball, jumping, ease in learning new motor skills, hitting a ball or birdie, planning an activity requiring motor coordination, and a tendency to avoid sports. The DCDQ correctly classified 68.1% of the total sample: 86.4% of the children with DCD, 44.1% of those with Suspect DCD, and 70.9% of the participants without DCD.

Factor Analysis

Based on the face validity of the test items, items were initially divided into five categories: gross motor, fine motor, general coordination, handwriting, and praxis. These categorizations of motor functions are commonly seen in clinical research and practice (Levine, 1994; Parker, Larkin, & Wade, 1997). Principal factor extraction with varimax rotation was performed to assist in determining the domains of the test, as demonstrated in the data, and to compare them to our original theoretical categories. Four distinct factors with eigenvalues > 1.0 emerged, explaining 63.4% of the variance. Loadings of items on factors and the labels assigned them are shown in Table 13.4. Control During Movement contained 5 items from the coordination and gross motor categories and 1 from praxis. All involved motor control when the child was in motion or when an object was in motion (caught or thrown). Fine Motor/Handwriting contained 4 items, 3 from the handwriting category and 1 from fine motor. Gross Motor/Planning contained 3 gross motor and 1 praxis

Table 13.4. Factor Loading for Principal Factors Extraction With Proposed Labels (Study 1)

Item	Factor 1 Control During Movement	Factor 2 Fine Motor/ Handwriting	Factor 3 Gross Motor/ Planning	Factor 4 General Coordination
1. Throw ball	.8175	.1934	.2556	.1044
2. Catch ball	.7996	.0785	.3166	.0160
3. Hit ball or birdie	.7939	.1295	.2596	.0134
4. Jump over	.7849	.1733	.0404	.1183
5. Run and stop	.7701	.1702	.0793	.2759
6. Plan activity	.5526	.3704	−.1151	.2965
7. Writing speed	.1182	.8446	.1656	−.0014
8. Writing legibly	.1653	.8275	.0552	.1879
9. Pencil pressure	.1705	.7964	.0353	.1648
10. Cutting	.3834	.5391	.0333	.2818
11. Team sports	.0310	.1594	.7176	−.0143
12. Avoids sports	.4524	.02924	.6416	.0235
13. Rides bicycle	.2148	−.1391	.5490	.2100
14. Learns skills	.3496	.2739	.4640	.2973
15. Bull in china shop	.0996	.1538	.1259	.7710
16. Awkward	.2068	.1309	.0568	.7607
17. Fatigues easily	−.0045	.2335	.4928	.5101
Eigenvalue	6.31	1.95	1.43	1.10
% Variance	37.1	11.5	8.4	6.4

item, and General Coordination contained 3 items that described the child as "a bull in a china shop," "slow and awkward," and easily fatigued.

Correlation of Factors

When items are combined additively to form an overall index, different patterns of response may lead to identical scores. For example, two similar total scores based on different combinations of item responses may reflect different motor abilities. For this reason, we examined the correlations between each of the factors and the subtests of the BOTMP and the Movement ABC (see Table 13.5). The number and patterns of significant correlations between the factors of the DCDQ and subtests of these motor measures support the validity of the factors outlined. As noted earlier, a negative correlation between the DCDQ and any score of the Movement ABC actually denotes a positive relationship, due to the reverse scoring procedure of the Movement ABC.

The Control During Movement factor correlated strongly with a large number of subtests that included measurement of the movement of an object and or the child. The Fine Motor/Handwriting factor demonstrated significant correlations with the manual dexterity subtest of the Movement ABC and the visual–motor control and bilateral coordination subtests of the BOTMP. Significant correlations were found between the Gross Motor/Planning factor and subtests measuring running speed and agility, bilateral coordination, strength, response speed, visual–motor control, and ball skills. The General Coordination factor was significantly correlated with balance (both tests) and visual–motor control.

Development of a DCDQ Impairment Score

The total possible score on the DCDQ was 85; the mean score for the entire sample was 65.9 (SD = 12.6, range 32–85). Using the same definition of motor impairment that we used earlier, we developed cutoff scores for each of the three categorizations of DCD: (1) 0–48, scores from 0–10th percentile, denoted as DCD; (2) 49–57,

Table 13.5. Pearson Product-Moment Correlations of DCDQ Factor Scores With Subtests of the BOTMP and Components of the Movement ABC (Study 1)

Subtest	Factor 1 Control During Movement (r)	Factor 2 Fine Motor/ Handwriting (r)	Factor 3 Gross Motor/ Planning (r)	Factor 4 General Coordination (r)
Running Speed and Agility	.3721****	− .1168	.1412*	.0101
Balance	.2124**	.0828	.0236	.2670****
Bilateral Coordination	.2387***	.1747*	.1409*	.1743*
Strength	.3902****	.0415	.1419*	− .0159
Upper-Limb Coordination	.3110****	.0732	.0935	.1076
Response Speed	.1624*	.0575	.1776*	− .0196
Visual–Motor Control	.2110**	.1751*	.3197****	.2436****
Upper-Limb Speed and Dexterity	.3110****	.0732	.0935	.1076
Manual Dexterity	− .3157**	− .2665**	− .1980	− .0511
Ball Skills	− .3828****	− .0535	− .3156**	.0587
Static and Dynamic Balance	− .1046	− .1665	− .1190	− .2798**

Note. BOTMP = Bruininks–Oseretsky Test of Motor Performance; DCDQ = Developmental Coordination Disorder Questionnaire; Movement ABC = Movement Assessment Battery for Children.

*$p < .05$. **$p < .01$. ***$p < .001$. ****$p < .0001$.

scores from 11th to 24th percentile, denoted as Suspect DCD; and (3) 58–85, scores from 25th to 100th percentile, denoted as non-DCD.

Study 2

As part of a different project whose purpose was to examine the interrater reliability of the BOTMP (Wilson, Kaplan, Crawford, & Dewey, 2000), the parents of 77 children completed a DCDQ at the same time that their children were tested on the Movement ABC and the BOTMP. This resulted in a further examination of the construct validity of the DCDQ, with a different population of children than those in studies 1 and 3.

Method

Participants

The 77 participants in this second study ranged in age from 7.28 to 14.25 years. They differed from the sample of Study 1 in that their diagnosis of learning disability (LD), ADHD, or DCD was based on parent, physician, or teacher, or all three, impressions, not on extensive testing and objective criteria. Some in this sample showed evidence of learning or attention problems or both ($n = 52$; 14 boys, 11 girls; average age = 9.87 years, $SD = 1.61$), and some showed no such problems ($n = 25$; 8 boys, 17 girls; average age = 9.29 years, $SD = 1.57$). No significant group difference was found for the children's age ($F(1, 76) = 2.21$, n.s.). However, there was a significant difference between the groups in gender ($\chi^2(1) = 16.01$, $p < .0001$), with more girls in the group with no known developmental problems and more boys in the group with learning and attention problems.

Using the same method of identifying children with DCD described for Study 1, the children were categorized into three groups: DCD, Suspect DCD, and non-DCD. Table 13.6 shows the ages and gender of the children in each of these

Table 13.6. Subject Characteristics (Study 2)

Group	Age (Years) M (SD)	No. of Boys/Girls	DCDQ Score M (SD)
DCD group (n = 13) 10 LD, 3 control	10.38 (1.85)	10 boys/ 3 girls	43.85 (9.46)
Suspect group (n = 13) 10 LD, 3 control	9.73 (1.41)	7 boys/ 6 girls	54.15 (11.28)
Non-DCD group (n = 51) 32 LD, 19 control	9.49 (1.58)	32 boys/ 19 girls	61.47 (10.63)
Total group (n = 77) 52 LD, 25 control	9.68 (1.61)	49 boys/ 28 girls	57.26 (12.36)

Note. DCD = developmental coordination disorder; DCDQ = Developmental Coordination Disorder Questionnaire; LD = learning disability.

three groups. When the three groups were compared, there was no significant group difference for the child's age ($F(2, 76) = 1.61$, n.s.). There was also no association between gender and group membership ($\chi^2(1) = 1.55$, n.s.). The child's age was not significantly correlated with the total DCDQ score ($r = -.0829$, n.s.), so age was not used as a covariate in the next analysis, which looked for group differences in the DCDQ score.

Results

There was a significant group difference in the DCDQ score ($F(2, 76) = 15.12$, $p < .0001$). Post hoc group comparisons using the Scheffe test revealed that the DCD group scored significantly lower than the non-DCD group. This supports the findings of the main study and demonstrates that the DCDQ discriminates between children with and without problems in motor skills.

The correlations between the DCDQ and the four composite scores of the BOTMP were similar to the correlations found in Study 1, ranging from $r = .57$ to $r = .66$ ($p < .001$). Correlations between the DCDQ score and the impairment

Table 13.7. Pearson Product-Moment Correlations of DCDQ Factor Scores With Subtests of the BOTMP and Components of the Movement ABC (Study 2)

Subtest	Factor 1 Control During Movement (r)	Factor 2 Fine Motor/ Handwriting (r)	Factor 3 Gross Motor/ Planning (r)	Factor 4 General Coordination (r)
Running Speed and Agility	.408***	.089	.325**	.127
Balance	.269*	.266*	.194	.311**
Bilateral Coordination	.259*	.329**	.247*	.339**
Strength	.391***	.173	.156	.193
Upper-Limb Coordination	.297**	.174	.204	.116
Response Speed	.224*	.298**	.101	.225*
Visual-Motor Control	.223	.440***	.218	.404***
Upper-Limb Speed and Dexterity	.325**	.346**	.273*	.322**
Manual Dexterity	− .352**	− .349**	− .190	− .344**
Ball Skills	− .329**	− .181	− .149	− .089
Static and Dynamic Balance	− .180	− .379**	− .107	− .236*

Note. BOTMP = Bruininks–Oseretsky Test of Motor Performance; DCDQ = Developmental Coordination Disorder Questionnaire; Movement ABC = Movement Assessment Battery for Children.

$*p < .05.$ $**p < .01.$ $***p < .001.$

score of the Movement ABC were also significant ($r = − .47$, $p < .001$). Table 13.7 shows the correlations between the three factors of the DCDQ and the subtests of the BOTMP and the Movement ABC. These significant correlations suggest that the DCDQ is measuring a similar function as other tests of motor coordination.

Study 3

The degree to which the DCDQ measures constructs clinically observed by occupational therapists was also examined. Forty-six of the motor assessments described in Study 1 were completed by one occupational therapist with more than 20 years of experience with children. The therapist was blind to the child's diagnosis of RD or ADHD at the time of testing but was aware that none of the children had been referred for DCD.

Method

The occupational therapist made her own diagnostic classification of each child whom she assessed while testing the children but before any

of the tests were scored. During the 2 1/2- to 3-hr assessment, she observed the child's abilities and judged whether the child demonstrated one of the three characteristics of motor functioning: (a) good coordination—no problems were apparent; (b) poor motor planning—the child appeared to have difficulty figuring out how to move, but once he or she learned or practiced the task, the coordination of the movement was acceptable; and (c) poor execution—the child appeared to know how to move his or her body to accomplish a task but had difficulty controlling the movements, and the motor response was slow, awkward, or inefficient.

Participants

In this convenience sample of 46 children assessed by this occupational therapist, there were 31 boys and 15 girls, ranging from 8.30 years to 14.09 years (average age = 11.23 years, $SD = 1.64$).

Results

Table 13.8 compares the identification made by the therapist with that made by the DCDQ.

Table 13.8. Comparison of the DCDQ and
Therapist Judgment (Study 3)

Category	Good Coordination	Poor Motor Planning	Poor Execution
Non-DCD	20	11	2
Suspect	1	2	3
DCD	0	2	5
Total	21	15	10

Note. DCD = developmental coordination disorder; DCDQ =
Developmental Coordination Disorder Questionnaire.

Agreement was 20 out of 21 (95%) for children who had no motor problems and 8 out of 10 (80%) for children who had difficulty executing (but not planning) movement. However, there was only a 27% (4/15) agreement between the therapist and the questionnaire for children who the therapist defined as having motor planning problems; the DCDQ did not identify children with planning problems as often as the therapist.

A series of ANOVAs was conducted to see if the three groups formed on the basis of clinical judgment showed any significant differences on the four factors that were generated from the DCDQ. Significant group differences emerged for the Control During Movement factor ($F(2,45) = 4.82$, $p < .05$) and for the Fine Motor/Handwriting factor ($F(2,45) = 3.52$, $p < .05$). For both of these factors, the group that the therapist identified as having good coordination scored significantly higher than the group that demonstrated poor execution of movement patterns.

Discussion

Several challenges have to be met when developing measures for use with children who exhibit DCD. The most difficult is that there is no "gold standard" for the identification of this condition (Dewey & Wilson, in press; Henderson & Barnett, 1998; Wright & Sugden, 1996). This is because there is no one test that is used extensively in the field and because of the apparent heterogeneity of the group of children that we collectively call "DCD." This heterogeneity is possibly suggestive of distinct populations within the group of DCD (Hoare, 1994; Macnab, Miller, & Polatajko, 1999; Miyahara & Mobs, 1995; Parker et al., 1997; Willoughby & Polatajko, 1995). If subgroups exist, it is not surprising that a child with DCD would score differently on different tests or exhibit a different profile on subtests within a test. In this study, we addressed the problem of identification of children with DCD by relying on a combination of the scores of two tests to identify children with DCD: the BOTMP, commonly used as a normative test to assess motor skills, and the Movement ABC, developed specifically for the identification of DCD.

The studies show that the psychometric qualities of the DCDQ appear to be sound. The scale is appropriate to use with either boys or girls, and the lack of correlation between test scores and age indicates that it can be used with confidence with children from 8 years to 14 years, 6 months of age. Internal consistency was very strong, with a high alpha coefficient for the test that did not change with the deletion of any item.

Assessment of the clinical validity of any measure occurs over time, with the continued use of a test. This will be true for the DCDQ as well, but the initial analysis reported here is encouraging. The questionnaire is significantly correlated with two tests of motor skills, indicating its effectiveness in assessing problems in motor skills through parent report. It is more highly correlated with the Movement ABC than with the BOTMP, which probably reflects the fact that the Movement ABC and the DCDQ were designed to identify motor problems, whereas the primary purpose of the BOTMP is to assess motor skills for educational placement and programming (Bruininks, 1978).

Using a scoring system that identified three groups (DCD, Suspect DCD, and non-DCD), the total score of the DCDQ accurately reflected the child's competency in motor skills. The questionnaire was most accurate in correctly classifying children with DCD (86% correct). Children without DCD were correctly identified 71% of the time; there were 29% of the children whose parents identified a movement problem but whose performance on standardized tests was not indicative of motor difficulties. Parents may have identified a problem in attention, aptitude, or motivation as difficulty in coordination, but assessments of motor skills did not confirm this. Conversely, the parent report of functional limitations of motor skills in their children may be the most accurate; and our current standardized tests did not identify the problems.

Participants whose motor skills were "suspect" were identified 44% of the time. This lowest percentage is not unusual considering that the motor difficulties of this group fall between a clearly defined presence or absence of the disorder; obtaining a score between 49 and 57 on the DCDQ suggests that the child should be examined further by a specialist in the field of children's motor skills, such as an occupational therapist. The specificity of the DCDQ is strong enough to recommend its use as a screening instrument. It was not developed to be a diagnostic index on its own or to replace existing tests but rather to provide the professional with the parent's perceptions of the children's functional skills outside of the clinic setting. Should the test score indicate a categorization of DCD or a suspicion of DCD, further testing of motor skills and functional performance is warranted.

The factor analysis largely supported our theoretical categorizations of the DCDQ, with some modifications. Four distinct factors explained 63% of the variance. To understand how these factors relate to different patterns of motor performance, we examined the correlation of these factors with the subtest scores of the two other tests used for identification of DCD. The existence of these factors is supported by the number

and patterns of moderately strong significant correlations between our factors and the subtests, which have items matching the motor function named. The most obvious example is that of the Fine Motor/Handwriting factor, which correlated significantly with the manual dexterity subtest of the Movement ABC and with the visual–motor control and bilateral coordination subtests of the BOTMP. The former two subtests are composed largely of visual–motor tasks and paper-and-pencil tasks, whereas the latter (bilateral coordination) has one paper-and-pencil item.

The Control During Movement factor is clearly related to almost all of the subtests of both the BOTMP and the Movement ABC, reflecting the fact that most of the items of these two tests involve control when the child is moving or when an object is being caught or thrown, as do these items on the DCDQ.

The General Coordination factor included three items of a very general nature. The association of subtests measuring balance with this factor supports clinical observations that there are children who exhibit low postural tone, are easily fatigued, are clumsy, and tend to have poor balance skills (Fisher, Murray, & Bundy, 1991).

It is interesting to note that the visual–motor control subtest of the BOTMP correlated significantly with all four factors, indicating how fine motor and handwriting problems can be related to many motor and perceptual functions: form and space perception, motor planning and motor memory, sequencing, and visuomotor coordination (Cermak, 1991). Handwriting is sometimes viewed as an "end-product" in the complex process of motor coordination, so its relation to many underlying factors is not surprising.

The discriminant function analysis revealed eight items that best predicted membership in the non-DCD group compared to the DCD or Suspect group. Of the eight items identified as the best predictors, six of them constituted one entire factor, the Control During Movement factor. These items measure children's motor skills when the child is moving, or an object is moving, or both are moving, which are higher level skills than activities that do not involve as much movement through space. If a child scores low in this factor, there is support for the identification of DCD. The usefulness of the DCDQ in discriminating between children with and without DCD was further supported through the results of two other studies, although the agreement between the therapist and the DCDQ was low for children whom the therapist saw as having problems in the planning of their movements. The fact that the DCDQ does not identify children with motor planning problems as readily as other types of problems could be related to the observation that the correlations between the Gross Motor/ Planning factor of the DCDQ and most subtests of the two motor tests were very low.

Current tests of motor abilities, as well as this questionnaire, appear to identify some children with motor problems but may "miss" those with planning difficulties (Hoare, 1994). Another possibility is that parents were able to identify problems in the execution and coordination of their children's motor skills but were less likely to be aware of difficulties in the planning component of movement. Finally, it is possible that there are too few items related solely to motor planning in this factor of the DCDQ, with most items being of a gross motor nature. It has been suggested that different tools are needed for the identification of developmental dyspraxia than for that of DCD (Miyahara & Mobs, 1995). This possibility is presently being investigated by some of the authors (Dewey, 1995; Dewey, Wilson, Crawford, & Kaplan, in preparation).

There were limitations inherent in the design of these three studies. One relates to a possible sampling bias in Study 1: The group of children we gathered data from was not representative of the entire population, in that they had more learning and attention problems. As described earlier, the sample used for the development of the DCDQ was children and families participating in a larger study of learning disabilities. This sample was also unique in that all the children involved were part of families who were willing to commit approximately 10 hours to a large research project; in families committed to supporting their children's learning, the parents may have been more familiar with the capabilities of their children than parents who did not volunteer to participate. Another possible sampling bias is that none of the children in Study 1 or 3 were referred because of their motor coordination problems. It is possible that children who are referred for DCD have a different type of problem from those who may be identified through other means (Missiuna, 1994; Wilson, Polatajko, Mandich, & Macnab, 1998). The final limitation lay in the initial design of the questionnaire, which allowed the parents to choose a "Don't know" response for any item. In a number of cases, this prevented us from calculating a total score, which in turn prevented us from determining the presence or absence of DCD. In retrospect, we realize that a "best guess" is more helpful to diagnosis than a nonanswer, and we have modified the questionnaire.

In summary, this chapter describes the development of a parent questionnaire and the examination of its reliability and validity. This questionnaire is succinct, is easy to administer and score, and provides information on the existence of motor difficulties in children. When used as a screening tool or in conjunction with a clinical assessment, the DCDQ could provide a valuable adjunct to measures used by occupational therapists.

Acknowledgments

We acknowledge the assistance of Cheryl Missiuna and Sheila Henderson in sharing their questionnaires, as well as their valuable contributions in the discussion of aspects of this study and the identification of DCD. We also thank the Alberta Children's Hospital Foundation and the Alberta Mental Health Research Unit Award for grant support.

The Office of Medical Bioethics, Faculty of Medicine, University of Calgary approved each of the studies described. The DCDQ is copyrighted in the United States and Canada. For more information about the DCDQ, contact the first author.

References

Achenbach, T. M. (1991). *Manual for the Child Behavior Check List 14–18 and 1991 Profile.* Burlington: University of Vermont.

American Psychiatric Association. (1994). *Diagnostic and statistical manual of mental disorders* (4th ed.). Washington, DC: American Psychiatric Association.

Ayres, J. A. (1989). *Sensory integration and praxis test.* Los Angeles, CA: Western Psychological Services.

Bayley, N. (1983). *Bayley Scales of Infant Development.* San Antonio, TX: Psychological Corporation.

Bruininks, R. H. (1978). *Bruininks–Oseretsky Test of Motor Proficiency: Examiner's manual.* Circle Pines, MN: American Guidance Service.

Burton, A. W., & Miller, D. E. (1998). *Movement skill assessment.* Champaign, IL: Human Kinetics.

Cantell, M. H., Smyth, M. M., & Ahonen, T. P. (1994). Clumsiness in adolescence: Educational, motor, and social outcomes of motor delay detected at 5 years. *Adapted Physical Activity Quarterly, 11,* 115–129.

Cermak, S. A. (1991). Somatodyspraxia. In A. G. Fisher, E. A. Murray, & A. C. Bundy (Eds.), *Sensory integration: Theory and practice* (pp. 137–170). Philadelphia: F. A. Davis.

Conners, C. K. (1991). *Conners' Rating Scales manual.* Toronto: Multi-Health Systems.

Costello, E. J., Edelbrock, C. S., & Costello, A. J. (1985). Validity of the NIMH Diagnostic Interview Schedule for Children: A comparison between psychiatric and pediatric referrals. *Journal of Abnormal Child Psychology, 13,* 579–595.

Dewey, D. (1995). What is developmental dyspraxia? *Brain and Cognition, 29,* 254–274.

Dewey, D., & Wilson, B. N. (in press). Developmental coordination disorder: What is it? *Physical and Occupational Therapy in Pediatrics.*

Dewey, D., Wilson, B. N., Crawford, S. G., & Kaplan, B. J. *Praxis and coordination: The same or different disorder?* Manuscript in preparation.

Faraone, S. F., Biederman, J., & Milberger, S. (1995). How reliable are maternal reports of their children's psychopathology? One-year recall of psychiatric diagnoses of ADHD children. *Journal of the American Academy of Child and Adolescent Psychiatry, 34,* 1001.

Fisher, A. G., Murray, E. A., & Bundy, A. C. (1991). *Sensory integration: Theory and practice.* Philadelphia: F. A. Davis.

Fox, M. A., & Lent, B. (1996). Clumsy children: Primer on developmental coordination disorder. *Canadian Family Physician, 42,* 1965–1971.

Glascoe, F. P., & Dworkin, P. H. (1995). The role of parents in the detection of developmental and behavioral problems. *Pediatrics, 95,* 829–836.

Henderson, S. E. (1987). The assessment of "clumsy children": Old and new approaches. *Journal of Child Psychology and Psychiatry, 28,* 511–527.

Henderson, S. E., & Barnett, A. L. (1998). The classification of specific motor coordination disorders in children: Some problems to be solved. *Human Movement Science, 17,* 449–470.

Henderson, S. E., & Sugden, D. A. (1992). *Movement Assessment Battery for Children.* Kent, UK: Psychological Corporation.

Hoare, D. (1994). Subtypes of developmental coordination disorder. *Adapted Physical Activity Quarterly, 11,* 158–169.

Jastak, S., & Wilkinson, G. S. (1984). *The Wide Range Achievement Test–Revised.* Wilmington, DE: Jastak Associates.

Kaplan, B. J., Dewey, D., Crawford, S., & Fisher, G. (1998). Deficits in long-term memory are not characteristic of ADHD. *Journal of Clinical and Experimental Neuropsychology, 20,* 518–528.

Kaplan, B. J., Wilson, B. N., Dewey, D. M., & Crawford, S. G. (1998). DCD may not be a discrete disorder. *Human Movement Science, 17,* 471–490.

Levine, M. (1994). *Educational care: A system for understanding and helping children with learning problems at home and in school.* Cambridge, MA: Educators Publishing Service.

Levine, M. D., Busch, B., & Aufseeser, C. (1982). The dimension of inattention among children with school problems. *Pediatrics, 3,* 387–395.

Levine, M. D., & Satz, P. (1984). *Middle childhood: Development and dysfunction.* Baltimore: University Park Press.

Losse, A., Henderson, S. A., Elliman, D., Hall, D., Knight, E., & Jongmans, M. (1991). Clumsiness in children: Do they outgrow it? A 10-year follow-up study. *Developmental Medicine and Child Neurology, 33,* 55–68.

Macnab, J. L., Miller, L. T., & Polatajko, H. J. (1999). *The search for subtypes of developmental coordination disorder: The impact of referral bias.* Paper presented at Developmental Coordination Disorder: From Research to Diagnostics and Intervention. Groningen, The Netherlands.

Maeland, A. F. (1992). Identification of children with motor coordination problems. *Adapted Physical Activity Quarterly, 9,* 330–342.

McConnell, D. (1995). Processes underlying clumsiness: A review of perspectives. *Physical and Occupational Therapy in Pediatrics, 15*(3), 33–52.

Missiuna, C. (1994). Motor skills acquisition in children with developmental coordination disorder. *Adapted Physical Activity Quarterly, 11,* 214–235.

Missiuna, C. (1996). *Keeping current in developmental coordination disorder.* Hamilton, Ontario: McMaster University, Faculty of Health Sciences.

Missiuna, C., & Polatajko, H. (1995). Developmental dyspraxia by any other name: Are they all just clumsy children? *American Journal of Occupational Therapy, 49,* 619–627.

Missiuna, C., & Pollock, N. (1995). Beyond the norms: Need for multiple sources of data in the assessment of children. *Physical and Occupational Therapy in Pediatrics, 15*(4), 57–71.

Miyahara, M., & Mobs, I. (1995). Developmental dyspraxia and developmental coordination disorder. *Neuropsychology Review, 5,* 245–268.

Parker, H. E., Larkin, D., & Wade, M. G. (1997). Are motor timing problems subgroup specific in children with developmental coordination disorder. *Australian Educational and Developmental Psychologist, 14*(1), 35–42.

Polatajko, H. J. (1999). Developmental coordination disorder (DCD); Alias the clumsy child syndrome. In K. Whitmore, H. Hart, & G. W. Willems (Eds.), *A neurodevelopmental approach to specific learning disorders* (pp. 119–133). London: MacKeith.

Pollock, N., & Stewart, D. (1998). Occupational performance needs of school-aged children with physical disabilities in the community. *Physical and Occupational Therapy in Pediatrics, 18,* 55–68.

Rosner, J., & Simon, D. P. (1971). The auditory analysis test: A paper. *Journal of Learning Disabilities, 4,* 384–392.

Schoemaker, M. M., & Kalverboer, A. F. (1994). Social and affective problems of children who are clumsy: How early do they begin? *Adapted Physical Activity Quarterly, 11,* 130–140.

Townsend, E., Stanton, S., Law, M., Polatajko, H., Baptiste, S., Thompson-Franson, T., et al. (1997). *Enabling occupation: An occupational therapy perspective.* Ottawa, Ontario: Canadian Association of Occupational Therapists.

Ulrich, B. (1985). *Test of Gross Motor Development.* Austin, TX: PRO-ED.

Williams, K. S., Ochs, J., Williams, J. M., & Mulhern, R. K. (1991). Parent report of everyday cognitive abilities among children treated for acute lymphoblastic leukemia. *Journal of Pediatric Psychology, 16,* 13–26.

Willoughby, C., & Polatajko, H. J. (1995). Motor problems in children with developmental coordination disorder: Review of the literature. *American Journal of Occupational Therapy, 49,* 787–793.

Wilson, B. N., Kaplan, B. J., Crawford, S. G., & Dewey, D. (2000). Interrater reliability of the Bruininks–Oseretsky Test of Motor Proficiency–Long Form. *Adapted Physical Activity Quarterly, 17,* 95–110.

Wilson, B. N., Polatajko, H. J., Mandich, A. D., & Macnab, J. J. (1998). *Standardized measures: How well do they identify children and adolescents with DCD?* Paper presented at the World Federation of Occupational Therapy, Montreal, Canada.

Woodcock, R. W., & Johnson, M. B. (1989). *Woodcock–Johnson Psychoeducational Battery–Revised.* Allen, TX: DLM Teaching Resources.

Wright, H. C., & Sugden, D. A. (1996). A two-step procedure for the identification of children with developmental coordination disorder in Singapore. *Developmental Medicine and Child Neurology, 38,* 1099–1105.

IV
Scholarship of Discovery:
Intervention
Outcomes

CHAPTER 14

Implicit Learning in Children With and Without Developmental Coordination Disorder

Catherine Candler and Harry Meeuwsen

Catherine Candler, PhD, OTR, BCP, *is assistant professor, Texas Woman's University, School of Occupational Therapy, 8194 Walnut Hill Lane, Dallas, TX 75231; Ccandler@twu.edu.*

Harry Meeuwsen, PhD, *is professor and program director, Department of Kinesiology, University of Texas at El Paso, College of Health Sciences, El Paso.*

Developmental coordination disorder is a condition that affects approximately 6% of all school-age children (Polatajko, 1999). The disorder presents as unexplained clumsiness and problems with tasks that require motor coordination. Of special concern to occupational therapists is the impact of this dysfunction on daily living tasks (American Psychiatric Association [APA], 1994). Children with developmental coordination disorder have trouble with skills such as writing, catching a ball, dressing, buttoning, tying shoes, or handling a spoon (Gordon & McKinley, 1980). These problems may translate into social and emotional challenges that can persist into the teen years (Cantell, Smyth, & Ahonen, 1994) and affect occupational choices made in adult life (Rasmussen & Gillberg, 2000).

Traditionally, occupational therapists have used treatment that is based on neuromaturational theories to address the occupational dysfunction of children with developmental coordination disorder. These treatments include sensory integration, process-oriented, and perceptual–motor programs. This bottom-up approach has been inconsistent with regard to improving occupational performance (Mandich, Polatajko, Macnab, & Miller, 2001). The challenge for children with developmental coordination disorder has recently been reconceptualized as one of motor skill acquisition (Missiuna, Mandich, Polatajko, & Malloy-Miller, 2001). This reconceptualization makes information about how children with developmental coordination disorder learn critical to intervention.

One crucial concept about motor skill acquisition is that a relationship must be forged between the learner and the task environment. Theories of motor learning that are based on the ecological approach forwarded by Gibson (1969) propose that certain aspects of the task environment are more important than others (Gentile, 1998). For example, an important perceptual cue to catching a ball is the angle of its descent. Children learn what the relevance of this cue is as they play catch. As the child gains experience in catching, finer discriminations

Originally published 2002 in *American Journal of Occupational Therapy,* 56, 429–435.

of angles that signal good versus difficult catches are learned (Lefebvre & Reid, 1998).

Although perceptual discrimination in motor learning presents as a very complex process, evidence suggests that it occurs without conscious direction or awareness. The classic experiment in this line of inquiry was published by Pew (1974). Pew conducted an experiment in which participants were asked to track a randomly oscillating line. The first and third portions of the line's path were random from trial to trial. The line's path on the middle third, however, remained constant. When the participants' performances were compared, all showed better accuracy for the middle portion, yet none reported any awareness of the consistency of the line pattern during the middle third of the path. The results of these experiments and others have led to the conclusion that it is not necessary to specifically and consciously direct a learner to the cues critical for successful task performance; these cues can be learned implicitly (Magill, 1998).

In addition to the contention that perceptual cues are best learned implicitly, some researchers have argued that calling conscious attention to task-relevant features actually impedes performance. Green and Flowers (1991) hypothesized that providing learners with explicit information about a task on a computer and thus inviting them to engage in conscious routes of learning would produce an informational processing load that would lead to poor performance. The task consisted of using a joystick to intercept an image of a ball with a paddle image at the bottom of a computer screen. On half of the trials, a glitch, or a visible wiggle, in the falling ball appeared during the first third of its path. On 75% of these glitch trials, the falling ball subsequently moved sharply to the right when it approached the catching zone at the bottom of the screen, called a fade. The fade made the ball harder to catch. Sometimes the glitch accurately predicted a fade; other

times, the glitch was a false predictor, and no fade appeared. Participants were divided into three groups: explicit, implicit, and control. Only the participants in the explicit group were informed about the glitch and fade probabilities.

At the end of practice, participants performed more poorly on trials involving a fade. The ball was harder to catch in the fade condition. However, participants produced less error when the glitch accurately predicted a fade and more error when the glitch was false and not followed by a fade. The participants had learned the relevance of the glitch cue. In addition, the participants in the explicit group demonstrated greater overall error under all conditions. Knowing in advance that the glitch predicted a fade impeded rather than improved the performances of the participants in the explicit learning group.

The benefits of implicit learning are not readily apparent in the skill acquisition of children with developmental coordination disorder. A characteristic of the motor performance of these children is an inability to learn from their own errors and the persistence of incorrect strategies (Goodgold-Edwards & Cermak, 1990). Knowing how children with developmental coordination disorder go about learning the tasks important to their occupational roles thus becomes critical for occupational therapy intervention planning. The purpose of this pilot study was to seek evidence about how children with developmental coordination disorder compare with their peers without the disorder in their ability to unconsciously discern and respond to a perceptual cue important to motor performance.

Method

This study used a split plot design (Maxwell & Delaney, 1990). Eleven children with developmental coordination disorder were matched to same-age peers without the disorder. The children played a computer game where they "caught" a descending ball image with a paddle on the screen. The dependent variable was accuracy of catch. On training trials, a visual cue that signaled the direction of the ball appeared 50% of the time. On probe trials, the visual cue was false. After completing the task, the children were interviewed about their conscious awareness of the cue.

Participants

Twenty-two children participated in this study. Eleven children met the criteria for inclusion in the developmental coordination disorder group, and 11 met the criteria for the control group. Ages ranged from 6 years to 11 years, 11 months. Two girls and 20 boys participated.

Developmental coordination disorder group. Sixteen children with developmental coordination disorder were recruited through referral from occupational therapists. Inclusion and exclusion criteria were based on the definition of developmental coordination disorder established by the APA (1994). Inclusion criteria were (a) a total score in the lower 15th percentile of the Movement Assessment Battery for Children (Movement ABC; Henderson & Sugden, 1992),

(b) dysfunction in daily living skills or educational tasks per therapist or educator report, (c) no discrete deficit or diagnosis known to directly affect motor coordination, and (d) receipt of instruction in a general education setting with same-age peers. Exclusion criteria were (a) presence of mental retardation, pervasive developmental delay, or autism as identified by therapist, educator, or parent report and (b) educational goals differing by more than one grade level from same-age peers. Eleven of the recruited children met the criteria (see Table 14.1).

Control group. Fourteen children without developmental coordination disorder were recruited from elementary school afternoon care programs and youth organizations. Inclusion criteria were (a) a total score above the 15th percentile of the Movement ABC, (b) receipt of instruction in a general education setting with same-age peers, and (c) age and gender match to that of a child in the developmental coordination disorder group. Eleven of the recruited children met the criteria (Table 14.1).

Parents of the identified children were contacted. The purpose, risks, and procedures of the study were explained to the parents in accordance with the recommendations of the Institutional

Table 14.1. Age and Movement Competence Scores

Developmental Coordination Disorder			Control		
	Movement ABC			Movement ABC	
Age (Months)	Score	Percentile	Age (Months)	Score	Percentile
142	15	3	143	15	23
134	10.5	13	140	7.5	65
129	12	8	129	5.5	40
120	18	1	120	2	79
107	23	2	107	1.5	93
106	20.5	3	100	0.5	49
101	13	6	95	0.5	93
81	33	1	75	3	45
81	23	1	80	5	84
77	17	3	80	4.5	89
72	14	9	74	6	36

Note. N = 22. Movement ABC = Movement Assessment Battery for Children. Higher scores on the Movement ABC denote larger movement deficits. Scores of 10 or above fall in the lower 15th percentile.

Review Board. Data collection was initiated on documentation of informed consent.

Instruments

The Movement ABC (Henderson & Sugden, 1992) is a standardized instrument that measures movement competence. It consists of eight tasks grouped under three headings: manual dexterity, ball skills, and static and dynamic balance. This assessment has been used extensively by researchers to identify children with developmental coordination disorder. The most frequent criterion for this identification is a movement impairment score below the 15th percentile (Barnett & Henderson, 1998). The test–retest reliability of the total impairment score ranges from 73% to 97% agreement over a 2-week period (Henderson & Sugden, 1992). The validity of the assessment has been compared with the Bruininks–Oseretsky Test of Motor Proficiency (Bruininks, 1978), with a resulting correlation coefficient of –.53 (Henderson & Sugden, 1992). More recently, Crawford, Wilson, and Dewey (2001) compared the identification abilities of the Movement ABC to that of the Bruininks–Oseretsky Test of Motor Proficiency of a sample of 34 children with and 38 children without developmental coordination disorder. They found that the Movement ABC tended to underidentify children with motor problems and had an overall decision agreement of 67%. The researchers concluded that identification of developmental coordination disorder must combine test results with clinical observations.

The instrument used for the experimental task in this study was the Implicit Learning Software Configuration. The parameters of this software were selected to allow the programming of variations of the task described by Green and Flowers (1991). The software was custom designed for the Department of Kinesiology,

Texas Woman's University, and used in other pilot work before the initiation of this project. The software program was installed on a 200 Hz Tangent microprocessor[1] with a 15-in. monitor, a keyboard, and a WingMan Attack joystick.[2] For this study, the image of a small red ball appeared at the top of the monitor screen. It descended the screen against a yellow background in an open reversed c-shaped curve, ending on the left. Descent time for the ball image was 2.5 sec.

On the monitor screen, a line twice as wide as the ball could be moved across the bottom of the screen by lateral manipulation of a joystick. The goal of the task was to "catch" the falling ball with this "paddle." The software program collected two measures of performance: feedback score and error score.

The feedback score was displayed on the computer monitor to each player. This score was measured in pixels (the points of light that together constitute the monitor screen image). A point system was used where 3 points were awarded for a catch at the center of the paddle, 2 points for catches 5 pixels from the center of the paddle, and 1 point for catches more than 10 pixels from the center of the paddle. Single-trial point scores were displayed after every trial. A total point score was given at the end of each session of practice. Error scores were recorded off screen and consisted of the number of pixels between the center of the paddle and the ball at the end of each trial.

Two features within this task were presented to the players. The first was a glitch that consisted of a color change of the ball image to white against the yellow background for 200 msec. The glitch was easily discernible to the viewer and occurred 1600 msec into the ball's descent. The second feature was a fade. The fade occurred 2000 msec into

---

[1]Tangent Computer, 197 Airport Boulevard, Burlingame, CA 94010.

[2]Logitech, 6505 Kaiser Drive, Fremont, CA 94555.

the ball's descent and during the 500 msec before the ball reached the bottom of the screen. The fade consisted of a shift in the ball's pathway sharply to the right.

The glitch and fade features were presented in controlled distributions. Each child completed five sessions of 100 trials each. Sessions 1, 2, and 4 were learning sessions. During the learning sessions on 50/100 trials, the glitch and fade were absent; this was the no-cue condition. On 50/100 trials, the glitch and fade were present; this was the cue condition. Sessions 3 and 5 were probe sessions. During the probe sessions, the no-cue condition was presented on 30/100 trials; the cue condition was presented for 35/100 trials. On the remaining 35 trials, the glitch was not followed by a fade; this was the false-cue condition.

Procedure

Data collection was conducted singly and lasted approximately 70 min per child. Motor performance testing for final group assignment (developmental coordination disorder or control) was conducted during the same session as the computer task. Thirty children completed the session. Eight did not meet inclusion criteria as defined by the Movement ABC, and their computer task performance data were not used in the study.

Data collection was conducted in a private room at the child's school or home as arranged with his or her parents. The child was seated in front of the computer monitor and joystick. Before initiating the computer program, the game was described. The children were told that the game was simple, without the detailed pictures seen in most computer games. They were cautioned that, although the game was simple, it was not always easy to catch the ball but not to worry because they would get better. The children were encouraged to place or hold the joystick in any manner they found comfortable. They were told that they would play the computer game five

times and that in between each session they would play a few of the researcher's games in a box.

Each child completed 5, 4.5-min, 100-trial sessions on the computer. A 5- to 10-min break was given between sessions. Testing for group membership confirmation was conducted simultaneously with data collection. During breaks between computer sessions, the children completed test items from the Movement ABC. During the first and second breaks, the examiner administered the manual dexterity portion of the Movement ABC. The ball skills portion of the Movement ABC was administered during the third break, and the balance skills portion was administered during the fourth break.

On completion of the five sessions, the children were asked four questions to determine whether they were consciously aware of any strategy:

1. How did you know how to catch the ball?
2. What would you tell another child to do to make a high score?
3. Did you have a secret way of knowing where the ball would land?
4. What was your secret?

Data Analysis

Sessions 1, 2, and 4 were learning sessions and contained only cue and no-cue trials. Sessions 3 and 5 were probe sessions, included false-cue trials, and contained a larger number of no-fade ball pathways. For this reason, data analysis was conducted separately for the learning and probe sessions. The performances of the children with and without developmental coordination disorder were analyzed with mixed factorial analysis of variance with repeated measures for trials (Maxwell & Delaney, 1990). Feedback scores reflected overall performance on the task. Error scores allowed comparison of performance among cue, no-cue, and false-cue trials. Because the fade made the ball harder to catch, the highest error was expected for cue trials. If the children were responding to the cue and anticipating the fade, then greater error would be expected on the false-cue trials than on the no-cue trials, neither of which contained a fade.

Results

Interview Data

During the exit interview, 6 children made statements indicating that they were consciously aware of the glitch cue within the game. These children were the oldest 5 from the control group and the oldest 1 from the developmental coordination disorder group. The remaining 16 children did not indicate any awareness of the relationship between the glitch cue and the direction of the ball's path. Chi-square analysis (group by awareness level) was not significant ($\chi^2 = 3.667$, $df = 1$, $p = .056$).

Feedback and Error Scores

Learning sessions. There was no significant difference between the performances of the children with and without developmental coordination disorder as measured by feedback scores, $F(1, 20) = 3.02$, $p = .097$, or error scores, $F(1, 20) = 1.54$, $p = .228$. There was evidence that all the children performed better with practice and were learning the computer game. A main effect for feedback scores for session, $F(2, 40) = 7.08$, $p = .002$, showed that the children's scores improved across sessions. Error score analysis also revealed improved performance as the children practiced the task, with a significant main effect for trials, $F(3.43, 68.60) = 2.66$, $p = .048$. A main effect for type of trial for error scores, $F(1, 20) = 12.87$, $p = .002$, revealed that the cue trials were indeed harder to catch. Error on cue trials ($M = 76.29$ errors) was significantly higher than error on no-cue trials ($M = 52.64$ errors).

Probe sessions. As in the learning sessions, no significant differences between the performances of the children with and without developmental coordination disorder were found for the probe sessions in feedback scores, $F(1, 20) = .057$, $p = .813$, or error scores, $F(1, 20) = .321$, $p = .577$. A main effect for type of trials was significant, $F(1.12, 22.49) = 27.27$, $p = .000$. Simple contrasts revealed a significant difference among the three types of trials. The cue trials that included a fade produced the most error ($M = 75.08$ errors); no-cue trials that contained neither cue nor fade produced the least amount of error ($M = 38.13$ errors); and the false-cue trials produced greater error than the no-cue trials ($M = 44.54$ errors).

Implicit Learning Analysis

In the exit interviews, 6 of the 22 children indicated they had conscious awareness of the relationship between the glitch and fade. To determine whether the performances of these children accounted for the greater error on the false-cue trials, a second analysis was conducted on the probe session error data. The error scores of the 6 children who demonstrated conscious awareness of the cue were dropped from the analysis. Because no group differences had been identified, group was removed as a factor. In this second analysis, again a main effect for type of trial was significant, $F(1.1, 16.65) = 13.01$, $p = .002$. Simple contrasts revealed significant differences among all types of trials, with cue trials showing the most error ($M = 69.53$ errors), no-cue trials showing the least error ($M = 41.94$ errors), and false-cue trials again showing greater error than the no-cue trials ($M = 46.57$ errors).

Discussion

The children with developmental coordination disorder in this study were able to recognize and use a perceptual cue to enhance their performance. This recognition occurred without conscious awareness in that, although the children's scores indicated they had learned that the glitch cue predicted a fade, the majority of the children themselves were unable to inform the examiner about the glitch–fade relationship. The ability to learn implicitly, therefore, is relevant to the occupational performances of children with developmental coordination disorder.

Although children with developmental coordination disorder frequently perform more poorly than their age-matched peers, this was not the case in this study. No group differences were identified in the analyses of feedback or error scores. One reason for this lack of group differences may have been the simplicity of the task. Motor differences between children with and without developmental coordination disorder may require a higher demand of task precision to be discernible. Further, this experiment used an artificial, two-dimensional task. How implicit learning proceeds for children with developmental coordination disorder in more complex and natural contexts requires further study. The task in this study, however, was not easy. Although the analysis of learning sessions indicated that the children made steady progress in the number and accuracy of their catches, the extent of their error on missed-catch trials remained large.

Several children indicated through the exit interviews that they had gained a conscious awareness of the relationship between the glitch cue and the path of the ball. Five of these children were from the control group and 1 from the developmental coordination disorder group. This distribution between groups was near significance when analyzed as nominal data. Age was also a factor in awareness of the relationship. Four of the 5 children from the control group older than the mean age of 8 years, 8 months, were consciously aware of the cue. Maturation may be influential

in the ability to consciously identify or verbalize cues used in motor performance. Only the child near 12 years of age in the developmental coordination disorder group was able to verbalize knowledge of the cue. The children in the developmental coordination group appeared to be at a disadvantage for this ability.

Purposefully directing learners to consciously think about their motor strategies is a technique currently being brought forward in occupational therapy treatment for children with developmental coordination disorder (Mandich, Polatajko, Missiuna, & Miller, 2001). It is important to note that the approach, called the cognitive orientation to daily occupational performance, does not recommend providing specific instruction and direction to the learner. Rather, the learner embarks on self-discovery of the parameters of the task through his or her own consciously mediated deliberation and self-talk.

This process of self-discovery is consistent with the methods suggested by Magill (1998, 2001). Magill stated that to enhance implicit routes of learning, detailed description of the perceptual cues inherent in the task should be avoided. Specifying cues is not necessary and, indeed, may impede learning. Children with developmental coordination disorder have difficulty learning nonhabitual motor tasks. Attempting to assist their learning with specific information about cues may have a detrimental effect. Instead, Magill has suggested that the learner's attention only should be drawn to the general area where the cues lie by using short verbal phrases, such as "look at the buttonholes" or "where are your legs?" Practice also should be structured, according to Magill, with cues relevant to the task in mind. Changing the context of an activity without changing the cue will assist in the recognition of the cue. For example, the angle of descent is a cue related to the likelihood that a falling object can be caught. Qualities of the descending object—size, color, speed—can be changed, leaving the relationship of the angle of descent to catch ability a constant to be discovered.

Conclusion

Children with developmental coordination disorder experience a significant challenge in learning new motor skills. This challenge has an immediate and direct impact on the occupational performance of these children in tasks basic to work, self-care, and play. The results of this study indicate that children with developmental coordination disorder can implicitly recognize and respond to environmental cues important to task performance. What this means to the occupational therapist providing intervention is that it may not be necessary and, further, may even be detrimental to provide specific and direct information about the environmental cues important to occupational outcome. Further study is needed to examine implicit learning capabilities in more complex and natural contexts.

Acknowledgments

This Chapter is based on the first author's doctoral dissertation from Texas Woman's University, Department of Kinesiology. This study was presented at the 2001 conference of the North American Society for the Psychology of Sport and Physical Activity.

References

American Psychiatric Association. (1994). Category 315.40. Developmental coordination disorder. In *Diagnostic and statistical manual of mental disorders* (4th ed., pp. 53–55). Washington DC: Author.

Barnett, A. L., & Henderson, S. E. (1998). *An annotated bibliography of studies using the TOMI/Movement ABC: 1984–1996*. London: Psychological Corporation.

Bruininks, R. H. (1978). *Bruininks–Oseretsky Test of Motor Proficiency*. Circle Pines, MN: American Guidance Service.

Cantell, M. H., Smyth, M. M., & Ahonen, T. P. (1994). Clumsiness in adolescence: Educational, motor, and social outcomes of motor delay detected at five years. *Adapted Physical Activity Quarterly, 11*, 115–129.

Crawford, S., Wilson, B., & Dewey, D. (2001). Identifying developmental coordination disorder: Consistency between tests. *Physical and Occupational Therapy in Pediatrics, 20*(2/3), 29–50.

Gentile, A. M. (1998). Implicit and explicit processes during acquisition of functional skills. *Scandinavian Journal of Occupational Therapy, 5*(1), 7–16.

Gibson, E. J. (1969). *Principles of perceptual learning and development*. Englewood Cliffs, NJ: Prentice Hall.

Goodgold-Edwards, S. A., & Cermak, S. (1990). Integrating motor control and motor learning concepts with neuropsychological perspectives on apraxia and developmental dyspraxia. *American Journal of Occupational Therapy, 44*, 431–440.

Gordon, N., & McKinley, I. (1980). *Helping clumsy children*. Edinburgh, UK: Churchill Livingstone.

Green, T. D., & Flowers, J. H. (1991). Implicit vs. explicit learning processes in a probabilistic, continuous fine motor catching task. *Journal of Motor Behavior, 23*, 293–300.

Henderson, S., & Sugden, D. (1992). *The Movement Assessment Battery for Children*. London: Saunders.

Lefebvre, C., & Reid, G. (1998). Prediction in ball catching by children with and without developmental coordination disorder. *Adapted Physical Activity Quarterly, 15*, 299–315.

Magill, R. A. (1998). 1997 McCloy Research Lecture: Knowledge is more than we can talk about: Implicit learning in motor skill acquisition. *Research Quarterly for Exercise and Sport, 69*, 104–110.

Magill, R. A. (2001). *Instruction and practice variables: What do we know about their influence on motor skill learning?* Paper presented at the meeting of the North American Society for the Psychology of Sport and Physical Activity, St. Louis.

Mandich, A. D., Polatajko, H. J., Macnab, C., & Miller, L. T. (2001). Treatment of children with developmental coordination disorder: What is the evidence? *Physical and Occupational Therapy in Pediatrics, 20*(2/3), 51–68.

Mandich, A. D., Polatajko, H. J., Missiuna, C., & Miller, L. T. (2001). Cognitive strategies and motor performance in children with developmental coordination disorder. *Physical and Occupational Therapy in Pediatrics, 20*(2/3), 125–143.

Maxwell, S., & Delaney, H. (1990). *Designing experiments and analyzing data: A model comparison perspective.* Pacific Grove, CA: Brooks/Cole.

Missiuna, C., Mandich, A. D., Polatajko, H. J., & Malloy-Miller, T. (2001). Cognition orientation to daily occupational performance (CO-OP): Part 1: Theoretical foundations. *Physical and Occupational Therapy in Pediatrics, 20*(2/3), 69–81.

Pew, R. W. (1974). Levels of analysis in motor control. *Brain Research, 71,* 393–400.

Polatajko, H. (1999). Developmental coordination disorder (DCD): Alias the clumsy child syndrome. In M. Bax, H. Hart, M. Pountney, & S. Miller (Eds.), *Clinics in developmental medicine* (pp. 119–133). London: Mac Keith Press.

Rasmussen, P., & Gillberg, C. (2000). Natural outcome of ADHD with DCD at age 22 years: A controlled, longitudinal, community-based study. *Journal of the American Academy of Child and Adolescent Psychiatry, 39,* 1424–1431.

CHAPTER 15

Effects of Occupational Therapy Services on Fine Motor and Functional Performance in Preschool Children

Jane Case-Smith

Jane Case-Smith, EdD, OTR/L, BCP, *is associate professor, Ohio State University, School of Allied Medical Professions, 1583 Perry Street, Columbus, OH 43210; Case-smith.1@osu.edu.*

Occupational therapists often provide services to preschool children with fine motor delays. These services have become an integral part of most preschool environments where children with disabilities are served. In intervention to improve preschoolers' fine motor skills, the occupational therapist often selects activities based on neurodevelopmental and sensory integration approaches (Couch, Deitz, & Kanny, 1998; Lawlor & Henderson, 1989; Swart, Kanny, Massagli, & Engel, 1997). Results of pediatric practice surveys indicate that occupational therapists emphasize a child's sensory motor performance components as a primary intervention to improve functional performance (e.g., self-care; Swart et al., 1997). However, the literature provides almost no empirical data relating performance components or intervention activities to functional outcomes. As a result, we have minimal evaluation data supporting an intervention focus on performance components or the use of specific activities or intervention approaches to enhance fine motor performance.

Relationship of Performance Components to Function

Many authors have theorized about the relationships between performance components and function (Case-Smith, 1995; Christiansen, 1991; Coster, 1998; Dunn, Brown, & McGuigan, 1994; Exner, 1995; Trombly, 1995), but these relationships have not been well researched. In one of the few studies, Case-Smith (1996) found moderate to strong relationships between performance components and functional skills in preschool children as measured by the Pediatric Evaluation of Disability Inventory (PEDI; Haley, Coster, Ludlow, Haltiwanger, & Andrellos, 1992). Self-care function significantly correlated with in-hand manipulation ($n = 26$; $r = -.62$) and motor accuracy ($r = .61$). Mobility scores correlated with in-hand manipu-

Originally published 2000 in *American Journal of Occupational Therapy, 54,* 372–380.

lation ($r = -.67$) and motor accuracy ($r = .43$). The correlation coefficients between these motor components and the Social Function Scale were not significant. Additional information regarding how performance components relate to functional performance is needed to guide selection of intervention activities. In addition to child variables that influence functional performance, contextual variables affect performance. Contextual variables include the objects and space available to the child and adult or peer support of performance. Occupational therapy intervention is one important support to the child's development of fine motor skills (Boehme, 1988; Exner, 1996; Swart et al., 1997).

Intervention for Fine Motor Problems in Preschool Children

Preparatory Activities With Emphasis on a Sensory Integration Approach

Specific frames of reference guide the therapist's activity selection and overall approach in intervention. In the initial part of an intervention session, preparatory activities may be implemented to improve the child's arousal, attentional focus, postural tone, and readiness for action. This initial phase may be guided by a sensory integration approach (Koomar & Bundy, 1991). For example, the therapist may provide vestibular and proprioceptive input to promote postural stability and behavioral organization as foundational elements to the child's performance. Specifically vestibular and proprioceptive input can enhance muscle tone and promote trunk stability related to the child's ability to use his or her hands in space (Danella & Vogtle, 1992; Exner, 1996; Parham & Mailloux, 1996). A sensory integration approach may also include activation or inhibition of the tactile system to increase the child's tolerance and perception of a variety of materials (Case-Smith & Berry, 1998; Exner, 1995; Miller & Heaphy, 1998). The hand's discrimination of an object's tactile qualities (i.e., haptic perception) is believed to be important to the expression of manipulation skill and may be an emphasis of this phase of intervention. Although clinical experience suggests that preparatory sensory activities enhance the child's performance, empirical evidence of this relationship is minimal.

Graded Motor Practice

A neurodevelopmental or motor learning approach often emphasizes graded movement experiences. In graded movement practice, the occupational therapist selects developmentally appropriate and challenging activities and provides sufficient support to the child so that he or she succeeds in the activities (Boehme, 1988; Exner, 1995). For example, the therapist plans a step-by-step sequence of motor activities to elicit isolated and controlled hand and arm movements, thereby improving manipulation skills, such as writing or cutting with scissors (Benbow, 1995; Exner, 1995). Neurodevelopmental approaches emphasize techniques to enhance the quality of movement, use the sequence of normal development to grade the activities presented, and include sensory (e.g., proprioceptive, tactile, kinesthetic) or cognitive (e.g., verbal) reinforcement of motor patterns (Benbow, 1995; Case-Smith, 1996; Exner, 1996; Exner & Henderson, 1995). Specific performance components are often the focus of intervention activities with the goal of improving related functional performance (Boehme, 1988). For example, activities to improve thumb stability can help the child develop precision grasp and in-hand manipulation for activities such as buttoning (Myers, 1992). Activities to improve isolated control of fingers can promote the child's play by increasing his or her ability to handle small objects such as Lego™[1] blocks and game or doll pieces. Therapy activities focused directly on fine motor goals provide the child with developmental movement experiences that challenge the child's skills. When children succeed in challenging motor activities, they are reinforced for their efforts.

Play and playful activities implemented in therapy sessions tend to elicit more participation, improve motivation, and increase learning (Bundy, 1991; Parham & Primeau, 1997). Whereas motor learning and sensory integration may be the focus of therapy and may determine the selection of activities, play is often the context for therapy (Mailloux & Burke, 1997).

Use of Play and Peer Interaction in Intervention

Object and social play interactions have been defined as both the mode and the method of intervention with children (Rast, 1986). Play can also be a goal of intervention (Parham & Primeau, 1997; Reilly, 1974). As an intervention mode, play activities maintain the child's attention, interest, and energy for the task (Blanche, 1997; Rast, 1986). A playful environment reinforces the child's efforts in therapy. As a means to therapeutic ends, it engages the child and motivates him or her to attempt the activity and to sustain the effort (Pierce, 1997). When playing, the child also experiences joy or pleasure and therefore associates positive affect with the activity at hand. Pleasurable experiences are ones that the child eagerly repeats and even initiates on another occasion; therefore, the skills associated with play are generalized and are likely to be practiced with peers and in other environments. Because play includes affective, social emotional

(e.g., with peers), and cognitive (e.g., imagination) components, as well as motor components, it provides opportunities for the child to integrate new skills into his or her repertoire of daily behaviors (Blanche, 1997; Bundy, 1991; Pierce, 1997). In addition to these variables that define in broad terms occupational therapy activities, intervention format and frequency likely affect child outcomes.

Intensity and Frequency of Services

Several studies have investigated how intensity of services is associated with differential gains in function (Jenkins & Sells, 1984; Law et al., 1997; Parette, Hendricks, & Rock, 1991). The question of whether more therapy produces better outcomes has not been completely answered (Hanft & Feinberg, 1997). In several studies of children with cerebral palsy, a greater intensity of service did not result in greater improvement in performance (e.g., Law et al., 1997). With inconclusive evidence about the benefit of greater frequency of services, additional data on the relative effects of this variable are needed. Therefore, this study was conducted to examine how performance components and variables in occupational therapy intervention influence fine motor and functional outcomes in preschool children. Two related research questions were investigated:

1. To evaluate the theoretical model that links (a) performance components, (b) skills, and (c) functional performance (Case-Smith, 1995; Coster & Haley, 1992; Dunn, et al., 1994): Do the performance components of visual perception, eye–hand coordination, and in-hand manipulation strongly correlate with fine motor skills and functional performance?

2. To explore the influence of intervention variables on performance outcomes:

---

[1]Kirkbi AG, Neuhofstrasse 21, CH–6340, Baar, Switzerland

Do (a) frequency of occupational therapy service and (b) frequency of specific intervention activities during occupational therapy sessions predict children's fine motor and functional performance outcomes?

Methods

Research Design

This multisite evaluative study examined fine motor and related functional performance before and after 8 months of occupational therapy services in preschool settings using a sample of children with fine motor delays. A descriptive rather than experimental design was used, in which the occupational therapy intervention was measured but not manipulated. By quantifying the intervention frequency and types of activities, outcome data could be correlated with the intervention variables. A research team of seven occupational therapists, with 14.2 years (range 5–20 years) of pediatric experience, performed the evaluations at the beginning and end of the academic year. Other collaborating therapists provided the intervention and recorded the type and amount of service provided during the 8 months.

Sample

A sample of children from 4 to 6 years of age who had fine motor delays and who attended preschool at least half-time was used for this study. They were recruited by the research team from their local school districts. Participants were volunteers who met the following criteria: Exclusion criteria for participants were (a) medical or educational diagnosis indicating central nervous system dysfunction (e.g., mental retardation, cerebral palsy, autism, traumatic brain injury), (b) severe sensory loss (i.e., visual or auditory impairment), and (c) serious health problems (requiring ongoing medical care). Inclusion criteria for the participants with fine motor delays included (a) scored 1.5 standard deviations or more below the mean on the Peabody Developmental Motor Scales–Fine Motor (PDMS–FM) (Folio & Fewell, 1983), (b) received weekly direct occupational therapy services, and (c) had at least one fine motor goal on his or her Individualized Education Program (IEP). Of the 48 children with fine motor delays who entered the study, 44 completed the end-of-the-year testing; two moved, one developed health problems, and one was unavailable at the end of the year. Table 15.1 presents demographic data about the participants.

Instruments

Functional performance and fine motor components of performance were measured at the beginning and end of the academic year, an

Table 15.1. Demographic Information About Participants (*N* = 44)

Variable	Summary Data
Age	
Mean age (months)	56.53
Age range (months)	44–72
Gender	
Girls	15
Boys	29
Ethnicity	
White	21
African-American	14
Hispanic	5
Other ethnic group	4
Parental education	
Mother's years of education (*M, SD*)	13.5 (2.5)
Father's years of education (*M, SD*)	14.0 (3.5)
Location of participants	
Columbus, Ohio	12
Rural Central Ohio	5
Cleveland, Ohio	6
Rural Illinois	6
Syracuse, New York	7
New York City, New York	3
Miami, Florida	3
San Antonio, Texas	2

interval of 8 months. For two of the standardized tests, only parts were administered to limit the amount of testing and the number of variables in the statistical analysis. The assessments and portions of assessments selected specifically measured targeted variables of the performance components–skills–functional performance model. Assessments were completed by the research team members in one to two observational testing sessions. Interviews of the parents were completed within 2 weeks of the observational testing.

Fine Motor Performance Components

In-hand manipulation. In-hand manipula-tion was assessed in translation and rotation tasks with five small pegs and a nine-hole pegboard. In the Rotation Test, the participant prehended a 1-in. peg from the pegboard and rotated it 180° in his or her fingertips, then returned it to its peg hole (see Case-Smith, 1994, 1995, for additional information regarding testing procedures). Each participant individually rotated the pegs with each hand, producing two timed scores. The number of drops and times the peg was stabilized on another surface were also recorded and summed. Using the means of these scores, a composite score based on the time (in seconds) and the number of drops was computed. In the Translation Test, the participant picked up two, three, four, and then five pegs from the pegboard, moving them into the palm and then back into the finger tips to return to the pegboard. The seconds required to complete each task and the number of drops were recorded and means calculated. A composite score of time and number of drops was used in the data analysis.

Eye–hand coordination. The Motor Accuracy test of the Sensory Integration and Praxis Tests (Ayres, 1989) was used to measure eye–hand coordination. In the testing task, the participant traced a long curved line, crossing the midline, with each hand. Accuracy was measured by using a map reader, and accuracy scores were adjusted for the time (in seconds) that was required to trace the line. The mean adjusted raw scores for both hands were computed for the data analysis.

Visual perception. Two subtests of the Developmental Test of Visual Perception (DTVP; Hammill, Pearson, & Voress, 1993) were used to measure visual perception. Position-in-Space measures the ability to recognize when forms have the same spatial orientation. Figure Ground requires identification of a figure hidden by lines or embedded within other lines and figures. This test is norm referenced, and high test–retest and interrater reliability are reported by the test authors (Hammill et al., 1993). Raw scores were used in the analysis because the children fell in the lowest categories of scaled and percentile scores, reducing sensitivity to score changes.

Measures of Skill

Fine motor. The PDMS–FM (Folio & Fewell, 1983) was administered to measure overall fine motor performance. This norm-referenced standardized test measures hand use, eye–hand coordination, and manual dexterity using typical preschool activities (e.g., cutting, building with blocks, lacing). Items are rated on a 3-point scale. Test–retest reliability for the PDMS–FM is good ($n = 38$, $r = .80$) and interrater reliability is excellent ($n = 35$, $r = .94$) (Folio & Fewell, 1983). Summed raw scores were used, because many of the participants fell into the lowest percentile group, where changes in scores were not reflected as changes in percentile.

Visual motor. Two subtests of the DTVP (Hammill et al., 1993) were used to measure visual motor skills. Both tests involve copying designs presented visually. In Spatial Relations, the child copies lines drawn on a grid made of dots, requiring analysis of forms and patterns. The test measures the ability to reproduce visually presented patterns. In Copying, the child copies forms of increasing complexity, which measures the ability to recognize the features of a design and to draw it from a model. Raw scores were used in the analysis.

The Draw-A-Person test was administered to measure integration of visual–motor skills (Short-DeGraff & Holan, 1992; Vane, 1967). Each participant was given a blank piece of paper and asked to draw a figure of himself or herself. Points were given for inclusion of facial features and various body parts. This simple scoring system did not account for the quality of the drawing because all lines that were intentionally drawn to represent body parts received credit. This scoring method has high interrater reliability ($n = 32$, $r = .93$) and concurrent validity with the Goodenough–Harris Draw-A-Person test ($n = 32$, $r = .64$) (Short-DeGraff & Holan, 1992).

Functional Performance

The functional scales of the Pediatric Evaluation of Disability Inventory (Haley et al., 1992) were administered by interviewing participants' parents. The interviews required between 30 and 40 min, using the standardized procedures for clarifying items and scoring. Two scales were used in the analysis; the Mobility Scale was not used because all of the participants were ambulatory and scored at the scale's ceiling. The Self-Care Scale includes items that rate the child's independence in feeding, dressing, bathing, fastening, and toileting. Many of these skills require some level of manipulation. The Social Function Scale measures the child's communication skills, self-identification skills, safety, participation in peer play and household chores, and ability to problem solve. Of particular interest were the child's play and problem-solving

skills. Haley et al. used both traditional analysis of their normative data and Rasch analysis to assist in interpreting test scores. Scaled scores based on the Rasch analysis that indicates item difficulty were used in the data analysis.

Intervention

Direct intervention was provided to the 44 participants by the 22 collaborating occupational therapy practitioners who were recruited by the research team members. The 17 occupational therapists and 5 certified occupational therapy assistants had a mean of 12 years, experience (7–23), with 9 (4–17) years in the public schools. The collaborating therapists used the form weekly to record the amount of time with the child, provision of consultation, use of group or individual format, and child's level of participation. Using a list of 20 possible intervention activities in four goal categories (sensory integration, motor/manipulation, self-care, and play/peer interaction), each therapist also recorded specific intervention activities included in the session. The data form was developed by the research team and was piloted by two team members. Evaluation of face validity by the collaborating therapists using a written questionnaire indicated that the form had adequate and sufficient categories to record their intervention activities (see Case-Smith et al., 1998).

Data Analysis

To create a reasonable number of variables for the analysis, the intervention activities recorded on the data forms were collapsed into 9 categories of related activities. Intervention activity data were combined only within the goal categories, and research team members concurred that collapsing the targeted activities did not result in lost information. Frequencies and percentages for the collapsed categories of goals and activities were computed to summarize the child's intervention over the year. Mean scores also were computed for intervention time and format. These scores and pretest and posttest scores for the 44 students were entered into a statistical computer program.

To validate the relationships among performance components, skills, and functional measures, Pearson correlation coefficients using year-end test scores for all participants were computed, followed by multiple regression analyses using the PEDI scores as the outcome variables.

To evaluate the influence of occupational therapy intervention variables on the fine motor outcomes, several steps of data analysis were completed. First, to establish whether participants made gains during the year, mean scores for the assessments at the beginning and end of the year were computed, and paired t tests were calculated. Then because each t test was significant, effect sizes (d values) were calculated, adjusting for the correlation coefficient between pretest and posttest scores. To determine the influence of intervention variables on outcomes, backward linear regression equations were computed for each outcome variable. The number of sessions, the pretest scores, and the percentages for the collapsed categories of intervention activities were entered in each equation.

Results

Description of Intervention

Occupational therapy intervention activities provided in the preschools are presented in Table 15.2. The frequencies of intervention goals and activities were quite varied despite similarities in the participants (i.e., all had mild to moderate fine motor delays). Some of the variation can be attrib-

Table 15.2. Percentage of Sessions That Included Specific Intervention Activities

Intervention Activities	M (%)	SD	Range
Vestibular/proprioceptive input	31.70	25.97	0–95
Tactile input/motor planning	40.36	25.33	0–83
Visual perception	58.57	26.61	4–100
Visual–motor integration	80.98	16.69	5–100
In-hand manipulation	64.98	15.74	24–100
Bilateral manipulation	51.02	22.73	3–92
Self-care (dressing)	13.02	14.66	0–61
Peer interaction	28.78	30.36	0–87
Play	15.95	25.12	0–87

uted to regional differences in services delivery models. The participants from New York received about 50% more intervention sessions than the participants in Ohio.

The 44 participants received a mean of 23.1 (SD = 6.01, range 12–43) sessions over the course of the year. Total time for intervention ranged from 408 to 1,824 min, with a mean of 825 min. The therapists consulted with teachers in 16.1% of their sessions and provided group intervention in 52.3% and individual intervention in 61.5% of the sessions (individual and group formats were combined in some sessions). Percentage of consultation and intervention session formats seemed to vary by therapist more than by region. However, regional differences in consultation percentages were found. Consultation was highest in rural Illinois, Texas, Florida, and Cleveland, where 87% to 100% of the children received some consultation during the year.

The high percentage of visual–motor and manipulation activities was anticipated given that the participants were selected because they had fine motor IEP goals. Infrequent use of sensory integration activities was expected because only two of the children had identified sensory integration problems; these activities were used in about a quarter of the sessions. The wide variance in application of sensory integration suggests that this approach was not used by some therapists and was extensively used by others. The variance in sensory integration activities may reflect that therapists with expertise in that approach frequently use activities that provide sensory input.

The participants made statistically significant gains in all eight measures over the course of the academic year. Table 15.3 presents beginning and end-of-the-year scores. Effect sizes are listed with pretest and posttest scores, and the mean effect size for the eight measures was 1.81.

Relationship Among Performance Components, Skills, and Functional Performance

The correlations between performance component and skill measures are listed in Table 15.4. The coefficients were moderate to high, suggesting a substantive relationship between the performance components and the fine motor skills examined. These results suggest that relationships are strongest at the bottom two levels of the performance components–skills–functional performance model.

Weaker correlations were expected between the component and skill measures and functional performance (i.e., PEDI scores). However, all coefficients, except visual perception

and self-care function, were statistically significant, suggesting that the parents' reports of their children's self-care and social function correlate with the fine motor and visual–motor skills measured (see Table 15.5). When regression equations were computed using the PEDI scores as outcome measures, specific skill measures predicted the functional performance outcomes. PEDI Self-Care scores were predicted by DTVP Visual Motor scores (ß = .450, p = .005). Social Function was predicted by the PDMS–FM scores (ß = .412, p = .001).

Outcome Measures Predicted by Occupational Therapy Intervention

To measure the effects of specific intervention activities in occupational therapy on fine motor outcomes, the percentage of sessions that included each category of intervention activities and the number of sessions were entered as independent variables in regression equations, with each of the fine motor skill and functional performance tests as the outcome variable. In each regression equation, the pretest score of the outcome variables was entered. By accounting for the participants' performance at the beginning of the year, the remaining variance in the year-end scores may be attributed to maturation and intervention. Backward linear regression equa-

Table 15.3. Pretest and Posttest Scores for the Performance Components

Category of Student	n	Beginning of Year M (SD)	End of Year M (SD)	Effect Size
In-hand manipulation	43	26.3 (7.7)	19.7 (5.5)*	2.01
Motor accuracy (adjusted score)	42	115.4 (15.7)	130.6 (13.3)*	1.99
DTVP–Visual Perception	42	5.4 (3.5)	8.7 (3.1)*	2.13
Draw-A-Person	43	3.32 (2.4)	6.7 (2.1)*	2.03
Peabody Fine Motor Scales	41	182.9 (12.1)	200.8 (12.6)*	1.87
DTVP–Visual Motor Integration	43	4.7 (5.8)	10.3 (8.0)*	1.83
PEDI Self-Care Function	36	67.5 (6.6)	76.1 (9.1)*	1.77
PEDI Social Function	36	63.83 (1.58)	69.47 (1.47)*	0.82

*Significant difference between pretest and posttest scores based on Tukey post hoc analysis.
Note. DTVP = Developmental Test of Visual Perception; PEDI = Pediatric Evaluation of Disability Inventory.

Table 15.4. Correlations Between Performance Components and Skill Measures (*N* = 44)

	Skills		
Performance Components	DTVP Visual Motor Scales r (p)	Draw-A-Person r (p)	Peabody Fine Motor Skills r (p)
DTVP–Visual Perception	.731 (.000)	.530 (.000)	.554 (.000)
Motor accuracy	.634 (.000)	.609 (.000)	.702 (.000)
In-hand manipulation	−.633 (.000)	−.559 (.000)	−.649 (.000)

Note. DTVP = Developmental Test of Visual Perception.

tions were computed to determine what intervention variables, if any, would predict the fine motor outcomes.

Of the nine collapsed variables defining the intervention activities, seven were entered into each equation. The variables included four intervention activities that were focused on performance component and skill levels (tactile input/motor planning, in-hand manipulation, visual–motor integration, bilateral coordination) and three that were focused on functional performance (self-care, play, peer interaction). Vestibular input and visual–perceptual activities were excluded from the regression analysis because the literature indicates that these variables are less related to fine motor skill acquisition than the seven selected (Fisher, 1991; Pehoski, 1995; Shumway Cook & Woollacott, 1995). The unique contributions of

these intervention activities provided by the occupational therapists to the participants' fine motor outcomes are presented in Table 15.6.

Of the descriptive variables, only play activities and peer interaction were predictive of the fine motor/visual–motor outcomes. The number of sessions was also predictive of DTVP Visual Motor Skills. The PEDI Self-Care Scale scores were predicted by inclusion of self-care (i.e., dressing) activities in the occupational therapy sessions. The participants' social function was predicted by the number of therapy sessions and by the percentage of sessions that included self-care and bilateral coordination activities.

Table 15.5. Correlations of Functional Performance With Skills and Performance Components (*N* = 44)

Performance Component Measures	Self-Care r (p)	Social Function r (p)
DTVP–Visual Perception	.232 (.075)	.298 (.021)
Motor accuracy	.450 (.000)	.472 (.000)
In-hand manipulation (composite of rotation and translation scores)	−.336 (.009)	−.407 (.002)
Skill measures		
DTVP–Visual–Motor Skills	.481 (.000)	.366 (.003)
Draw-A-Person	.482 (.001)	.400 (.001)
Peabody Fine Motor Scale	.473 (.000)	.553 (.000)

Note. DTVP = Developmental Test of Visual Perception.

Table 15.6. Intervention Variables That Predict Fine Motor and Functional Performance Outcomes

Outcome Variable[a]	Intervention Predictor Variable	b	p
Visual–motor skills	% of sessions with play activities	.207	.015
	No. of sessions	.170	.043
Peabody Fine Motor Scale	% of sessions with peer interaction activities	.399	.013
Draw-A-Person	% of sessions with play activities	.292	.034
Self-care function	% of sessions with self-care activities	.266	.035
Social function	No. of sessions	.225	.044
	% of sessions with self-care activities	.324	.004
	% of sessions with bilateral coordination activities	.215	.071

[a]In each analysis, the posttest score was the dependent variable after controlling for the pretest score.

Discussion

Relationships Between Performance Components and Child's Function

The motor components measured accounted for a large portion of the variance in skills and functional performance. As predicted, performance components (including visual–perception and motor accuracy) had a strong relationship to fine motor and visual–motor skills. These correlations support the findings of others that visual–perceptual and eye–hand skills are measured in the Draw-A-Person test (Short-DeGraff & Holan, 1992) and that eye–hand coordination is measured in the PDMS–FM (Folio & Fewell, 1983). The strong correlation coefficients between performance components and skill measures are similar to those found in Case-Smith (1996).

As expected, the correlation between observed measures of performance components and skill and parent reports of functional performance were low to moderate. Although most of the correlation coefficients were significant, the lower relationships reflect that roles and function are influenced by variables other than standard measures of performance components and skills. Roles and function are strongly influenced by the environment and the opportunities provided to the child (e.g., to demonstrate independence in dressing or bathing) as well as skill. The moderate correlation coefficients of motor accuracy and visual motor skill to self-care function suggest the importance of those skills to the child's abilities in self-feeding, hygiene, and dressing. The correlation between fine motor skill and social function is more difficult to interpret. Several items on the PEDI Social Function Scale require fine motor skills (e.g., those that measure play skills). An alternative interpretation is that the correlation coefficients reflect the influence of a third variable, for example, cognition or language. The PDMS–FM in particular has items that require receptive language and cognitive skill. Therefore, the shared variance between these measures may suggest that children with higher level motor skills have higher level cognitive and communication skills and, by extension, social function (Odom, McConnell, & McEvoy, 1992).

In general, the relationships expressed validate the performance components–skills–functional performance model used to evaluate the children and support the hierarchy of performance that links components to skills to function and roles. As in Case-Smith (1995, 1996), the relationships are strongest between performance components and skills and are more tenuous but significant when skills are related to the functional performance of the child as reported by the parent.

Influence of Intervention Variables

Intervention activities as recorded by the collaborating therapists were entered into regression equations to measure their influence on fine motor outcomes. It was expected that the child's year-end fine motor skills would relate to the frequency that fine motor and manipulation activities were implemented in the sessions, to validate the belief that practice of skill relates to improved performance (Pehoski, 1995; Schmidt, 1982). However, the percentage of sessions with fine motor manipulation, as well as visual–perception activities, did not significantly relate to fine motor outcomes. In addition, activities that provided sensory input (e.g., tactile) did not uniquely contribute to fine motor outcomes. Although the relationships between number of sessions and outcome measures were positive, frequency of intervention was predictive of only two outcomes. Participants who received more occupational therapy sessions improved more in visual–motor skills and social function.

The most surprising finding was that the therapist's use of play and peer interaction predicted the fine motor outcomes and that among the intervention variables, play and peer interaction were the only significant predictors. Almost half of the sessions used small groups, and about 30% of the sessions included peer interaction goals. This finding suggests that occupational therapists do address social function and that positive effects may be derived from this intervention focus (Case-Smith, 1997; Davidson, 1996; Davidson & LaVesser, 1998). Their focus on development of childrens' social function is inherent in their holistic approaches but is not always reported (i.e., occupational therapy may not be listed as a service provided to meet psychosocial goals) (Case-Smith, 1997; Davidson & LaVesser, 1998).

The influence of play activities on fine motor outcomes can be interpreted a number of ways. Play may be an effective means to motivate and engage children so that they become more focused or make greater efforts to attempt fine motor activities (Pierce, 1997). Couch et al. (1998) found that 91% of the 202 occupational therapists they surveyed used play to motivate the child. A second interpretation is that the play activities gave the participants a comfortable, enjoyable context to practice their fine motor skills in other environments at other times. Because children play in all environments, use of play activities that enhance fine motor skills enabled the children to generalize their skills to other settings and other play opportunities (Parham & Primeau, 1997; Reilly, 1974). A third interpretation of this relationship suggests that the therapists who reported use of play were more skillful and creative in motivating children to achieve fine motor and functional performance goals. Occupational therapists who create a playful environment not only motivate children but also generally provide the "just-right" challenges in which children can succeed and master the environment. When therapists succeed in engaging a child in play, the selected activities are more likely to be effective in improving performance (Gliner, 1985; Reilly, 1974). It is important to note that the therapists who reported using play also used sensory and motor activities, suggesting that the performance component objectives were embedded in play or congruent with the play activities.

Limitations

Although the therapists reported which activities and goals they used in intervention, the recording forms did not provide space to explain the rationale or details of their activities. The amount of time of each activity was also not recorded. More precise measurement of the occupational therapy sessions is recommended for future study.

Summary

Fine motor and functional performance outcomes of preschool children after 8 months of regular occupational therapy intervention were correlated with performance components. An evaluation model that links fine motor performance components, skills, and functional performance was supported. As in previous studies, foundational components and skills are highly related, and skills are moderately related to roles and functional performance. Specific performance outcomes were predicted by the frequency of sessions and the percentage in which specific activities were implemented. Occupational therapists' use of play activities and use of peer interaction were important predictors of skill levels at the end of the year. These results support the importance of therapeutic use of play in intervention.

Acknowledgments

I thank the research team for their dedicated work in evaluating the participants, gathering the data, and interpreting the results: Barrie Galvin; Terri Heaphy, MS; Vera Koch, MS; Debbie Marr, MS; Marcie Good-Ellis, MS; and Irma Perez. This study was funded by the American Occupational Therapy Foundation in coordination with American Occupational Therapy Association Special Interest Sections. The efforts of the collaborating occupational therapists in maintaining records of their therapy sessions also are appreciated.

References

Ayres, A. J. (1989). *Sensory Integration and Praxis Tests*. Los Angeles: Western Psychological Services.

Benbow, M. (1995). Principles and practices of teaching handwriting. In A. Henderson & C. Pehoski (Eds.), *Hand function in the child* (pp. 255–281). St. Louis, MO: Mosby YearBook.

Blanche, E. (1997). Doing with—Not doing to: Play and the child with cerebral palsy. In D. Parham & L. Fazio (Eds.), *Play and occupational therapy with children* (pp. 202–218). St. Louis, MO: Mosby YearBook.

Boehme, R. (1988). *Improving upper body control*. Tucson, AZ: Therapy SkillBuilders.

Bundy, A. (1991). Play theory and sensory integration. In A. Fisher, E. Murray, & A. Bundy (Eds.), *Sensory integration: Principles and theory* (pp. 46–68). Philadelphia: F. A. Davis.

Case-Smith, J. (1994). Efficacy of occupational therapy services related to hand skills development in preschool children. *Physical and Occupational Therapy in Pediatrics, 14*(3/4), 31–57.

Case-Smith, J. (1995). The relationships among sensorimotor components, fine motor skills, and functional performance in preschool children. *American Journal of Occupational Therapy, 49*, 645–652.

Case-Smith, J. (1996). Fine motor outcomes in preschool children who receive occupational therapy services. *American Journal of Occupational Therapy, 50*, 52–61.

Case-Smith, J. (1997). Variables related to successful school-based practice. *Occupational Therapy Journal of Research, 17*, 133–153.

Case-Smith, J., & Berry, J. (1998). Preschool hand skills. In J. Case-Smith (Ed.), *Occupational therapy: Making a difference in school-based practice*. Bethesda, MD: American Occupational Therapy Association.

Case-Smith, J., Heaphy, T., Galvin, B., Marr, D., Koch, V., Good-Ellis, M., et al. (1998). Fine motor and related functional performance outcomes in preschool children. *American Journal of Occupational Therapy, 52*, 788–796.

Christiansen, C. (1991). Occupational therapy: Intervention for life performance. In C. Christiansen & C. Baum (Eds.), *Occupational therapy: Overcoming human performance deficits* (pp. 3–44). Thorofare, NJ: Slack.

Coster, W. (1998). Occupational-centered assessment of children. *American Journal of Occupational Therapy, 52*, 337–344.

Coster, W., & Haley, S. M. (1992). A conceptual model of disablement in childhood. *Infants and Young Children, 4*, 11–22.

Couch, K. J., Deitz, J. C., & Kanny, E. M. (1998). The role of play in pediatric occupational therapy. *American Journal of Occupational Therapy, 52*, 111–118.

Danella, E., & Vogtle, L. (1992). Neurodevelopmental treatment for the young child with cerebral palsy. In J. Case-Smith & C. Pehoski (Eds.), *Development of hand skills in the child* (pp. 92–110). Rockville, MD: American Occupational Therapy Association.

Davidson, D. A. (1996). Programs and services for children with psychosocial dysfunction. In J. Case-Smith, A. Allen, & P. Pratt (Eds.), *Occupational therapy for children* (3rd ed., pp. 796–807). St. Louis, MO: Mosby YearBook.

Davidson, D. A., & LaVesser, P. D. (1998). Facilitating adaptive behaviors in elementary school-aged children. In J. Case-Smith (Ed.), *Occupational therapy: Making a difference in school-based practice*. Bethesda, MD: American Occupational Therapy Association.

Dunn, W., Brown, C., & McGuigan, A. (1994). The ecology of human performance: A framework for considering the effect of context. *American Journal of Occupational Therapy, 48*, 595–607.

Exner, C. E. (1995). Remediation of hand skill problems in children. In A. Henderson & C. Pehoski (Eds.), *Hand function in the child* (pp. 197–222). St. Louis, MO: Mosby YearBook.

Exner, C. E. (1996). Development of hand skills. In J. Case-Smith, A. Allen, & P. Pratt (Eds.) *Occupational therapy for children* (pp. 268–306). St. Louis, MO: Mosby.

Exner, C., & Henderson, A. (1995). Cognition and motor skill. In A. Henderson & C. Pehoski (Eds.), *Hand function in the child* (pp. 93–111). St. Louis, MO: Mosby YearBook.

Fisher, A. (1991). Vestibular–proprioceptive processing and bilateral integration and sequencing deficits. In A. Fisher, E. Murray, & A. Bundy (Eds.), *Sensory integration: Principles and theory* (pp. 71–107). Philadelphia: F. A. Davis.

Folio, R. M., & Fewell, R. (1983). *Peabody Developmental Motor Scales.* Austin, TX: Pro-Ed.

Gliner, J. (1985). Purposeful activity in motor learning theory: An event approach to motor skill acquisition. *American Journal of Occupational Therapy, 20,* 251–252.

Haley, S., Coster, W., Ludlow, L. H., Haltiwanger, J. T., & Andrellos, P. J. (1992). *Pediatric Evaluation of Disabilities Inventory.* San Antonio, TX: Psychological Corporation.

Hammill, D. D., Pearson, N. A., & Voress, J. K. (1993). *Developmental test of visual perception* (2nd ed.). Austin, TX: Pro-Ed.

Hanft, G. E., & Feinberg, E. (1997). Toward the development of a framework for determining the frequency and intensity of early intervention services. *Infants and Young Children, 10*(1), 27–37.

Jenkins, J. R., & Sells, C. J. (1984). Physical and occupational therapy: Effects related to treatment frequency and motor delay. *Journal of Learning Disability, 17,* 88–95.

Koomar, J., & Bundy, A. C. (1991). The art and science of creating direct intervention from theory. In A. Fisher, E. Murray, & A. Bundy (Eds.), *Sensory integration: Principles and theory* (pp. 251–317). Philadelphia: F. A. Davis.

Law, M., Russell, D., Pollock, N., Rosenbaum, P., Walter, S., & King, G. (1997). A comparison of intensive neurodevelopmental therapy and a regular occupational therapy program for children

with cerebral palsy. *Developmental Medicine and Child Neurology, 39,* 664–670.

Lawlor, M. C., & Henderson, A. (1989). A descriptive study of the clinical practice patterns of occupational therapists working with infants and young children. *American Journal of Occupational Therapy, 43,* 755–764.

Mailloux, Z., & Burke, J. P. (1997). Play and the sensory integrative approach. In L. D. Parham & L. S. Fazio (Eds.), *Play and occupational therapy for children* (pp. 112–125). St. Louis, MO: Mosby YearBook.

Miller, H., & Heaphy, T. (1998). Sensory processing in preschool children. In J. Case-Smith (Ed.), *Occupational therapy: Making a difference in school-based practice.* Bethesda, MD: American Occupational Therapy Association.

Myers, C. A. (1992). Therapeutic fine-motor activities for preschoolers. In J. Case-Smith & C. Pehoski (Eds.), *Development of hand skills in the child* (pp. 47–62). Rockville, MD: American Occupational Therapy Association.

Odom, S. L., McConnell, S. R., & McEvoy, M. A. (1992). Peer-related social competence and its significance for young children with disabilities. In S. L. Odom, S. R. McConnell, & M. A. McEvoy (Eds.), *Social competence of young children with disabilities* (pp. 3–36). Baltimore: Brookes.

Parette, H. P., Hendricks, M. D., & Rock, S. L. (1991). Efficacy of therapeutic intervention intensity with infants and young children with cerebral palsy. *Infants and Young Children, 4*(2), 8–11.

Parham, L. D., & Mailloux, Z. (1996). Sensory integration. In J. Case-Smith, A. Allen, & P. Pratt (Eds.), *Occupational therapy for children* (pp. 307–352). St. Louis, MO: Mosby YearBook.

Parham, L. D., & Primeau, L. (1997). Play and occupational therapy. In L. D. Parham & L. Fazio (Eds.), *Play in occupational therapy for children* (pp. 2–22). St. Louis, MO: Mosby YearBook.

Pehoski, C. (1995). Cortical control of skilled movements of the hand. In A. Henderson & C. Pehoski (Eds.), *Hand function in the child* (pp. 3–15). St. Louis, MO: Mosby YearBook.

Pierce, D. (1997). The power of object play for infants and toddlers at risk for developmental delays. In D. Parham & L. Fazio (Eds.), *Play in occupational therapy for children* (pp. 86–111). St. Louis, MO: Mosby YearBook.

Rast, M. (1986). Play and therapy, play or therapy. In *Play, a skill for life—Monograph project of the Developmental Disabilities Special Interest Section of the American Occupational Therapy Association* (pp. 29–41). Rockville, MD: American Occupational Therapy Association.

Reilly, M. (1974). *Play as exploratory learning.* Beverly Hills, CA: Sage.

Schmidt, R. (1982). *Motor learning and performance.* Champaign, IL: Human Kinetics.

Short-DeGraff, M., & Holan, S. (1992). Self-drawing as a gauge of perceptual–motor skill. *Physical and Occupational Therapy in Pediatrics, 12*(1), 53–68.

Shumway Cook, A., & Woollacott, M. (1995). *Motor control: Theory and practical application.* Baltimore: Williams & Wilkins.

Swart, S. K., Kanny, E. M., Massagli, T. L., & Engel, J. M. (1997). Therapists' perceptions of pediatric occupational therapy interventions in self-care. *American Journal of Occupational Therapy, 51,* 239–296.

Trombly, C. (1995). Occupation: Purposefulness and meaningfulness as therapeutic mechanisms [1995 Eleanor Clarke Slagle Lecture]. *American Journal of Occupational Therapy, 49,* 960–972.

Vane, J. R. (1967). An evaluation of the Harris revision of the Goodenough Draw-A-Man test. *Journal of Clinical Psychology, 23,* 375–377.

CHAPTER 16

Occupational Therapy Effects on Visual–Motor Skills in Preschool Children

Heather L. Dankert, Patricia L. Davies, and William J. Gavin

Heather L. Dankert, MS, OTR, *is director of occupational therapy, Jamestown Community College, Jamestown, NY.*

Patricia L. Davies, PhD, OTR, *is assistant professor, Department of Occupational Therapy, Colorado State University, Fort Collins, CO 80521; pdavies@lamar.colostate.edu.*

William J. Gavin, PhD, *is research associate professor, Department of Speech, Language, and Hearing Sciences, University of Colorado, Boulder.*

Evidence-based practice is becoming increasingly important to occupational therapy and other health professions in this current climate of health reform (Law & Baum, 1998; Tickle-Degnen, 1999). Given this climate it has become of paramount importance for practicing occupational therapists to conduct effectiveness studies in the field. This present study examines the effectiveness of occupational therapy on enhancing the visual–motor skills in preschool children.

Visual–motor skills have been defined as "the ability to integrate the visual image of letters or shapes with the appropriate motor response" (Schneck, 1996, p. 370). While visual–motor skills may be seen as isolated motor responses, these skills have been demonstrated as being highly associated with other functional activities such as handwriting. For example, scores from tests of visual–motor skills and fine motor accuracy have been shown to correlate positively with handwriting ability scores (e.g., Cornhill & Case-Smith, 1996; Tseng & Murray, 1994). Thus, visual–motor skills can be thought of as being multifaceted and influenced by a number of factors (e.g., pencil grip, fine motor skills, eye–hand coordination, kinesthesia, motor planning, and visual–perceptual skills) as described by Schneck (1996).

While each of these factors may have an impact on the visual–motor skills necessary to succeed in pre-academic and academic settings, the research on the effects of each of these factors individually on visual–motor ability is inconclusive (e.g., Levine, Oberklaid, & Meltzer, 1981; Schneck, 1991; Ziviani & Elkins, 1986). However, if visual–motor skills are a product of the interaction of multiple factors, then it would be reasonable to assume that only multifaceted intervention would produce results with positive outcomes in visual–motor skills.

A few studies investigating the impact of intervention on visual–motor skills have been reported for both preschool-age and school-age children. In one of the studies, Kannegieter (1970) provided "normal" preschool children with a "perceptual–cognitive–learning program" and evaluated the impact of 3 months

Originally published 2003 in *American Journal of Occupational Therapy, 57,* 542–549.

of training on their ability to replicate geometric drawings at 3 time periods—once prior to treatment (pretest), immediately following the treatment period (posttest), and 4 weeks following treatment completion (follow-up test). Fifty-eight preschool participants were randomly assigned to an experimental group (perceptual–cognitive training) and a control group (no perceptual–cognitive training). Both groups performed equally well on the visual–motor posttest immediately following intervention. However, the experimental group performed significantly better than the control group on the follow-up test 4 weeks later. Kannegieter suggested that the time between the posttest and follow-up test allowed generalization to occur in the treatment group. Given the short duration of intervention (less than 3 months) and the significant differences between the treatment group and the no-treatment group that occurred at follow-up, one might speculate that a longer intervention period may result in even greater improvement.

In a study with a longer intervention period, Parush and Markowitz (1997) compared the effects of two types of therapy, gross motor (large space treatment) and fine motor (restricted place treatment), on 53 preschool children with perceptual–motor dysfunction. For both groups, treatment was provided for 7 months at an intensity of 1.5 hours per week in a group setting of 4–6 children. Participants in both the treatment groups showed significant improvements in perceptual–motor functioning. There were no significant differences between the two therapy groups.

In an earlier study of school-age students, Oliver (1990) combined occupational therapy treatment with a supplementary program implemented by parents and staff, in which both interventions emphasized sensorimotor activities. Outcome measures were related to writing readiness. Three groups of elementary students were

included in the study: (a) students without disabilities, (b) students who demonstrated a verbal IQ at least 15 points above performance IQ, and (c) students who were placed in special education classes. All groups received direct treatment one time per week for 30 minutes and also participated in the supplemental program three times per week. The duration of treatment for students in all three groups was 5–8 months. Students with discrepancies between verbal and performance IQ made the most gain in visual–motor skills, as measured by the Developmental Test of Visual Motor Integration (VMI; Beery, 1982), followed by the students in special education. Students without disabilities made gains; however, the gains were not as marked as the other two groups. Unfortunately, tests for neither statistical significance nor effect sizes were reported in this study.

The results of Parush and Markowitz (1997) and Oliver (1990) suggest that intervention can improve visual–motor skills for school-age students with cognitive deficits and preschool children with perceptual–motor deficits. However, the results of these studies are confounded by maturation effects; that is, the observed changes may be due to the fact that the children gained skills due to maturation alone during the period between assessments.

Rationale for the Study

The relationship between visual–motor skill performance and academic success is unmistakable. With pencil-and-paper activities being one of the primary focuses of instruction in early education, the role that visual–motor skills can have on pre-academic and academic success (i.e., copying shapes and handwriting) is self-evident. In addition, a number of investigations support the notion that good visual–motor skill development is a precursor to performing well in kindergarten and early primary grades (Beery, 1967; Solan & Mozlin, 1986; Weil & Amundson, 1994).

The VMI (Beery, 1967, 1982, 1989, 1997), a standardized test, is an assessment tool that has been used in a number of these studies, as well as the studies that have evaluated the effectiveness of intervention on visual–motor skills discussed previously. Duffey, Ritter, and Fedner (1976) found that the VMI and the Goodenough–Harris Draw-A-Man test (Vane, 1967) were predictors of future academic success. Weil and Amundson (1994) found that children who were able to copy the first nine designs on the VMI performed better on letter-copying activities than those children who copied fewer than nine forms. In addition, Klein (1978) demonstrated that the VMI was a consistent predictor of academic performance through second grade, as well as a "reliable instrument to be used with a young preschool population" (p. 461). Maeland (1992) compared clumsy, dysgraphic, and "normal" children and concluded that "handwriting was significantly related to visuomotor integration, visual form perception, and tracing in the total group" (p. 1,207). Together the results of these studies demonstrate that the score on the VMI is a good predictor of academic performance. The use of the VMI in occupational therapy intervention effectiveness studies is justified. However, the use of the VMI as an outcome measure should be consistent with the intervention approach being assessed. For example, the VMI may be considered as an appropriate outcome measure if the acquisitional frame of reference (Royeen & Duncan, 1999) is guiding the intervention in a preschool setting, where imitating and copying represent some of the skills that the children are learning.

Purpose of This Study

The purpose of this study was to evaluate the assumption that occupational therapy provided to preschool children with developmental delays and preschool children without disabilities will significantly improve their visual–motor skills. The following research questions guided the study:

1. Do preschool children with developmental delays demonstrate significant improvements in visual–motor skills as shown by the ability to copy a greater number of forms on the VMI following occupational therapy for 1 school year when compared to their performance on the VMI prior to therapy?
2. Will preschool children with developmental delays exhibit a rate of gain consistent with typical peers by obtaining a standard score following occupational therapy for 1 school year that is equal to or greater than the standard score obtained prior to therapy?

Method

Design

A quasi-experimental, two-factor mixed design was used. The three groups of preschool children differing in disability level and the amount of therapy received across 8 months represented the first factor—a between factor. The three repeated measurements of the participants' visual–motor skills that were assessed, pre-, mid-, and post-therapy, constituted the second factor—a within factor. The research questions were evaluated statistically using a series of planned comparisons (a priori t tests) between the groups' visual–motor skills pre- and post-therapy.

Participants

The participants, preschool children with developmental delays and preschool children without disabilities, were selected via a convenience sample. All students were enrolled in a 1/2-day preschool program. The group of preschool children with developmental delays (G1: $n = 12$, including 8 boys) were selected based on the following criteria: (a) were served by the same county Board of Cooperative Educational Services (BOCES; 50-mile radius); (b) were 3–6 years of age (M = 53.34 months, SD = 10.04); (c) had parental consent to participate in the study; (d) demonstrated normal hearing and visual acuity as measured by the preschool screening and preschool files; and (e) qualified for occupational therapy services (all demonstrated delays in fine motor and visual–motor skills) and received services as directed by their individualized educational plan (IEP). None of the children in this study had specific medical diagnoses (e.g., Down syndrome or cerebral palsy). Students with severe physical limitations (i.e., could not use their arms functionally) or those with profound retardation (in accordance with psychological testing) were excluded from the study.

Preschool children without disabilities were selected according to the following criteria: (a) all were residents within one rural western New York school district included in the above-mentioned BOCES with varied socioeconomic backgrounds; (b) all candidates had parental consent to participate in the study; (c) children were 3–6 years of age; and (d) children were free from disability as indicated by a regularly conducted screening using the Screening Test for Educational Prerequisite Skills (Smith, 1990). At the beginning of the school year an informational meeting with all parents of these preschool children was held to explain the purpose of the study and to inform them that their child may or may not receive occupational therapy. Parents made an informed consent knowing their child would be randomly assigned to either the treatment or no treatment (control) group. For the purpose of deriving two research control groups, random sampling was used to place these preschool children into the treatment group (G2: n = 16, including 5 boys; M = 52.63 months, SD = 4.10) and control group (G3: n = 15, including 8 boys; M = 53.40 months, SD =

2.88). Members of these two groups were equally distributed between the two preschool classrooms housed in one school.

Instrumentation

The VMI (Beery, 1997), a standardized test, served as the principal assessment instrument. The VMI has 24 geometric forms that are developmentally sequenced and measures visual–motor skills by examining the child's drawings that attempt to replicate the geometric stimulus. Rating criteria are provided for accurate scoring of the drawings. The highest possible raw score is 50. The mean standard score is 100, with a standard deviation of 15. Reliability and validity for the VMI have been reported across age groups (De Mers, Wright, & Dappen, 1981; Klein, 1978). Rykman and Rentfrow (1971) reported the split-half reliability of the VMI in 2nd, 4th, and 6th grade to be r = .74. Test–retest reliability was established between two independent scorers within a 1-week time interval and were .62 and .84 for each scorer, respectively (Rykman & Rentfrow, 1971).

The most recent version of the VMI (Beery, 1997) includes two supplemental tests (Visual Perception and Motor Coordination) in addition to the principal visual–motor test. These supplemental tests were added to assist in separating out the components of visual perception and motor coordination from the primary visual–motor test that assesses both components as an integral skill (Beery, 1997). The total possible raw score that can be achieved on each of the supplemental tests is 27. Each supplemental test also has a standard score mean of 100 with a standard deviation of 15.

Procedures

Assessment. All students were given the VMI individually three times during the school year— in September, in December, and at the end of May. All testing was administered by a registered occupational therapist (the first author) in accordance to the guidelines in the VMI manual. The VMI tests were scored by two occupational therapy graduate students who were trained in scoring the VMI and blind to both the purpose of the study and the group membership of the participants. Twenty-five percent of the tests were scored by an additional registered occupational therapist blind to the groupings to establish interrater reliability. A high correlation coefficient ($r = .97$) was found when the scoring outcomes of the graduate students were compared to the scoring outcomes of the registered occupational therapist, indicating a strong interrater reliability in this study.

The VMI is one of several assessments that can be used by occupational therapists to evaluate pre-academic skills in preschool children. Children included in this study received other evaluations and observations to plan the individualized interventions according to guidelines outlined in the Individuals With Disabilities Education Act (IDEA, 1999) and recommendations in relationship to occupational performance (for an extended discussion, see Coster, 1998). The VMI was used as an outcome measure in this research because all of the children with developmental delays in this study displayed visual–motor deficits.

Occupational therapy intervention. The acquisitional and developmental frames of reference guided the occupational therapy intervention. Within the acquisitional frame of reference, the therapist shapes behaviors that contribute to skills acquisition, the goal of intervention (Royeen & Duncan, 1999). The developmental frame of reference emphasizes the continuous modification and emergence of skills with age (Law, Missiuna, Pollock, & Stewart, 2001). In keeping with the developmental frame of reference, all activities were designed based on the children's chronological and developmental ages.

Children in Group 1 (G1) received direct occupational therapy consisting of at least one 30-minute individual and one 30-minute group session per week. Individual therapy sessions for children with developmental delays addressed all areas of need as defined on their IEPs except for visual–motor skills. Needs in the visual–motor domain were addressed in the group therapy sessions only. Therapy commenced following pretest administration of the VMI (3rd week of September) and lasted through the end of May.

Children in Group 2 (G2) received direct occupational therapy services consisting of one 30-minute group session per week. The group therapy sessions for G2 consisted of the same visual–motor activities as G1 group sessions. Thus, the two treatment groups (G1 and G2) received the same amount and type of therapy in the visual–motor domain, although the children in G2 did not have developmental delays.

The following types of activities were included in the group therapy: (a) fine motor activities, such as arts and crafts, finger plays, and small manipulatives; (b) gross motor activities, such as obstacle course, music, dancing; and (c) visual–motor and visual perception activities, such as drawing, cutting, and assembly. These activities required visual–motor skills and were carefully designed so as not to teach to the outcome measure (i.e., VMI) by using alternative geometric lines and shapes for drawing activities.

Children in Group 3 (G3) served as the control group. These children did not have developmental delays and did not receive occupational therapy. Given that children in G2 and G3 were in the same preschool room, all group therapy was provided in a room outside the preschool classroom to ensure that children in the no-treatment control group did not participate. All intervention was conducted by an occupational therapist (i.e., the first author).

Data Analysis

Because the research questions were posed as a series of planned comparisons between groups, analysis of variance (ANOVA) procedures employing a 3×3 mixed design were conducted using SPSS for Windows (Version 10.0, 2001) to obtain an unbiased error term for the a priori Tukey *t* tests (Kirk, 1995, pp. 118–119). The three treatment groups (G1, G2, and G3) represented the between factor, and the three assessment periods (the September, the December, and the June assessments) constituted the within factor. These ANOVAs were conducted using both the raw scores and the standard scores of the VMI and the Visual Perception and Motor Coordination tests. The data met the assumptions for ANOVA; that is, the data

were found to be normally distributed and homogeneous (Bartlett's Box's M ranged from $F = 0.50$, $p = .92$ to $F = 1.68$, $p = .07$; Green, Salkind, & Akey, 2000, pp. 200–203). To preserve the experimentwise error rate of alpha $= .05$ for the study, the testwise rate for each ANOVA was set to alpha $= .008$ using a technique similar to the Dunn/Bonferroni procedure (i.e., dividing the experimentwise alpha level by the number of analyses (.05/6; Kirk, 1995, p. 120). The results of these ANOVAs are presented in Table 16.1.

Because the multiple a priori Tukey *t*-test procedures (Kirk, 1995) that were used to evaluate the planned comparisons were conducted based on these ANOVAs, no further adjustment of the alpha level was needed (Sheskin, 1997, p. 341).

Table 16.1. Results of the Six 3×3 Mixed ANOVA Designs Conducted to Derive Unbiased Error Terms for Raw Scores and the Standard Scores of the VMI Total, the Visual Perception, and the Motor Coordination Measures

Scale and Measure	Source	Mean Squares	df	F	p
Raw Scores					
VMI Total					
	Groups	58.408	2, 40	11.242	<.0005
	Time	74.567	2, 80	40.361	<.0005
	Time*Group	1.717	4, 80	.929	.451
Visual Perception					
	Groups	74.700	2, 40	11.600	<.0005
	Time	151.418	2, 80	19.605	<.0005
	Time*Group	.836	4, 80	.108	.979
Motor Coordination					
	Groups	76.009	2, 40	11.332	<.0005
	Time	67.501	2, 80	13.942	<.0005
	Time*Group	4.334	4, 80	.895	.471
Standard Scores					
VMI Total					
	Groups	1,521.069	2, 39	10.676	<.0005
	Time	129.550	2, 78	1.990	.144
	Time*Group	96.492	4, 78	1.482	.216
Visual Perception					
	Groups	2,312.590	2, 40	10.188	<.0005
	Time	438.167	2, 80	1.975	.145
	Time*Group	112.164	4, 80	.506	.732
Motor Coordination					
	Groups	1,318.207	2, 40	9.010	.001
	Time	370.918	2, 76	2.175	.121
	Time*Group	126.501	4, 76	.742	.567

Note. ANOVA = analysis of variance; VMI = Developmental Test of Visual–Motor Integration.

*$p < .005$ (i.e., that the obtained *t* value is statistically significant).

To allow direct comparisons of the gains across tests and groups, effect sizes were computed for the obtained t scores and were adjusted for correlation between the pre- and posttest (Cohen, 1988, pp. 538–539). A pooled estimated sigma obtained from the mean squared error term of the ANOVA and an r value pooled across groups were used to calculate the effect size. Any effect size greater than .80 is considered large and meaningful (Cohen, 1988).

Results

Planned comparisons of the post-therapy (3rd administration) mean raw scores on the VMI (M = 7.75) to the pre-therapy (1st administration) mean raw scores (M = 4.83) revealed that preschoolers with developmental delays (G1) demonstrated statistically significant improvement in VMI scores, $t(80) = 5.71$, $p < .0005$. Significant gains in performance were also found on the Visual Perception supplemental test, $t(80) = 3.98$, $p < .0005$. However, the gains observed on the Motor Coordination supplemental test were not significant, $t(80) = 2.21$,

when evaluated against the adjusted alpha level of .008. Children without disabilities (G2 and G3) also had statistically significant gains on the VMI and the Visual Perception supplemental test though smaller effect sizes than the children with developmental delays (G1). On the Motor Coordination supplemental test, children without disabilities demonstrated statistically significant larger gains than those exhibited by the children with developmental delays (see Table 16.2).

To further evaluate the effects of therapy on children with developmental delays (G1), comparisons between their performance and the performance of children without disabilities who did not receive therapy (G3) were made. As expected, at the first administration prior to therapy, significant differences existed between these two groups on the raw scores of the VMI total, Visual Perception, and Motor Coordination measures ($t(2,80) = 4.14$, $p < .0005$; $t(2,80) = 3.20$, $p < .005$; $t(2,80) = 3.15$, $p < .005$, respectively). Significant differences between the two groups continued to exist on all three measures after therapy as well ($t(2,80) = 3.73$, $p < .0005$;

Table 16.2. Mean Performance as Measured by the Raw Scores on the VMI, the Visual Perception Supplemental Test, and the Motor Coordination Supplemental Test for Each Group Before and After Therapy

Scale and Group	Mean (SD) Pre-Therapy	Mean (SD) Post-Therapy	Gain	Tukey t value	Effect Size
VMI Total					
G1 (n = 12)	4.83 (3.04)	7.75 (2.63)	2.92	5.71**	3.31
G2 (n = 16)	7.81 (1.87)	10.31 (2.15)	2.50	4.98**	2.84
G3 (n = 15)	8.73 (2.55)	11.27 (3.33)	2.54	4.96**	2.88
Visual Perception					
G1 (n = 12)	5.67 (3.08)	9.83 (2.59)	4.16	3.98**	1.54
G2 (n = 16)	9.94 (3.68)	13.81 (2.97)	3.87	3.70**	1.44
G3 (n = 15)	10.40 (4.12)	13.67 (3.77)	3.27	3.13*	1.21
Motor Coordination					
G1 (n = 12)	5.17 (3.83)	7.00 (3.79)	1.83	2.21	.95
G2 (n = 16)	7.75 (2.93)	10.94 (2.95)	3.19	3.85**	1.66
G3 (n = 15)	9.20 (3.00)	11.27 (2.40)	2.07	2.49*	1.08

Note. Differences between group means pre- and post-therapy (i.e., gain) were evaluated using one-tailed, a priori t tests where df = 80. *VMI* = Developmental Test of Visual–Motor Integration; G1: Group with developmental delays receiving treatment; G2: Group without disabilities receiving treatment; G3: Group without disabilities and not receiving treatment.
*p < .005 (i.e., the obtained t value is statistically significant).
**p < .0005 (i.e., the obtained t value is statistically significant).

t (2, 80) = 2.60, p < .005; t (2, 80) = 3.34, p < .005, respectively).

To assess whether or not preschool children with developmental delays exhibited a rate of gain consistent with children without disabilities, the mean standard scores following therapy were compared to the mean standard scores obtained prior to therapy for all three measures. The results of these comparisons and the effect sizes are shown in Table 16.3. The comparison of the mean standard scores of the VMI following occupational therapy to the mean performance on the VMI prior to therapy revealed that preschool children with developmental delays (G1) made a positive gain of 7.09 standard scores. However, while this mean gain is large compared to the gains of the other two groups, it is not statistically significant, t (78) = 2.29, when evaluated against the adjusted alpha level of .008. In contrast, the children without disabilities exhibited only small positive gains on the VMI (see Table 16.3). Comparisons of the standard scores of the Visual Perception supplemental test and the standard scores of the Motor Coordination supplemental test also showed that children with developmental delays demon-

strated small positive gains (2.91 and 2.0, respectively). Children without disabilities exhibited larger gains than the children with developmental delays on these two supplemental tests, although these gains were not statistically significant.

Discussion

This study found that occupational therapy might be beneficial to preschool children with visual–motor skill delays. As discussed below, the results provide evidence not only that preschool children with developmental delays who received occupational therapy made significant gains on the VMI after 8 months of therapy, but also that these gains were acquired at a rate that exceeded typical development.

In answering the first research question, preschool children with developmental delays (G1) did demonstrate significant improvements in visual–motor skills as shown by their ability to copy a greater number of forms on the VMI following occupational therapy when compared to their performance on the VMI prior to therapy. This study did not provide evidence that chil-

Table 16.3. Mean Performance as Measured by the Standard Scores on the VMI, the Visual Perception Supplemental Test, and the Motor Coordination Supplemental Test for Each Group Before and After Therapy

Scale and Group	Mean (*SD*) Pre-Therapy	Mean (*SD*) Post-Therapy	Gain	Tukey *t* value	Effect Size
VMI Total					
G1 (*n* = 12)	78.64 (10.25)	85.73 (11.65)	7.09	2.29	1.15
G2 (*n* = 16)	96.0 (9.32)	96.56 (9.84)	.56	.18	.09
G3 (*n* = 15)	100.8 (17.57)	101.8 (19.06)	1.00	.32	.16
Visual Perception					
G1 (*n* = 12)	74.17 (21.59)	77.08 (23.64)	2.91	.52	.24
G2 (*n* = 16)	94.50 (16.28)	105.12 (16.40)	10.62	1.89	.89
G3 (*n* = 15)	98.33 (20.34)	104.07 (21.61)	5.74	1.02	.48
Motor Coordination					
G1 (*n* = 12)	75.00 (13.24)	77.00 (19.46)	2.00	.57	.13
G2 (*n* = 16)	86.50 (16.86)	92.06 (13.67)	5.56	1.09	.35
G3 (*n* = 15)	91.0 (17.30)	95.20 (12.67)	4.20	.82	.27

Note. Differences between group means pre- and post-therapy (i.e., gain) were evaluated using one-tailed, a priori *t* tests where *df* = 80. All differences were found to be nonsignificant. VMI = Developmental Test of Visual–Motor Integration; G1: Group with developmental delays receiving treatment; G2: Group without disabilities receiving treatment; G3: Group without disabilities and not receiving treatment.

dren who received therapy (G1 and G2) gained significantly more skills than the children without disabilities who did not receive therapy (G3). Because the group of preschool children without disabilities and no therapy also demonstrated the ability to copy significantly more forms during the posttest when compared to the pretest, the gains of G1 may be attributed to maturation. However, the group of children with delays that received therapy (G1) did obtain effect sizes that exceeded the preschool group without disabilities that received no therapy (G3) for the VMI and the Visual Perception tests, although not the Motor Coordination test. These larger effect sizes do provide evidence to address the effectiveness of therapy.

The second research question asked whether preschool children with developmental delays exhibit a rate of gain consistent with typical peers by obtaining a standard score following therapy that is equal to or greater than the standard score obtained prior to therapy. Note that statistical significances pre- to post-therapy in standard scores are not necessarily expected or necessary for children with developmental delays to have a rate of gain similar to typically developing peers (see Davies and Gavin, 1999, for further discussion of interpreting standard scores).

In the present study, the preschool children with developmental delays treatment group (G1) showed a substantial, but not statistically significant, improvement from the pretest VMI standard scores ($M = 78.64$) to the posttest standard scores ($M = 85.73$). This finding suggests that the preschool children with developmental delays who received treatment (G1) developed visual–motor skills at a rate that exceed typically developing peers when compared to either the standardization sample of the VMI or the groups of preschool children without disabilities included in this study. The preschool children without disabilities who received treatment (G2) had similar

VMI standard scores at the pretest ($M = 96.0$) and the posttest ($M = 96.6$), suggesting that they obtained visual–motor skills at a rate similar to the standardization sample. The preschool children without disabilities who received no occupational therapy (G3) also demonstrated similar pretest standardized scores ($M = 100.8$) to posttest standardized scores ($M = 101.8$), suggesting that they also gained skills at a rate similar to the standardization sample. Only the group of preschool children with developmental delays who received occupational therapy showed a substantial increase in standard score, thus moderately lessening the gap that existed at the beginning of the study between this group and the groups of children without disabilities (see Table 16.3).

The intervention approach used in this study, guided by two frames of reference (acquisitional and developmental), resulted in improvements in visual–motor skill, especially in the group of children with developmental delays. Including a variety of activities in the group therapy sessions (i.e., not training to specific drawing skills) is consistent with recent ideas about the development of tool use, such as writing tools. Lockman (2000) has recently proposed a perception–action perspective on tool use development. He suggested that the interaction between tools (e.g., pencil and paper, mallet and wooden block) and the actions used may be as important in the development of tool use as the ability to hold or manipulate the tool itself. He further suggested that early movement patterns (i.e., actions) lay the foundation for later tool use. This supports the idea of using multiple intervention strategies in early intervention and preschool environments that include movement patterns without tools to develop foundations for the use of drawing and writing tools.

The use of the VMI as an outcome measure in studies involving preschool children is supported by some recent research by Adi-Japha and Freeman (2001). Adi-Japha and Freeman provided evidence suggesting that in preschool-age children, the same motor and thinking process is used whether they are writing letters or drawing geometric figures. Alternatively, starting around 6 years of age, separate mechanisms and processes for drawing and writing begin to emerge, and by 12 years of age the separation of the two processes is well developed. This timing is similar to that reported by Vinter (1999), who suggested that around 8 to 9 years of age there is a transition from drawing being driven by geometric rules to drawing being driven or influenced by meaning. Thus, the use of the VMI, a test of drawing geometric figures, may be more appropriate in effectiveness studies involving younger children than in studies involving older children (i.e., older than 6 years of age) if the outcomes of interest are academic or handwriting function.

Beyond the research questions posed, this study further contributes to the field of occupational therapy by providing evidence for the use of the VMI with the preschool population. The VMI standard scores of the preschool children without disabilities in this present study ranged from 75 to 125, with a mean of 100.8, and these results agree with the findings of the VMI standardization sample (Beery, 1997). These findings support use of the standardized scores for the VMI in rural preschool settings such as the one in which this study was conducted. More importantly, data from this study show that the VMI and supplemental tests are sensitive to detecting change due to intervention or development, as seen by the significant gains in raw scores achieved by all preschool children in this study.

Due to some limitations of this study, the results reported here should be interpreted cautiously. First, the VMI does not provide equal interval scores, so the raw scores were used to indicate gains in visual–motor skills. Although raw scores determined in a manner such as the VMI may not be true equal interval measures, if the obtained data meet the assumptions of parametric procedures (e.g., normalcy and homogeneity), statistical analysis of the raw scores can be used to reflect gain in skills, although the term "gain in skills" here does assume that each additional VMI form scored is more complex than the previous one (see Davies & Gavin, 1999). Second, the person administering the assessments and providing the therapy was not blinded to the study purpose or group membership. Third, although the amount and type of group therapy emphasizing visual–motor skills was identical for the two treatment groups, the children with developmental delays received additional therapy to address needs other than visual–motor. Thus, the total amount of therapy provided to the two treatment groups was not identical; consequently, the comparison of the different outcomes of these two groups should be interpreted with caution because the difference in gain could be due to the difference in therapy amount. Finally, the sample size was relatively small, but the effect sizes reported suggest that even with the small sample size, the results have clinical significance.

In summary, the primary finding of this study is encouraging in that children with developmental delays were able to maintain their standings with the two groups of preschool children without disabilities and even showed an effect size on VMI standard scores greater than one and exceeded that of the other two groups. The results of this study demonstrate that intervention, including occupational therapy, can effectively improve visual–motor skills in preschool-age children.

Acknowledgments

We would like to thank the children who participated in this study and their parents for their support. We appreciate the effort and support offered by teachers and school administrators of a school district and BOCES in rural western New York. We thank Machico Tomita, PhD, for her feedback on an earlier write-up of this study. We appreciate the help of graduate students Theri Woods and Tipa Pragnant, who scored the VMI tests.

References

Adi-Japha, E., & Freeman, N. H. (2001). Development of differentiating between writing and drawing systems. *Developmental Psychology, 17,* 101–114.

Beery, K. (1967). *The Developmental Test of Visual–Motor Integration: Administration and scoring manual.* Chicago: Follett.

Beery, K. (1982). *The Developmental Test of Visual–Motor Integration: Administration, scoring, and teaching manual* (2nd ed.). Chicago: Follett.

Beery, K. (1989). *The Developmental Test of Visual–Motor Integration: Administration, scoring, and teaching manual* (3rd ed.). Cleveland, OH: Modern Curriculum Press.

Beery, K. (1997). *The Developmental Test of Visual–Motor Integration: Administration, scoring, and teaching manual* (4th ed.). Cleveland, OH: Modern Curriculum Press.

Cohen, J. (1988). *Statistical power analysis for the behavioral sciences* (2nd ed.). Hillsdale, NJ: Erlbaum.

Cornhill, H., & Case-Smith, J. (1996). Factors that relate to good and poor handwriting. *American Journal of Occupational Therapy, 50,* 732–739.

Coster, W. (1998). Occupation-centered assessment of children. *American Journal of Occupational Therapy, 52,* 337–344.

Davies, P. L., & Gavin, W. J. (1999). Measurement issues in treatment effectiveness studies. *American Journal of Occupational Therapy, 53,* 363–372.

De Mers, S. T., Wright, D., & Dappen, L. (1981). Comparison of scores on two visual–motor tests for children referred for learning or adjustment difficulties. *Perceptual and Motor Skills, 53,* 863–867.

Duffey, J. B., Ritter, D. B., & Fedner, M. (1976). Developmental Test of Visual–Motor Integration and the Goodenough Draw-A-Man Test as predictors of academic success. *Perceptual and Motor Skills, 43,* 543–546.

Green, S. B., Salkind, N. J., & Akey, T. M. (2000). *Using SPSS for windows: Analyzing and understanding data* (2nd ed.). Upper Saddle River, NJ: Prentice Hall.

Individuals With Disabilities Education Act Final Regulations of 1999, Pub. L. 1205-17, 34 C.F.R. Part 300.

Kannegieter, R. (1970). The results of a perceptual–motor–cognitive learning program designed for normal preschool children. *American Journal of Occupational Therapy, 24,* 208–214.

Kirk, R. E. (1995). *Experimental design: Procedures for the behavioral sciences* (3rd ed.). Pacific Grove, CA: Brooks/Cole.

Klein, A. E. (1978). The validity of the Beery Test of Visual Motor Integration in predicting achievement in kindergarten, first, and second grades. *Educational and Psychological Measurement, 38,* 457–461.

Law, M., & Baum, C. (1998). Evidence-based occupational therapy practice. *Canadian Journal of Occupational Therapy, 65,* 131–135.

Law, M., Missiuna, C., Pollock, N., & Stewart, D. (2001). Foundations for occupational therapy practice with children. In J. Case-Smith (Ed.), *Occupational therapy for children* (pp. 39–70). St. Louis, MO: Mosby.

Levine, M. D., Oberklaid, F., & Meltzer, L. (1981). Developmental output failure: A study of low productivity in school-aged children. *Pediatrics, 67,* 18–25.

Lockman, J. J. (2000). A perception–action perspective on toll use development. *Child Development, 71*(1), 137–144.

Maeland, A. F. (1992). Handwriting and perceptual–motor skills in clumsy, dysgraphic, and "normal children." *Perceptual and Motor Skills, 75,* 1207–1217.

Oliver, C. E. (1990). A sensorimotor program for improving writing readiness in elementary-age children. *American Journal of Occupational Therapy, 44,* 111–116.

Parush, S., & Markowitz, J. (1997). A comparison of two group settings for group treatment in promoting perceptual–motor function of learning disabled children. *Physical and Occupational Therapy in Pediatrics, 17,* 47–57.

Royeen, C. B., & Duncan, M. (1999). Acquisition frame of reference. In P. Kramer & J. Hinojosa (Eds.), *Frames of reference for pediatric occupational therapy* (2nd ed., pp. 377–400). Philadelphia: Lippincott Williams & Wilkins.

Rykman, D. B., & Rentfrow, R. K. (1971). The Beery Developmental Test of Visual–Motor Integration: An investigation of reliability. *Journal of Learning Disabilities, 4,* 48–49.

Schneck, C. M. (1991). Comparison of pencil-grip patterns in first graders with good and poor writing skills. *American Journal of Occupational Therapy, 45,* 701–706.

Schneck, C. M. (1996). Visual perception. In J. Case-Smith, A. S. Allen, & P. Pratt (Eds.), *Occupational therapy for children* (3rd ed., pp. 357–386). St. Louis, MO: Mosby.

Sheskin, D. J. (1997). *Handbook of parametric and nonparametric statistical procedures.* Boca Raton, FL: CRC.

Smith, F. S. (1990). *Screening Test for Educational Prerequisite Skills.* Los Angeles: Western Psychological Services.

Solan, H. A., & Mozlin, R. (1986). The correlations of perceptual–motor maturation to readiness and reading in kindergarten and the primary grades.

Journal of the American Optometric Association, 57, 28–35.

SPSS for Windows. (2001). (Version 10.1) [Computer software]. Chicago: SPSS Inc.

Tickle-Degnen, L. (1999). Evidence-based practice forum: Organizing, evaluating, and using evidence in occupational therapy practice. *American Journal of Occupational Therapy, 53,* 537–539.

Tseng, M., & Murray, E. A. (1994). Differences in perceptual–motor measures in children with good and poor handwriting. *Occupational Therapy Journal of Research, 14,* 19–36.

Vane, J. R. (1967). An evaluation of the Harris revision of the Goodenough Draw-A-Man test. *Journal of Clinical Psychology, 23,* 375–377.

Vinter, A. (1999). How meaning modifies drawing behavior in children. *Child Development, 70*(1), 33–49.

Weil, M. J., & Amundson, S. J. C. (1994). Relationship between visual–motor and handwriting skills in children in kindergarten. *American Journal of Occupational Therapy, 48,* 982–988.

Ziviani, J., & Elkins, J. (1986). Effect of pencil grip on handwriting speed and legibility. *Educational Review, 38,* 247–257.

CHAPTER 17

Powered Mobility and Preschoolers With Complex Developmental Delays

Jean Deitz, Yvonne Swinth, and Owen White

Jean Deitz, PhD, OTR/L, FAOTA, *is professor and graduate program coordinator, Department of Rehabilitation Medicine, Box 356490, University of Washington, Seattle, WA 98195; deitz@u.washington.edu.*

Yvonne Swinth, PhD, OTR/L, *is associate professor, University of Puget Sound, School of Occupational Therapy, Tacoma, WA.*

Owen White, PhD, *is professor, College of Education, University of Washington, Seattle.*

Often, children with disabilities have physical limitations that prevent them from independently interacting with their environments. This lack of independence relates to three interconnected concepts: learned helplessness (Abramson, Seligman, & Teasdale, 1978; Maier & Seligman, 1976), contingency learning (Sullivan & Lewis, 1993), and self-efficacy (Hildebrand, 1988). Maier and Seligman's (1976) *learned helplessness* hypothesis is that "when events are uncontrollable the organism learns that its behavior and outcomes are independent and that this learning produces the motivational, cognitive, and emotional effects of uncontrollability" (p. 3). These theorists further stated that belief in uncontrollability undermines incentive to initiate responses. This belief relates to what Sullivan and Lewis (1993) referred to as *contingency learning*, or the process of becoming aware of "response–outcome relations and actively controlling or exploring them" (p. 59). According to Sullivan and Lewis, contingency learning promotes motivational, attentional, and cognitive development and has implications for infants with disabilities because they have reduced probability of experiencing a clear relationship between self-generated actions and environmental consequences. Drawing on the work of Bandura (1977), Hildebrand (1988) described *self-efficacy* as the individual's belief in his or her ability to perform a behavior and suggested that success with one task tends to generalize to other tasks.

Because disabilities compromise some children's abilities to interact with and control their environments, it is hypothesized that these children have an increased tendency to develop learned helplessness, to have fewer opportunities for contingency learning, and to have a lower sense of self-efficacy. Therefore, methods of providing these children with options for controlling their environments merit exploration.

One way that children who are typically developing learn the effects of their actions on their environment is through self-initiated locomotor activities

Originally published 2002 in *American Journal of Occupational Therapy, 56*, 86–96.

(e.g., creeping, walking, riding tricycles). Through participation in these activities, children are able to experience consistent relationships between their behavior and environmental consequences and, thus, learn that their world is controllable (Brinker & Lewis, 1982). These experiences may foster further attempts to control environmental events (Brinker & Lewis, 1982). In addition to the potential to help overcome learned helplessness and deficits in motivation, independent mobility also may affect children's cognitive and social–emotional development (Campos, Kermoian, & Zumbahlen, 1992; Kermoian, 1998).

Independent mobility seems to increase children's sensitivity to objects and events beyond arm's reach and changes their goal orientation (Kermoian, 1998). Further, both research studies and theoretical articles suggest that independent mobility may affect children's spatial understanding (Butler, 1986; Kermoian, 1997, 1998; Telzrow, Campos, Shepherd, Bertenthal, & Atwater, 1987).

The development of independent locomotion also contributes to socialization, transformations in child–adult interactions, and the sense of independence and competence (Campos et al., 1992; Kermoian, 1997). Children with disabilities who gained independent mobility by using powered mobility devices demonstrated better social–emotional skills than when they did not have independent mobility (Butler, 1986, 1997; Douglas & Ryan, 1987; Paulsson & Christofferson, 1984). Further, parents of children who use powered mobility reported that independence in mobility stimulated their children's social and emotional skills and intellectual behaviors (Butler, Okamoto, & McKay, 1983; Paulsson & Christofferson, 1984). For some children with disabilities, the use of powered mobility devices improved self-initiated behaviors (Butler, 1986).

The question of when young children with mobility impairments should be introduced to powered mobility is not new. Both the theoretical and the research literature have supported the use of powered mobility for young children with disabilities (Butler, 1986, 1997; Chiulli, Corradi-Scalise, & Donatelli-Schultheiss, 1988; Kermoian, 1997; Paulsson & Christofferson, 1984; Tefft, Furumasu, & Guerette, 1997; Wright-Ott, 1997). Some literature indicates that preschool-age children have learned to use powered mobility devices (Butler, 1986; Butler et al., 1983; Paulsson & Christofferson, 1984). Further, devices specific to very young children have been designed, developed, and clinically implemented. Two examples are (a) the Transitional Power Mobility Aid for children as young as 18 months of age (Wright-Ott, 1997) and (b) an electric cart for an 11-month-old with multiple limb deficiencies (Zazula & Foulds, 1983).

In summary, the literature supports the use of powered mobility with young children with disabilities as well as its usefulness related to motivational, cognitive, and social–emotional gains. As described by Snell and Balfour (1997), "mobility is no longer seen as a luxury for the person with a disability, but as an important contributor to lifestyle and self-development" (p. 23).

In most of the existing literature and research on powered mobility, the children studied either were developing typically or had disabilities that primarily affected their mobility (e.g., spina bifida, arthrogryposis, spinal cord injuries, limb deficiencies). The usefulness of powered mobility has not been adequately examined for children who have complex developmental delays that affect not only their mobility but also other functional skills, speech, and cognitive development. Because the assumption often is made that such children cannot benefit from powered mobility, therapists and families need information regarding its use to make informed decisions.

Purpose

This study extended existing research on powered mobility for young children to children with complex developmental delays who are facing the challenges of severe neuromotor impairments, speech impairments, substantial limitations in functional skills, and cognitive skills assessed to be below chronological age. Specifically, the purpose of this study, which focused on two young children with complex developmental delays, was to explore the effects of a powered mobility riding toy during free play (recess or gym class) on three dependent variables: (a) self-initiated movement; (b) initiation of contact with others (target child initiations directed to adults, target child initiations directed to peers, peer initiations directed to target child, adult initiations directed to target child), and (c) affect. We hoped that powered mobility use would increase self-initiated movement and contacts initiated by other children as well as by the target children. Further, we expected that if target child-initiated behavior increased, a decrease would be observed in adult-initiated contacts with the target children. Finally, we anticipated that the intervention would lead to increases in the target children's positive affect.

Method

Participants

By contacting community occupational therapists, two children were recruited for this study, and informed consent was obtained from their parents. Both children had spastic quadriplegia and no previous experience with powered mobility. Both had sufficient cognitive ability to play simple cause-and-effect games, both were able to follow one-step commands, and neither had been identified as having uncorrected visual deficits. The two children attended different public schools and were in classes for children with disabilities. Before this study, neither child had been

considered for powered mobility use, with limiting factors being the complexity of their disabilities and the costs of powered mobility.

Diane (pseudonym), a 5-year-old girl, had spastic quadriplegia and developmental delay. According to school records, Diane scored at the 1-month level on the Fine Motor scale of the Peabody Developmental Motor Scales (Folio & Fewell, 1983) when she was 43 months of age. Her school records contained no other standardized testing information. She could indicate yes and no with gestures but had no oral language. She used her left fist to touch or point at a picture icon for most of her communication. In conversation, Diane was persistent in pursuing her topic and ensuring that her communication partner understood her. She was dependent in all self-care skills, wore diapers, and had mobility skills that were limited to rolling from prone to supine and supine to prone and pivoting when positioned in either prone or supine. She often was positioned in a wheelchair with a custom foam seat. Diane's assets included her ability to focus on a task and her effective use of nonverbal communication, such as facial expressions and gross hand movements. Diane's peers appeared to like her, as evidenced by comments they made to her and the frequency with which they spontaneously brought her objects. She frequently was excluded from an activity during free time if it was not specifically set up for her to be involved. Diane had ankle-foot orthoses but often came to school without them. For trunk support, she wore a short-sleeved neoprene suit that extended to mid-thigh. As part of her educational program, Diane received occupational therapy, physical therapy, and speech therapy.

John (pseudonym), a boy with spastic quadriplegia and developmental delay, reached 5 years of age during the study. According to school records, his scores at age 4 on the Battelle Developmental Inventory (Newborg,

Stock, Wnek, Guidubaldi, & Svinicki, 1984) were more than 2 standard deviations below the mean. His scores on the Sequenced Inventory of Communication Development–Revised (Hedrick, Prather, & Tobin, 1984) were reported as 2 standard deviations below the mean for expressive language and 3 standard deviations below the mean for receptive language. Functionally, John was able to move from sitting to sidelying, could roll from supine to prone and prone to supine, and could sit independently. He was not able to crawl or creep. When engaged in activities, he tended to use his left hand almost exclusively, with his right hand often in a fisted position. Relative to self-care skills, John drank from a two-handled cup with assistance, self-fed finger foods, used a spoon with some spilling, and wore diapers. He effectively used gestures, facial expressions, some signing, and two-word and three-word combinations to communicate. His primary assets were his sunny personality and parents who were supportive and committed to him. John often wore a neoprene vest to assist with trunk support, a neoprene sleeve splint over the right elbow to limit flexion, and ankle-foot orthoses. Although he used bifocal glasses and had undergone surgery for strabismus, his therapist believed that his visual problems had been corrected and would not compromise his use of powered mobility.

The staff in John's preschool program included one teacher, aides, an occupational therapist, a physical therapist, and a speech–language pathologist. In addition, parents volunteered in the classroom, and student helpers and an adapted physical education teacher aided regular classroom staff in the physical education setting. At the beginning of the study, John was learning to ride an adapted tricycle. He had difficulty initiating pedaling movement, but once started, he could sustain a maximum of three to four consecutive rotations.

Procedure and Research Design

The first two authors collected data at the children's schools either during gym class or at recess during playground activities. All sessions in baseline and intervention phases were videotaped with a Panasonic VHS Professional/Industrial Camera.[1] The camera operator, either a research assistant or one of the researchers, started each 10-min taping session after the child was positioned appropriately (e.g., on a mat or swing during phases when the powered mobility device was not used or in the powered mobility device in phases when it was used). The camera operator stayed approximately 10 ft to 20 ft from the side or front of the child. Neither child appeared to attend to the camera.

Our original plan was to use an ABAB single-subject withdrawal design to examine the effects of powered mobility on several dependent variables. However, an extended training period, vacations, and illnesses required that we drop the last B phase for John. Baselines (A phases) reflected typical gym class and outdoor recess routines. The intervention (B phases) consisted of using the powered mobility riding toy (a car) during these times. For each child, training in using the riding toy followed the initial baseline phase.

Training was individualized and occurred within each child's school environment. No other children were present during training, which provided the study children with the ability to start and stop the car, turn the car on command, and move 5 ft or more in one direction spontaneously or on request. The children's occupational therapists and a researcher were directly involved in the training. For John, his mother and teacher also were involved. After one training session, Diane met all training criteria. During the initial training sessions, John spent much of his time turning in circles and laughing. After five training sessions,

---

[1]Panasonic, www.panasonic.com.

ranging in length from approximately 15 min to 30 min, the car was introduced into John's school routine. Even though his performance was inconsistent, he appeared to have adequate control to operate the car with supervision.

Independent Variable

The powered mobility riding toy was a Boss battery-operated ride-on car (see Figure 17.1).[2] Controls[3] were (a) digital electronic controls for less jerking when the car was started and (b) adjustable-speed controls for slower maximum speeds for training purposes and indoor environments and faster speeds for outdoor environments. A remote-control device[4] with an override switch enabled the supervising adult to control the car if necessary for safety.

The first two authors, working collaboratively with each child's therapist, adapted the seating and controls. Using individualized inserts made from medium-density foam, the children were positioned in long-leg sitting with the knees abducted and slightly flexed. The inserts provided support laterally to slightly above waist height for Diane and behind the back to above shoulder height for both Diane and John. Lap belts provided further stabilization for both children. Diane used the Slik Stik[TM5] joystick, whereas John used the Proportional Joystick[TM6] because he was unsuccessful with the Slik Stik. For both children, the joystick was positioned slightly less than 4 in. above its normal midline position.

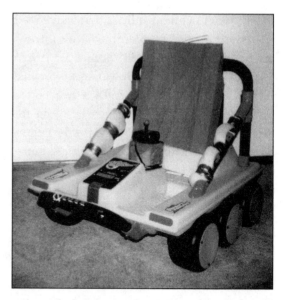

Figure 17.1. Powered mobility riding toy with foam inserts and adapted positioning of joystick for John.

Dependent Variables

The dependent variables were measured during baseline and intervention. They were divided into three categories: child-initiated movement, initiation of contact with others, and affect.

Child-initiated movement. Movement occurrences were defined as any displacement of the body in one direction (e.g., rolling, pivoting 90° or more, riding a toy) with no physical assistance given by another person. A series of movements of one type and in one direction were considered a single occurrence if they occurred with no greater than a 3-sec pause between movements. For example, if the car moved for 10 sec with a 2-sec pause and then moved again in the same direction for 6 sec, it was recorded as one movement occurrence. Alternatively, if the child changed the type or direction of movement (e.g., rolling to pivoting; going straight, then turning right), each type or direction of movement was counted as one movement occurrence (e.g., rolling to pivoting was counted as two occurrences).

---

[2]Innovative Products Inc., 830 48th Street, Grand Forks, ND 58201. Similar battery-operated riding toys are available from toy stores and other vendors.

[3]Innovative Products Inc., 830 48th Street, Grand Forks, ND 58201.

[4]Innovative Products Inc., 830 48th Street, Grand Forks, ND 58201.

[5]Suncom Technologies, 6400 West Gross Point Road, Niles, IL 60648.

[6]Part #950001, PML Flightlink Limited, Bordon Trading Estate, Oakhanger Road, Bordon, Hampshire GU35 9HY United Kingdom.

During baseline, frequency counts of movement occurrences were determined by viewing videos of the sessions. For Diane's intervention condition, a counter attached to the car and configured to count movement occurrences was used. Either the research assistant or one of the researchers started the counter at the beginning and stopped the counter at the end of each 10-min taping session. The intent was to use the counter for both children. However, although it was reliable for Diane, it provided inconsistent data on the outdoor playground at John's school. Consequently, videotapes were used to collect frequency data during John's intervention phase.

Initiation of contact with others. Target child–initiated contacts with others were counted whenever two conditions were met: (a) The target child (Diane or John) initiated the contact with another individual without any observable prompting or initiating behavior on the part of another person, and (2) the target child independently vocalized (with either comprehensible words or other vocalizations, including shouting, laughing, grunting) or physically pointed to, touched, or indicated that he or she wanted something from another individual. Target child–initiated contacts and vocalizations were divided into two categories— peer directed and adult directed—and further categorized as positive or negative. Examples of positive contacts included saying comprehensible words, laughing, and using gestures to indicate desires. Examples of negative contacts were crying and screaming.

Other-initiated contacts with the target child also were divided into two categories: contacts by peers and contacts by adults. Peer-initiated contacts were defined as any child initiating any type of contact with the target child (e.g., talking to the child, touching the child or the mobility device the child was using, giving a toy or item to the child, taking a toy or item away from the

child). Playing in proximity of the target child was not included unless contact occurred between the children. Adult-initiated contacts with the target child were (a) carrying, moving, or otherwise touching the child or the device in which the child was seated (e.g., swing, wheelchair, toy car); (b) talking to the child or giving him or her a toy or item; or (c) taking a toy or item away from the child. Contact with the target child by another individual was coded as positive if it appeared positive or neutral (e.g., asking a question, sharing a toy). The contact was coded as negative if it involved something that could be judged as potentially aversive, such as name-calling or commands such as "Stop that!"

Affect. Affect was coded as positive, negative, or neutral. Positive affect was defined as clearly smiling, laughing, or squealing happily, whereas negative affect was defined as crying, throwing a tantrum, frowning, abruptly turning away from another person, or pouting. Neutral affect was defined as anything between those two extremes. Readers should note that just because affect or a contact was coded as negative, it was not necessarily a negative outcome for the child.

Data Collection

For each baseline session for Diane and each baseline and intervention session for John, the raters counted the number of movement occurrences while watching the 10-min videotape of the session. For Diane's intervention sessions, the person videotaping recorded the number of movement occurrences indicated on the counter at the end of each session. Sessions were timed with a stopwatch.

For all initiation of contact variables, partial interval recording was used whereby a rater viewed videotapes of the 10-min sessions and recorded every 15 sec whether a targeted behavior occurred at any time during that 15-sec period. For example, in the middle of a 15-sec interval, if an adult initiated a 3-sec contact with the child, the rater recorded it as adult-initiated contact, even though the contact did not extend throughout the interval. For affect, momentary time sampling was used whereby every 15 sec, at the moment of a beep, the rater rated affect as positive, negative, or neutral. For each initiation of contact and affect variable within the 10-min data collection session, it was possible to record a maximum of 40 occurrences. In instances when a child was obstructed from view, the rater indicated that obstruction on the recording form, and data from that interval were not included in the analyses. Obstructed view only occurred for affect.

One physical therapy graduate student served as the primary rater for all variables for Diane. Five senior occupational therapy students served as primary raters for John. All were blind to the purpose of the study. Five additional occupational therapy students and the first two authors conducted agreement checks on dependent variable evaluation both before and during data collection. For Diane, interrater agreement was determined for 7 of the 18 sessions; for John, interrater agreement was examined for all sessions. For movement occurrences, the percentage of agreement for overall behavior counts was used. For all other variables, point-by-point percent agreement across observation intervals was calculated (Ottenbacher, 1986). For both children, average interrater agreement was 98% or above for all variables except affect, where it was 91% for Diane and 94% for John.

Results

Movement Occurrences

In the A phases (no car), Diane either did not initiate movement or did so only one to three times during a given session (see Figure 17.2[1]). Each movement consisted of one laborious roll from either prone to supine or supine to prone. After only minimal training, Diane's movement in the B phases (car) increased to between 44 and 87 movement occurrences per 10-min session. John's frequency of self-initiated independent movement occurrences also increased, going from 0 to 19 during the two A phases to 28 to 65 movement occurrences during the B phase (see Figure 17.2[2]).

Initiation of Contact With Others

Diane demonstrated no negative initiations of contact with adults or other children. Although her rates of positive initiations were very low, she did have some positive initiations with others during 3 of the 6 intervention sessions across two phases. By contrast, Diane initiated contact with others during only 1 of the 12 sessions in the two baseline phases (see Figure 17.3[1]). Conversely, John had more positive initiations with adults during the two baseline phases as opposed to the intervention phase (see Figure 17.3[2]).

Adults initiated numerous positive contacts and no negative contacts with Diane, regardless of the experimental condition (see Figure 17.3[3]). Of the 40 possible recording intervals per session, the number of intervals per session reflecting positive contacts by an adult ranged from 1 to 38 (median = 7) during baseline and from 7 to 33 (median = 22) during intervention.

Although adults initiated positive contacts with John during all phases, they generally initiated more negative contacts with him during the intervention phase than during the baseline phases (see Figure 17.3[4]). The median number of intervals in which positive contacts were recorded was 40 (100%) for each baseline phase and 26 (65%) for the intervention phase. Adults made no negative contacts with John during the first baseline phase. During 4 of the 5 days of intervention, however, the number of intervals reflecting negative adult contact

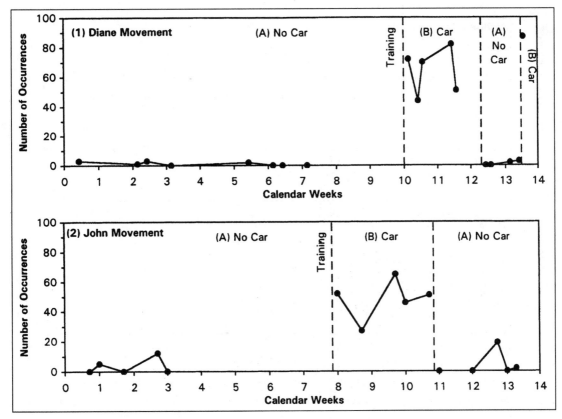

Figure 17.2. Child-initiated movement occurrences.

ranged from 1 to 3. In the final baseline phase, the same pattern occurred as during the first baseline, except on the day John rode an adapted tricycle and negative adult contact was coded in 5 intervals.

Other children initiated interactions with both target children during all conditions (see Figures 17.3[3]–17.3[4]). For Diane, the number of intervals reflecting positive contact initiated by another child ranged from 1 to 34 (median = 4.5) during baseline and from 0 to 11 (median = 3) during intervention. Children made positive contact with John during more intervention sessions (4 out of 5) than during baseline sessions (1 out of 10). The only negative contact by another child occurred during John's third intervention session.

Affect

Affect data are presented in percentages because the number of moments in which affect could be coded reliably varied from one day to the next. This variation occurred because the child's face sometimes could not be seen when the child moved quickly or when other children blocked the view. For Diane, the percentages of moments for which positive affect was recorded in baseline were highly variable, ranging from 6 to 50 (see Figure 17.4[1]). Less variability occurred during the intervention phases, with percentages ranging from 15 to 36. The percentage of moments reflecting John's positive affect also were highly variable (see Figure 17.4[2]). Negative affect occurred on 2 days: (a) the 2nd day of intervention during 3 (11%) of the 27 moments in which affect could be observed and

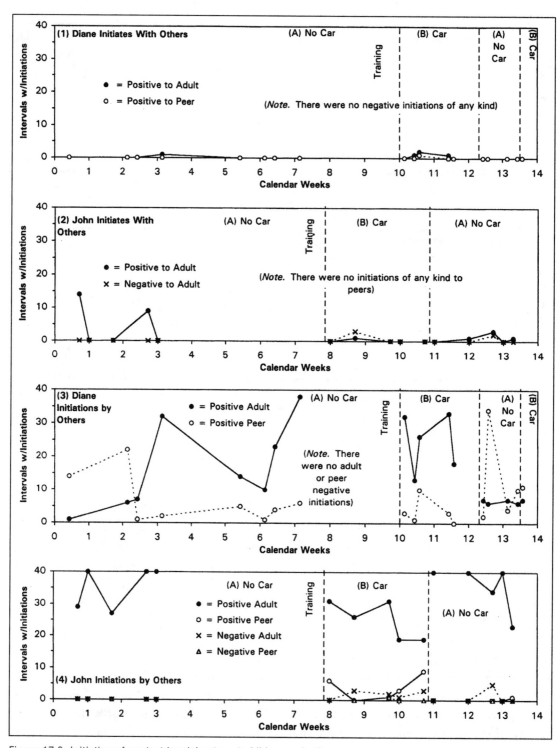

Figure 17.3. Initiation of contact involving target children and others.

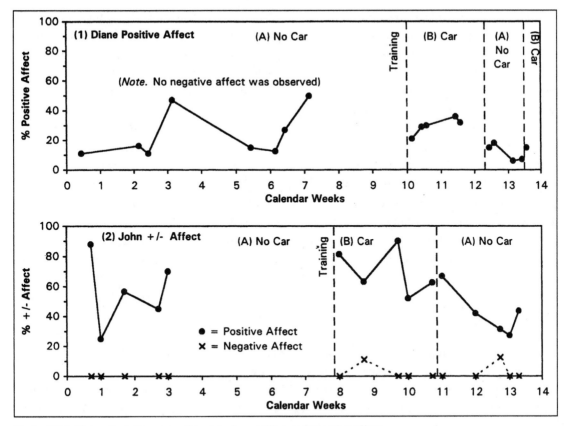

Figure 17.4. Momentary time-sampling data for positive and negative affect.

(b) the 3rd day of the second baseline phase during 2 (13%) of the 16 moments in which affect could be observed. The latter was when he was playing on an adapted tricycle.

Findings From Interviews and Experiences Associated With the Study

Interviews with school staff and the parent of one child and a record of the researchers' experiences associated with the use of the powered mobility riding toy in the school environment provided additional information. First, several positive characteristics of the intervention were identified. Therapists mentioned that the powered mobility device used in this study looks like a toy, was a source of interest to other children, and could be used to enable mobility play for children who, because of their disabilities, cannot otherwise independently participate in playground and gym activities. Further, therapists found that the car was easy to adapt with foam inserts to support sitting and to meet the unique needs of the individual children. Coupled with its low cost compared with most powered mobility devices, adaptability makes the device a useful evaluation and early training tool when therapists and the child's family are trying to determine whether the child can benefit from powered mobility. Therapists also identified the adjustable-speed setting as helpful during this process, because the lower speeds could be used when the child was first learning to control the device and when the child needed to maneuver in congested areas.

Negative characteristics of the intervention also were identified. First, the car was loud. Teachers and other staff members commented about the noise, and the first author attempted to minimize it by greasing the bearings and putting rubber tubing on the wheels. Despite the modifications, staff reported that the car was disruptive when used indoors. Second, the car was challenged by rough surfaces, and the children sometimes became stuck in small potholes, on the grass, or up inclines on the playground. Third, therapists noted that the large turning radius made the car impractical for use in most classrooms and other small or crowded spaces. Fourth, frequent, but solvable, breakdowns were encountered.

Discussion

This study demonstrated that two young children with complex developmental delays, including severe neuromotor impairments, could learn to drive a powered mobility riding toy and use it during adaptive physical education or recess successfully. The primary finding for both children was that use of the riding toy had a reliable and clinically important impact on initiation of movement occurrences. After introducing the intervention, both children had immediate and substantial changes in movement occurrence data, with immediate returns to baseline levels when the intervention was withdrawn. Further, use of the riding toy appeared to have some effect on initiation of contacts with others but did not have a clear impact on amount of positive affect.

The type and magnitude of changes observed in both children are impressive considering the short duration of the intervention and the fact that neither child typically would be considered a candidate for powered mobility. Combined total training and intervention time was slightly less than 3 hr divided over 7 sessions (1 training, 6 intervention) for Diane and less than 4 hr divided over 10 sessions (5 training, 5 intervention) for John. Having only intermittent use of the power mobility riding toy, each child was successful in learning to use the device and demonstrated some changes in other developmentally appropriate behavior. These results suggest that, even if it is not possible to obtain powered mobility for a child for full-time use, a child with complex developmental delays may benefit from using a device part-time during his or her school program. However, if one device is purchased for use by multiple children, we suggest using a proportional joystick and having an alternative switch-access control system to try with children who are unsuccessful with joystick control.

Consistent with the work of Sullivan and Lewis (1993) and the importance of a clear relationship between self-generated actions and environmental consequences, both children had substantially higher frequencies of self-initiated movement occurrences when using the powered mobility riding toy. However, the data related to the dependent measure of movement occurrences communicate only part of the story. Both children seemed to value the ability to direct their own movement in their respective environments. John often headed out a door or toward distant parts of the playground away from his classmates, resisting teacher and parental efforts to direct him back to the group. He was persistent about pursuing his own goals, many of which involved vestibular and proprioceptive stimulation, including (a) repeatedly turning in circles over a playground drainage grate, resulting in both circular movement and up and down bumping; (b) going over holes and other irregularities in the pavement; and (c) bumping into walls. The latter often appeared to be purposeful in that John would stop 1 ft to 2 ft from the wall, look at the adults, smile, and then push the joystick forward. He seemed to enjoy the crash. Thus, for John, the riding toy seemed to become the primary object of play rather than a mobility device for reaching other persons or play objects in the environment.

John's occupational therapist also commented that after using the car John did better with the adapted tricycle and seemed to have a clearer understanding of movement. This change is consistent with the data in that his maximum number of baseline movement occurrences happened during the second baseline when he was using the adapted tricycle. Possibly, his increased success with the adapted tricycle reflects Hildebrand's (1988) suggestion that success with one task tends to generalize to other tasks or to Kermoian's (1998) contention that independent mobility changes the children's goal orientation.

Diane's patterns of movement provide further support for the importance of a clear relationship between self-generated behavior and environmental consequences (Sullivan & Lewis, 1993). Although she was able to roll over, she seldom used this skill to move from one place to another, possibly because it was labor intensive and provided little in terms of environmental consequences. By contrast, when in the riding toy, she was almost always in motion, intent on planning her next movement or positioning the car so she could observe her peers' activities. Unlike John, she rarely bumped into things. Often it appeared that if Diane believed she might bump another person or an object, she would not move at all. For example, she was told that another child was in a blind spot behind her, so she did not move for 2 to 3 min. She started moving only after she was told that the other child was no longer there. This level of caution was typical of Diane's performance.

The findings related to initiation of contact with others were more variable. Although little difference was observed in the numbers of intervals in baseline versus intervention reflecting peer initiations with Diane, qualitative differences existed. Diane's play during the intervention phases appeared more mature than during the baseline phases. For example, when she was on the mat in the gym, her peers often placed an object near her or in her hand in much the same way children play with infants. The initiation of this type of interaction appeared to be consistent with the overt behaviors Diane exhibited because she did not speak and could not move efficiently. The placement of an object did encourage some arm movement toward the object, but her ability to manipulate the object was limited, and no developmentally appropriate play was observed. This situation is contrasted by two situations of her play in the car. First, a common activity observed during preschool gym class and recess when riding toys were available was that the children drove in circles or lines, following each other. As Diane appeared to become comfortable with the powered mobility riding toy, she began to join in this activity. Second, on one occasion in the car (the last session), one child in a group of several had a caterpillar. She put it on the car within Diane's visual field, and the children giggled and made eye contact with Diane. Then Diane took the caterpillar for a ride with the other children chasing after her. These occurrences were the only clear examples of developmentally appropriate interactive play, and it appeared that the use of the car increased Diane's opportunities to participate meaningfully. Because these occurrences were toward the end of the intervention, we might have seen more of this type of play with longer periods using the car. Neither child used the car to access or retrieve objects.

The results related to adult initiations were mixed relative to our hypothesis that adult initiations would decrease during intervention. The findings somewhat supported this hypothesis for John, whose school environment had a high adult-to-child ratio. John almost always had an adult available to help him, and his data reflect almost continuous adult initiations during some baseline sessions. In this situation, although he was positioned on swings and moved around the environment by adults, he had limited control. When John was in the car, although adults maintained a high level of contact with him, adult initiations generally were lower than during baseline sessions. In contrast, the findings for Diane provided no support for the hypothesis.

As expected, both children exhibited considerable laughter and smiling during the initial training. This affective response was transitory, with the data during intervention being less variable than during baseline. For future research, we question the usefulness of this dependent measure. In reviewing the videotapes, several observers noted the children's intense concentration and attention to the environment during the intervention phases. This attending behavior seemed to reflect the children's engagement in the playground or gym experience. A datum that focuses specifically on those behavioral characteristics might prove more useful than general affect data.

Some of the findings related to John's affect parallel the findings of Lloyd, Kermoian, and Campos (1994), who studied a group of locomotor 8-month-old infants and a group of prelocomotor infants of the same age. These researchers reported that locomotor infants expressed more negative affect when their goal-directed activity was blocked than did prelocomotor infants. John was noted as being a generally positive, compliant child. However, both a classroom aide and his therapist commented that he was saying "no" more often and being more assertive once the car was introduced into his program. This observation was consistent with the data in that he exhibited no negative affect during the first baseline phase but displayed negative affect during the 2nd day of intervention and during the second baseline on a day when he was using the adapted tricycle, a toy that allowed self-initiated mobility. In parallel, John asserted himself by initiating negative contacts with adults on these same days. The possible impact of self-initiated movement on assertiveness merits further study as related to the introduction of mobility technology to children with complex developmental delays.

Use of the powered mobility riding toy in the protected school environment had advantages. When the children ran into things, either accidentally or on purpose, they experienced the consequences of their actions. For example, adults admonished John for running into walls, "running away," or not moving with the group. Additionally, when John bumped into another child on a tricycle, the bumped child took it in stride and sped off, admonishing, "Watch where you're going!" Free play during gym class and outdoor recess provided learning opportunities in an environment where bumps are common occurrences and others in the environment provide appropriate feedback. Compared with John, Diane had a more cautious approach. She soon learned how much space she took up in the car and how to maneuver without bumping into things. She carefully waited for clearings in the preschool traffic, sometimes taking more time than would be desirable for efficient movement. Thus, Diane was able to develop skills at her own pace in the free-play environment.

Conclusion

Despite the two children's differing approaches, our experiences with them suggest that powered mobility play on the playground or in the gym provided developmentally appropriate mobility education that we predict will facilitate the transition to wheelchair use in the larger community. We need additional research to verify this prediction and increase our understanding of the effects of powered mobility on children with complex developmental delays. As a next step, single-subject studies should be extended over longer periods and meet the conditions required for application of inferential statistics. Further, efforts should be made to extend this research by using dependent variables related to developmental levels of play, self-assertiveness, and attention to the environment. Finally, longitudinal studies of children with complex developmental delays who use powered mobility riding toys could determine the extent to which powered mobility play facilitates the transition to powered mobility use in the community.

Acknowledgments

We thank the Association for Retarded Citizens for providing funding for this project; Jim Steinky and Innovative Products Inc. for contributions to the electronic systems used in the study; Marvin Soderquist for assistance with the technology and for troubleshooting; Susan Chalcraft, PT, Lisa Duits, and the senior occupational therapy students for assistance with either videotaping or data coding; "John's" mother, Voski Sprague, OTR/L, and Barbara Forney, MOT/L, for assisting us with this research; the teachers, therapists, and aides at two schools in Washington State for their support; and "Diane" and "John" for their cooperation, unfailing interest, and smiles.

References

Abramson, L. Y., Seligman, M. E. P., & Teasdale, J. D. (1978). Learned helplessness in humans: Critique and reformulation. *Journal of Abnormal Psychology, 87,* 49–74.

Bandura, A. (1977). *Social learning theory.* Englewood Cliffs, NJ: Prentice Hall.

Brinker, R. P., & Lewis, M. (1982). Discovering the competent handicapped infant: A process approach to assessment and intervention. *Topics in Early Childhood Special Education, 2*(2), 1–16.

Butler, C. (1986). Effects of powered mobility on self-initiated behaviors of very young children with locomotor disability. *Developmental Medicine and Child Neurology, 28,* 325–332.

Butler, C. (1997). Wheelchair toddlers. In J. Furumasu (Ed.), *Pediatric powered mobility: Developmental perspectives, technical issues, clinical approaches* (pp. 1–6). Arlington, VA: RESNA.

Butler, C., Okamoto, G. A., & McKay, T. M. (1983). Powered mobility for very young disabled children. *Developmental Medicine and Child Neurology, 25,* 472–474.

Campos, J., Kermoian, R., & Zumbahlen, M. (1992). Socioemotional transformations in the family system following infant crawling onset. In N. Eisenberg & R. Fabes (Eds.), *New directions for child development: No. 55. Emotion and its regulation in early development* (pp. 25–40). San Francisco: Jossey-Bass.

Chiulli, C., Corradi-Scalise, D., & Donatelli-Schultheiss, L. (1988). Powered mobility vehicles as aids in independent locomotion for young children. *Physical Therapy, 68,* 997–999.

Douglas, J., & Ryan, M. (1987). A preschool severely disabled boy and his powered wheelchair: A case study. *Child: Care, Health, and Development, 13,* 303–309.

Folio, R. M., & Fewell, R. R. (1983). *Peabody Developmental Motor Scales and Activity Cards.* Allen, TX: DLM/Teaching Resources.

Hedrick, D., Prather, E., & Tobin, A. (1984). *Sequenced Inventory of Communication Development–Revised.* Seattle: University of Washington P.

Hildebrand, V. (1988). Young children's self-care and independence tasks: Applying self-efficacy theory. *Early Child Development and Care, 30,* 199–204.

Kermoian, R. (1997). Locomotion experience and psychological development in infancy. In J. Furumasu (Ed.), *Pediatric powered mobility: Developmental perspectives, technical issues, clinical approaches* (pp. 7–21). Arlington, VA: RESNA.

Kermoian, R. (1998). Locomotor experience facilitates psychological functioning: Implications for assistive mobility for young children. In D. Gray, L. Quatrano, & M. Lieberman (Eds.), *Designing and using assistive technology: The human perspective* (pp. 251–268). Baltimore: Brookes.

Lloyd, R., Kermoian, R., & Campos, J. (1994, June). *Effects of locomotor experience on emotional display during a manual detour search task.* Paper presented at the Ninth International Conference on Infant Studies, Paris.

Maier, S. F., & Seligman, M. E. P. (1976). Learned helplessness: Theory and evidence. *Journal of Experimental Psychology: General, 105,* 3–46.

Newborg, J., Stock, J., Wnek, L., Guidubaldi, J., & Svinicki, J. (1984). *The Battelle Developmental Inventory.* Allen TX: DLM/Teaching Resources.

Ottenbacher, K. (1986). *Evaluating clinical change: Strategies for occupational and physical therapists.* Baltimore: Williams & Wilkins.

Paulsson, K., & Christofferson, M. (1984). Psychosocial aspects on technical aids: How does independent mobility affect the psychosocial and intellectual development of children with physical disabilities? In *Proceedings of the 2nd International Conference on Rehabilitation Engineering* (pp. 282–286). Washington, DC: RESNA.

Snell, E., & Balfour, L. (1997). Pediatric powered mobility: Service delivery and associated research. In J. Furumasu (Ed.), *Pediatric powered mobility: Developmental perspectives, technical issues, clinical approaches* (pp. 23–32). Arlington, VA: RESNA.

Sullivan, M. W., & Lewis, M. (1993). Contingency, means–end skills, and the use of technology in infant intervention. *Infants and Young Children, 5*(4), 58–77.

Tefft, D., Furumasu, J., & Guerette, P. (1997). Pediatric powered mobility: Influential cognitive skills. In J. Furumasu (Ed.), *Pediatric powered mobility: Developmental perspectives, technical issues, clinical approaches* (pp. 70–82). Arlington, VA: RESNA.

Telzrow, R. W., Campos, J. J., Shepherd, A., Bertenthal, B. I., & Atwater, S. (1987). Spatial understanding in infants with motor handicaps. In K. M. Jaffe (Ed.), *Childhood powered mobility: Developmental, technical, and clinical perspectives: Proceedings of the RESNA First Northwest Regional Conference* (pp. 62–69). Washington, DC: RESNA.

Wright-Ott, C. (1997). The transitional mobility aid: A new concept and tool for early mobility. In J. Furumasu (Ed.), *Pediatric powered mobility: Developmental perspectives, technical issues, clinical approaches* (pp. 58–69). Arlington, VA: RESNA.

Zazula, J. L., & Foulds, R. A. (1983). Mobility device for a child with phocomelia. *Archives of Physical Medicine and Rehabilitation, 64,* 137–139.

CHAPTER 18

A Comparison of Consultative Model and Direct–Indirect Intervention With Preschoolers

Diann S. Dreiling and Anita C. Bundy

Diann S. Dreiling, MS, OTR, *is school therapist, Douglas County School District, Castle Rock, CO. At the time of the study, she was graduate student, Occupational Therapy Program, Colorado State University, Fort Collins. Mailing address: 1478 S. Moline, Aurora, CO 80012; ddotr@aol.com.*

Anita C. Bundy, ScD, OTR, *is professor and chair, School of Occupation and Leisure Sciences, University of Sydney, Sydney, Australia. At the time the study was completed, she was professor, Department of Occupational Therapy, Colorado State University, Fort Collins.*

Originally published 2003 in *American Journal of Occupational Therapy,* 57, 566–569.

Occupational therapists who work in early childhood education provide interventions that support the programming for students with developmental delays. Currently approximately 50% of therapists in the school systems use a direct service model, including a combination of individual and group intervention (Davies & Gavin, 1994). In addition to direct service, other models of intervention include indirect service (also known as monitoring) and consultation.

An increasing number of therapists in the schools are using consultation for various reasons (Dudgeon & Greenberg, 1998). Some therapists choose consultation because they feel that support in the classroom will benefit the child more than direct service once a week. Sometimes this model of service is not chosen by the therapist or determined in response to the individual education plan (IEP) but is dictated by special service administrators in the hope of increasing caseloads of the occupational therapists. However, consultation is a complex process and can take as much or more time as direct service (Hanft & Place, 1996). Further, when the consultation model is used, it is important to emphasize that students who need hands-on therapy must still receive direct services from an occupational therapist (Hanft & Place, 1996).

Even though some authors have suggested that models of service delivery may be differentially responsive to different types of goals (Davies & Gavin, 1994; Dunn, 1988; Kemmis & Dunn, 1996), recent research has found no statistically significant differences between the results of direct, indirect, and consultative models of intervention for preschoolers with motor delays (Davies & Gavin, 1994; Dunn, 1988; Kemmis & Dunn, 1996). Dunn compared the three models and demonstrated, with three students ages 6, 9, and 17 years, that all models can be effective for accomplishing goals. Davies and Gavin compared progress in two groups of 10 preschoolers ages 3 to 5 years using consultation with one group and direct intervention with the other. Dunn and

Davies and Gavin have all suggested that further study should be done to define use of consultation in schools.

The purpose of this study was to compare outcomes for students with motor delays who were served through either direct–indirect intervention or consultation to parents and preschool staff.

Method

Design

A between-group design was used for this study. One group of children received a consultative model of intervention, and the second group received direct–indirect intervention.

Participants

Participants were children who were evaluated through a county child assessment program. The children were assigned to one of 23 integrated preschool classrooms within the county based on the results of their developmental assessment. Each classroom had 10 typically developing students and five or six students with special needs.

Twenty-two boys and girls from 12 classrooms who met the following criteria participated: (a) were between 3 and 5 years of age; (b) had gross or fine motor–visual motor delays defined as scores at least one standard deviation below their age norms on one standardized measure of motor skill (i.e., Peabody Developmental Motor Scales [Folio & Fewell, 1983], Learning Accomplishment Profile [LAP–D] [Nehring, Nehring, Bruni, & Randolph, 1992], Developmental Test of Visual–Motor Integration [VMI] [Beery, 1997]); (c) had a current IEP requiring occupational therapy; and (d) were not receiving private occupational therapy or physical therapy during the time of the study. The participants did not have a medical diagnosis (e.g., attention deficit disorder, muscular dystrophy, cerebral palsy) recorded in their school

records or by parent report and were not taking medication on a regular basis. They did not have significant cognitive or emotional delays, but some of the participants did have speech or language delays.

The children were assigned to one of two groups for the study, consultation or direct–indirect, depending on the model already in place in their classrooms. Students in the consultation group ($n = 11$; 7 boys, 4 girls; $M_{age} = 4.5$ years) were selected from 6 of 8 classrooms in the district using the consultative model for occupational therapy. These classrooms were selected for this study because the staff was the most experienced and the occupational therapist demonstrated the greatest understanding and use of consultation. Although these specialists all had worked for at least 3 years in Douglas County, the team members had not previously worked together (see Figure 18.1).

Students in the direct–indirect intervention group ($n = 9$; 5 boys, 4 girls; $M_{age} = 4.7$) were selected from 3 classrooms (3 morning classes and 3 afternoon classes) being served by one special education team. The classes were also chosen for the experience of the special education team including the occupational therapist, who had been part of this team previous to the study (see Figure 18.1).

The parents were an integral part of the therapy teams in both groups. They agreed to participate during the entire study, including implementing all home programs, although no measure of compliance was used for the parents in the study.

Instrumentation

Goal Attainment Scaling (GAS) (Carr, 1979) was used to determine the efficacy of each model of intervention. Using GAS, we measured the degree to which goals were achieved regardless of the intervention. The goals used as outcome measures

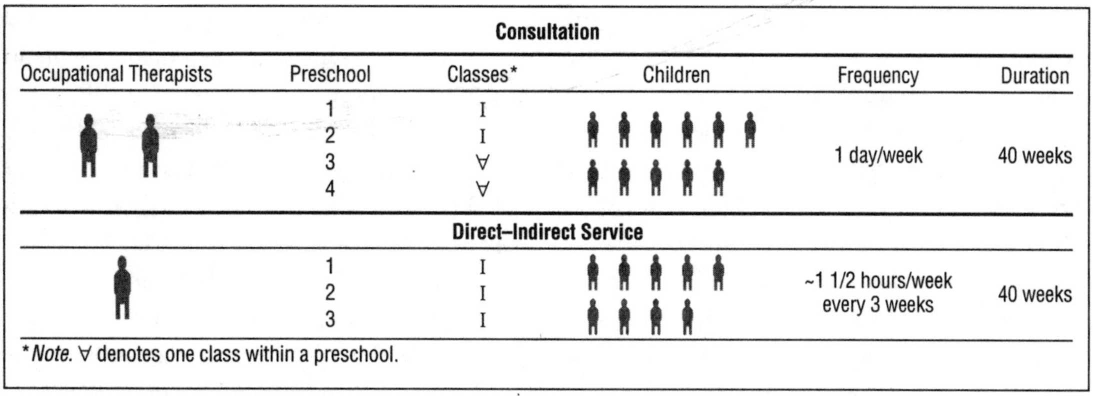

Figure 18.1. Schematic representation of therapists, preschools, classes, and children.

for this study were drawn from the IEP of each student.

Procedure

Before beginning the study, parents signed informed consent forms for both their child's and their own participation. In addition, the two therapists (one in each group) who provided intervention participated in one training session with the first author to record the intervention data and prioritize goals.

We followed eight steps described by Ottenbacher and Cusick (1990) for Goal Attainment Scaling. The first author and two occupational therapists from a county assessment program (different from the therapists providing the intervention) completed the initial evaluation of all the children prior to their placement in preschool. The therapists providing intervention evaluated students who had been in the preschool program for a year. Following testing, the therapists set goals to address the specific motor needs of each student tailored to the preschool environment and educational expectations.

The two primary therapists, who provided consultative intervention (including the first author, who was the only therapist to take part in both initial evaluation and intervention), and the one primary therapist, who provided

direct–indirect intervention, determined the expected levels of performance as well as the weights for each goal. Input from parents, teachers, and special educators was considered when setting the expected levels and weights (Ottenbacher & Cusick, 1990).

Data were recorded for a total of 39 goals (M = 3.55, range = 2–6) for students receiving intervention through a consultation model and 56 goals (M = 6.22, range = 2–10) for students receiving services through direct–indirect intervention. The number of goals for each student varied based on his or her needs, parents' input, and the determinations of the team assigning the goals. The results for this study are based on completion of goals. For both models of service, the special education team collected data regarding goal attainment weekly on all students as per the protocol for the district. Data for both groups used in this study were kept for the final 4 months of the study. The occupational therapists reviewed the data weekly and discussed the success of the strategies with staff or parents or both. If the strategies were not effective, they were modified.

Intervention

Two occupational therapists provided consultation services (see Figure 18.1). Each therapist consulted to one different preschool team.

They spent 1 full day a week during the 40-week school year in each of their assigned classrooms observing the students during various activities and consulting with the staff regarding therapeutic strategies used for the students' needs in gross motor, fine motor, or visual–motor skills and student progress; they also met with the full preschool team for 1 half-day twice a month during the school year. In addition, the occupational therapists met with parents on an as-needed basis for consultation and to review home activities. At the beginning of the year, the consulting occupational therapists spent additional time in the schools to build rapport with team members, set and review role expectations, educate, and collaborate on strategies. Toward the end of the study, their time was spent primarily on evaluating and modifying ongoing treatment strategies.

One occupational therapist worked on a transdisciplinary team and provided the direct–indirect model of intervention to another 9 children for a full week every 3 weeks for the 40-week school year (see Figure 18.1). The occupational therapist provided direct services daily in the classroom during her week's rotation; each child received an average of an hour and a half of service per week to address the students' needs in gross motor, fine motor, or visual–motor skills. The occupational therapist instructed the team in how to implement the intervention in her absence. She also participated in a half-day planning session weekly with the team.

Data Analysis

At the completion of the intervention period, T scores were computed on the goal-related data for each student using the formula for GAS (Kiresuk & Sherman, 1968). The formula is

$$T = 50 + \frac{(10\sum W_i X_i)}{\sqrt{(1-r)\sum W_i^2 + r(\sum W_i)^2}}$$

where W_i represents the weighting for a particular goal and X_i represents the outcome score for each behavior (i.e., a value from -2 to $+2$). The r value in the formula reflects the estimated average intercorrelation for the outcome scores. An r value of .30 was suggested as a constant by Kiresuk and Sherman (1968) and Maloney, Mirrett, Brooks, and Johannes (1978); the latter felt that the r value yielded a standard deviation of 10 units around 50. The T value is a standardized score with a mean of 50 and standard deviation of 10.

Results

Both models of intervention were found to help students meet their goals ($M_{consult} = 48.25$, $M_{dir.svc} = 49.69$) at approximately the rate expected ($M_{expected} = 50$, $SD = 10$). Students in the consultation group met or exceeded expectations (levels 0 to +2) on 22 of their 39 (56%) goals, whereas students in the direct–indirect intervention group met or exceeded expectations on 28 of the 56 (50%) goals. A t test for independent samples revealed no significant difference between the outcomes for students receiving intervention in the consultative model and those receiving direct–indirect intervention ($t = .359$, $df = 18$, $p = .724$). The small difference between groups was supported by a small effect size ($d = .16$).

Discussion

The results of this study indicate that a consultative model of intervention and a direct–indirect intervention model were equally effective for addressing goals related to improved motor performance for preschoolers in this study. This finding supports recent research that found no statistically significant difference in outcomes for different types of service delivery (Davies & Gavin, 1994; Kemmis & Dunn, 1996). These results also support the beliefs of many (e.g., Donaldson &

Christiansen, 1990; Kemmis & Dunn, 1996) regarding the efficacy of consultation.

Because many of the goals in this study were similar for students regardless of the type of service they received, these results challenge theorists' suggestions that some kinds of goals are better met with a specific type of intervention (Bundy, 1993; Dunn, 1988; Hanft & Place, 1996). Given that the goals were primarily to improve motor skill, it might have been logical to assume that direct–indirect service would be the best service approach because the occupational therapist is the best trained to observe a child's performance and alter the nature of a therapeutic task to ensure success. In indirect service, the occupational therapist would teach a caregiver to do particular activities with the child, thus providing the child with many opportunities for practice. However, the consulting therapists in this study were able to help other caregivers insert motor activities into their routines in particularly clever ways. Many preschool teachers use preacademic activities when transitioning from one activity to another (e.g., "children with red shirts, go line up"), whereas preschool teachers in the present study paired that with a movement activity (e.g., "children with red shirts, hop like a bunny to line up"). With these preschool-age children who had relatively minor disabilities, consultation provided opportunities for repetition of motor skills in the natural context of the preschool classroom or at home. This may explain some of the reason for the success of this model.

Another reason for the success of both models of intervention could be that the preschool teams met regularly and agreed to work collaboratively to establish and carry out suggested strategies. That is, the fit of each model to the beliefs and skills of each of the teams was particularly good. Adequate time for consultative teams to meet regularly has been considered by many authors to be necessary to the success of consulta-tion (e.g., Kemmis & Dunn, 1996). In fact, Kemmis and Dunn (1996) indicated that remedial and compensatory interventions were equally successful within a consultative framework when the therapist and teacher met 1 hour weekly to collaborate. Although administrators often see the consultative model as a way of increasing therapists' caseloads, the results of this study suggest that the required time for consultation is initially just as much or more than that of direct intervention, but as the year progresses the amount of time required decreases. This pattern occurs because initially the consultant is spending more time building rapport with, educating, and planning strategies with the teams and observing the students. As the year progresses, the team typically becomes more effective at solving their own problems (i.e., determining which strategies work in their classrooms and carrying out those strategies) and need less time for education. Future studies could evaluate the exact amount of time that is spent in consulting versus direct intervention to give a more accurate assessment of the difference in time spent and, thus, shed light on the relative cost-effectiveness of each model.

Interestingly, the therapist in this study who administered direct–indirect service created significantly more objectives ($M = 6.2$, $SD = 1.3$) for the children on her caseload than the therapists who utilized consultation ($M = 3.7$, $SD = 2.8$, $p_{equal\ variances\ not\ assumed} = .03$). The reason for this is unclear. Perhaps when therapists collaborate with colleagues to create plans that will be carried out by the others, they consider very carefully the number of objectives that seems reasonable. Each objective requires the insertion of one or more strategies into the school day. This can be very time consuming with five or six children with special needs in each classroom. Thus, more objectives actually may mean less success at meeting them and, consequently, less progress for each child.

A small sample size and the use of one geographic region limit the ability to generalize the results of this study beyond the sample. Variability of special needs among the participants may have influenced the intervention outcomes. Although all students had delays in motor skills and no diagnosable condition, other areas of development (i.e., cognitive or behavioral) were not well controlled. For future studies, participants could be limited to children with delays in motor skills with all other developmental areas within the limits of typical development. The extent to which parents implemented home programs also was a variable that was not specifically examined. As a member of a county assessment team providing the initial assessments as well as part of one of the preschool teams, the first author both evaluated and provided intervention for four of the children receiving consultation, a factor that may have influenced the results. Finally, differential amounts of experience working together among the various teams also may have affected the success of their interventions.

Conclusion

Eleven students who received a consultation model of intervention achieved 22 of 39 (56%) goals addressing improved motor performance, while the nine students in the direct intervention model met or exceeded expectations on 28 of their 56 (50%) goals. The results of this study support the conclusion that consultation is a viable model of intervention in preschool settings and is just as effective as direct–indirect interventions.

References

Beery, K. E. (1997). *The Beery–Buktenic Developmental Test of Visual–Motor Integration*. Parsippany, NJ: Modern Curriculum Press.

Bundy, A. (1993). Will I see you in September? A question of educational relevance. *American Journal of Occupational Therapy, 47,* 848–850.

Carr, R. (1979). Goal attainment scaling as a useful tool for evaluating progress in special education. *Exceptional Children, 46,* 88–95.

Davies, P. L., & Gavin, W. J. (1994). Comparison of individual and group: Consultation treatment methods for preschool children with developmental delays. *American Journal of Occupational Therapy, 48,* 155–161.

Donaldson, R., & Christiansen, J. (1990, Winter). Consultation and collaboration: A decision-making model. *Teaching Exceptional Children,* pp. 22–25.

Dudgeon, B. J., & Greenberg, S. L. (1998). Preparing students for consultation roles and systems. *American Journal of Occupational Therapy, 52,* 801–809.

Dunn, W. (1988). Models of occupational therapy service provision in the school system. *American Journal of Occupational Therapy, 42,* 718–723.

Folio, M. R., & Fewell, R. R. (1983). *Peabody Developmental Motor Scales and activity cards.* Austin, TX: PRO-ED.

Hanft, B. E., & Place, P. A. (1996). *The consulting therapist.* San Antonio, TX: Therapy SkillBuilders.

Kemmis, B. L., & Dunn, W. (1996). Collaborative consultation: The efficacy of remedial and compensatory intervention in school contexts. *American Journal of Occupational Therapy, 50,* 709–717.

Kiresuk, T., & Sherman, R. (1968). Goal attainment scaling: A general method of evaluating comprehensive mental health programs. *Community Mental Health Journal, 4,* 443–453.

Maloney, P. F., Mirrett, P., Brooks, C., & Johannes, K. (1978). Use of the goal attainment scale in the treatment and ongoing evaluation of neurologically handicapped children. *American Journal of Occupational Therapy, 32,* 505–511.

Nehring, A. D., Nehring, E. F., Bruni, J. R., Jr., & Randolph, P. L. (1992). *Learning accomplishment profile—Diagnostic standardized assessment.* Lewisville, NC: Kaplan Press.

Ottenbacher, K. J., & Cusick, A. (1990). Goal Attainment scaling as a method of clinical service evaluation. *American Journal of Occupational Therapy, 44,* 6, 519–524.

CHAPTER 19

Effects of a Weighted Vest on Attention to Task and Self-Stimulatory Behaviors in Preschoolers With Pervasive Developmental Disorders

Doreen Fertel-Daly, Gary Bedell, and Jim Hinojosa

Doreen Fertel-Daly, MA, OT, BCP, *is occupational therapist, Challenge Infant Developmental Center, Brooklyn, NY.*

Gary Bedell, PhD, OT, *is postdoctoral research fellow, Boston University, Center for Rehabilitation Effectiveness, Sargent College of Health and Rehabilitation Sciences, Boston. At the time of this study, he was adjunct associate professor, New York University.*

Jim Hinojosa, PhD, OT, FAOTA, *is professor, New York University, 35 West 4th Street, 11th Floor, New York, NY 10011; jim.hinojosa@nyu.edu.*

Deep pressure, a form of tactile sensory stimulation, is believed to have a calming effect on adults and children with pervasive developmental disorders (PDD) (Edelson, Edelson, Kerr, & Grandin, 1999; Grandin, 1992; McClure & Holtz-Yotz, 1991). Deep pressure often is provided by holding, stroking, hugging, and swaddling (Grandin, 1992). Researchers have hypothesized that deep pressure calms children by modulating their central nervous system processing of sensory information (Grandin, 1992; McClure & Holtz-Yotz, 1991). Recently, occupational therapists have been using weighted vests (e.g., AliMed,[1] Sammons,[2] Therapy SkillBuilders[3]) as an intervention modality to provide deep pressure while children are engaged in routine daily activities; however, no studies were found in the literature that examined the effectiveness of using weighted vests as part of an intervention approach.

Limited evidence from anecdotal case studies indicates that deep pressure has an effect on attentional behaviors and reduces self-stimulatory behaviors in children with autism (Edelson et al., 1999; Joe, 1998; McClure & Holtz-Yotz, 1991; Zissermann, 1992). Joe (1998) reported that children with developmental disabilities and autism demonstrated a decrease in self-stimulatory behaviors, became less distractible, and demonstrated increased attention to a task while wearing weighted vests. McClure and Holtz-Yotz (1991) reported reduced self-stimulatory and self-injurious behaviors in one child with autism when deep pressure was applied to the upper extremities in the form of splinting and padding. Changes in behavior were based on reported observations from the hospital staff. The child exhibited an increased ability to interact with others, a calmer behavioral state, and an apparent strong desire to wear the pressure materials.

Originally published 2001 in *American Journal of Occupational Therapy,* 55, 629–640.

[1]AliMed, Inc., 2917 High Street, Dedham, MA 02026.
[2]Sammons Preston, 4 Sammons Court, Bolingbrook, IL 60440-4989.
[3]Therapy SkillBuilders, 555 Academic Court, San Antonio, TX 78204.

Zissermann (1992) observed an 11.8% decrease in instances of self-stimulatory behavior when a child with autism wore bilateral long arm gloves made from support pantyhose. Data were compared based on observations of self-stimulatory behaviors when the pressure garments were applied and removed.

Edelson et al. (1999) reported on a pilot study that supports the use of deep pressure with children with autism. The experimental group used a hug machine to administer deep pressure evenly across the lateral parts of the body, and a placebo group did not apply deep pressure. The results indicated a significant reduction in behavioral indicators of anxiety and a marginal reduction in physiological indicators of anxiety in the experimental group.

Children with PDD, which includes autism, often engage in self-stimulatory behaviors and have difficulty attending to tasks. Severe impairment in social interaction skills and communication, with the presence of stereotyped behaviors (e.g., repetitive, stereotyped mannerisms such as rocking, twirling, spinning, arm flapping, tapping, and squinting), interferes with their ability to attend to tasks and learn (American Psychiatric Association, 1994; Lovaas, 1981, 1987). Attention is a state that reflects a person's receptivity to information and occurs because a task needs to be accomplished (Ruff & Lawson, 1991). Kientz and Dunn's (1997) comparison of children with and without autism revealed that 75% of their subjects with autism had difficulty paying attention. Self-stimulation is a major problem that often interferes with attention to a task. King and Grandin (1990) suggested that self-stimulating behaviors may be the child's attempt to calm and modulate his or her arousal level during times of general overarousal. Additionally, Lovaas (1987) found that the children's attention problems appeared worse when they self-stimulated.

A child's inability to adequately modulate sensory input manifests itself as either a lack of responsiveness or an exaggerated reaction to sensory stimulation (Ayres & Tickle, 1980; Kimball, 1999; Ornitz, 1985). Ayres and Tickle (1980) concluded that children with autism have difficulty registering sensory stimuli. Research on children with PDD indicates that they prefer and often seek out sensory stimulation (e.g., sounds, visual stimuli, touching, being sandwiched between mats) (Ayres, 1987; Kootz, Marinelli, & Cohen, 1981). Some treatment approaches for behaviors associated with PDD have been based on the use of general sensory stimulation to modulate sensory information processing (Ayres, 1987; Dunn & Fisher, 1983). A slow, steady application of pressure has been reported to have a calming effect on a person, whereas sudden, jerky motions tend to cause hyperarousal (Grandin, 1992).

The study presented here resulted from personal observations in a clinical setting. Although it is common practice for occupational therapists to use weighted vests to provide deep pressure stimulation to children with PDD, to date minimal research has been conducted to examine the effects of this practice. Accordingly, this study systematically examined the effects of wearing a weighted vest on attention to task and self-stimulatory behaviors of five preschool children with PDD.

Method

The single-subject ABA reversal design (Kazdin, 1982; Ottenbacher, 1986) was selected to examine the effects of wearing a weighted vest on attention to task and self-stimulatory behavior of five preschool children with PDD. This design allowed for systematic measurement of individual changes in each participant with and without the weighted vests. The study was conducted within a self-contained classroom that included six children, one teacher, and six assistants; five of the six children participated in the study. Each child in the classroom worked one-on-one with an assistant. All participants were observed at a table during a fine motor task for 15 sessions over a 6-week period.

Participants

The five participants ranged from 2 years to 4 years of age, were diagnosed with PDD, had reported difficulties in attention to task, and were not currently being treated with a weighted vest. Participant 5 had been further diagnosed with autism. Participant 1 had been treated with a weighted vest for a short time 1 year before the study. All participants attended a 5-day-a-week preschool program in New York City for 3 hr each day. The program used an applied behavioral analysis approach for behavior management (Lovaas, 1987). All participants received speech and occupational therapy services. The consent procedure required that a letter be sent to all of the parents whose children attended the applied behavioral analysis program and had been diagnosed with PDD. Parents who were interested in having their child participate in the study returned a signed consent form to the classroom teacher and were assured that assent procedures would be followed. Five consent forms were returned. The study was approved by the New York University Office of Sponsored Programs, University Committee on Activities Involving Human Subjects, and the appropriate personnel in the institution where the data were collected.

Participant 1 was a 2-year, 7-month-old girl who was the smallest of all the participants, weighing 25.5 lb. At the time of this study, she was nonverbal and required assistance to walk. Her mother and teacher were concerned about her decreased attention span. Observations confirmed that Participant 1 engaged in the self-stimulatory behaviors of biting, staring at her

hands, and repetitive verbal humming. She avoided eye contact and seldom responded to a play object. She would repeatedly throw herself out of her chair and push objects off the table when required to participate in fine motor activities.

Participant 2 was a 2-year, 10-month-old boy who weighed 32 lb. During baseline observations, he engaged in a few self-stimulatory behaviors (hand biting, perseverative verbal humming and singing). Although he remained seated at the table with minimal cuing, his teacher reported that he needed his attention to be redirected continuously when attempting fine motor activities. He was observed to be easily distracted by background auditory sounds and needed to be constantly redirected to do fine motor activities.

Participant 3 was a 3-year, 1-month-old boy who was the largest of all the participants, weighing 37 lb. His mother reported that he was active and preferred gross motor activities to fine motor tasks. His teacher reported that he required continuous prompts and redirection to get him to engage in fine motor activities. During observations, he appeared to become frustrated easily and would have a tantrum or walk away from the table when the activity became difficult. When engaged in an activity, Participant 3 would look away from the task toward auditory and visual stimuli. He often twirled objects, rolled his eyes, repetitively clicked his tongue, and sang the same phrases. He responded to his name with brief eye contact that he could not sustain.

Participant 4 was a 2-year, 9-month-old girl who weighed 33 lb. Both her teacher and mother were concerned about her lack of play skills and her inability to attend to fine motor activities. During observations, she repeatedly engaged in self-stimulatory behaviors of rocking, twirling and tapping objects, and repetitive verbal chanting when a fine motor activity was presented. Distractible behaviors observed included recurrent tantrums, throwing herself on the floor, and frequently turning her head away from the direction of the activity. She also directed her attention toward background noises and visual stimuli. If not physically prompted to remain seated at the table, she would get out of her chair and move around the room.

Participant 5 was a 2-year, 10-month-old boy who weighed 27 lb. He demonstrated spontaneous eye contact and verbalized simple phrases when he wanted something. He voluntarily sat at the table and appeared to enjoy fine motor activities; however, he did not play appropriately with the materials. When presented with a fine motor activity, he repetitively twirled the task materials and required his attention to be redirected toward the activity. He also continuously turned his head to visual and auditory stimuli. He would occasionally engage in verbal and oral self-stimulation.

Procedure

A measurement procedure was developed to record the duration of focused attention to task, number of distractions, and duration and type of self-stimulatory behaviors during a 5-min fine motor activity. Duration of focused attention to task was measured by recording the length of time a child looked at and simultaneously engaged in some deliberate manipulation of fine motor objects or materials related to the activity (Ruff & Lawson, 1991) within the 5-min period. The number of distractions was the number of times the participant turned his or her head or eyes away from the task within a 5-min interval. Finally, the type and the summed duration of self-stimulatory behaviors observed within a 5-min period were recorded. Self-stimulatory behaviors were defined as a variety of repetitive, stereotyped mannerisms, such as rocking, spinning objects, twirling, arm flapping, gazing, tapping, hand biting, flicking ears, crossing eyes, rolling eyes, squinting, or repetitive and monotonous vocalizations (Lovaas, 1981).

The fine motor activities observed in these children were part of the applied behavioral analysis program. The children were familiar with the activities presented during the data collection. Activities included scribbling and imitating crayon strokes, building with blocks, imitating block patterns, putting pegs into a pegboard, stringing beads, snipping with scissors, and pointing to objects.

The first author collected all data. Another rater measured the behaviors on three occasions during the baseline phase of the study to ensure that data were collected in a reliable and consistent manner. Interobserver agreement on attending and self-stimulatory behaviors was determined by comparing the scores of the first author with the second rater using the frequency formula described by Kazdin (1982). Interobserver agreement for the number of distractions was 100%. The interobserver agreement was 97% for duration of focused attention to task and duration and type of self-stimulatory behaviors.

Intervention Protocol

Because a published protocol for the use of weighted vests was unavailable, anecdotal reports from colleagues and Wilbarger's (1995) brushing protocol suggested that weighted vests were most effective when worn for 2 hr and then removed for 2 hr before being worn again. This protocol was also consistent with Takagi and Kobayasi's (1955) animal studies, where it was determined that an initial surge in arousal before calming occurred when deep pressure was worn for 2 hr. A multipocketed denim vest sized to fit each participant was used for this study. Each weighted vest contained four pouches—two in the front and two in the back—with a .25-lb weight in each pouch (The Kiddie Vest™4). During the inter-

---

[4]Kiddie Vest™, 501 W. Richwoods Boulevard, Peoria, IL 61604.

vention phase (B), the first author or the teacher put the weighted vests on the children shortly after they arrived at school in the morning, and the vests were worn for 2 hr. The applied behavioral analysis programs continued as usual throughout the school day.

Data Collection

Before data collection, the participants' teachers and therapists were informed of the nature of this study. They were encouraged to keep the existing therapy programs consistent throughout the duration of this study and inform the researcher if any changes occurred. This study consisted of three phases: initial baseline phase (A), intervention phase (B), and intervention withdrawal phase (A). The observations and data collection for all phases occurred while the participants were engaged in a structured fine motor activity in the classroom with their teacher. Three separate 5-min observation periods for each participant were used to record the three measures investigated in this study. Accordingly, three observation sessions, one for each measure, per participant, and per phase, resulted in a total of nine observation periods for each participant across all phases. A timer was used to mark the 5-min intervals. The number of distractions was recorded on the data sheet and totaled at the end of the 5-min interval. A stopwatch was used to record the summed total duration of focused attention and self-stimulatory behaviors. The time of day for data collection for each participant remained consistent throughout the study.

The initial baseline measures for the number of distractions, duration of focused attention, and duration of self-stimulatory behaviors were taken in the baseline phase (A). Initial baseline observations for all 5 participants began within a 48-hr period. Participants were observed 3 days each alternating over a 5-day period for the 1st week and 2 days each alternating over a 4-day period for

the 2nd week. Within 2 weeks, baseline data were collected for all 5 participants on all three measures.

Data collection for the intervention phase (B) began in the 3rd week of the study. The weighted vests were worn three times a week for a 2-week period. Data were collected after the participant had worn a weighted vest for 1.5 hr. During the final 2 weeks of the intervention phase, data collection was staggered for three times over a 4-day period for the 3rd week and two times in the 4th week for a total of five sessions.

Intervention was discontinued in the 5th week of the study, the intervention withdrawal phase (A), and the weighted vests were not worn during the final 2 weeks of the study. Data for the intervention withdrawal phase were collected in same manner as in the baseline and intervention phases. Data collection was staggered, with each participant observed five times during the 5th and 6th week for a total of five sessions.

Data Analysis

The duration of focused attention, the number of distractions, and the duration of self-stimulatory behaviors were recorded on the data collection sheets. Data for each session were graphed separately for each participant using Microsoft Excel for Windows 95 (Microsoft Corporation, 1995) throughout the three phases of the study. Data analysis included the visual inspection of the slope, height, and direction of the trend line for each phase and the calculation of mean performance for each of the three measures per phase (Ottenbacher, 1986).

Results

Figure 19.1 includes three graphs that document duration of focused attention, number of distractions, and duration of self-stimulatory behaviors for Participant 1 for each 5-min obser-

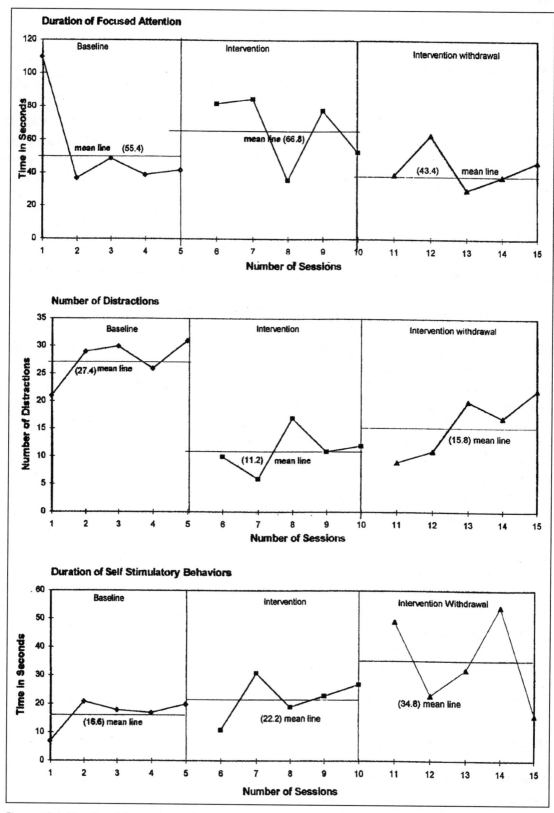

Figure 19.1. Duration of focused attention, number of distractions, and duration of self-stimulatory behaviors for Participant 1.

vation. Focused attention to task, with a mean of 55.4 sec in the baseline phase, increased during the intervention phase (M = 66.8 sec) and decreased in the intervention withdrawal phase (M = 43.4 sec). Number of distractions, with a mean of 27.4 during the baseline phase, decreased substantially during the intervention phase (M = 11.2) and increased in the intervention withdrawal phase (M = 15.8). Duration of self-stimulatory behaviors, with a mean of 16.6 sec in the baseline phase, increased in the intervention phase (M = 22.2 sec) and increased again during the intervention withdrawal phase (M = 38.4 sec).

Figure 19.2 represents the data taken for Participant 2. Focused attention to task, with a mean of 84.6 sec during the baseline phase, increased during the intervention phase (M = 97.6 sec) and declined in the intervention withdrawal phase (M = 64 sec). Number of distractions, with a mean of 17.6 during the baseline phase, decreased during the intervention phase (M = 7.2) and increased during the intervention withdrawal phase (M = 10.4). Duration of self-stimulatory behavior, with a mean of 8.2 sec in the baseline phase, decreased in the intervention phase (M = 5.2 sec) and increased in the intervention withdrawal phase (M = 22.4 sec).

Figure 19.3 represents the data for Participant 3. Focused attention to task, with a mean of 115 sec in the baseline phase, increased in the intervention phase (M = 140 sec) and decreased in the intervention withdrawal phase (M = 105.8 sec). Number of distractions, with a mean of 17.2 during the baseline phase, decreased during the intervention phase (M = 7.2) and increased in the intervention withdrawal phase (M = 11.2). Duration of self-stimulatory behaviors, with a mean of 17.6 sec in the baseline phase, decreased during the intervention phase (M = 8.6 sec) and increased in the intervention withdrawal phase (M = 10.2 sec).

Figure 19.4 represents data for Participant 4. Focused attention to task, with a mean of 65.4 sec in the baseline phase, increased in the intervention phase (M = 101.8 sec) and decreased during the intervention withdrawal phase (M = 10.2 sec). Number of distractions, with a mean of 17.4 in the baseline phase, decreased in the intervention phase (M = 6.8) and gradually increased during the intervention withdrawal phase (M = 9.6). Duration of self-stimulatory behavior, with a mean of 227.6 sec in the baseline phase, decreased in the intervention phase (M = 99 sec) and decreased further during the intervention withdrawal phase (M = 75.8 sec).

Figure 19.5 represents data for Participant 5. Focused attention, with a mean of 95.2 sec in the baseline phase, increased in the intervention phase (M = 131.8 sec) and decreased during the intervention withdrawal phase (M = 92.2 sec). Number of distractions, with a mean of 14.2 in the baseline phase, decreased during the intervention phase (M = 3.8) and increased during the intervention withdrawal phase (M = 5.2). Duration of self-stimulatory behavior, with a mean of 61.6 in the baseline phase, decreased during the intervention phase (M = 19.2 sec) and remained low during the intervention withdrawal phase (M = 16.2 sec).

Visual analysis of Figures 19.1 through 19.5 supports the clinical observation that a weighted vest had a positive effect on at least two measures of attention for all five participants. The participants appeared less distractible and demonstrated fewer self-stimulatory behaviors. All showed an increase in the duration of focused attention while wearing a weighted vest, although the extent that a weighted vest influenced duration of focused attention varied among them. The mean value for the duration of focused attention during the intervention phase for Participant 2 would have been greater if not for a gap in the data for Session 10, a day when he went home ill. A weighted vest

(*text continues on page 226*)

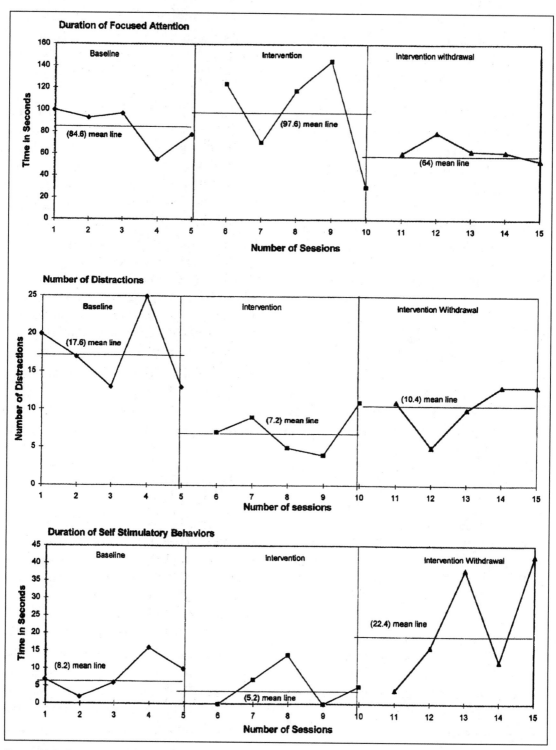

Figure 19.2. Duration of focused attention, number of distractions, and duration of self-stimulatory behaviors for Participant 2.

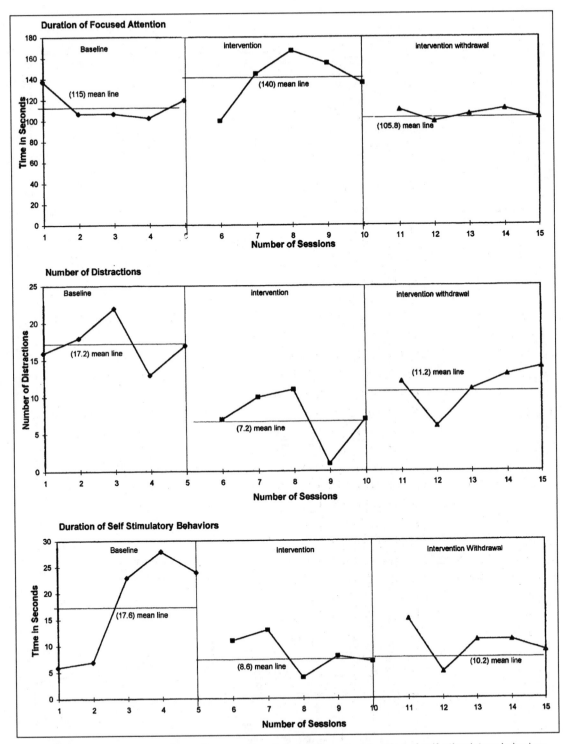

Figure 19.3. Duration of focused attention, number of distractions, and duration of self-stimulatory behaviors for Participant 3.

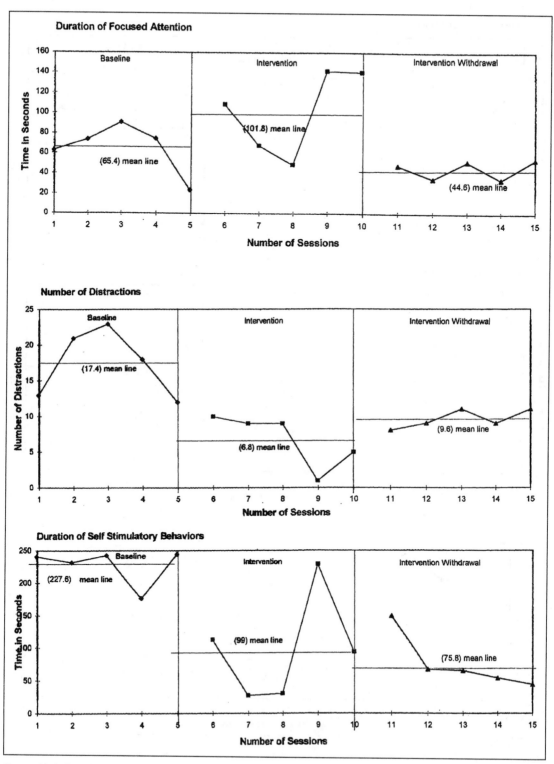

Figure 19.4. Duration of focused attention, number of distractions, and duration of self-stimulatory behaviors for Participant 4.

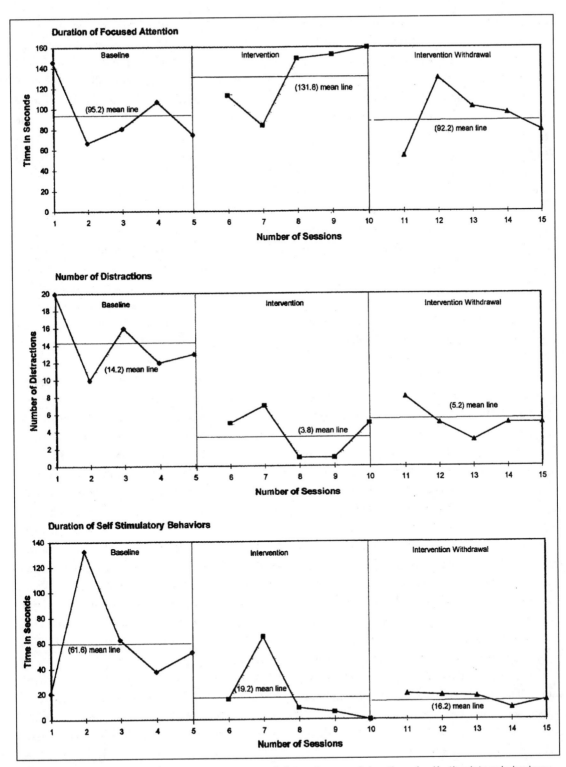

Figure 19.5. Duration of focused attention, number of distractions, and duration of self-stimulatory behaviors for Participant 5.

appeared to have the greatest impact on duration of focused attention for Participants 4 and 5 as well as on decreasing substantially the duration of their self-stimulatory behaviors.

The increase in the duration of focused attention that occurred during the intervention phase was not sustained when a weighted vest was removed. All five participants demonstrated a decrease in duration of focused attention during the intervention withdrawal phase; however, the duration of focused attention to task was less in the intervention withdrawal phase than in the initial baseline phase. After a weighted vest was removed, four participants demonstrated abrupt decreases in the duration of focused attention to task. This abrupt change was revealed through visual inspection of the data at Session 11 (the first session in which data were collected after the removal of a weighted vest). Although this information strengthens the support for the use of a weighted vest to increase duration of focused attention, it does not provide support for long-term effects once a vest is removed.

All the participants demonstrated a decrease in the number of distractions while wearing a weighted vest. Although distractibility varied among them, a weighted vest had the greatest impact on this measurement of attention to task. The most notable decrease in the number of distractions occurred for Participant 1, who was the smallest of the participants in this study. This finding could be an indication that the larger participants would have benefited from more weight in the vest. Although the number of distractions increased in the intervention withdrawal phase, this number never returned to the initial baseline values. This result may suggest that a weighted vest has some lasting effects, although the greatest effects were demonstrated during the intervention phase while the vest was worn.

It is also worth noting the immediate impact that a weighted vest had on the number of dis-

tractions. Visual inspection of Figures 19.1 through 19.5 demonstrates an abrupt drop in the number of distractions during the first session of the intervention phase for all participants. Participants 3 and 4 also demonstrated an abrupt decrease in the number of distractions in the fourth session. Participants 2, 3, 4, and 5 all displayed the lowest number of distractions during the fourth session. This finding may be important because data during the fourth session were collected after a weekend. One tentative explanation for this finding may be that the participants became accustomed to wearing the weighted vest after 3 days during the first week, thus reducing the vest's purported effects on decreasing distractibility. Further, the novelty of wearing the vest again after a weekend without wearing it may have renewed its initial effects on decreasing the number of distractions.

Four participants demonstrated a decrease in the duration of self-stimulatory behaviors while wearing a weighted vest. Participant 4, who during the initial baseline phase displayed the greatest frequency and duration of self-stimulatory behaviors, demonstrated the greatest reduction during the intervention phase. A weighted vest did not appear to have much of an impact on the duration of self-stimulatory behaviors for Participant 1, although the nature of the self-stimulatory behaviors changed and became less self-abusive for this child. While wearing a weighted vest, Participant 1 demonstrated less hand biting and no longer engaged in twirling objects, but the hand-staring behaviors increased.

On removal of a weighted vest, self-stimulatory behaviors increased for all participants. Although Participants 3, 4, and 5 demonstrated an increase in the duration of self-stimulatory behaviors during the intervention withdrawal phase compared with the intervention phase, this increase did not reach initial baseline levels.

Parents and teachers reported positive effects of a weighted vest. The classroom teacher indicated that Participant 1 was able to remain in her seat for longer periods while wearing the vest and that Participant 2's tantrums appeared to increase when the study was over. Two teachers reported that Participant 3 showed a decrease in aggressive behavior while wearing the weighted vest and an increase in aggressive behaviors during the period after it was removed. Informal observations and documentation from the teachers who worked with Participant 4 revealed a reduction in self-stimulatory behaviors during fine motor activities. The teachers and parents of Participant 5 reported an improvement in upright sitting posture while wearing a weighted vest.

The decrease in the duration of self-stimulatory behaviors, drop in the number of distractions, and increase in the duration of focused attention suggest that a weighted vest may be an effective intervention tool for clinicians, teachers, and parents of children with PDD. The observed changes in behavior (i.e., fewer aggressive episodes, self-stimulatory behaviors, and tantrums) are clinically significant. The reduction of these behaviors can improve the child's activity performance and participation in the classroom, community, and home.

Discussion

A weighted vest appeared to be beneficial for clinical use with five children with PDD who had difficulty attending to tasks and who exhibited self-stimulatory behaviors. The results of this study support parent and clinician observations that wearing a weighted vest produced calming effects and positive changes in attending behaviors for these children. However, additional research is necessary to establish more specific guidelines for intervention.

Questions arose about the amount of weight to use in the vest in relation to the children's weight. An association between the proportion of weight of the child and the effects of a weighted vest was apparent. For example, all participants' vests were weighted the same, and yet the smallest participant demonstrated the greatest decrease in the number of distractions.

The abrupt changes in behaviors and increased attention to task that occurred after a weekend may be related to the children being in a calmer, more structured environment after a possibly unstructured weekend at home. It is also important to note that Participant 4 demonstrated an increase in duration of focused attention that was accompanied by an increased duration of self-stimulatory behaviors. This latter finding may suggest that engaging in self-stimulatory behaviors may have supported or influenced the greater degree of focused attention demonstrated by Participant 4.

The results from this study cannot be generalized to a larger population because it was conducted with a small number of participants in one particular context. We suggest that a longer data collection period be used in future research. The addition of another intervention phase and a longer withdrawal phase could be useful in better determining lasting effects once a weighted vest is removed. On the basis of visual inspection of the data graphs, no positive latent effects were found from a weighted vest during the intervention withdrawal phase for duration of focused attention; however, beneficial latent effects in relation to the number of distractions were apparent. We also suggest that interobserver agreement be examined in all phases of the study to control for observer drift. Because of constraints in time and resources for the first author, interobserver agreement could be examined only during the baseline phase of this study.

One limitation of this study was the use of an ABA instead of a multiple baseline design because some behaviors did not exhibit reversibility or did not return to the baseline after the intervention phase (Kazdin, 1998; Ottenbacher, 1986). Based on clinical experience and with no contrary literature to state otherwise, we believed that the behaviors would return to baseline. Despite this design limitation, the results suggest positive outcomes from the use of a weighted vest for increasing the duration of attention to task and decreasing the number of distractions. Additional research is necessary to build a consensus about the effectiveness of wearing a weighted vest to increase attention to task and decrease self-stimulatory behaviors. Replicating this study in other contexts or examining other guidelines for the use of a weighted vest can do this.

Conclusion

The results from this single-subject study provide preliminary support for the use of the weighted vest with children with PDD who have difficulty attending to tasks and exhibit self-stimulatory behaviors. All participants exhibited a decrease in the number of distractions and an increase in focused attention while wearing the weighted vest. All but one participant demonstrated a decrease in the duration of self-stimulatory behaviors while wearing the vest. Additional research is needed to examine further the effectiveness of wearing the weighted vest to increase attention to task and decrease self-stimulatory behaviors.

Acknowledgments

We thank Howard Kaplan, PhD; Dawn Leger, PhD; Anne Buckley Reen and Virginia Clark for The Kiddie Vest™; and the participants, their families, and the staff from Challenge Infant Developmental Center. This study was partially funded by the U.S. Department of Health and Human Services, Maternal and Child Health Grant MCJ369289.

This chapter was completed as part of the first author's requirements for the master of arts degree in the School of Education at New York University.

References

American Psychiatric Association. (1994). *Diagnostic and statistical manual of mental disorders* (4th ed.). Washington, DC: Author.

Ayres, A. J. (1987). *Sensory integration and the child.* Los Angeles: Western Psychological Services.

Ayres, A. J., & Tickle, L. S. (1980). Hyper-responsivity to touch and vestibular stimuli as a predictor of positive response to sensory integration procedures by autistic children. *American Journal of Occupational Therapy, 34,* 375–381.

Dunn, W., & Fisher, A. G. (1983). Sensory registration, autism, and tactile defensiveness. *Sensory Integration Special Interest Newsletter, 6*(2), 3–4.

Edelson, S. M., Edelson, M. G., Kerr, D. C. R., & Grandin, T. (1999). Behavioral and physiological effects of deep pressure on children with autism: A pilot study evaluating the efficacy of Grandin's hug machine. *American Journal of Occupational Therapy, 53,* 145–152.

Grandin, T. (1992). Calming effects of deep pressure in patients with autistic disorder, college students, and animals. *Journal of Child and Adolescent Pharmacology, 2,* 63–72.

Joe, B. E. (1998, May 21). Are weighted vests worth their weight? *OT Week, 12,* pp. 12–13.

Kazdin, A. E. (1982). *Single case research designs: Methods for clinical and applied settings.* New York: Oxford University Press.

Kazdin, A. E. (1998). *Research designs in clinical psychology* (3rd ed.). Needham Heights, MA: Allyn & Bacon.

Kientz, M. A., & Dunn, W. (1997). A comparison of the performance of children with and without autism on the Sensory Profile. *American Journal of Occupational Therapy, 51,* 530–537.

Kimball, G. J. (1999). Sensory integration frame of reference: Theoretical base, function/dysfunction continua, and guide to evaluation. In P. Kramer & J. Hinojosa (Eds.), *Frames of reference for pediatric occupational therapy* (2nd ed., pp.119–168). Baltimore: Lippincott Williams & Wilkins.

King, L. J., & Grandin, T. (1990). *Attention deficits in learning disorders and autism: A sensory-integrative treatment approach.* Workshop presented at the conference of the Continuing Education Programs of America, Milwaukee, WI.

Kootz, J. P., Marinelli, B., & Cohen, D. J. (1981). Sensory receptor hypersensitivity in autistic children. *Archives of General Psychiatry, 38,* 271–273.

Lovaas, I. O. (1981). *Teaching developmentally disabled children: The me book.* Austin, TX: PRO-ED.

Lovaas, I. O. (1987). Behavioral treatment and normal educational and intellectual functioning in young autistic children. *Journal of Consulting and Clinical Psychology, 55,* 3–9.

McClure, M. K., & Holtz-Yotz, M. (1991). Case Report—The effects of sensory stimulatory treatment on an autistic child. *American Journal of Occupational Therapy, 45,* 1138–1142.

Microsoft Corporation. (1995). Microsoft Excel for Windows 95 (version 7.0) [Computer software]. Roselle, WA: Author.

Ornitz, E. M. (1985). Neurophysiology of infantile autism. *Journal of American Academy of Child Psychiatry, 24,* 251–262.

Ottenbacher, K. (1986). *Evaluating clinical change: Strategies for occupational and physical therapists.* Baltimore: Williams & Wilkins.

Ruff, H. A., & Lawson, K. R. (1991). Assessment of infant's attention during play with objects. In C. E. Schaefer, K. Gitlin, & A. Sandgrund (Eds.), *Play diagnosis and assessment* (pp. 115–129). New York: Wiley.

Takagi, K., & Kobayasi, S. (1955). Skin pressure vegetative reflex. *Acta Medica et Biologica, 4,* 31–57.

Wilbarger, P. (1995, June). The sensory diet: Activity programs based on sensory processing theory. *Sensory Integration Special Interest Section Newsletter, 18,* pp. 1–4.

Zissermann, L. (1992). Case Report: The effects of deep pressure on self-stimulating behaviors in a child with autism and other disabilities. *American Journal of Occupational Therapy, 46,* 547–551.

CHAPTER 20

The Effects of Hands-on Occupation Versus Demonstration on Children's Recall Memory

Beth A. Hartman, Barbara Kopp Miller, and David L. Nelson

Beth A. Hartman, MOT, *is occupational therapist, First Step Autism Program, Fond du Lac, WI. She was an occupational therapy student at the Medical College of Ohio, Toledo, at the time of this study.*

Barbara Kopp Miller, PhD, *is associate professor, Medical College of Ohio, 3015 Arlington Avenue, Toledo, OH 43614-5803; bkoppmiller@mco.edu.*

David L. Nelson, PhD, OTR/L, FAOTA, *is professor, Medical College of Ohio, Toledo.*

The eminent American philosopher and educator John Dewey (1916/1966, p. 202) advocated the use of "active occupations," including play as well as work, as the best means for promoting learning and education in healthy children and other citizens. Dewey valued active, hands-on occupations that are "carried on for their own sake" (p. 205) as contexts for students to obtain skill and information. Dewey stated that the powers of observation and recollection depend on occupation. Observation leading to learning takes place when the person "has something to do which can be accomplished successfully only through intensive and extensive use of hand and eye" (p. 66). In a learning occupation, "each earlier act prepares the way for later acts, while these take account of and reckon with the results already attained" (p. 337). Learning is an outcome of the enhanced sensation provided by occupation, as well as the observed changes wrought in the occupational process. Dewey argued that the occupational approach to learning is superior to the traditional educational method of training the mental faculties through "monotonously uniform exercise" (p. 66).

Dewey's thoughts concerning occupation and learning in healthy citizens influenced the founders of occupational therapy, who were attempting to use active occupations for the betterment of persons with impairments and disabilities. Tracy (1910, p. 13) explicitly cited the philosophy of John Dewey in describing the power of occupation in improving the recovery of hospitalized persons. Later, Slagle (1922) also cited Dewey's ideas as influential to the field of occupational therapy (see also Breines, 1986, for a description of the work relationships between early occupational therapists and associates of Dewey).

From the beginning of the profession of occupational therapy, the benefits of occupation were seen as extending to both the mind and the body (Kidner, 1930; Slagle, 1922). In 1925, a committee of the American Occupational Therapy Association stated that one of the principal psychological aims of occupation used with patients was to improve "concentration of attention" (Dunton, Adams, Carr,

Originally published 2000 in *American Journal of Occupational Therapy,* *54,* 477–483.

& Robinson, 1925). Dunton (1928) was explicit in noting the relationships between occupation and the mental processes of observation, concentration, and memory. Tracy (1910) had called for the use of occupations in the treatment of persons with mental deficiencies, whether developmental or acquired. Therapeutic occupation could simultaneously be an intervention for improving movement, emotional well-being, and the processes of thinking. As Meyer (1922, p. 5) stated, "It is the use that we make of ourselves that gives the ultimate stamp to our every organ."

Given the profession's commitment to occupation as a context for learning, it is ironic that little research can be identified in the occupational therapy literature that directly addresses this issue. In his Eleanor Clarke Slagle lecture, Nelson (1997) recognized this:

> For decades, occupational therapists have used common, everyday occupational forms and hands-on doing to enhance what Dunton (1945, p. 11), one of the founders, called the "mental processes of reasoning or judgment or remembering." Recently, cognitive researchers, mainly psychologists, have developed a body of knowledge concerning the effects of "subject-performed tasks," or SPTs, on human cognition (for example, please see Backman, 1985). The basic idea of SPTs is that hands-on doing, with its added sensory input and opportunity for feedback, is a greater cognitive stimulant than demonstration or other teaching techniques not involving hands-on experience. The problem is that the cognitive psychologists pursuing this line of research have not cited occupational therapy authors, who have advocated this principle since the beginning of the profession. Our problem here is that we have not done the research necessary to establish our special expertise in the area of hands-on doing, or occupation.

Nelson (1988, 1994) defined *occupation* as a special relationship between occupational form and occupational performance. *Occupational form* is the physical and sociocultural situation external to the person. Depending on the person's developmental structure, an occupational form can become subjectively meaningful for a person. This may lead to a sense of purposefulness and active, voluntary occupational performance. In the very act of doing something with meaning and purpose, the person adapts, or changes. The person also changes the world (impact) (see Figure 20.1).

Dewey and the early occupational therapists suggested that the opportunity for transforming materials in socioculturally recognizable ways is a key component for learning. We can think of this opportunity as part of the occupational form of an occupation. A therapist or an educator is viewed as an opportunity giver, as opposed to someone who imparts information by talking. As the learner pursues the opportunity with meaning and purpose, active occupational performance results in impacts. These products of the changing occupational form provide opportunities for feedback (evolving meanings). Two types of feedback are involved: sensory/perceptual meanings originating potentially in each of the sensory systems and symbolic meanings involving judgments as to the ongoing success of the occupation. A judgment of sociocultural success is the degree to which the impact matches sociocultural norms, whereas the judgment of personal success is the degree to which the impact matches one's own purposes (Nelson, 1994).

An occupational form involving the opportunity for transforming materials is theorized to be more meaningful to many people than other kinds of instruction because of the sensory/perceptual and symbolic feedback. As the person transforms materials, tactile and proprioceptive inputs (and sometimes vestibular, olfactory, or gustatory inputs) are experienced in combination with visual and auditory inputs in ways that are not possible when attending a lecture or a demon-

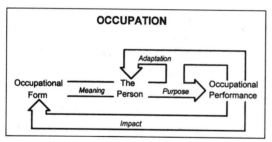

Figure 20.1. Occupation.
Note. Copyright © D. Nelson, 1994. Reprinted with permission.

stration. In addition, it is theorized that the experience of success through one's own active doing makes the occupation memorable.

Occupational therapists have done little to demonstrate the effects of occupation on verbal learning and memory. An exception is the research by Yuen, Nelson, Peterson, and Dickinson (1994), who studied the learning of a novel motor task. In this study, an occupational form providing feedback to movement was compared with a free-movement condition within the context of mastering an upper extremity training prosthesis. The researchers theorized that the added affordance provided by the feedback was responsible for the superior learning documented in the study.

Those outside the field of occupational therapy who have studied the effects of subject-performed tasks (tasks performed by the individual) include Backman (1985); Karlsson et al. (1989); Larsson and Ronnberg (1987); Hutton, Sheppard, Rusted, and Ratner (1996); Zimmer and Saathoff (1997), and Vakil, Hoffman, and Myzliek (1998). In general, these studies have found that individuals who engage in subject-performed tasks recall more than those engaged in passive learning. For example, Larsson and Ronnberg (1987) reported that subject-performed tasks elicited considerably higher levels of both immediate and long-term recall than passive

learning situations. Vakil et al. (1998) found that active learning left relatively durable traces in memory and resulted in an enhanced ability to solve an advanced problem related to the training task.

Only three prior experiments have addressed the issue of active versus passive learning from an occupational therapy perspective. Warner (1989) coined the term "hands-on occupation" as a label that recognized the historical importance of work with the hands within the profession of occupational therapy. Twenty-nine older women with moderate mental impairments were randomly assigned to either a demonstration with a hands-on occupation or a demonstration-only occupation. The demonstration-only group observed the researcher making ice cream, while the hands-on group both observed the researcher and practiced making ice cream. At the end of the occupation, both groups were given a written task-related quiz designed as a measurement of memory retention. The questions were based on information that could have been learned through the occupation in either condition (e.g., Should the ice cream custard be cooked over low, medium, or high flame?) A *t* test supported the hypothesis that participants in the hands-on occupation had higher memory retention than participants in the demonstration-only occupation.

Eakman and Nelson (in press) continued this line of research by comparing the effects of hands-on occupation with verbal training on free recall. Thirty men (mean age = 29.6) who had sustained brain injuries were randomly assigned to two experimental conditions. Individuals in the hands-on occupation received step-by-step verbal instructions on how to make meatballs as well as hands-on practice of each step; participants in the verbal training received step-by-step instructions only. After the final step for both groups, participants were asked to recall the steps involved in making meatballs in their proper order. A Mann–

Whitney *U* test supported the hypothesis that participants in the hands-on occupation recalled significantly more task steps in their proper order than participants in the verbal occupation.

Buddelmeyer (1995) extended the work of Eakman and Nelson (in press). Sixty children with learning disabilities between 8 and 13 years of age were randomly assigned in subgroups to either a hands-on occupation or to verbal training. Children in the hands-on occupation received step-by-step verbal instructions on how to make a modeling compound as well as hands-on practice of each step. Children in the verbal training condition received step-by-step instructions only. After the final step for both groups, the children were asked to recall the steps involved in making the compound in their proper order. A *t* test supported the hypothesis that children in the hands-on occupation group had higher memory retention than children in the verbal training condition.

Continued studies with children in the area of hands-on learning are needed in the occupational therapy profession. Occupational therapists play a critical role in the provision of educational services and, as authorized by law, their role in the school system is to provide services that are directly related to helping students meet their educational needs (Drummond, 1996; Sarracino & Hanft, 1996). Learning and retaining new information are primary educational needs, and occupational therapists can play an important role in assisting students to meet these needs. One way in which occupational therapists can enhance student learning is by modifying methods of instruction to best match individual learning styles.

In contrast to previous studies, the current study focuses on children without impairments or disabilities. While one study in occupational therapy focused on children with learning disabilities (Buddelmeyer, 1995), no published study has compared hands-on occupation versus demonstration in terms of healthy children's verbal recall ability. The participants in the current study were 3rd-grade children between 7 and 9 years of age. This age was chosen based on the literature of cognitive development. While recognition memory is well developed by the end of the preschool years, recall memory occurs after the development of recognition memory. At approximately 7 years of age, a child progresses to the concrete-operations level of cognitive development (Piaget, 1981), when recall memory development begins to occur (Ginsberg & Opper, 1988).

In previous studies of hands-on learning, the dependent variable involved a combination of the number of instructions recalled and the correctness of the order of recall. In the current study, it was decided to treat these two factors as separate dependent variables. It is possible that hands-on learning affects the two variables differently.

In the current study, it was important to select an occupational form that would provide an appealing learning situation to 3rd-grade children. An informal survey of six grade school teachers indicated that school-age children often found science experiments meaningful and enjoyable. Based on this information and a review of science curriculum literature, the construction of an "erupting volcano" was chosen. Building a model of a volcano was educationally relevant to a science curriculum while providing an opportunity to experience either hands-on learning or passive instruction via demonstration.

Based on occupational therapy principles and prior studies supporting the use of hands-on occupation to enhance learning, two directional hypotheses were made. It was hypothesized that participants engaged in a hands-on teaching method embedded in a meaningful and purposeful occupation would have a greater recall score than participants engaged in a demonstration teaching method. It also was hypothesized that participants who engaged in a hands-on teaching method would recall more task steps in their proper order than participants who engaged in a demonstration teaching method.

Method

Participants

Administrators of five midwestern schools were invited to participate in the study; three expressed interest. Of these three, one was excluded from participation because the children had recently completed a science unit that involved building models of volcanoes. A packet of information including a consent form, a brief description of the study, and a letter of support from school officials was distributed to all children enrolled in the 3rd grade at the two participating schools. Participants were required to be free from developmental disorders, to be between 7 and 9 years of age, and to have no previous experience with making a model of a volcano.

Eighty-three children (39 boys and 44 girls) turned in permission slips and were allowed to participate in the study (60 children from one school and 23 children from the second school). Ten children did not meet the study's requirements, and although they were allowed to participate in making the volcano, their results were not included in the data analysis. Eight of the 10 children became ineligible after the testing was under way (one became sick, one did not want to be recorded, six reported making volcanoes in the past). Testing of the participants occurred over an 8-week period.

Materials

The following materials were used in both the hands-on and the demonstration conditions: 10 lb of sand, 9 in. by 11 in. foil roasting pan, small plastic sandbox shovel, 18 oz aluminum can, empty 18 oz plastic tumbler, 8 in. plastic spoon, 8 oz plastic measuring cup, plastic mea-

suring cup (1/4 cup), plastic measuring cup (1/3 cup), 16 oz box of baking soda, 20 oz plastic bottle of dishwashing liquid, 20 oz plastic bottle of white vinegar, 1 oz plastic bottle of red food coloring, 16 oz plastic cup filled with lukewarm water, eyedropper, and plastic tablecloth. In both conditions, a digital kitchen timer was used to regulate the allotted response time, and a tape recorder and cassette tape were used to record participant recall.

Procedure

Informed consent was obtained from all participants and their parents or legal guardians before they were allowed to participate. Students were randomly assigned to the hands-on condition ($n = 42$) or the demonstration condition ($n = 41$). Each participant was seen individually by the researcher. In both conditions, the participant was seated at a table, directly across from the investigator. Participants in the demonstration condition observed the investigator making a model of a volcano, while participants in the hands-on condition made a model of a volcano by themselves (the investigator did not make a volcano in the hands-on condition). Immediately before each of the 11 steps in making the volcano (see Appendix), the investigator read aloud the instructions printed on a 5 in. by 7 in. note card. Participants verbally repeated each instruction within 5 sec before proceeding. Both the investigator in the demonstration condition and the participants in the hands-on condition had 30 sec to complete each step, which proved adequate. Each condition lasted approximately 15 min.

In both conditions, the materials were kept out of sight until they were needed. Once materials were used and were no longer needed, they were removed from view. Following both conditions, the investigator asked three distractor questions to divert participants from rehearsing the steps. Next, each participant was given an opportunity to be excused if he or she did not want to be tape recorded. If the participant agreed to be tape recorded, he or she was asked to state the exact steps involved in making the volcano. None of the students exceeded the 210 sec allotted for a response. If the participant indicated that he or she could not remember any more steps, recording was stopped. If the participant was silent for 10 sec, the participant was instructed to try to remember the steps. If the participant remained silent for an additional 10 sec, the participant was asked if he or she could remember any more steps. If the participant responded no, the recording ended. If the participant responded yes, he or she was prompted to tell them. If the participant failed to respond to this verbal prompt within 10 sec, the recording ended. Prompts were neutral and consistent across both conditions.

Scoring

The participants' responses were transcribed and scored by the investigator. A research assistant coded the cassette tapes so that the investigator was unaware of the condition being scored. The steps presented to the participants were divided into syntactical units, with each unit having a value of one point. A syntactical unit was defined as a verb, an object of a verb, or a prepositional phrase (e.g., "Make/hill/with sand" equaled three syntactical units and therefore three possible points). See the Appendix for the 11 steps and the analysis of syntactical units. Substitution of functional synonyms was allowed. For the dependent variable free recall, the score was the number of syntactical units recalled correctly. The total possible score for free recall was 41. For order, a point was rewarded if a task step was recalled in its correct slot of order. For a step to be considered recalled, at least two of its syntactical units had to be recalled. The total possible score for order was 11.

Results

Data analysis was based on the results of 73 children, with 36 children (17 boys and 19 girls) participating in the hands-on condition and 37 children (14 boys and 23 girls) participating in the demonstration condition.

Interrater Reliability

To test for interrater reliability, a research assistant who was blind to the purpose, hypotheses, and conditions of the study was recruited to rescore 25 randomly selected tape recordings of the participants. The Shrout and Fleiss (1979) intraclass correlation coefficient for fixed effects was used. This procedure assesses interrater agreement between a specified set of raters (in this case, two raters). A .990 agreement was found for free recall scores, and a .994 agreement was found for order scores.

Hypotheses Testing

An alpha level of .05 was used for all statistical tests. Participants in the hands-on condition had a mean recall score of 22.81 (SD = 6.87), while participants in the demonstration condition had a mean recall score of 17.97 (SD = 8.68). A one-tailed t test confirmed that hands-on occupation led to significantly more recall than the demonstration condition, t (71) = 2.63, p < .005. The effect size d equaled .62, a moderate effect according to Cohen (1988).

Participants in the hands-on condition had a mean order score of 4.17 (SD = 3.36), and participants in the demonstration condition had a mean order score of 3.32 (SD = 3.47). The task step order scores were not normally distributed and lacked variance; therefore, a Mann–Whitney U test was used. No statistically significant difference was found between the two conditions. Effect size was not calculated because of problems with this measurement.

Discussion

The results for the recall variable of the current study are consistent with the results of past studies involving the effects of hands-on learning on children's recall ability (Buddelmeyer, 1995; Vessey, 1988). Vessey (1988) found that an approach involving oral presentations and hands-on student participation led to greater recall and recognition scores than either a demonstration approach or a control group. Buddelmeyer (1995) found that children with learning disabilities who participated in hands-on learning remembered more than those who learned by demonstration. The results of the current study also are consistent with the results of prior studies involving healthy adults of various ages (Vakil et al., 1998) as well as adults with cognitive impairments (Eakman & Nelson, in press; Warner, 1989).

These results support traditional principles and practices within occupational therapy as well as the principles of pragmatism as espoused by Dewey (1916/1966). Learning by doing is characteristic of occupational therapy. The question is, what are the components of hands-on learning that make it more effective than passive styles of learning? The occupational form of volcano making provides an excellent example of the special potentials of hands-on learning. Occupational analysis (Nelson, 1994) suggests that the making of a volcano provided the child with special opportunities for two types of feedback: sensory/perceptual meanings as well as symbolic meanings. The sensory/perceptual meanings included the tactile, proprioceptive, and visual experiences enjoyed as the child made a mound out of the sand and dug a hole in the middle of the sand. Sand has a gritty texture, sticks to the hands, and provides some resistance to digging. The measuring of items such as baking soda, soap, vinegar, water, and food coloring provided proprioceptive and tactile sensations of

weight that are integrated with visual information. In contrast, the demonstration condition provided no special tactile and proprioceptive perception, and the visual and auditory inputs of the demonstration and instructions were not integrated with somatosensory input. In like manner, the smell of the vinegar was present in both experimental conditions, but it could be integrated with tactile and proprioceptive input only in the hands-on condition.

The other type of meaning that was possible in the hands-on condition was symbolic in nature. In the hands-on condition the child had the opportunity to experience success at each stage of the occupation (each suboccupation). The child was able to see that his or her own occupational performance resulted in a product (an impact) that matched the rules for this occupational form, as represented in the instructions. The final reward for hands-on doing was the visually striking image of an erupting volcano. This repeated subjective experience of personal success was not possible in the demonstration condition where the child could only observe the success of an adult.

Prior research in the area of subject-performed tasks has emphasized the sensory/perceptual meanings of hands-on occupation. For example, Vessey (1988) discussed the importance of the multisensory nature of active learning. However, the importance of symbolic meaning is also important. The sense of personal efficacy that one gets by doing something well (according to personal and sociocultural criteria) is an additional component to hands-on learning. The question arises, which type of meaning—sensory/perceptual or symbolic—is more responsible for memory and recall? Is there a difference depending on what is being learned? Is there a difference depending on the duration of the learning, or the capacity of the person to transfer the learning to increasingly complex situations? These are important areas for future research, but it will be difficult to separate the sensory/perceptual aspects of an occupation from the symbolic aspects, because the two are typically found in hands-on learning. As with many occupational phenomena, hands-on learning is naturally multidimensional.

In the current study, the results for the order variable were ambiguous. This ambiguity may reflect a problem in how the order variable was scored. If a participant skipped a step, the remaining steps were automatically in the incorrect order slots. A review of raw data revealed that many of the participants in both conditions had difficulty remembering the fourth step; therefore, they received scores of three or less. This resulted in skewness and lack of variance for the order variable. Therefore, the statistical test of order may not reflect participants' actual memory of order. The authors continue to believe that the separate study of order has potential value, because successful completion of many occupations depends on order. For example, careful attention to proper order is necessary for safety and independence in wheelchair mobility and transfers. Further study of hands-on occupation should operationalize order in a way that does not excessively penalize errors early in the sequence.

Limitations

The present study had several limitations. One limitation was that the principal investigator administered the experiment. To help control against bias, the investigator followed a strict protocol for administration and scoring of the results. When scoring the tape recordings, the investigator was blind to experimental condition. Additionally, a research assistant independently scored 25 of the tape recordings for interrater reliability.

Another limitation was the limited number of schools that participated. While five schools were invited to participate, only two schools took part. The two schools used in the study were

diverse in nature, but a larger, more heterogeneous sample could have improved the representativeness of the sample. Another problem was that different testing settings were used at each school, and all of the participants were tested at different times and days of the week.

A final limitation was the use of a tape recorder to score the participant's responses. The tape recorder was an unnatural aspect of the occupational form and may have affected some of the participants' responses. Some of the participants appeared hesitant and nervous to be tape recorded, which may have had a negative effect on their recall performance. However, this was balanced across the two experimental conditions.

In addition to correcting the above limitations and developing a better way to score the task step order variable, future studies could examine the effects of hands-on doing on long-term recall performance. Participants could be scored once at the completion of the task and then again after a specified time period. Another idea would be to test procedural memory by measuring how well subjects complete the task after some specified time period (as opposed to asking them to state verbally the steps involved). Future studies may also include other age groups, especially older persons, and may incorporate different occupations from the one utilized in this study. Almost all the clinical populations seen by occupational therapists, whether with cognitive impairments or not, need to learn multistep procedures. Do they learn more effectively through hands-on occupation than by other methods?

Conclusion

The results demonstrated that participants were able to recall more information when engaged in a hands-on teaching method versus a demonstration method. The findings of this study have important implications for both education and occupational therapy. Active learning and participation in meaningful occupation have been at the core of occupational therapy since its inception. This study contributes to the establishment of a valid base of research supporting the principle of hands-on learning.

Acknowledgments

The authors thank the students, parents, and staff of St. Joseph School in Sylvania, Ohio, and Ottawa River Elementary School in Toledo, Ohio. The first author thanks the Student Research Grant Program at the American Occupational Therapy Foundation and the Graduate School Research Award Program at the Medical College of Ohio for providing the funding for this project. The first author also offers special thanks to Beth Samuelson-Schultz, OTR/L, and Liz Jorling, OTR/L, for their encouragement, help, and support.

Appendix

Instructions and Syntactical Units

Make/hill/with sand. (3)
Remove/sand/from top and center/of hill. (4)
Place/can/in center/of hill. (4)
Measure/baking soda. (2)
Put/baking soda/in can. (3)
Measure/soap,/vinegar,/and water. (4)
Add/soap,/vinegar,/and water/to plastic cup. (5)
Stir/soap,/vinegar,/and water/with spoon. (5)
Add/three drops/of red food coloring/to the
    plastic cup/with the eyedropper. (5)
Stir/with spoon. (2)
Pour/mixture/into can/in sand. (4)

References

Backman, L. (1985). Further evidence for the lack of adult age differences on free recall of subject-performed tasks: The importance of motor action. *Human Learning, 4,* 79–85.

Breines, E. (1986). *Origins and adaptations: A philosophy of practice.* Lebanon, NJ: Geri-Rehab.

Buddelmeyer, S. L. (1995). *Hands-on versus verbal occupation: The effect on free recall in learning disabled children.* Unpublished master's project, Medical College of Ohio, Toledo.

Cohen, J. (1988). *Statistical power analysis for the behavioral sciences* (2nd ed.). Hillsdale, NJ: Erlbaum.

Dewey, J. (1966). *Democracy and education.* New York: Macmillan. (Original work published 1916).

Drummond, C. W. (1996). Inclusion and school-based occupational therapy. *School System Special Interest Section Newsletter, 3*(3), 1–3.

Dunton, W. R., Jr. (1928). *Prescribing occupational therapy.* Springfield, IL: Charles C Thomas.

Dunton, W. R., Jr. (1945). *Prescribing occupational therapy* (2nd ed.). Springfield, IL: Charles C Thomas.

Dunton, W. R., Jr., Adams, B. W., Carr, B. W., & Robinson, G. C. (1925). An outline of lectures on occupational therapy to medical students and physicians. *Occupational Therapy and Rehabilitation, 4,* 277–292.

Eakman, A. M., & Nelson, D. L. (in press). The effect of hands-on occupation on recall memory in men with traumatic brain injury. *Occupational Therapy Journal of Research.*

Ginsberg, H., & Opper, S. (1988). *Piaget's theory of intellectual development* (3rd ed.). Englewood Cliffs, NJ: Prentice Hall.

Hutton, S., Sheppard, L., Rusted, J. M., & Ratner, H. H. (1996). Structuring the acquisition and retrieval environment to facilitate learning in individuals with dementia of Alzheimer type. *Memory, 4*(2), 113–130.

Karlsson, T., Backman, L., Herlitz, A., Nilsson, L. G., Winblad, B., & Osterlind, P. O. (1989). Memory improvements at different stages of Alzheimer's disease. *Neuropsychologia, 27*(5), 737–742.

Kidner, T. B. (1930). *Occupational therapy: The science of prescribed work for invalids.* Stuttgart, Germany: W. Kohlhammer.

Larsson, C., & Ronnberg, J. (1987). Memory disorders as a function of traumatic brain injury. *Scandinavian Journal of Rehabilitation Medicine, 19,* 99–104.

Meyer, A. (1922). The philosophy of occupational therapy. *Archives of Occupational Therapy, 1,* 1–10.

Nelson, D. L. (1988). Occupation: Form and performance. *American Journal of Occupational Therapy, 42,* 633–641.

Nelson, D. L. (1994). Occupational form, occupational performance, and therapeutic occupation. In C. B. Royeen (Ed.), *AOTA Self-Study Series: The practice of the future: Putting occupation back into therapy* (Lesson 2, pp. 9–48). Rockville, MD: American Occupational Therapy Association.

Nelson, D. L. (1997). Why the profession of occupational therapy will continue to flourish in the twenty-first century [1996 Eleanor Clarke Slagle Lecture]. *American Journal of Occupational Therapy, 51,* 11–24.

Piaget, J. (1981). *The psychology of intelligence.* Totowa, NJ: Littlefield, Adams & Co.

Sarracino, T., & Hanft, B. (1996). Developing state guidelines for school-based therapy. *School System Special Interest Section Newsletter, 3*(1), 1–4.

Shrout, P. E., & Fleiss, J. L. (1979). Intraclass correlations: Uses in assessing rater reliability. *Psychological Bulletin, 86,* 420–428.

Slagle, E. C. (1922). Training aides for mental patients. *Archives of Occupational Therapy, 1,* 11–17.

Tracy, S. E. (1910). *Studies in invalid occupation: A manual for nurses and attendants.* Boston: Whitcomb & Barrows.

Vakil, E., Hoffman, Y., & Myzliek, D. (1998). Active versus passive procedural learning in older and younger adults. *Neuropsychological Rehabilitation, 8*(1), 31–41.

Vessey, J. A. (1988). Comparison of two teaching methods on children's knowledge of their internal bodies. *Nursing Research, 37,* 262–267.

Warner, D. A. (1989). *Hands-on purposeful activity and short-term memory retention in elderly patients with cognitive deficits.* Unpublished master's thesis, Western Michigan University, Kalamazoo.

Yuen, H. K., Nelson, D. L., Peterson, C. Q., & Dickinson, A. (1994). Prosthesis training as a context for studying occupational forms and motoric adaptation. *American Journal of Occupational Therapy, 48,* 55–61.

Zimmer, H. D., & Saathoff, J. (1997). The influence of enactment on short-term recognition. *Acta Psychologia, 95*(1), 85–95.

CHAPTER 21

Children With Burn Injuries

Purposeful Activity Versus Rote Exercise

Kim Melchert-McKearnan, Jean Deitz, Joyce M. Engel, and Owen White

Kim Melchert-McKearnan, MS, OTR/L, *is research consultant, University of Washington, and occupational therapist, Harborview Medical Center, Seattle. At the time of this study, she was a graduate student, Department of Rehabilitation Medicine, University of Washington, Seattle. Mailing address: 1022 North 48th Street, Seattle, WA 98103.*

Jean Deitz, PhD, OTR, FAOTA, *is professor, Department of Rehabilitation Medicine, University of Washington, Seattle.*

Joyce M. Engel, PhD, OTR, FAOTA, *is associate professor, Department of Rehabilitation Medicine, University of Washington, Seattle.*

Owen White, PhD, *is professor, Department of Education, University of Washington, Seattle.*

Originally published 2000 in *American Journal of Occupational Therapy,* 54, 381–390.

Historically rooted in the foundations of occupational therapy is the premise that purposeful and meaningful activities may be used to evaluate, improve, or maintain a person's ability to participate in occupations. *Purposeful activity* is the term most often used in occupational therapy literature to identify the therapeutic activities that are goal directed and characterized by purpose and meaning as determined by the person participating in the activity (American Occupational Therapy Association [AOTA], 1993, 1995; Katz, Marcus, & Weiss, 1994). Both purposefulness and meaningfulness are thought to increase effort and time spent pursuing an activity because cognitive, social, and emotional sources of motivation are accessed through added purpose and meaning. Additionally, the engaged person receives immediate feedback regarding the application of such activities in daily life (Dutton, 1989; Trombly, 1995). Although a number of studies have specifically focused on the effectiveness of using purposeful activity versus rote exercise or nonpurposeful activity (Hsieh, Nelson, Smith, & Peterson, 1996; Katz et al., 1994; Nelson et al., 1996; Van der Weel, van der Meer, & Lee, 1991; Wu, Trombly, & Lin, 1994), only one of these studies (Van der Weel et al., 1991) concentrated on this issue using pediatric participants.

Occupation has been defined as "an individual's active participation in self-maintenance, work, leisure, and play" (AOTA, 1994, p. 912). Play is often recognized as the primary occupation of children and is designated as a developmental phenomenon that contributes to the evolution of other occupations such as work, activities of daily living, and leisure (Knox, 1993; Pratt, 1989). Play has been described as a developmentally appropriate and powerful medium for evaluation of occupational performance skills and for interventions to improve or maintain these skills (Knox, 1993; Pratt, 1989). Play, as used in therapy, may vary depending on the age and motivation of the player, the theoretical perspective of the therapist, the environment, and the purpose (Burke, 1993;

Knox, 1993). Play may be used as a modality to assess and promote sensorimotor, cognitive, and psychosocial function or to address the occupational behaviors of play (Burke, 1993; Pratt, 1989). Play also has been postulated to be an effective nonpharmacological intervention for pain relief in children (McGrath, 1990).

Pain may be defined as "an unpleasant sensory and emotional experience associated with actual or potential tissue damage, or described in terms of such damage" (Merskey, 1986, p. 5217) and is noted as invariably subjective in nature. In addition to these immediate neurophysiological, emotional, and psychological elements associated with the perception of a noxious stimulus, Parker and Cinciripini (1984) also noted the ensuing behavior problems and subjective reports of discomfort and distress that often accompany a pain experience. The formulation of an operational definition for pain is further complicated when addressing pain in children. This is due to developmental factors such as a limited vocabulary, which may affect the ability to describe a pain experience (Tyler, 1990; Varni, 1983).

The evaluation of pain has included the measurement of physiological responses, self-report, and the observation of overt behaviors (Sanders, 1979). Several physiological responses have been examined for their relation to pain, including heart rate, blood pressure, palmar sweating, oxygenation changes, and endocrine responses (Carter, 1994; Marvin, 1995; McGrath, 1990). It is difficult, however, to identify pain as the sole impetus for these physiological changes. Other stress responses to noxious stimuli, such as anxiety, may contribute to these changes. Therefore, physiological responses may not be accurate measures of pain (Hester, 1993; McGrath, 1990).

Covert pain behaviors are measured via self-reports. Examples of such measures are the Oucher (Beyer, Villarruel, & Denyes, 1995), the Poker Chip Tool (Hester, 1979), the "pain ther-mometer" (Jay, Ozolins, Elliott, & Caldwell, 1983), and the Eland Color Tool (Eland, 1985). These instruments are limited in that they address only pain intensity and, because they are self-report measures, they may be influenced by familial factors, environmental cues, and anxiety or fear (McGrath, 1990).

Overt responses often associated with pain include observable motor behaviors indicative of discomfort or distress, such as crying (Jay & Elliot, 1984), and observable pain responses, including recorded intake of pain medication (Engel, 1988). Because pain and anxiety are difficult to separate in the clinical setting, the term *behavioral distress* is used to capture the verbal, behavioral, and physiological indications of the inseparable elements of pain and anxiety (Katz, Kellerman, & Siegel, 1980; McGrath, 1990). Examples of pediatric pain assessments that are designed to measure overt behavioral distress are the Children's Hospital of Eastern Ontario Pain Scale (CHEOPS; McGrath et al., 1985), the Observational Scale of Behavioral Distress (OSBD; Jay et al., 1983), and the Procedural Rating Scale, Revised (Katz et al., 1980). Discernible pain responses are frequently recorded in pain diaries, which serve as a vehicle to compile information regarding medication intake, daily activities, and therapy measures (Engel, 1988; Turnquist & Engel, 1994). However, overt behaviors may not always accurately reflect a child's pain experience.

Because the assessment of pain is complicated, multidimensional evaluation is advisable. Self-reports coupled with periodic observations of overt and physiological pain behaviors by a trained person appear warranted to determine the impact of pain experiences.

The role of occupational therapists in pediatric pain management is emerging. In a survey of 129 occupational therapists, Turnquist and Engel (1994) found that occupational therapists working with children lacked sufficient knowledge about pain in children. The authors suggested that further research and education on pediatric pain as it relates to the delivery of comprehensive occupational therapy services were warranted. Information concerning pain control might be especially pertinent for occupational therapists working with children who have sustained burn injuries, due to the universal presence of pain after burn injuries.

The role of the occupational therapist on a burn unit is multifaceted and somewhat variable depending on the specific protocols and policies established by the facility. A few of the traditional roles include (a) splinting and pressure treatments to prevent deformity (e.g., contracture, hypertrophic scarring) while maximizing proper positioning; (b) facilitation and adaptation of activities of daily living, including provision of adaptive equipment and instruction in its use as appropriate; (c) use of psychosocial therapeutic interventions to address the emotional well-being of the child; and (d) provision of developmentally appropriate treatment activities to address range of motion, strength, and functional gross and fine motor coordination deficits (Doane, 1989; Fader, 1988). The pain from therapeutic activities may exacerbate the existing pain caused by the initial injury (Choiniere, Melzack, Rondeau, Girard, & Paquin, 1989; Szyfelbein, Osgood, & Carr, 1985). Therefore, it is often easier to attain maximal cooperation from the child when play (Doane, 1989; Helvig, 1993; Nothdurft, Smith, & LeMaster, 1984) or other multistrategy interventions (e.g., predictability, relaxation, distraction, hypnosis, visual imagery, developmentally appropriate active participation, positive reinforcement) are incorporated into the activity (Elliot & Olson, 1983; Fader, 1988; Kavanagh, 1983; Kelley, Jarvie, Middlebrook, McNeer, & Drabman, 1984).

Continued research concerning the efficacy of purposeful activity versus rote exercise in occupational therapy assessments and interventions, especially with regard to the pediatric population, is warranted. Because play is considered the primary occupation of children (Knox, 1993; Pratt, 1989), it is reasonable that purposeful activities used in pediatric therapy include play activities. Play also was noted to be one of the strategies for pain management in children (McGrath, 1990).

The current study was designed to examine the differences in participation, overt pain behaviors, pain perceptions, and personal satisfaction with the overall experience of a therapeutic activity when children with burn injuries were engaged in a play activity versus rote exercise.

For each participant, the following research questions were addressed:

1. Does the number of repetitions of a therapeutic movement differ when the participant is engaged in a purposeful activity versus rote exercise?
2. Does the number of overt distress behaviors (as measured by the OSBD [Jay et al., 1983]) exhibited by the participant differ when engaged in a purposeful activity versus rote exercise?
3. Do a participant's self-report measures of pain intensity (measured by the Oucher [Beyer et al., 1995]) differ during purposeful activities versus rote exercise?
4. Do a participant's reports of overall enjoyment as measured on a Likert-type Fun Scale differ when engaged in purposeful activity versus rote exercise?

Method

Participants

The participants in this study were two 6-year-old boys who both had sustained a second-degree to third-degree (indeterminate to deep) burn injury involving one or more extremities with potential for impaired mobility in at least one joint. Participant 1 sustained an 11% total body surface area (TBSA) intermediate to deep gasoline flame burn to the nondominant, left side of his body. The dorsal aspect and palmar surface of his hand were burned, including all digits, dorsal wrist, medial/posterior aspect of the forearm and upper arm (noncircumferential), and a portion of the pectoral area of his chest. He underwent one surgical procedure for a split thickness skin graft to the left hand, arm, and chest, with the donor site being the right side of his back and his left buttock.

Participant 2 was right hand dominant and was admitted for hospitalization as a result of a 16.5% TBSA intermediate to deep gasoline flame burn to the right face and right arm (noncircumferential). Included were the posterior forearm and fingers but not the palm, right posterior/medial lower extremity (noncircumferential), and left lower extremity (primarily the posterior calf). He required surgery for excision and autografting of his right upper extremity, hand, and lower extremity, with his back as the donor site. Early in his rehabilitation, participant 2 also underwent two anesthesia-assisted procedures for staple removal, wound care, and dressing changes.

Coincidentally, both participants were Hispanic, and their primary language was English. The participants were recruited from the inpatient burn unit at a medical center on the West Coast. After review of each child's medical chart, it was determined that both had had an unremarkable past medical history. Neither had a record of a previous serious painful injury or illness. Both boys had a referral for therapy services that included range of motion to improve functional performance. Both were medically stable and were postsurgery a minimum of 72 hr before initiation of the research protocol.

Alternate Treatment Conditions

Condition 1. The first treatment condition consisted of therapeutic activities deemed *purposeful* (i.e., playing a game that was identified by the child as an activity that he enjoyed doing). Each child and his parent(s) were interviewed before initiation of the study to determine which play activities were purposeful and meaningful to the child. This interview included a parent or guardian questionnaire developed by the first author. For each child, the principal investigator designed or modified between 8 and 10 of the identified play activities to promote mobility so that individual range-of-motion goals could be established during the initial occupational therapy assessment. At the beginning of each treatment session in which a purposeful activity condition was applied, the child was given a choice of three play activities. The decision as to which three choices to offer the child each session was based on availability of the toy or game, prior success with the activity (e.g., the child had completed the desired number of repetitions while doing the activity in another session or had reported enjoying the activity), and where the activity was to take place (i.e., gym vs. patient room). The child was then given instructions related to the game or play activity and told the expectations for repetitions of movements within the set range-of-motion goal.

Condition 2. The second condition involved using rote exercise to promote range of motion. In these therapy sessions, the child was instructed to perform a certain number of repetitions of a range-of-motion exercise corresponding to the range-of-motion goals determined during the initial occupational therapy evaluation.

Research Design

A single-subject, multiple-treatment, randomization design was implemented to compare the effectiveness and perceptions of purposeful activity versus rote exercise. An initial baseline phase was not necessary because the two treatment conditions were compared with one another in rapid alternation (Kazdin, 1982). The two conditions were randomly selected over a 2-day block of time so that each condition occurred twice in the 2 days but did not necessarily alternate during the course of 1 day. This design was chosen to reduce the predictability of treatment conditions for any given therapy session, which is an important consideration because a child's ability to predict a treatment activity may influence his or her level of anxiety, willingness to participate, or perception of pain before initiation of the session. Three such treatment blocks (6 days) were completed for one child. To get a clearer picture of outcomes, one additional block of trials (8 days total) was completed with the second child.

Measures

The following measures were recorded for both participants on each day when therapy was provided during the study:

Repetitions. One repetition was defined as movement through the desired active range of motion. The number of repetitions was tallied by the primary investigator during the activity.

OSBD score. The OSBD is a revised version of the Procedural Behavior Rating Scale (Katz et al., 1980). This assessment comprises eight operationally defined behaviors that have been shown to indicate pain, anxiety, or both in children (Jay et al., 1983)—crying, screaming, physical restraint, verbal resistance, requesting emotional support, verbal pain, flailing, and information seeking. Each behavioral category is assigned a weighted score from 1 to 4 according to intensity. A weighted score of 1 indicates a lower intensity of distress (e.g., information seeking), whereas a score of 4 implies a more intense indicator of distress (e.g., screaming or

physical restraint). The OSBD is designed to record behaviors in 15-sec intervals throughout the observed procedure or activity.

Jay et al. (1983) examined interrater reliability using pediatric participants undergoing bone marrow aspirations. The Pearson product-moment correlations ranged from .72 to .99. The validity of the OSBD also was examined in the same study by Jay et al. (1983), as well as in subsequent studies by Jay and Elliot (1984) and Elliot, Jay, and Woody (1987). The authors in each of these studies recognized the potential influences of a number of factors (i.e., complexity of the phenomenon of pain, parental presence, habituation to the procedure or noxious stimuli, cognitive level of the child) on the experience, overt display of distress, and reporting of pain. However, the authors concluded that the OSBD is an acceptably reliable and valid measure of distress in children who are undergoing potentially painful medical procedures.

Oucher score. The Oucher is a self-report tool for children 3 to 12 years of age (Beyer et al., 1995). There are three ethnic versions: white or Caucasian, black or African-American, and Hispanic. It comprises an ordinal scale denoting 20-unit intervals from 0 to 100 and an ordinal scale composed of six pictures of children in various expressions of pain. When the child is initially introduced to the Oucher, he or she is asked to count from 1 to 100 by ones, choose which of two numbers is greater, and sequence six equilateral triangles (or squares or circles) of increasing size. These questions determine whether the child is cognitively mature enough to use the Oucher and, if so, which scale to use. If the child is able to complete all these tasks, he or she uses the numerical scale. Otherwise, if the child is able to complete only the task of sequencing the shapes from smallest to largest, then the child is instructed to use the pictures to identify the level of his or her pain. Both children in this study used the Hispanic version and the photographic scale.

The directions further explain that 0 or the bottom picture is the *least amount of hurt* the child has ever experienced, whereas 100 or the top picture is the *most hurt* the child has ever had. During the course of the current study, a number on a scale of 0 to 5 was recorded both before and after each activity depending on which picture the participant identified as indicative of the amount of hurt he was experiencing. In other words, if the child chose the picture immediately above the bottom picture on the scale as reflective of how much hurt he was having, then a score of 1 was recorded in the participant's journal.

Content validity of the original Oucher was examined by Beyer and Aradine (1986) in a study where 78 Caucasian children, 3 to 7 years of age, from three sites were asked to sequence six photographs. A concordance coefficient of .73 ($p < .01$) was revealed using Kendall's coefficient of concordance. The content validity of the Hispanic version was later examined (Marshall, 1988, as cited in the Oucher manual; Villarruel & Deynes, 1991). The agreement according to Kendall's coefficient of concordance was .65, $p < .0001$. The construct validity of the original Oucher also was evaluated (Aradine, Beyer, & Tompkins, 1988; Beyer & Aradine, 1987, 1988). In addition, as reported in the Oucher manual technical report (Beyer et al., 1995), the construct validity, including both convergent and discriminant validity, of the African-American and Hispanic versions of the Oucher was examined.

Fun Scale score. For the purposes of the current study, the first author developed the Fun Scale. The number associated with the face chosen by the child as indicative of the amount of fun he had during the activity was recorded as the Fun Scale score for that session (see Figure 21.1). Although this scale appears to have face validity,

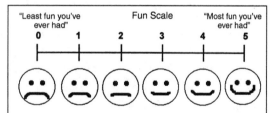

Directions for Administering the Fun Scale

Present the Fun Scale to the child by setting it in front of him or her on the table.

Orient the child to the scale by saying, "See these numbers and faces? We are going to use them to help you tell me how much fun you had doing the activity we just did. Five or the smiley face is the MOST fun you have ever had. Zero or the sad face is the LEAST fun you have ever had." Repeat this orientation sequence as often as needed.

Ask the child to rate his or her enjoyment of the therapy activity he or she just participated in by saying, "How much fun did you have just now?" The child may also be cued with phrases such as "Was it the MOST fun you've ever had? Was it the LEAST fun you've ever had? Was it somewhere in between?"

If the child used faces to rate his or her pain on the Oucher, then instruct the child to "Pick the face that shows how much fun you had." If the child used numbers to rate his or her pain on the Oucher, then instruct the child to "Pick the number that shows how much fun you had."

Record the child's answer in his or her journal noting the date, time, and session activity.

Figure 21.1. Fun Scale: A self-report tool to measure fun experienced during therapy.

Note: The Fun Scale was developed specifically for this study and allowed each participant to rate his overall enjoyment of the therapeutic activity.

no formal reliability or validity studies were conducted.

Data Collection

After the participants had been recruited, informed consent obtained, and an initial assessment completed, data collection began. During the initial assessment, the primary investigator obtained standardized range-of-motion measurements using the goniometer (Trombly, 1995) and appropriate active range-of-motion goals were established, including the goal used for the purposes of this study. The goal for the first participant was 10 repetitions of 0–80° active left shoulder abduction. Ten repetitions of 0–90° of active right shoulder flexion was the research-oriented goal for the second participant. The goal motion for this study was based on the participants' ability to actively range the joint and the appropriateness of a twice-a-day therapy regimen for range of motion of this joint. The number of desired repetitions was established on the basis of common clinical practice in the burn unit at the medical center in addition to the primary investigators' clinical judgment regarding attainable therapeutic goals. Additionally, during the initial assessment, both participants were introduced to the Oucher and were administered the outlined procedure for determining which form to use (Beyer et al., 1995). It was concluded that both participants would use the ordinal (photographic) form in the Hispanic ethnic version.

Materials required for data collection included

1. A video camera with tripod stand;
2. A camera that develops photos instantly;
3. A universal goniometer;
4. The Parent or Guardian Play Questionnaire, which was designed to gather information regarding their child's play interests (this questionnaire, which is available from the first author, included toys or games appropriate for children 5 to 12 years of age that were available on the burn unit);
5. The Child Play Interview, which was similar to the Parent or Guardian Play Questionnaire but was intended to gather information from the child's perspective;
6. Age-appropriate toys and games;
7. The Oucher (Beyer et al., 1995);
8. The OSBD (Jay et al., 1983); and
9. The Fun Scale (see Figure 21.1).

Data were collected in the occupational therapy–physical therapy clinic of the medical center burn unit or the participant's room. The video camera was set up in a static position to tape the therapeutic activity. Therapy was scheduled Monday through Sunday as needed and appropriate. Timing of daily sessions was determined on an individualized basis, taking into account established medication, procedures or wound care, and mealtime schedules. As common practice dictates, an attempt was made to arrange therapy sessions to coincide with the maximum effectiveness of medication for pain relief by consulting with the pharmacist and nursing staff. In addition, therapy sessions were scheduled at times when the participant was adequately rested.

Both the morning and afternoon therapy sessions began with the participant rating his pain intensity on the Oucher (Beyer et al., 1995). This was immediately followed by the videotaped therapeutic activity. Directly after the activity, the participant (a) again rated his pain intensity on the Oucher and (b) rated his overall experience on the Likert-type Fun Scale. After completing the desired minimum number of repetitions of the therapeutic activity (or after the child's refusal to continue participating) and the self-report rating tasks, the video camera was turned off and the therapy session continued as appropriate to meet intervention goals (including more repetitions of the therapeutic activity being researched if the child chose to do so after being asked whether he wanted to continue).

To determine whether the range-of-motion goal was achieved during both the rote exercises and purposeful activities, trained occupational therapists (one specializing in burn rehabilitation and one specializing in adult physical disabilities) were asked to view randomly selected 1-min clips of video from each of the taped sessions. Next, each therapist was instructed to determine whether the goal was met or not as compared to an instant photo of the participant positioned at the goal angle of range of motion determined in the initial occupational therapy evaluation. After reviewing the 1-min clips of each videotaped session for both participants, the raters agreed that the respective therapeutic goals were met in each of the sessions.

Finally, overt distress behaviors were scored on the OSBD (Jay et al., 1983) by the principal investigator and one other pediatric occupational therapist. Once data collection was completed for the study, the videotaped therapy activities were re-recorded in random order and an auditory signal (i.e., a beep) was superimposed onto the videos at 15-sec intervals. The two raters viewed the videotapes simultaneously while seated out of view of one another and recorded any of the eight behaviors occurring at the moment each 15-sec interval ended. The frequencies of behaviors were observed during each activity. Next, the frequency for each category was divided by the number of intervals, resulting in a mean interval score. The mean interval score for each behavioral category was then multiplied by the assigned weighted score for that category, which resulted in a weighted mean interval score. Lastly, the weighted mean interval scores for each category were added, yielding the total OSBD score for that activity (Jay et al., 1983).

Reliability

Interrater reliability on the OSBD (Jay et al., 1983) was calculated using *kappa* (*k*) (Kazdin, 1982). This statistic was chosen to correct for chance due to the low rate of occurrence and high rate of nonoccurrence of distress behaviors when scoring the video clips using the OSBD (Jay et al., 1983).

The interobserver agreement on scoring the eight behavioral categories of the OSBD (Jay et al., 1983) for the therapeutic activities recorded on video ranged from $k = .79$ to 1, implying a level of interrater reliability significantly over and above that which might have occurred by chance.

The point-by-point agreement ratio (Kazdin, 1982) also was computed and yielded ratios from 99% to 100% for the eight behavioral categories on the OSBD for both participants.

Results

Figures 21.2 to 21.4 present the results obtained with each subject on each measure. The figures were constructed to show the entire range of scores possible on each measure to make it easier for readers to discriminate how the participants performed relative to those scales. Results for the two therapy sessions completed on any given day are plotted closer to one another than are the results for adjacent days, enabling readers to discriminate when during the day (AM or PM) each session was conducted. Regression lines are also

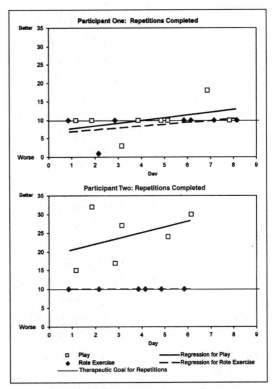

Figure 21.2. Number of repetitions completed by the first participant (top box) and the second participant (bottom box).

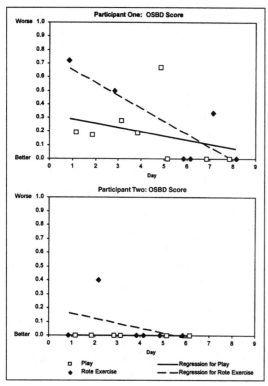

Figure 21.3. Scores on the Observational Scale of Behavioral Distress (Jay et al., 1983) received by the first participant (top box) and the second participant (bottom box).

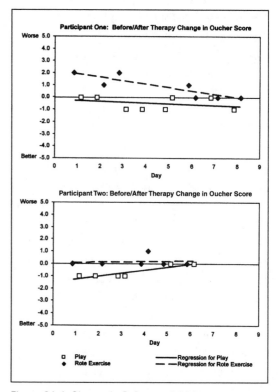

Figure 21.4. Change in Before and After scores on the Oucher (Beyer, Villarruel, & Denyes, 1995) received by the first participant (top box) and the second participant (bottom box).

plotted to summarize the change in scores over time for each condition.

Repetitions

The first participant generally chose to stop performing when the target number of repetitions (10) was reached (see Figure 21.2). On two occasions, he stopped well short of the target (Day 2, PM, rote exercise, and Day 3, PM, play) and once exceeded the target by nearly a factor of 2 (Day 7, AM, play). Overall, it would appear that neither the time of day nor the experimental condition exerted differential influences on the number of repetitions completed by the first participant.

The second participant demonstrated a strong reaction to the experimental conditions. When exposed to rote exercise, he always completed the

target number of repetitions but never exceeded it. The number of repetitions completed with play therapy, on the other hand, always exceeded the target and generally increased over time.

OSBD Score

Higher scores on the OSBD indicate greater numbers of observed overt distress behaviors. For the first 4 days of the study, the first participant displayed fewer distress behaviors during play than during rote exercise (see Figure 21.3). By the end of the experiment, however, overt signs of distress behaviors had generally disappeared for both conditions.

The second participant displayed overt distress behaviors on only one day (Day 2, PM, rote exercise). Without more variance in the results, no conclusions can be drawn about the relative effects of experimental conditions on the distress of this child.

Change in Oucher Scores

The data presented in Figure 21.4 reflect the difference between the pre-therapeutic activity and post-therapeutic activity Oucher scores for any given session. For example, on the first day of rote exercise, the first participant reported an Oucher score of 1 before the therapy began and an Oucher score of 3 at the end of therapy. The difference between those scores is 2 (3 − 1 = 2). As with the OSBD scores, a higher score is worse, reflecting an increase in pain over the course of the session.

During the early part of the experiment, the first participant always recorded an increase in pain after rote exercise; however, after play, he reported either no change or a decrease in pain. The advantage of play diminished over time, however, and was generally gone by the end of the experiment (see Figure 21.4).

The second participant also demonstrated more favorable results with play during the early part of the experiment. He had either no change or an increase in self-reported pain in response to rote exercise, whereas he had either no change or a decrease in self-reported pain after play. As with the first participant, those differences generally were absent by the end of the experiment.

Fun Scale

The first participant rated play as the "most fun he'd ever had" after 6 of the 8 sessions but never rated rote exercise higher than 3 on the 5-point scale. Generally, however, rote exercise was being rated more highly as time progressed.

The second participant always rated play as the "most fun he'd ever had." Like the first participant, he never rated exercise higher than 3 on the 5-point scale, and although the regression for rote exercise was ascending, the change over time was very modest.

Discussion

The most important finding of this study was that scores on the four dependent measures (i.e., number of repetitions of therapeutic exercise completed, number and type of overt distress behaviors displayed, scores on self-report scales of pain intensity and "fun") generally were better for play activities than for rote exercise. Visual inspection of the graphs of OSBD scores, Fun Scale scores, and especially Oucher scores suggests that, as time progresses after trauma, the differences in reports of pain intensity and enjoyment between the two conditions (purposeful activity and rote exercise) become less pronounced. These results suggest directions for intervention. For example, range of motion embedded in play activities may be the most effective use of therapy time early in the rehabilitation process because the child may experience less pain intensity, perform more repetitions, and enjoy the activity more. However, later in the rehabilitation process, rote exercise may be equally effective and take less time (average of 1–2 min vs. the average of 7–8 min it took to complete the exercises embedded in a play activity). Alternatively, once the child is demonstrating few pain behaviors, the child may be self-motivated to engage in therapeutic play with parental monitoring and indirect therapist supervision. To make informed decisions regarding transitioning from therapist-monitored therapeutic play to either rote exercise or family-monitored play, the post-injury progression of pain in children needs to be monitored.

Clinical Observations and Implications

The Oucher and the Fun Scale both appeared to have clinical utility. Both discriminated between the two experimental conditions, were simple to administer, and were well received by the participants. The Oucher easily could be incorporated into the delivery of improved therapy services and nursing care, including wound and medication management. Parents of the children expressed appreciation for having a tool to use to help their children describe the amount of hurt they were experiencing. Similarly, the Fun Scale facilitated communication. The participants willingly rated how much fun they had during therapy and were not reluctant to express boredom or dislike. Fun Scale scores were helpful in treatment planning. Activities that the child identified as "most fun" were used as viable choices for future treatment sessions, whereas activities with lower ratings, with the exception of range of motion, were not repeated. Additionally, activities rated as 5 (most fun) were often noted as activities in which the participant did more repetitions and reported less intense pain. This same procedure easily could be replicated in other clinical settings.

During the course of the study, the first participant had a clear downward trend in the frequency of distress behaviors as measured by the OSBD. Because pain behavior regulation was not part of the treatment intervention, the gradual decline of overt pain behaviors for Participant 1 may reflect the healing process. As tissue regeneration naturally occurred, it is likely that improved well-being and pain reduction were experienced and that this resulted in a decrease in overt distress behaviors as measured by the OSBD. However, because a lack of overt pain behaviors cannot be equated with the absence of pain (Engel, 1988), it is recommended that practitioners monitor children's reports of pain and overt behaviors (e.g., activity levels, pain behaviors such as medication use, facial grimacing) when establishing and modifying therapeutic interventions. Increased pain intensity may occur several hours after physical exercise; therefore, it may be important to have the child complete pain diaries at regular intervals throughout the day.

Clinical observations suggested that play (a) distracted participants' attention from their pain complaints and increased enjoyment of the therapeutic activity and (b) resulted in more fluid, spontaneous movement. Additionally, quality movement in two or more joints simultaneously occurred more often during play than during rote exercise, where movement typically was focused on one joint at a time. These benefits may carry over into other functional activities and compliance with target behaviors. Although this is beneficial, practitioners need to be aware that it may be tempting to exceed therapeutic physical activity quotas. Research by Fordyce (1976) suggested that when adults exceed pre-established activity quotas, it may result in exacerbated pain states, usually delayed by several hours. This pain, in turn, may result in consequent activity avoidance, distress (e.g., anxiety), increased pain medication use, and lack of motivation for additional physical retraining. If future research demonstrates that this finding is valid for children, then pacing of activity may be important. Therefore, to appropriately assist in the rehabilitation of children who are reinforced by accelerated activity, instruction in a pacing regimen may be beneficial for the children, their parents, and professionals working with the children.

Future Research

The current study suggests that children voluntarily engage in more repetitions when involved in a play activity as compared to when involved in rote exercise. Although findings suggested no increase in reported pain intensity immediately after intervention, in view of the previously cited research by Fordyce (1976), it is important to study the effects of more repetitions on pain perception one or more hours after intervention.

This study also highlighted the need for the development of a measure of overt distress designed for children with burn injuries. The

OSBD proved to be less than an ideal measure for several reasons. First, because many of the distress behaviors that occurred fell between the 15-sec scoring intervals, the OSBD was not sensitive enough to accurately depict the degree of overt distress being demonstrated by the participants. It would appear that shorter intervals or whole interval recording procedures might be warranted (Kazdin, 1982). Second, the OSBD does not include many behaviors that were demonstrated by the participants that may be indicative of distress (e.g., facial grimacing, touching wounds). Third, the OSBD does not take into account well behaviors exhibited by the participants (e.g., smiling, positive verbalizations). Due to these identified limitations of the OSBD and the complexity of pain, a new multidimensional measure needs to be developed for use with children with burn injuries.

Experiences with the Fun Scale were positive and point to the need for more research directed at further developing this measure. Results from this study identified possible clinical use of the Fun Scale in facilitating communication and in discriminating between children's perceptions of different activities. However, before recommending widespread use of this measure, rigorous examination of its psychometric properties is indicated.

Last, the impact of volition on therapeutic outcomes needs to be determined. The greater impact of play versus rote exercise on outcomes may have resulted from the child's personal causation and interests (Neville, Kielhofner, & Royeen, 1985). In this study, the child was given the opportunity to select the play activity but not the rote exercise. This opportunity may have resulted in the child having more feelings of control and enjoyment, which may have resulted in improved Oucher, OSBD, and Fun Scale scores.

Occupational therapy is based on the idea that purposeful activity may be used to evaluate,

improve, or maintain functional performance skills required for activities of daily living, work, and play or leisure. The current study suggests that the use of play in therapy with children with burn injuries can yield results that are equal to and often better than those achieved using rote exercise in terms of repetitions, overt distress behaviors, self-reported pain intensity, and self-reported enjoyment of the activity.

Acknowledgments

The principal investigator acknowledges the U.S. Department of Education for supporting her graduate education in part via Grant 84-029F, "Preparation of Related Service Personnel; Preservice Training of Occupational Therapists to Provide Services to Children with Emotional and Behavioral Disorders."

This study was conducted in partial fulfillment of the first author's requirements for a master of science degree, Department of Rehabilitation Medicine, University of Washington, Seattle.

References

American Occupational Therapy Association. (1993). Position paper: Purposeful activity. *American Journal of Occupational Therapy, 47,* 1081–1082.

American Occupational Therapy Association. (1994). Uniform terminology for occupational therapy (3rd ed). *American Journal of Occupational Therapy, 45,* 912–916.

American Occupational Therapy Association. (1995). Position paper: Occupation. *American Journal of Occupational Therapy, 49,* 1015–1018.

Aradine, C., Beyer, J., & Tompkins, J. (1988). Children's pain perceptions before and after analgesia: A study of instrument construct validity. *Journal of Pediatric Nursing, 3,* 11–23.

Beyer, J. E., & Aradine, C. R. (1987). Patterns of pediatric pain intensity: A methodological investigation of a self-report scale. *Clinical Journal of Pain, 3,* 130–141.

Beyer, J. E., & Aradine, C. R. (1988). Convergent and discriminant validity of a self-report measure of pain intensity for children. *Children's Health Care, 14,* 233–241.

Beyer, J. E., Villarruel, A. M., & Denyes, M. J. (1995). *The Oucher: A user's manual and technical report.* Bethesda, MD: Association for the Care of Children's Health.

Burke, J. P. (1993). Play: The life role of the infant and young child. In J. Case-Smith (Ed.), *Pediatric occupational therapy and early intervention* (pp. 198–224). Boston: Andover Medical.

Carter, B. (1994). Assessment and measurement of pain. In B. Carter (Ed.), *Child and infant pain: Principles of nursing care and management* (pp. 22–43). London: Chapman & Hall.

Choiniere, M., Melzack, R., Rondeau, J., Girard, N., & Paquin, M. J. (1989). The path of burns: Characteristics and correlates. *Journal of Trauma, 29,* 1531–1539.

Doane, C. B. (1989). Children with severe burns. In P. N. Pratt & A. S. Allen (Eds.), *Occupational therapy for children* (2nd ed., pp. 524–534). St. Louis, MO: Mosby.

Dutton, R. (1989). Guidelines for using both activity and exercise. *American Journal of Occupational Therapy, 43,* 573–580.

Eland, J. M. (1985). The role of the nurse in children's pain. In K. King (Ed.), *Recent advances in nursing* (pp. 29–45). Edinburgh, Scotland: Churchill Livingstone.

Elliot, C. H., Jay, S. M., & Woody, P. (1987). An observation scale for measuring children's distress during medical procedures. *Journal of Pediatric Psychology, 12,* 543–551.

Elliot, C. H., & Olson, R. A. (1983). The management of children's distress in response to painful medical treatment for burn injuries. *Behaviour Research and Therapy, 21,* 675–683.

Engel, J. M. (1988). *Pediatric pain.* Athens, GA: Elliott & Fitzpatrick.

Fader, P. (1988). Preserving function and minimizing deformity: The role of the occupational therapist. In H. F. Cavajal & D. H. Parks (Eds.), *Burns in children: Pediatric burn management* (pp. 324–344). Chicago: Year Book Medical.

Fordyce, W. E. (1976). *Behavioral methods for chronic pain and illness.* St. Louis, MO: Mosby.

Helvig, E. (1993). Pediatric burn injuries. *AACN Clinical Issues in Critical Care Nursing, 4,* 433–442.

Hester, N. O. (1979). The preoperational child's reaction to immunization. *Nursing Research, 28,* 250–252.

Hester, N. O. (1993). Pain in children. *Annual Review of Nursing Research, 11,* 105–142.

Hsieh, C.-L., Nelson, D. L., Smith, D. A., & Peterson, C. Q. (1996). A comparison of performance in added-purpose occupations and rote exercise for dynamic standing balance in persons with hemiplegia. *American Journal of Occupational Therapy, 50,* 10–15.

Jay, S. M., & Elliott, C. (1984). Behavioral observation scales for measuring children's distress: The effects of increased methodological rigor. *Journal of Consulting and Clinical Psychology, 52,* 1106–1107.

Jay, S. M., Ozolins, M., Elliott, C. M., & Caldwell, S. (1983). Assessment of children's distress during painful medical procedures. *Health Psychology, 2,* 133–148.

Katz, E. R., Kellerman, J., & Siegel, S. E. (1980). Behavioral distress in children with cancer undergoing medical procedures: Developmental considerations. *Journal of Consulting and Clinical Psychology, 48,* 356–365.

Katz, N., Marcus, S., & Weiss, P. (1994). Purposeful activity in physical rehabilitation. *Critical Reviews in Physical and Rehabilitation Medicine, 6,* 199–218.

Kavanagh, C. (1983). A new approach to dressing change in the severely burned child and its effect on burn-related psychopathology. *Heart and Lung, 12,* 612-619.

Kazdin, A. E. (1982). *Single-case research designs: Methods for clinical and applied settings.* New York: Oxford University Press.

Kelley, M. L., Jarvie, G. J., Middlebrook, J. L., McNeer, M. F., & Drabman, R. S. (1984). Decreasing burned children's pain behavior: Impacting the trauma of hydrotherapy. *Journal of Applied Behavior Analysis, 17,* 147–158.

Knox, S. H. (1993). Play and leisure. In H. L. Hopkins & H. D. Smith (Eds.), *Willard and Spackman's occupational therapy* (8th ed., pp. 260–268). Philadelphia: Lippincott.

Marshall, C. (1988). *A nursing study: Perception of pain in black children.* Unpublished master's thesis, Wayne State University, Detroit.

Marvin, J. A. (1995). Pain assessment versus measurement. *Journal of Burn Care and Rehabilitation, 16,* 348–357.

McGrath, P. A. (1990). *Pain in children: Nature, assessment, and treatment.* New York: Guilford.

McGrath, P. J., Johnson, G., Goodman, J. T., Schillinger, J., Dunn, J., & Chapman, J.-A. (1985). CHEOPS: A behavioral scale for rating postoperative pain in children. In H. L. Fields, R. Dubner, & F. Cervero (Eds.), *Advances in pain research and therapy* (Vol. 9, pp. 395–402). New York: Raven Press.

Merskey, H. (Ed.). (1986). Classification of chronic pain: Descriptions of chronic pain syndromes and definitions of pain terms. *Pain, 24*(3), 5217.

Nelson, D. L., Konosky, K., Fleharty, K., Webb, R., Newer, K., Hazboun, V. P., et al. (1996). The effects of an occupationally embedded exercise on bilaterally assisted supination in persons with hemiplegia. *American Journal of Occupational Therapy, 50,* 639–646.

Neville, P., Kielhofner, G., & Royeen, C. B. (1985). Childhood. In G. Kielhofner (Ed.), *A model of human occupation* (pp. 82–98). Baltimore: Williams & Wilkins.

Nothdurft, D., Smith, P. S., & LeMaster, J. E. (1984). Exercise and treatment modalities. In S. V. Fisher & P. A. Helm (Eds.), *Comprehensive rehabilitation of burns* (pp. 96–147). Baltimore: Williams & Wilkins.

Parker, L. H., & Cinciripini, P. M. (1984). Behavioral medicine with children: Applications in chronic disease. *Progress in Behavior Modification, 17,* 136–165.

Pratt, P. N. (1989). Play and recreational activities. In P. N. Pratt & A. S. Allen (Eds.), *Occupational therapy for children* (2nd ed., pp. 295–310). St. Louis, MO: Mosby.

Sanders, S. H. (1979). A trimodal behavioral conceptualization of clinical pain. *Perceptual and Motor Skills, 48,* 551–555.

Szyfelbein, S. K., Osgood, P. F., & Carr, D. B. (1985). The assessment of pain and plasma B-endorphin immunoactivity in burned children. *Pain, 22,* 173–182.

Trombly, C. A. (1995). Occupation: Purposefulness and meaningfulness as therapeutic mechanisms [1995 Eleanor Clarke Slagle Lecture]. *American Journal of Occupational Therapy, 49,* 960–972.

Turnquist, K. M., & Engel, J. M. (1994). Occupational therapists' experiences and knowledge of pain in children. *Physical and Occupational Therapy in Pediatrics, 14,* 35–51.

Tyler, D. C. (1990). Pain in infants and children. In J. J. Bonica (Ed.), *The management of pain* (2nd ed., pp. 538–551). Philadelphia: Lea & Febiger.

Van der Weel, F. R., van der Meer, A. L. H., & Lee, D. N. (1991). Effect of task on movement control in cerebral palsy: Implications for assessment and therapy. *Developmental Medicine and Child Neurology, 33,* 419–426.

Varni, J. W. (1983). *Clinical behavioral pediatrics: An interdisciplinary biobehavioral approach.* New York: Pergamon.

Villarruel, A., & Deynes, M. (1991). Pain assessment in children: Theoretical and empirical validity. *Advances in Nursing Science, 14,* 31–39.

Wu, C., Trombly, C. A., & Lin, K. (1994). The relationship between occupational form and occupational performance: A kinematic perspective. *American Journal of Occupational Therapy, 48,* 679–687.

CHAPTER 22

Playfulness in Children With and Without Disability

Measurement and Intervention

Ann Mari Okimoto, Anita Bundy, and Jodie Hanzlik

Ann Mari Okimoto, MS, OTR, *is occupational therapist, 1309 Maleko Street, Kailua, HI 96734.*

Anita Bundy, ScD, OTR, *is professor, Occupational Therapy Department, Colorado State University, Fort Collins.*

Jodie Hanzlik, PhD, OTR, *is professor and head, Occupational Therapy Department, Colorado State University, Fort Collins.*

The primary occupation of young children is play (Parham & Primeau, 1997). When a child has a physical disability, playfulness can be diminished. Research suggests that young children with cerebral palsy are often limited in their expression of playfulness due, in part, to suboptimal interactions that take place with their caregivers. It is important, therefore, to look at the ways mothers interact with their children during play and to intervene when necessary. It also is important to examine the effectiveness of such intervention.

Literature Review

Many areas of infant development depend on active, dynamic interactions between mothers and infants (Connor, Williamson, & Siepp, 1978; Hanzlik, 1989b; Holloway, 1997). These playful interactions promote the child's physical and cognitive development and emotional well-being (Connor et al., 1978). Sutton-Smith (1980) argued that children's playfulness and play skills are derived from the early play routines between mother and infant beginning in the infant's second month of life. These routines involve imitation, turn taking, manipulating a play activity to increase enjoyment, and determining the outcome of the game.

When an infant has a physical disability, such as cerebral palsy, many of the dynamics between the infant and the caregiver are different from those between a caregiver and an infant who is typically developing (Connor et al., 1978). Hanzlik (1989b) suggested that

> if one of the infant–mother dyads is unable to demonstrate or elicit behaviors that promote joint regulation of interactions, maladaptive behaviors may result, and the dyad may be at risk for interactional behavioral anomalies that can affect the development of the infant. (p. 35)

Originally published 2000 in *American Journal of Occupational Therapy, 54,* 73–82.

The development of typical play routines also may be at risk for a young child with a physical disability. Hanzlik (1986) compared the social interactions of infants who were typically developing and their mothers with those of infants with cerebral palsy and developmental delays and their mothers. Each dyad was observed as they engaged in free play, and both participants' behaviors were recorded. Hanzlik found that mothers of infants with cerebral palsy were more verbally and physically directive, engaged in more physical contact, and had fewer face-to-face interactions with their infants. In turn, infants with cerebral palsy were more compliant, less responsive, and less independent than their peers who were typically developing.

Other researchers who compared similar mother–infant dyads found that mothers with infants who had disabilities displayed more maternal-directed behaviors (e.g., mother controls infant's physical response by moving infant's body; mother makes direct commands or statements to the infant) toward their infants, engaged in more social play involving physical contact, were warmer in affection, and initiated interactions more frequently than mothers of infants who were typically developing. In turn, infants with disabilities engaged in less eye contact, less vocalization, and less independent play than their peers who were typically developing (Barrera & Vella, 1987; Brooks-Gunn & Lewis, 1984; Eheart, 1982; Hanzlik & Stevenson, 1986; Kogan & Tyler, 1973; Lieberman, Padan-Belkin, & Harel, 1995).

Subsequently, Hanzlik (1989a) implemented an intervention for mothers that addressed appropriate ways to increase positive and decrease negative verbal and nonverbal interactions with their infants who had cerebral palsy. Hanzlik studied the effects of the intervention and found that, compared with mothers who did not receive the intervention, the mothers in the experimental group were able to decrease their physical contact and directiveness and increase their face-to-face contact with their infants. The infants also engaged in less physically directed compliance and increased their voluntary responsiveness to their mothers.

According to Missiuna and Pollock (1991), the interaction characteristics that were improved in Hanzlik's (1989a) follow-up study are important features of an infant–caregiver play session. These characteristics may increase the infant's independence and motivation, which, in turn, are key to infant exploration. Not coincidentally, motivation is also an element recognized by Bundy (1997b) and others (Lieberman et al., 1995; Rubin, Fein, & Vandenberg, 1983) as contributing to the playfulness of a child.

Bundy (1997a) suggested that a child who is more playful has more internal control, is more intrinsically motivated, is freer from some constraints of reality, and is better able to give and receive interactional cues than a child who is less playful. On the basis of these beliefs, Bundy (1997b) developed the Test of Playfulness (ToP). A list of the items on this instrument and their descriptions are found in Table 22.1.

One purpose of this study was to determine whether the ToP (Version 3) was a reliable and valid instrument to assess young children. Once validity and reliability were established, we used the ToP to compare the playfulness of young children with cerebral palsy and developmental delays with that of peers who are typically developing. Finally, we used the ToP to compare the effect of an intervention aimed at improving mother–infant interactions with that of neurodevelopmental treatment (NDT) on the children's playfulness. In regard to the latter purpose, we compared gain scores of the two groups and examined differences within each group at pretest and

Table 22.1. Test of Playfulness (Version 3) Item Descriptions

Item	Description
Is actively engaged.	1. Extent: Proportion of time the child is involved in activities rather than aimless wandering or other nonfocused activity or temper tantrums. 2. Intensity: Degree to which the child is concentrating on the activity or playmates. 3. Skill: Child's ability to stay focused on activity.
Decides what to do.	4. Extent: Proportion of time during which the child actively chooses to do what he or she is doing. Activity does not have to be purposeful, and purposeful activity does not have to be the child's idea.
Maintains level of safety sufficient to play.	5. Extent: Proportion of time during which the child feels safe enough to continue to play. If necessary, the child may alter the environment.
Demonstrates obvious exuberance, manifests joy.	6. Extent: Proportion of time during which the child exhibits outward and obvious signs of having fun; being gleeful.
Tries to overcome difficulties, barriers, or obstacles to persist with an activity.	7. Intensity: Degree to which the child perseveres in order to overcome obstacles to continuing the activity.
Modifies activity to maintain to challenge or make it more fun.	8. Skill: Ease with which the child actively changes the requirements or complexity of the task in order to vary the challenge or degree of novelty.
Engages in playful mischief or teasing.	9. Extent: Proportion of time during which the child is involved in teasing or razzing or minor infractions of the rules. Neither mischief nor teasing is done out of a spirit of meanness. 10. Skill: The adeptness with which the child creates or carries out the mischief or teasing.
Engages in activity for sheer pleasure (process) rather than primarily for the outcome.	11. Extent: Proportion of time during which the child seems to want to do the activity simply because he or she enjoys it rather than to attain a particular outcome.
Pretends.	12. Extent: Proportion of time during which there are overt indicators that the child is assuming different character roles, pretending to be doing something, pretending something is happening that is not, or pretending that an object or person is something other than what it actually is. 13. Skill: The degree to which the performance is convincing.
Incorporates objects or other people into play in novel, imaginative, unconventional, creative, or variable ways.	14. Extent: Proportion of time during which the child (a) uses objects commonly thought of as toys in ways other than those the manufacturer clearly intended, (b) incorporates objects not classically thought of as toys into the play (e.g., bugs, jars, cans, table legs), or (c) uses one toy or object in a number of different ways.
Negotiates with others to have needs or desires met.	15. Skill: Ease and finesse with which the child verbally or nonverbally asks for what he or she needs.
Engages in social play.	16. Extent: Proportion of time during which the child interacts with others involved in the same or similar activity. 17. Skill: The level of social play.
Supports play of others.	18. Skill: Ease with which child supports play of others (encouragement, scaffolding).
Enters a group already engaged in an activity.	19. Skill: Ease with which the child does something to become part of a group already engaged in an activity; the action is not disruptive to what is going on.
Initiates play with others.	20. Skill: Ease with which the child initiates a new activity.
Clowns or jokes with others.	21. Extent: Proportion of time during which the child tells jokes or funny stories or engages in exaggerated, swaggering behavior (usually for the purpose of gaining others' attention).
Shares (toys, equipment, friends, ideas).	22. Extent: Proportion of time during which the child allows others to play with toys, personal belongings, or playmates or on equipment the child is currently using; or during which the child shares ideas.
Gives clear understandable cues (facial and body) that say, "This is how you should act toward me."	23. Extent: Proportion of time during which the child acts in a way to give out clear messages about how others should interact with him or her.
Responds to others' cues in a way that furthers play.	24. Extent: Proportion of time during which the child acts in accord with others' play cues, and the response results in play.

posttest. The hypotheses for the present study were as follows:

1. The ToP is a reliable and valid instrument to assess young children.
2. Young children with typical development would score significantly higher on the ToP than young children with cerebral palsy and developmental delays before intervention.
3. The ToP scores of young children with cerebral palsy and developmental delays whose mothers were given information on improving their verbal and nonverbal communication patterns would increase significantly more than those of young children with cerebral palsy and developmental delays who received direct NDT designed to improve their developmental motor skills.
4. Young children with cerebral palsy and developmental delays whose mothers were given information on improving their verbal and nonverbal communication patterns would score significantly higher on the ToP at posttest than before the intervention.

Method

Participants

The participants in the present study originally were videotaped for a study conducted by Hanzlik (1986). Hanzlik's study was organized into two phases (see the "Procedure" section for explanation of phases). Unfor-tunately, the tapes from one session in Phase 1 and three sessions from Phase 2 were lost in the intervening years. Therefore, the participants for the first phase of this study were two matched groups of 19 Caucasian mother–infant pairs (data from the child paired with the child on the lost tape also were

eliminated). One group (*n* = 19) consisted of mothers and their young children with cerebral palsy and developmental delays, and the second group (*n* = 19) consisted of mothers and their young children with no cerebral palsy or developmental delays. Gender, age, conditions, and severity classification information of both groups of participants appear in Table 22.2. Developmental status was determined using Cruickshank's (1976) classification for severity.

According to the Bayley Scales of Mental Development (Bayley, 1969), the mental age for each child with cerebral palsy and developmental delay was at least one standard deviation below the mean for the child's chronological age. The two groups of children were matched for gender and mental age. The mother–child pairs in which the children had no developmental delays volunteered to participate in the study by answering an advertisement in the newspaper, whereas the mother–child pairs in which the children had

Table 22.2. Gender, Age, Conditions, and Developmental Status of Participants in Phase 1

Characteristic	Children With No Delays (*n* = 19)	Children With Cerebral Palsy (*n* = 19)
Gender		
Male	13	13
Female	6	6
Mean chronological age (months)	9	18
Chronological age range (months)	3–18	8–32
Mean mental age (months)	9	9
Mental age range (months)	3–18	3–18
Condition		
Hemiplegia	—	5
Diplegia	—	3
Quadriplegia	—	11
Developmental status		
Mild impairments	—	7
Moderate impairments	—	4
Moderately severe impairments	—	6

cerebral palsy and developmental delays were recruited through various intervention programs in Wisconsin and Iowa.

The same mother–child pairs in which the child had cerebral palsy and developmental delays from Phase 1 participated in Phase 2. The mother–infant pairs were randomly assigned either to a group in which the mothers received intervention to improve mother–child interactions ($n = 10$) or a group where the children received NDT while their mothers assisted ($n = 6$). Gender, age, conditions, and severity classification information for the participants in the second phase appear in Table 22.3. The present study was approved by the Human Research Committee at Colorado State University.

Instrument

The ToP, Version 3 (Bundy, 1997b), consists of 24 items scored on a 4-point (0–3) scale. Each score reflects extent (proportion of time observed), intensity (degree), or skillfulness (ease of performance observed) relative to specific behaviors. Bundy, Metzger, Brooks, and Bingaman (in press) reported evidence of preliminary validity and reliability with Version 2 of the ToP. Data from 95% of the items, 96% of the children ($n = 400$; age range = 6 months–14 years), and 100% of the raters ($n = 73$) conformed to the expectations of the Rasch measurement model. Children with disabilities, including 28 children with cerebral palsy, were included in this analysis (Bundy, 1997b). Reliability and validity estimations of Version 3 have not been published but do not differ markedly from Version 2 (A. Bundy, personal communication, September 1997). From its inception, ongoing revisions to the ToP have been made to more accurately reflect the true playfulness of children taking the test, including children with disabilities. Table 22.1 contains a description of ToP Version 3 items.

Procedure

As previously noted, participants who were videotaped for Hanzlik's (1986) study were used for the current research purpose of scoring the playfulness of young children using the ToP. Hanzlik's (1986) original study was done in two phases. In Phase 1, 38 videotaped segments of mothers and their young children (19 were typically developing, 19 had cerebral palsy and developmental delays) were made while each dyad engaged in a 15-min free play session at home. A standard box of toys (ball, doll, busy box, shape box, puppet, pegs and hammer, squeeze toys, weighted rocking bear, radio, pull truck, stacking rings, telephone, 1-in. colored blocks, rattle) was provided during each taping. Mothers were instructed to act as naturally as possible while playing with their young children.

Phase 2 was scheduled 2 weeks after Phase 1. During Phase 2, a 1-hr intervention designed to

Table 22.3. Gender, Age, Conditions, and Developmental Status of Participants (Children With Cerebral Palsy and Developmental Delay) in Phase 2

Characteristic	Intervention Group ($n = 10$)	Control Group ($n = 6$)
Gender		
Male	8	3
Female	2	3
Mean chronological age (months)	16	21
Chronological age range (months)	8–25	12–32
Mean mental age (months)	9	8
Mental age range (months)	3–18	4–15
Conditions		
Hemiplegia	2	2
Diplegia	1	1
Quadriplegia	7	3
Developmental status		
Mild impairments	3	2
Moderate impairments	2	2
Moderately severe impairments	4	1
Severe impairments	1	1

improve verbal and nonverbal communication between mothers and infants was given to 10 of the mothers whose children had cerebral palsy and developmental delays, whereas the other 6 children received NDT with their mothers assisting. Because four tapes (one from Phase 1, three from Phase 2) from Hanzlik's (1986) study were lost in the intervening years, the numbers of participants in the two groups in this study was uneven. The mother–infant dyads were randomly assigned either to the intervention to improve mother–child interactions or to the NDT group.

The intervention to improve mother–child interaction consisted of (a) discussing mothers' concerns regarding play with their children and research on mother–infant interaction and cerebral palsy, (b) modeling specific (verbal and nonverbal) interaction and positioning techniques, and (c) demonstrating maternal interaction styles (see Table 22.4 for Hanzlik's [1998] intervention techniques). Mothers then received a handout to

Table 22.4. Mother–Child Interaction Intervention Techniques

Technique	Instructions
Parent–child turn taking during interaction.	Initiate interaction, wait 5–10 sec for child's response. If there is no response: (1) Signal the child to take a turn with nonverbal cues (e.g., nodding the head, pointing at child). Wait 5–10 sec. If no response, (2) physically or verbally, or both, prompt the child to take a turn depending on the context of the situation. Or, (3) if the child has not responded, initiate a new interaction.
Parental imitation of child behavior.	Take short turns. Imitate all verbal and nonverbal actions of child.
Face-to-face interaction.	Find a position with or without adaptive equipment that allows face-to-face interaction.
Use of adaptive positioning and adaptive equipment that includes face-to-face positioning.	Use therapeutically appropriate positions whether you use equipment that also facilitates mother–child face-to-face interaction.
Verbal directives should not be used exclusively during interaction.	Make statements and exclamations, give praise, and imitate the child as you communicate with him or her. Try not to verbally direct your child all the time. For example, if the child is looking at the ball, say, "The ball is red," and wait for the child's response. Make your next comment after the child responds or after you wait for 10 sec for the child to respond.
Decrease physical directives.	When playing with toys with your child, give him or her a chance to physically respond to the toys independently before you assist the child in manipulating them. For example, before you show your child a toy, make sure that he or she is in a good position that allows maximum control. Then allow the child to play with the toy. If the child does not respond in 10 sec or so, demonstrate how the toy works. If the child does not respond again, physically prompt him or her and wait for a response. If still no response, physically assist the child in playing with the toy.
Use "wh" questions (who, where, what) that continue the established topic of conversation and are developmentally appropriate.	To focus on verbal reciprocity during interaction, use questions that are directed toward the child's production of familiar behavior. To focus on specific linguistic responses, use questions that ask the child to demonstrate advanced linguistic skills. (This technique should not be used to the point that it discourages the child's reciprocal interaction level.)
Interactive match.	Interactions should be paced to maintain the child's tempo. Interactions should only occasionally challenge or stretch the child's skills. For the most part, statements and questions referring to the play activity should be at the child's current level of functioning.

Note. Reprinted from *Pediatric Occupational Therapy and Early Intervention*, J. R. Hanzlik, "Parent–Child Relations: Interaction and Intervention," pp. 213–215, Copyright 1998, with permission from Elsevier.

take with them, summarizing what they were taught during the session.

NDT was provided to the children by an occupational therapist certified in NDT. Treatment focused on such areas as sitting balance and normalizing muscle tone through facilitation of normal developmental movement patterns. In contrast with the intervention to improve mother–child interaction, no social interaction techniques were addressed with the NDT group. Mothers were present during the sessions, but their involvement was limited to activities such as holding a toy while the occupational therapist facilitated the infant's reaching for the toy.

After the interventions, both groups of mother–infant dyads were videotaped again for 15 min of free play in their homes. The same conditions, instructions, and toys provided in Phase 1 were provided again in Phase 2. Taped segments of children with cerebral palsy and developmental delays from Phase 1 were considered "pretest" tapes, and segments of children after either the intervention or the NDT sessions were considered "posttest" tapes.

For the present study, the 54 videotaped segments of mother–infant play (38 from Phase 1, 16 from Phase 2) were placed in random order so that the raters would be naive to the phase. Each of the 54 tapes was then scored using the ToP. The tapes were viewed by three trained raters who had been previously calibrated to score the ToP. (All of the raters were occupational therapy students from Colorado State University; the principal investigator was a professional master's student, and the other two raters were senior undergraduates.) Calibration involved scoring videotapes previously scored by trained raters and examining the data for goodness-of-fit.

Data Analysis

ToP scores from both phases of the study were analyzed using the Rasch analysis computer program FACETS (Linacre, 1989–1994). Rasch analysis generates two types of statistics. One is fit statistics that determine goodness-of-fit of the items, raters, and children to the Rasch measurement model. The second is measure scores, on which subsequent analyses are performed. The measure scores represent the raw scores converted from ordinal to interval data; in this study, measure scores reflect the relative playfulness of the children, severity of the raters, and difficulty of the items on the ToP.

Three assumptions of Rasch must be met by a scale for the data to conform to the expectations of the model. For the ToP scale, these assumptions are that

1. Easy items are easier for all participants;
2. More playful participants are more apt to get higher scores on harder items than are less playful participants; and
3. Lenient raters are more apt to give high scores than are severe raters (Wright & Stone, 1979).

When all assumptions are met, the data are said to "fit the model" (goodness-of-fit).

To answer the question regarding the validity and reliability of the ToP to test playfulness in young children with cerebral palsy and developmental delays (Hypothesis 1), goodness-of-fit was analyzed using the fit statistics generated by Rasch analysis. Goodness-of-fit is determined through mean square (MnSq) and t statistics. Ideally, the MnSq value should be 1.0 and the t value 0. However, values 0 ± 2.0 for t and 1 ± 0.4 for MnSq are acceptable. Rasch analysis generates two t values and two MnSq values. One set reflects "infit" statistics pertaining primarily to items, raters, and subjects in the middle of the scale. The second set reflects "outfit" statistics pertaining primarily to items, raters, and subjects at the extremes of the scale. Only when both statistical values (MnSq and t) fall outside of the acceptable range for either infit or outfit do the data for the item, rater, or subject fail to conform to the expectations of the model.

To answer the question regarding the differences in playfulness in young children with cerebral palsy and young children with no developmental delays (Hypothesis 2), we subjected the measure scores generated by Rasch analysis to a paired *t* test. To answer the question regarding the change in playfulness in young children with cerebral palsy and developmental delays whose mothers received the intervention

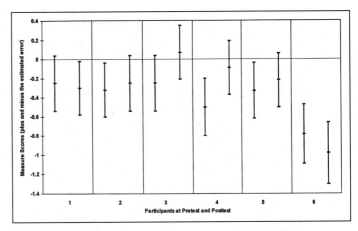

Figure 22.1. Neurodevelopmental treatment group's Test of Playfulness pretest and posttest measure scores plus and minus the estimated error. *Note.* The first bar in each column represents the participant's pretest score. The second bar represents the posttest score.

compared with young children with cerebral palsy and developmental delays who received NDT at posttest (Hypothesis 3), we originally planned to use an analysis of covariance. Despite random assignment to intervention groups, however, the mean pretest score of the NDT group was significantly higher than that of the intervention group ($t = -3.23$, $p = .006$). Thus, we subjected the gain scores (posttest – pretest) in Phase 2 to an independent *t* test (Gliner & Morgan, 1996). Because we were interested in individual differences that would otherwise be masked in the group analysis, we also graphically plotted each participant's pretest and posttest measure scores plus and minus the estimated error (see Figures 22.1 and 22.2). In cases in which the resulting pretest and posttest bands did not overlap (such as with Participants 6 and 8 in Figure 22.2), we considered that person's scores to be significantly different (Silverstein, Kilgore, & Fisher, 1989). Finally, to answer the question regarding the differences in playfulness in young children with cerebral palsy before

and after the intervention (Hypothesis 4), we subjected the measure scores generated by Rasch analysis in Phase 2 to a paired *t* test. Because of the small sample size and the exploratory nature of the study, all significance levels were set at $p = .10$.

Results

The data from 100% of the participants conformed to the expectations of the Rasch measurement model. That is, fit statistic *t* values ranged

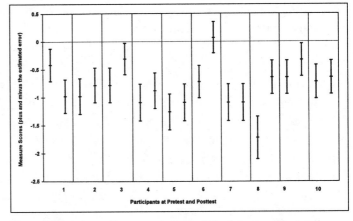

Figure 22.2. Intervention group's Test of Playfulness pretest and posttest measure scores plus and minus the estimated error. *Note.* The first bar in each column represents the participant's pretest score. The second bar represents the posttest score.

between ≤ 2 and ≥ –2 and MnSq values between .6 and 1.4. Data from all three raters also conformed to the expectations of the model. Of the 1,296 scores assigned (24 items × 54 tests), Rasch analysis determined that only 33 ratings (2.5%) were unexpected. Twenty-two of these were for the item Shares, and seven were for the item Decides. Therefore, we concluded that the ToP is a valid and reliable instrument to test playfulness in young children, and Hypothesis 1 was supported. The significance of the unexpected ratings on Shares and Decides will be discussed in subsequent sections.

The results of the paired *t* test indicated that the mean score of the children who were typically developing was significantly higher on the ToP than the mean score of their matched counterparts with cerebral palsy and developmental delays (*t* = –3.938, *p* = .0005). Hypothesis 2 was, therefore, supported. However, Hypothesis 3 was not supported. The results of a *t* test on the gain scores indicated that there was no significant difference between the mean gain score of the children whose mothers received the intervention and that of the children who received NDT (*t* = .562, *p* = .583). Finally, the results of a paired *t* test comparing the mean pretest and posttest scores of the children whose mothers received the intervention revealed significant differences (*t* = 1.615, *p* = .062), thereby supporting Hypothesis 4. This occurred despite the mean pretest score of the NDT group being significantly higher than that of the intervention group (*t* = –3.23, *p* = .006); no significant differences were found between pretest and posttest of the NDT group using a similar paired *t* test (*t* = –1.188, *p* = .144). Table 22.5 illustrates the results associated with Hypotheses 3 and 4.

Discussion

The primary purpose of this investigation was to examine playfulness in young children. Using the

Table 22.5. Mean ToP Scores by Intervention Group at Pretest and Posttest (by Hypothesis) and *t* Test Results

Hypothesis[a]	Mean ToP Scores		*t*	*p*
	NDT	M–C Interaction		
3 (Posttest)	–.295	–.681	0.562	.583
4 (Pretest)		–.924		
4 (Posttest)		–.681	1.625	.062*

Note. ToP = Test of Playfulness; NDT = neurodevelopmental treatment; M–C = mother–child.

[a]Hypothesis 3 stated that the ToP scores of young children with cerebral palsy and developmental delays whose mothers were given the intervention would increase significantly more than those of young children with cerebral palsy and developmental delays who received direct NDT. Hypothesis 4 stated that young children with cerebral palsy and developmental delays whose mothers were given information on improving their verbal and nonverbal communication patterns would score significantly higher on the ToP at posttest than before the intervention.

*Significant mean difference (*p* < .10).

ToP (Bundy, 1997b), we examined (a) differences in playfulness among children who were typically developing and children who had cerebral palsy and developmental delays and (b) the effect of an intervention to improve verbal and nonverbal communication patterns between mothers and children with cerebral palsy and developmental delays.

Before any further analysis could be done, reliability and validity of the ToP needed to be established for this population. The data from all of the children and the raters were found to conform to the expectations of the Rasch measurement model, providing evidence that the ToP was indeed a reliable and valid measurement tool to assess this population. This finding is of particular interest because four of the children had mental ages of less than 6 months. Although the ToP previously has been shown to be a reliable and valid tool for children with disabilities, these results suggest that the ToP is also a reliable and valid tool for children with cognitive deficits and children as young as 3 months of age. It is important to note, however, that the measure scores for all of the children in the present study were relatively low.

Forty-eight (89%) of the 54 taped mother–child play sessions yielded measure scores that were below average (0.0). Only two of the children with cerebral palsy had measure scores that were above average, both of them at posttest (one in the intervention group, one in the NDT group). These results suggest that either these children were not particularly playful or many of the characteristics of playfulness, as measured by the ToP, are not readily seen in very young children. Future research is needed to examine the stability of ToP scores over time with very young children.

As expected, young children with cerebral palsy and developmental delays scored significantly lower on the ToP than their matched counterparts who were typically developing. These findings support previous research regarding playfulness and mother–young child interaction patterns of children with physical disabilities (Barrera & Vella, 1987; Brooks-Gunn & Lewis, 1984; Hanzlik, 1989b; Missiuna & Pollock, 1991). Over the years, researchers and theorists have argued the importance of turn taking and cuing to an infant's development (Connor et al., 1978; Hanzlik, 1998; Papousek & Papousek, 1975). These skills also contribute to a child's playfulness. One important element reflected in the ToP is *framing,* the ability of the child to give and read social cues. This element is represented in the ToP on the items Gives Cues and Responds to Cues.

We found that the raw scores on these two items tended to be higher for children who are typically developing. For Gives Cues, 79% of the children with no delays spent more than half the play session giving appropriate cues to their mothers, compared with only 37% of children with cerebral palsy and developmental delays. Likewise, for Responds to Cues, 47% of the children with no delays spent their play session responding appropriately to cues from their mothers, whereas only 21% of the children with cerebral palsy did the same.

Hanzlik (1986) found that young children with cerebral palsy and developmental delays displayed less voluntary responsive behavior and more physically directed compliant behavior when interacting with their mothers than young children with no developmental delays. These same young children also scored similarly on items of the ToP that required the young child to advocate for his or her needs—items such as Shares and Decides.

There were 33 unexpected ratings of the 1,296 assigned scores. Interestingly, 22 of those 33 scores were on the item Shares. In addition, 17 of the 22 unexpected ratings for Shares came from young children with cerebral palsy, and the remaining 5 were from young children with typical development who were younger than 5 months of age. The latter suggests that Shares, as it is currently described, is not developmentally appropriate for children that young.

According to the ToP scoring guidelines (Bundy, 1997b), Shares is scored on the extent to which the "player allows others to use toys, personal belongings, or equipment. Generally, if the player is not protesting the others' use of possessions or interactions with playmates, consider that the player is sharing" (p. 32). All 22 unexpected ratings for Shares resulted because the child scored higher on this item than expected. Children were given high ratings for this item because they did not protest when toys were taken away from them. In fact, these 22 children did not seem to notice and gave no response to their mothers' actions. This suggests that the scoring criteria for the item Shares should be revised because one of the core assumptions of Rasch analysis has been violated. That assumption—easier items are easier for all people—did not hold true on this item for 22 of the 54 children scored.

Along with Shares, the item Decides also yielded unexpected ratings for seven children, five of whom had cerebral palsy. The ToP manual (Bundy, 1997b) defines Decides as the "proportion of time during which the player actively chooses to do what [he or] she is doing" (p. 26). In contrast with Shares, scores on Decides were unexpectedly low. These unexpected ratings occurred because the young children's mothers made most of the decisions in terms of what toys to play with and what to do next. In fact, the children on 52 of the 54 taped play sessions scored 1 or 0 on this item, meaning that they had spent less than 50% of their time deciding what to do during the play session. The fact that this item was especially low for children with cerebral palsy and developmental delays confirms Missiuna and Pollock's (1991) suggestion that young children with physical disabilities can be deprived of opportunities to explore the environment because their caregivers anticipate their needs. It also supports Marfo's (1992) belief that mother intrusiveness is associated with suboptimal interactions between infant and mother.

The hypothesis that children whose mothers had the intervention would score significantly higher on the ToP after intervention than before intervention also was supported. This finding also is in accord with previous researchers' findings that when mother directiveness is tempered by increased maternal sensitivity (which is what the intervention encouraged), the child is more apt to initiate and persist with activities (Hanzlik, 1998).

In Hanzlik's (1986) study, the greatest improvement after intervention was in mother–infant nonverbal communication skills. Specifically, mothers engaged in less directive physical guidance, more face-to-face contact, and less physical contact with their young children. In turn, their infants engaged in less physically directed compliance and more voluntary responsiveness. We noted similar changes in children's abilities to give and respond to cues. This result is particularly compelling, given that the intervention lasted only

1 hr. However, because of its short duration, the results of this study do not tell us whether the gains were maintained over time. Further research should be aimed at long-term benefits associated with intervention.

As noted, the mothers in the intervention group had less physical and more face-to-face contact with their young children at posttest. These actions may have resulted in increased scores on the cuing items because their relative positions and the physical distance between them allowed the children to read cues and respond to them more effectively. In addition, the fact that the mothers were able to change some of their nonverbal communication in Hanzlik's (1986) study and then effect a change in their young children's response patterns also may have contributed to facilitating increased ability of the children to give and respond to cues.

Although the differences in playfulness for children in the intervention group at pretest and posttest were significant, the difference in playfulness between children whose mothers received intervention and those who received NDT was not significant. This is in apparent contrast with Hanzlik's (1989b) results, in which she found that children's voluntary responsiveness increased while physical compliance decreased. Although voluntary responsiveness is necessary to demonstrating playfulness, playfulness is a much larger construct. Further, most of what Hanzlik coded as voluntary responsiveness we scored as Gives Cues and Responds to Cues (J. Hanzlik, personal communication, April 1999). Giving and responding to cues were the most likely playfulness behaviors to change. However, those alone were not always sufficient to change the child's overall ToP score significantly.

Several additional points should be considered. First and most importantly, the small sample size minimized the power to detect differences if such differences, in fact, do exist. Although not significant, the mean change of the intervention group was slightly greater than that of the NDT group.

Second, although the differences between pretest and posttest mean gain scores were significantly different for the group whose mothers received intervention, they were not different for the NDT group. Examination of the individual changes in measure scores (see Figure 22.1) revealed that only two children's scores improved significantly; both were in the group whose mothers received the intervention. In retrospect, the most obvious differences for those two children resulted from their positioning relative to their mothers. For the posttest, both children were placed in adaptive seating devices per Hanzlik's (1989b) intervention suggestion. This change facilitated more eye contact and more time for the dyad to give and respond to each other's cues, as evidenced by better scores for both children on the cuing items on the ToP. This finding demonstrates the importance of altering the environment to maximize children's performance.

Finally, despite random assignment to the groups, more children with moderately severe impairments and quadriplegia were in the group whose mothers received intervention than in the NDT group. However, it must be noted that one of the two children whose scores changed significantly was a child with very severe impairment; his mental age, according to the Bayley scales, was 2.62 standard deviations below the mean for his chronological age. Therefore, despite his severe impairment, this child was able to benefit from the effects of the intervention.

Clearly, the effectiveness of a short-term intervention designed to improve mother–child interactions lies in its power to enable children to demonstrate their inherent capabilities (in this case, playfulness). Thus, in many respects, it is not surprising that children with major developmental delays who received 1 hr of NDT aimed at improving their motor skills were not as likely to demonstrate increased playfulness. Perhaps with more long-term intervention, these children might have gained skills underlying play. However, the findings suggest that intervention aimed at improving parent–child interactions should be coupled with (and perhaps take precedence over) direct intervention aimed at improving a child's developmental motor skills.

Further study clearly is needed. To maximize potential differences, the intervention should be ongoing and of longer duration; it also should be aimed at the specific needs of the dyad, as typically would be the case in a child's therapy program, rather than a standardized intervention as administered in this study. The long-term effects of intervention also should be monitored. Further, although nonverbal communication skills were significantly changed in Hanzlik's (1986) study, verbal ones did not change. With more intervention, mothers would have increased time to focus on improving verbal communication skills. A larger sample size also would increase the power of the study, specifically by increasing the chances of getting more homogeneous groups through random assignment.

Conclusion

As expected, we found the ToP to be a reliable and valid instrument to assess playfulness with young children with cerebral palsy. We also found significant differences in playfulness between young children with cerebral palsy and developmental delays and young children with no developmental disabilities. As predicted, we found that the intervention that Hanzlik (1986) used to improve mother–infant nonverbal communication skills also significantly improved the level of playfulness of children in that group. Graphic analysis of individual scores revealed that two children in the intervention group, but no children in the NDT group, had significant improvement in their ToP scores. However, despite group and individual differences, the mean gain score of children in the group whose mothers received the intervention was not significantly higher than that of the NDT group. Greatly diminished power from the small sample size likely contributed to the failure to find significant differences in gain scores between groups. Clearly, there is a need for further study.

Young children with cerebral palsy and developmental delays face many more challenges than their peers who are typically developing, secondary to physical limitations and limitations perceived by caregivers and playmates. When caregivers are helped to effectively support children's abilities, children respond in more playful ways. Altering the environment is another important part of intervention aimed at improving mother–child interactions. Small changes, such as changing the relative positioning of the dyad during play, are effective for enabling children to demonstrate their capabilities. Thus, occupational therapists and others who work with young children with disabilities and their families should consider the full range of possibilities for facilitating mother–child interaction through intervention.

Acknowledgments

We thank Jennifer Ierna, OTR, and Brad Quinn, OTR, for their assistance with scoring the tapes and Jeff Gliner, PhD, for his statistical advice. This study was done in partial fulfillment of the first author's requirement for a master's degree in occupational therapy from Colorado State University.

References

Barrera, M. E., & Vella, D. M. (1987). Disabled and nondisabled infants' interactions with their mothers. *American Journal of Occupational Therapy, 41,* 168–172.

Bayley, N. (1969). *Bayley Scales of Infant Development.* New York: Psychological Corporation.

Brooks-Gunn, J., & Lewis, M. (1984). Maternal responsivity in interaction with handicapped infants. *Child Development, 55,* 782–793.

Bundy, A. C. (1997a). Play and playfulness: What to look for. In L. D. Parham & L. S. Fazio (Eds.), *Play in occupational therapy for children* (pp. 52–66). St. Louis, MO: Mosby.

Bundy, A. C. (1997b). *Test of Playfulness (ToP) Manual, Version 3.4.* Fort Collins: Colorado State University.

Bundy, A. C., Metzger, M., Brooks, L., & Bingaman, K. (in press). Reliability and validity of a test of playfulness. *Occupational Therapy Journal of Research.*

Connor, F. P., Williamson, G. G., & Siepp, J. M. (Eds.). (1978). *Program guide for infants and toddlers with neuromotor and other developmental disabilities.* New York: Teacher's College.

Cruickshank, W. (1976). *Cerebral palsy: A developmental disability.* New York: Syracuse University.

Eheart, B. K. (1982). Mother–child interactions with nonretarded and mentally retarded preschoolers. *American Journal on Mental Deficiency, 87,* 20–25.

Gliner, J. A., & Morgan, G. A. (1996). *Research design and analysis in applied settings.* Fort Collins: Colorado State University.

Hanzlik, J. R. (1986). *Interaction and intervention with mothers and their cerebral-palsied infants.* Doctoral dissertation, Iowa State University, Ames.

Hanzlik, J. R. (1989a). The effect of intervention on the free-play experience for mothers and their infants with developmental delay and cerebral palsy. *Physical and Occupational Therapy in Pediatrics, 9,* 33–51.

Hanzlik, J. R. (1989b). Interactions between mothers and their infants with developmental disabilities: Analysis and review. *Physical and Occupational Therapy in Pediatrics, 9,* 33–47.

Hanzlik, J. R. (1998). Parent–child relations: Interaction and intervention. In J. Case-Smith (Ed.), *Pediatric occupational therapy and early intervention* (pp. 207–292). Woburn, MA: Butterworth-Heinemann.

Hanzlik, J. R., & Stevenson, M. B. (1986). Interaction of mothers with their infants who are mentally retarded, retarded with cerebral palsy, or non-retarded. *American Journal of Mental Deficiency, 90,* 513–520.

Holloway, E. (1997). Fostering parent–infant playfulness in the neonatal intensive care unit. In L. D. Parham & L. S. Fazio (Eds.), *Play in occupational therapy for children* (pp. 171–183). St. Louis, MO: Mosby.

Kogan, K. L., & Tyler, N. (1973). Mother–child interaction in young physically handicapped children. *American Journal of Mental Deficiency, 77,* 492–497.

Lieberman, D., Padan-Belkin, E., & Harel, S. (1995). Maternal directiveness and infant compliance at one year of age: A comparison between mothers and their developmentally-delayed infants and mothers and their nondelayed infants. *Journal of Child Psychology and Psychiatry, 36,* 1091–1096.

Linacre, J. M. (1989–1994). *Facets: Computer program for many-faceted Rasch measurement.* Chicago: MESA.

Marfo, K. (1992). Correlates of maternal directiveness with children who are developmentally delayed. *American Journal of Orthopsychiatry, 62,* 219–233.

Missiuna, C., & Pollock, N. (1991). Play deprivation in children with physical disabilities: The role of the occupational therapist in preventing secondary disability. *American Journal of Occupational Therapy, 45,* 882–888.

Papousek, H., & Papousek, M. (1975). Cognitive aspects of preverbal social interaction between human infants and adults. *CIBA Foundation Symposium: Vol. 33, Parent–Infant Interaction* (pp. 241–269). Amsterdam: Associated Scientific.

Parham, L. D., & Primeau, L. A. (1997). Play and occupational therapy. In L. D. Parham & L. A. Fazio (Eds.), *Play in occupational therapy for children* (pp. 2–21). St. Louis, MO: Mosby.

Rubin, K., Fein, G. G., & Vandenberg, B. (1983). Play. In P. H. Mussen (Ed.), *Handbook of child psychology* (4th ed., pp. 693–774). New York: Wiley.

Silverstein, B., Kilgore, K., & Fisher, W. (1989). *Implementing patient tracking systems and using functional assessment scales.* Wheaton, IL: Marianjoy Rehabilitation Center.

Sutton-Smith, B. (1980). A sportive theory of play. In H. B. Schwartzman (Ed.), *Play and culture* (pp. 10–19). West Point, NY: Leisure.

Wright, B. D., & Stone, M. H. (1979). *Best test design.* Chicago: MESA.

CHAPTER 23

Classroom Seating for Children With Attention Deficit Hyperactivity Disorder

Therapy Balls Versus Chairs

Denise Lynn Schilling, Kathleen Washington,
Felix F. Billingsley, and Jean Deitz

Denise Lynn Schilling, MS, PT, *was a graduate student at the time of this study in the master's of science program, Department of Rehabilitation Medicine, University of Washington, Seattle. Mailing address: 4210 258th Avenue, SE, Issaquah, WA 98029; missdeesg@aol.com.*

Kathleen Washington, PhD, PT, *is clinical assistant professor, Department of Rehabilitation Medicine, University of Washington, Seattle.*

Felix F. Billingsley, PhD, *is professor and chair, Special Education, University of Washington, Seattle.*

Jean Deitz, PhD, OTR/L, FAOTA, *is professor and graduate program coordinator, Department of Rehabilitation Medicine, University of Washington, Seattle.*

Originally published 2003 in *American Journal of Occupational Therapy,* 57, 534–541.

Attention deficit hyperactivity disorder (ADHD) is the most frequently diagnosed neurobehavioral disorder in childhood (Kauffman, 2001). Current estimates indicate the prevalence of ADHD in the United States ranges from approximately 4% to 6% of school-age children (Jaksa, 1998; Rosenblum, 2000) to as high as 13% in America's inner cities (Goldman, Genel, Bezman, & Slanetz, 1998; Meaux, 2000). According to Mulligan (2001), children diagnosed with ADHD often experience significant academic and sensory motor problems that make typical school activities a challenge. Goldstein and Goldstein (1992) identified sitting and paying attention as problems for these children in the classroom, and Barkley (1990) noted that children with ADHD often fail to complete assignments or underperform academically.

As a result of the increasing numbers of children with ADHD and the identified problems, Mulligan (2001) made two recommendations. First, she maintained that there is an increased need for therapists to be knowledgeable about ways of managing the classroom behaviors of children with ADHD; second, she identified the need for strategies designed to enhance the school performance of these children. These recommendations seem especially important, as many children with ADHD experience a wide range of secondary behavioral and emotional problems at school (Goldstein & Goldstein, 1992), and more than one-third of students with ADHD drop out of school (Rosenblum, 2000).

Mulligan (2001) suggested that sensory modulation deficits might be a factor in children who demonstrate attention deficits. According to Miller and Lane (2000), *sensory modulation* "reflects an adjustment in ongoing physiological processes to ensure internal adaptation to new or changing sensory information" (p. 3). Furthermore, Hanft, Miller, and Lane (2000) noted that, because interactions among tasks, environments, and people continually change, a person's responses may fluctuate considerably, not only day to day but also within an activity. Therefore, it seems that one potential intervention approach to address the behavioral problems of children with ADHD at school is to adapt the environment to meet the children's needs.

Occupational therapy literature has specifically suggested the implementation of sensory modulation strategies in classrooms for the purpose of improving the classroom performance of children with ADHD (Kimball, 1999; Mulligan, 1996). One possible strategy of using therapy balls for seating was suggested by back-health studies. Incidental to these studies, researchers commented that children using therapy balls in the classroom appeared to improve in attention, sustained sitting, and school performance (Illi, 1994; Witt & Talbot, 1998). These behaviors are compatible with Ayres's suggestion that an overexcited child may be calmed by gently rocking on a ball (Ayres, 1977). Although these reports and the literature, either directly or indirectly, suggested the use of therapy balls for classroom seating for children with ADHD, prior to the current study no studies had systematically examined the use of this strategy for such children.

Therefore, the purpose of this study was to examine the use of therapy balls for classroom seating as an intervention for children with ADHD. Two specific research questions were addressed. First, what effect does using therapy balls as chairs have on in-seat behavior? Second, what effect does sitting on balls have on legible word productivity? In addition, social validity was examined to evaluate the teacher's and students' opinions regarding the acceptability and viability of the intervention. Schwartz and Baer (1991) recommended that social validity assessment be a standard part of applied behavioral research, because it is possible for an intervention to result in positive changes in dependent variables while simultaneously being identified by research participants as unacceptable.

Method

This study used a single-subject, ABAB interrupted time series design (Kazdin, 1982) across three students with ADHD. During baseline phases (A), participants and all other members of the class used chairs during language arts; during intervention phases (B), participants and all other members of the class sat on therapy balls during language arts. The language arts period was chosen because it occurred at the same time daily (immediately after lunch recess) and it was a time in the children's daily schedules when they were regularly involved in producing written assignments. The total study was 12 weeks in length; each phase was 3 weeks long.

Participants

A convenience sample was used from a 4th-grade classroom in a public school in Washington state. Three children with a diagnosis of ADHD participated in this study; however, all 24 students in the classroom used the balls and chairs. Study procedures were approved by a university human subjects review committee and met the requirements of the school district where the study was implemented.

The participants, 1 girl and 2 boys, were ages 9 years, 11 months; 9 years, 11 months; and 9 years, 8 months, respectively. Each had a physician's diagnosis of ADHD. In addition, one boy had a concomitant diagnosis of oppositional defiant disorder and the other boy a concomitant diagnosis of severe behavior disorder. All were of average intelligence or above as defined by a score equal to 80 or above on the Wechsler Intelligence Scale for Children (Wechsler, 1991). Each participant was taking Clonidine, Ritalin, or Adderall. Medications remained constant throughout the study. Prior to the study, all participants regularly demonstrated out-of-seat behavior during the language arts period and required repeated verbal reminders or physical prompts or both from the teacher.

Independent Variable

The therapy balls selected for classroom use had molded feet (Sit 'n' Gym™ by Gymnic) that extended when the ball was not in use to prevent rolling away. Therapy balls were individually fitted for each student in the classroom for a diameter that assured the student could sit comfortably with his or her feet flat on the floor with knees and hips flexed at 90 degrees.

Dependent Variables

In-seat behavior. In-seat behavior (chair) was defined as behavior that occurred when any portion of a participant's buttocks was in contact with the seat portion of the chair (Sugai & Rowe, 1984) and the four legs of the chair were in contact with the floor. In-seat behavior (ball) was defined as behavior that occurred when any portion of a participant's buttocks was in contact with the ball, the ball was in contact with the floor, and a minimum of one foot of the participant was in contact with the floor. These criteria were measured using momentary real-time sampling (Richards, Taylor, Ramasamy, & Richards, 1999), whereby following each 10-second interval of the observation, the rater scored the participant's behavior as either in-seat or out-of-seat. Because each participant was observed each session for five 2-minute periods, this resulted in 60 observations per session per participant. To determine percentage of in-seat behavior, the number of observations of in-seat behavior was divided by the total number of possible observations that occurred within that session. Therefore, if a session included all 60 observations and if a participant was recorded as being in seat during 20 observations, his or her percentage of in-seat behavior for that session was 33% (20/60).

Legible word productivity. Legible word productivity was defined as the percentage of difference between the participant's legible word production and the class mean for legible word production on the same assignment. The percentage difference between the participant's legible word production and the class mean (excluding the study participants) on the same assignment was used because of the high variability in the type and length of writing assignments from one day to the next (e.g., fill-in-the-blank assignments, story writing). Although assignments varied from day to day, all students were given the same assignment on the same day. A method described by Hasbrouck, Tindal, and Parker (1994) was used to assess legibility of produced words. This involved using a window card to expose only one word at a time starting at the end of the document and progressing to the beginning so that words were read out of context.

Procedures

After consent and assent were obtained and prior to the first baseline session, all students in the class were individually fitted for therapy balls. Each ball was labeled to ensure that each student used the ball sized specifically for him or her. An introductory session followed in which the primary investigator answered questions and developed classroom rules, with input from the students, for ball use. Students then had 30 minutes to sit on the balls and independently explore movement and balance. Throughout the study, the teacher was instructed to give no positive or negative feedback on sitting behavior and to intervene only if a student exhibited a behavior deemed by her to be dangerous or destructive. Students were not told the purpose of the study or which members of the class were being observed.

Following the first phase of the study, all students used the balls for 1 week during the language arts period to allow for novelty effects. During this time, no data were collected.

During all baseline and intervention phases, data collection on in-seat behavior (chair and ball) occurred during the middle 40 minutes of the 60-minute language arts session. This allowed for 10 minutes at the beginning of the class for a potential late start and 10 minutes at the conclusion of class for early lesson completion. To collect observational data and address reliability, two pediatric therapists were used. Employing momentary real-time sampling, these two therapists independently and simultaneously observed and scored the in-seat behavior of the same participant. Each therapist wore a wireless headset to hear a preprogrammed tape that announced which participant to record at each 10-second interval. Raters heard the signals and instructions at the exact same moment. Each participant was observed for five 2-minute periods, thus resulting in 60 observations per participant per session. A 30-second break occurred following each 2-minute recording period to ease the data collection process for the raters and to allow time for raters to reposition for observation of the next participant in the rotation pattern. The order in which participants were observed each day was randomly selected from a list of six potential patterns (e.g., Pattern 1: John, Emily, Mike; Pattern 2: Mike, Emily, John [pseudonyms]). Once a pattern had been selected for a session, it was used five times during that session and not used again in subsequent sessions until all patterns had been used.

Prior to beginning data collection and periodically throughout the study, interrater agreement was examined. The minimum standard was set at 80 percent (Kazdin, 1982).

For out-of-seat–off-of-ball, in-seat–on-ball, and in-seat–asleep behaviors, interrater point-by-point agreement (Kazdin, 1982) ranged from 95% to 100% ($M = 98\%$). When a difference in scores between the two raters occurred, the mean score of the two raters was used because it is more reliable than scores of a single rater when the reliability between the two raters is high (Tuckman, 1988). Although data were collected for 12 sessions during each phase, during some phases some participants had fewer data points because of classroom absences.

To assess legible word productivity, five writing samples were randomly selected per phase for each participant. The primary investigator evaluated all selected samples for word productivity using the process described under dependent variables. To assess reliability, a second evaluator, blind to the study, evaluated two randomly selected papers per phase per participant. Average interrater agreement (using the formula for percent agreement) was 94%.

The primary investigator checked procedural reliability once weekly with the day randomly selected (Billingsley, White, & Munson, 1980). She used a checklist describing the classroom environment (e.g., levels of feedback to the students from the teacher, consistency of staff in the classroom, daily schedule, and absence of discussion regarding potential study outcomes). Procedural reliability was 100%, thus suggesting that the environment and the teacher's management style and expectations remained constant during the study.

At the completion of phases 2, 3, and 4, during class time, the teacher and all 24 students completed social validity questionnaires. The teacher and student questionnaires had nine and six questions, respectively. Three choices (ball, chair, and no difference) followed each question. Topics covered in the questionnaires included classroom behavior and assignment completion. Sample teacher questions were "Students had better attention to task when sitting on ___." "Students remained seated longer when sitting on ___." "Students were least disruptive to peers when sitting on ___." Sample student questions were "I finish my work better sitting on ___." "I can listen and pay attention better sitting on ___." Prior to implementation, a physical therapist, an occupational therapist, and an educator reviewed the questions for relevance and potential for biasing results.

At the end of the study, the teacher and the students were all given blank sheets of paper and asked to write about their overall perceptions regarding using balls, chairs, or both. Instructions were to "Write a sentence or two on how you felt about sitting on balls. It can be what you liked or didn't like."

Results

In-Seat Behavior

Figure 23.1 indicates that improvements in sitting behavior were evident for all the participants when using therapy balls for seating. John displayed in-class sleeping behavior in addition to his disruptive out-of-seat activities during Phases 1 and 3, when seated on a chair. During Phases 2 and 4, when seated on the ball, there were no sessions in which John was asleep.

Emily, the participant with no coexisting conditions, displayed consistent patterns of behavior on the chair and on the ball. During chair phases she was in constant motion and often out-of-seat. During therapy ball phases she remained in her seat appearing still and steady.

As noted in Figure 23.1, Mike presented differently from the other two participants. During baseline he was in-seat approximately 75% of the time, considerably more than the other participants were. However, observations revealed that when Mike was out of his seat, he spent his time talking with classmates, removing items from other students' desks, and frequently interrupting the teacher. When seated quietly in his chair he would often read a pleasure book and not participate in class activities. Mike frequently left the class and would not return for prolonged periods and often left school early. As a result, Mike was not present for the ball introduction and the five-session novelty phase. After the first week of intervention, which served as Mike's novelty phase, his in-seat behavior on the ball was consistently above his behavior on the chair.

Legible Word Productivity

It was hypothesized that if students with ADHD increased their in-seat behavior when sitting on balls versus chairs, the amount of written work they produced would also increase. As noted in Figure 23.2, productivity percentage of difference from the class mean for five randomly selected assignments per phase indicated that all three participants' legible word productivity was generally higher when seated on therapy balls. Note that when a participant was present in class but completed no written work, that participant received a score of 0.

Social Validity

All three participants with ADHD reported preferring balls to chairs for comfort, writing, and productivity. In addition, 21 other students in the class reported via questionnaire that they believed the therapy balls were more comfortable, improved their writing, and increased their ability to listen and finish class work. Of this group, 17 students reported that they preferred balls, 2 preferred chairs, and 2 had no preference.

At the conclusion of the study, all students also were given an opportunity to put in writing their opinions of sitting on balls in the classroom. Students could write more than one comment. Of the 30 responses made by the students, 26 were positive in support of sitting on balls and 4 were negative. The 4 negative responses were reports of back discomfort, with 2 of the 4

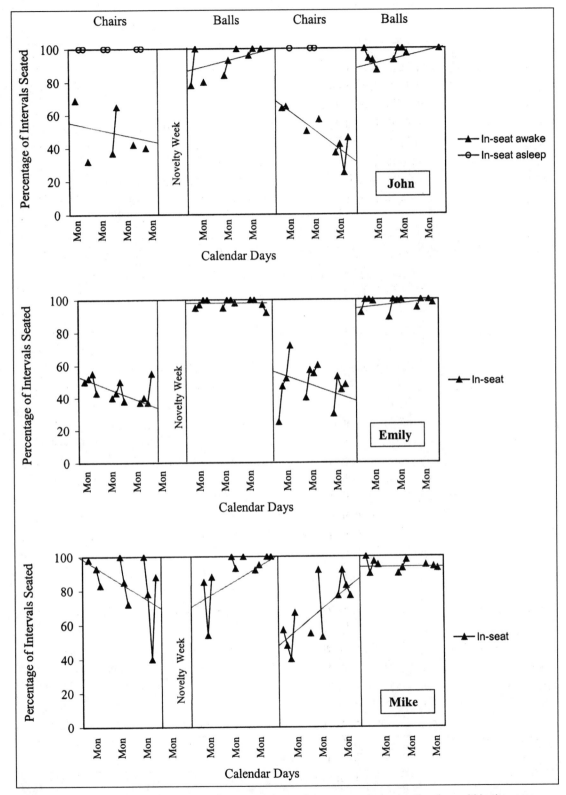

Figure 23.1. In-seat behavior by session. Connected data points represent consecutive days within the same week. Variability in the number of data points was the result of a non–school day or student absence from class.

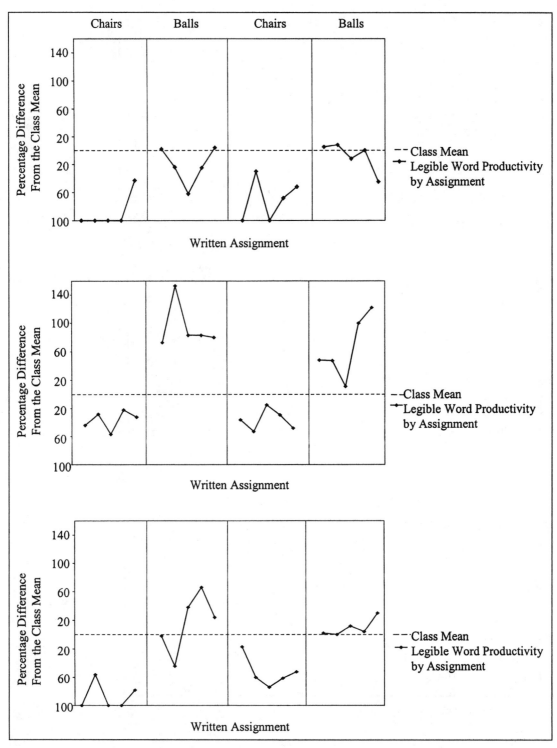

Figure 23.2. Comparison of legible word productivity to the class mean. Each participant's productivity on each paper was based on the percentage of difference between his or her word production and that of the class mean on the same assignment.

disliking the lack of a backrest. Additionally, John reported "a downside of balls is being unable to sleep in class." Of the 26 positive responses in support of sitting on balls, 13 reported increased back comfort or improved posture, 6 reported increased freedom of movement, 4 reported increased attention, and 3 reported improved handwriting. A sampling of the positive written comments regarding sitting on balls were "You can keep your brain active even when you're bored" (typical child), "My posture improves" (Mike), "I can get my work done better" (Emily), and "Writing is funner than ever" (typical child).

The teacher's responses also supported the use of balls for classroom seating. Sample teacher comments included, "Although students are bouncing, they are more focused on what I am saying," "The noise level immediately decreases," "Following the use of the balls the students seem to remain calmer and focus better for about 30 to 45 minutes," and "For some students work production has dramatically improved." At the completion of this study, the teacher continued to use therapy balls for seating for the children with ADHD and ordered additional balls for other students, thus further supporting the social validity of this intervention.

Discussion

Findings of this study support the use of therapy balls for students with ADHD as an alternative classroom seating option. For all participants, both in-seat behavior and legible word productivity improved when seated on the therapy balls. This study demonstrated that the intervention was effective with three students with ADHD who varied in terms of gender, concomitant diagnoses, and medications. This provides some support for the generality of the findings and is important as ADHD often co-

exists with other disorders (Barkley, 1990; Mulligan, 2001; Silver, 1990). In addition, the teacher's and students' general preferences for therapy balls for seating supported the social validity of the intervention.

Therapists and the teacher reported observing substantial student differences in movement patterns (e.g., b ouncing, gently rocking) while seated on the therapy balls. One explanation could be self-modulation of personal sensory needs by each student to maintain an optimal state of arousal (Dunn, 2000; Kimball, 1999; Mulligan, 2001; Williams & Shellenberger, 1994). An example of an individual student's variation in movement pattern was observed in Mike who, at the beginning of a session, gently rocked on the therapy ball and vigorously bounced toward the conclusion of the same session. This variation in movement patterns may reflect responses to changing sensory needs, possibly explained by the theory that a person's sensory needs continually change as they are affected by interactions with tasks, environments, and people (Brown, Tollefson, Dunn, Cromwell, & Filion, 2001; Cohn, Miller, & Tickle-Degnen, 2000; Dunn, 1997; Dunn & Brown, 1997; Mulligan, 2001).

For Emily, the use of the ball immediately addressed safety issues. On the chair she was in constant movement, often out-of-seat, and when seated, she generally assumed extreme postures that were potentially dangerous (e.g., tipping her chair and balancing on the top of the backrest). By contrast, on the ball, she needed to keep at least one foot in contact with the floor to maintain sitting balance, thus minimizing classroom disruption and safety concerns.

For John, therapy balls for seating decreased in-class sleeping behavior. It appeared that when John attempted to sleep, slight movement of the ball would alert him, and he would immediately sit up. This was further supported by John's comment regarding his inability to sleep when seated on the therapy ball.

According to Mulligan (2001), a common function of the school-based therapist is collaborating with teachers to develop strategies to improve behavior and classroom performance of students with ADHD. She further identified the need to evaluate the effectiveness of such strategies. The current study addressed this need and exemplified the use and evaluation of a strategy involving collaboration with a teacher for both implementation and success.

Limitations

Limitations of the study included the short duration of the study (12 weeks), the sample size, the use of a single classroom, and the fact that quality of written work was not assessed. Although the teacher reported improvements in class work for the participants when seated on the balls versus chairs, no formal assessments were performed on the written assignments regarding spelling, sentence structure, or content.

Directions for Future Research

Therapists in school system practice need to continue to study the use of therapy balls in the classroom for the purpose of helping students succeed. Three directions for future research are warranted. First, the longitudinal effects of using therapy balls for classroom seating for children with ADHD should be studied. Second, the use of therapy balls for children with other diagnoses (e.g., autism, Down syndrome) merits investigation. Last, future research should include dependent variables such as classroom noise levels, classroom behaviors (e.g., raising hand, verbal outbursts), peer relationships, quality of word production, and student performance in a variety of academic areas.

Conclusion

This study suggests that the use of therapy balls for classroom seating is one strategy that therapists in school systems practice might consider when working with children with ADHD who are having difficulty meeting school expectations of staying on task and remaining seated. Additionally, this intervention strategy was found to be compatible with inclusive educational practice and interdisciplinary teaming.

Acknowledgments

This research was funded in part by a grant from the U.S. Department of Health and Human Services, Maternal and Child Health Bureau to the University of Washington, Center for Leadership in Pediatric Physical Therapy Education. We thank the students and families who made this research possible and the teachers, administrators, and coworkers who provided resources and assistance.

References

Ayres, A. J. (1977). *Sensory integration and learning disorders.* Los Angeles: Western Psychological Services.

Barkley, R. (1990). *Attention deficit hyperactivity disorder: A handbook for diagnosis and treatment.* New York: Guilford.

Billingsley, F., White, O., & Munson, R. (1980). Procedural reliability: A rationale and an example. *Behavioral Assessment, 2,* 229–241.

Brown, C., Tollefson, N., Dunn, W., Cromwell, R., & Filion, D. (2001). The Adult Sensory Profile: Measuring patterns of sensory processing. *American Journal of Occupational Therapy, 55,* 75–82.

Cohn, E., Miller, L., & Tickle-Degnen, L. (2000). Parental hopes for therapy outcomes: Children with sensory modulation disorders. *American Journal of Occupational Therapy, 54,* 36–43.

Dunn, W. (1997). The impact of sensory processing abilities on the daily lives of young children and their families: A conceptual model. *Infants and Young Children, 9,* 23–35.

Dunn, W. (2000). Habit: What's the brain got to do with it? *Occupational Therapy Journal of Research, 20,* 6s–20s.

Dunn, W., & Brown, C. (1997). Factor analysis on the Sensory Profile from a national sample of children without disabilities. *American Journal of Occupational Therapy, 51,* 490–495.

Goldman, L., Genel, M., Bezman, R., & Slanetz, P. (1998). Diagnosis and treatment of attention deficit/hyperactivity disorder in children and adolescents. *JAMA, 279,* 1100–1107.

Goldstein, S., & Goldstein, M. (1992). *Hyperactivity—Why won't my child pay attention?* New York: Wiley.

Hanft, B., Miller, L., & Lane, S. (2000, September). Toward a consensus in terminology in sensory integration theory and practice: Part 3. Observable behaviors: Sensory integration dysfunction. *Sensory Integration Special Interest Section Quarterly, 23,* pp. 1–4.

Hasbrouck, J., Tindal, G., & Parker, R. (1994, Winter). Objective procedures for scoring student's writing. *Teaching Exceptional Children,* pp. 18–22.

Illi, U. (1994). Balls instead of chairs in the classroom? *Swiss Journal of Physical Education, 6,* 37–39.

Jaksa, P. (1998). *Fact sheet on attention deficit hyperactivity disorder.* Retrieved October 18, 2002, from www.add.org/content/abc/factsheet.htm

Kauffman, J. (2001). *Characteristics of emotional and behavioral disorders of children and youth* (7th ed.). Columbus, OH: Merrill/Prentice Hall.

Kazdin, A. E. (1982). *Single-case research design.* New York: Oxford University Press.

Kimball, J. (1999). Sensory integration frame of reference: Postulates regarding change and application to practice. In P. Kramer & J. Hinojosa (Eds.), *Frames of reference for pediatric occupational therapy* (2nd ed., pp. 169–204). Philadelphia: Lippincott Williams & Wilkins.

Meaux, J. (2000). Stop, look, and listen: The challenge for children with ADHD. *Issues in Comprehensive Pediatric Nursing, 23,* 1–13.

Miller, L., & Lane, S. (2000, March). Toward a consensus in terminology in sensory integration theory and practice: Part 1. Taxonomy of neurophysiological processes. *Sensory Integration Special Interest Section Quarterly, 23,* pp. 1–4.

Mulligan, S. (1996). An analysis of score patterns of children with attention disorders on the Sensory Integration and Praxis Tests. *American Journal of Occupational Therapy, 50,* 647–654.

Mulligan, S. (2001). Classroom strategies used by teachers of students with attention deficit hyperactivity disorder. *Physical and Occupational Therapy in Pediatrics, 20,* 25–44.

Richards, S., Taylor, R., Ramasamy, R., & Richards, R. (1999). *Single subject research: Applications in educational and clinical settings.* San Diego: Singular.

Rosenblum, G. (2000). *Your child and ADHD.* Singapore: Creative Publishing International.

Schwartz, I., & Baer, D. (1991). Social validity assessments: Is current practice state of the art? *Journal of Applied Behavior Analysis, 24,* 189–204.

Silver, L. (1990). Attention deficit hyperactivity disorder: Is it a learning disability or a related disorder? *Journal of Learning Disabilities, 23,* 394–397.

Sugai, G., & Rowe, P. (1984, February). The effect of self-recording on out-of-seat behavior of an EMR student. *Education and Training of the Mentally Retarded,* pp. 23–28.

Tuckman, B. (1988). *Conducting educational research* (3rd ed.). San Diego: Harcourt Brace Jovanovich.

Wechsler, D. (1991). *Manual for Wechsler Intelligence Scale for Children* (3rd ed). San Antonio, TX: Psychological Corporation.

Williams, M., & Shellenberger, S. (1994). *How does your engine run?* Albuquerque, NM: Therapy Works.

Witt, D., & Talbot, R. (1998, February). Let's get our kids on the ball. *Advance for Physical Therapists,* pp. 27–28.

CHAPTER 24

Testing the Effect of Kinesthetic Training on Handwriting Performance in First-Grade Students

Pimjai Sudsawad, Catherine A. Trombly,

Ann Henderson, and Linda Tickle-Degnen

Pimjai Sudsawad, ScD, OTR, *is assistant professor, Department of Occupational Therapy, University of Wisconsin–Milwaukee, PO Box 413, Milwaukee, WI 53201; pimjais@uwm.edu.*

Catherine A. Trombly, ScD, OTR, *is professor emeritus, Department of Occupational Therapy, Boston University, Boston.*

Ann Henderson, PhD, OTR, *is professor emeritus, Department of Occupational Therapy, Boston University, Boston.*

Linda Tickle-Degnen, PhD, OTR, *is associate professor, Department of Occupational Therapy, Boston University, Boston.*

Originally published 2002 in *American Journal of Occupational Therapy, 56,* 26–33.

Learning to write is one of the major occupations of childhood (Amundson, 1992; McHale & Cermak, 1992). Children's handwriting performance is of concern to occupational therapists, educators, and parents because it is an essential skill required to participate in educational activities successfully. Difficulties with handwriting can be resistive to change even after several years of formal handwriting education (Alston & Taylor, 1987; Rubin & Henderson, 1982).

Kinesthesis is a sense of movement and position of the limbs that arises from information from the muscles, joints, and skin (McClosky, 1978). On the basis of their closed-loop theory of motor control, Laszlo and Bairstow (1984) proposed that kinesthetic feedback is essential to handwriting development. They proposed that kinesthetic information has two functions in the performance and acquisition of handwriting: It provides ongoing error information, and it is stored in memory to be recalled when the writing is repeated. Error information leads to error correction programming, and the upgraded program generates its own kinesthetic input when executed. Storage of this input leads to improved programming in subsequent attempts at handwriting and is responsible for improvement in handwriting skill. Therefore, if kinesthetic information cannot be perceived or used, efficient programming cannot occur. A child with kinesthetic impairment will find writing difficult and will be unable to improve his or her writing performance through practice because lack of kinesthetic error detection and error correction lead to inability to improve motor programs necessary for writing (Laszlo & Bairstow, 1984).

Laszlo and Bairstow (1983, 1985b) proposed a kinesthetic intervention with the underlying assumptions that kinesthesis can be changed through training and that improvement in kinesthesis will lead to improvement in motor performance, including writing. This kinesthetic training program consists of intensive daily training of 2 weeks or less to improve motor performance by improving two aspects of kinesthesis: *kinesthetic acuity,* or the ability to discriminate between relative positions and movements of two upper limbs, and *kinesthetic perception and memory,* or the ability to perceive and recall movement patterns of an upper limb.

The effectiveness of this kinesthetic training program in improving handwriting in children has been investigated in a few studies with varied results. In a study of 30 schoolchildren 5 to 7 years of age, Harris and Livesey (1992) found that the children who received kinesthetic training showed significantly greater improvement in handwriting than the children who received handwriting practice. Escribano (1991)[1] further investigated the relationship between the kinesthetic training program and handwriting performance in 23 children 7 to 8 years of age and found no significant handwriting improvement in either the kinesthetic training group or the no-treatment group. Sims, Henderson, Hulme, and Morton (1996) studied 20 children 8 to 9 years of age who were clumsy and found no significant improvement of handwriting immediately after treatment in either the kinesthetic training group or the no-treatment group. However, the children in both groups showed improvement at follow-up approximately 3 months after the treatment. In a second study of 36 children 6 to 10 years of age who were clumsy, these researchers found that both the kinesthetic training group and the alternative treatment group (activities not related to kinesthetic training) did not show significant improvement in handwriting at either posttest or 4-month follow-up as judged by blinded raters (Sims, Henderson, Morton, & Hulme, 1996). Only the Parents/Teachers Checklist, a measure of parents' and teachers' judgment, showed improvement in handwriting at follow-up for both study groups.

Based on the studies reviewed, the effect of kinesthetic intervention on handwriting performance has not been clearly established. One of the reasons for lack of agreement could be several methodological issues found in those studies. The present study was intended to address these methodological problems, including small sample size, lack of screening of either kinesthetic impairment or handwriting difficulties before training, use of only subjective judgment of handwriting, lack of control for experimenter bias in test administration and scoring, and omission of standardized procedures for kinesthetic testing. This study also investigated the effect of kinesthetic training on handwriting speed because speed is an important aspect of handwriting performance (Alston & Taylor, 1987; Amundson, 1995; Mojet, 1991). Levine (1987) proposed that kinesthetic impairment in children might lead to decreased speed of handwriting because of either the excessive pressure needed for kinesthetic feedback or the slower visual feedback used to substitute for kinesthetic feedback.

The purpose of this study, therefore, was to investigate whether kinesthetic training would lead to improvement in kinesthesis and handwriting performance in first-grade students. Handwriting performance included both handwriting legibility and handwriting speed. The hypothesis was that children who received kinesthetic training would show significantly more improvement in both kinesthesis and handwriting performance than children who received either handwriting practice or no treatment.

Method

Design

This study used a randomized–blinded three-group research design. The three groups were a kinesthetic training group, a handwriting practice group, and a no-treatment group. Each child was tested on three occasions: pretest within 1 week before treatment, posttest within 1 week after

---

[1]This study was conducted after Harris and Livesey's (1992) study. The date discrepancy was due to publication delay.

treatment, and follow-up at 4 weeks after posttest. Both the evaluators and the teachers were blinded to the treatment conditions. In addition, the children were not aware of the study hypothesis.

Instruments

Kinesthetic Sensitivity Test (KST). Laszlo and Bairstow (1985a) developed the KST to measure kinesthetic sensitivity while eliminating the confounding factor of motor control on test performance by using passive movements during testing. The KST provides normative data for 5-year-old to 12-year-old children and for adults. The KST contains two subtests, the Kinesthetic Acuity subtest (Runway task; see Figure 24.1) and the Kinesthetic Perception and Memory subtest (Pattern task; see Figure 24.2). The test–retest reliability coefficients of the Runway task were reported to be .69 for 6-year-olds and .52 for 7-year-olds, whereas those of the Pattern task were .38 for 6-year-olds and .16 for 7-year-olds. To combine the scores of both subtests to obtain a valid overall score of kinesthesis, each raw score was transformed into a Z score based on the norm for each age group provided by the test manual.

Kinesthetic Acuity subtest (Runway task). The Runway task equipment consists of two

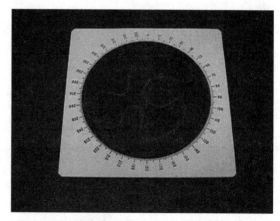

Figure 24.2. Kinesthetic Perception and Memory subtest (Pattern task).

tabletop runways that can be adjusted independently from 0° to 22° from the horizontal. Each child was required to discriminate the relative heights of the two runways set at different degree angles while vision was obstructed with a masking box. The child's hands (each holding onto a peg at the base of each runway) were passively moved simultaneously up and down the runways, and the child was asked to indicate which hand went up higher. The degree differences were presented according to the standardized testing procedures. The score of the Runway task for each child is the number of correct responses from 32 trials.

Kinesthetic Perception and Memory subtest (Pattern task). For the Pattern task, a stylus, which the child held with the hand normally used for writing, was passively guided to trace each of four stencil patterns while the child's vision was obstructed with a masking box. The experimenter then rotated the pattern from its original position. The masking box was removed, and the child was asked to reorient the pattern to its original position with the aid of vision. The score of the Pattern task is the average degree angle of the absolute errors (deviation from the correct orientation) from four trials.

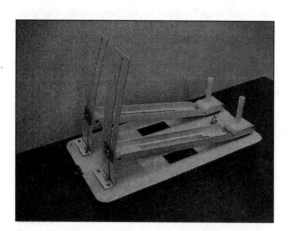

Figure 24.1. Kinesthetic Acuity subtest (Runway task).

Evaluation Tool of Children's Handwriting (ETCH). Designed for use with 6-year-olds to 12-year-olds, the ETCH (Amundson, 1995) is composed of assessments for two types of handwriting: manuscript and cursive. Only the assessment for manuscript was used in this study. This test measures both handwriting legibility and handwriting speed using six evaluation tasks that resemble tasks required during classroom participation: writing the alphabet from memory, writing numbers from memory, copying from a near-point model, copying from a far-point model, writing from dictation, and composing a sentence. Three total legibility scores—total letter legibility, total word legibility, and total numeral legibility—were calculated for each child. Each total legibility score came from the number of legible letters, words, and numbers from all tasks combined and then transformed into percentages based on the possible letters, words, and numbers, respectively. A higher percentage represented a higher level of legibility. For speed, a stopwatch was used to time the children during the copying tasks and composition task.

The test–retest reliability coefficients of this test for first-grade and second-grade students are .63 for total numeral legibility, .77 for total letter legibility, and .71 for total word legibility (Diekema, Deitz, & Amundson, 1998). The test administration time for the ETCH was approximately 15 min to 20 min per child.

Teacher questionnaire. This tool was developed for this study. The questionnaire was used to obtain teachers' judgments of the children's handwriting legibility during classroom activities compared with other children in the same class. Teachers were asked to indicate whether the child's overall handwriting legibility in the classroom setting was much below average, below average, slightly below average, average, slightly above average, above average, or much above average. A score was assigned to each choice, ranging from –3 for much below average to 3 for much above average.

Participants

A power analysis (Cohen, 1988) with a desired power of .80 at a significance level of .05 using an estimated effect size (r) of .43 indicated a required number of 15 children per group. Therefore, 45 first-grade students were recruited for this study. First-grade students were selected because children in first grade had demonstrated greater improvement in handwriting than children in kindergarten who had less experience with formal handwriting in a previous study (Harris & Livesey, 1992). The estimated effect size was obtained from Harris and Livesey's (1992) study, which had the greatest internal validity of the studies reviewed.

Each child met the following inclusion criteria: (a) kinesthetic deficit as determined by KST scores at or below the 25th percentile in one or both subtests, (b) handwriting difficulties during classroom activities as indicated by the classroom teacher, (c) normal or corrected vision and hearing as indicated by the classroom teacher, (d) full passive range of motion and normal muscle tone of both arms as determined by the first author or research assistants, and (e) appropriate attention span within the classroom setting as observed and indicated by the classroom teacher. Because studies have indicated no gender difference in kinesthesis (Bairstow & Laszlo, 1981; Laszlo & Bairstow, 1985b; Livesey & Intili, 1996), an equal number of boys and girls was not sought. Studies also have found that right-handed and left-handed children were not significantly different in their kinesthetic abilities (Bairstow & Laszlo, 1981; Laszlo & Bairstow, 1985b); therefore, both left-handed and right-handed children were included. The only exclusion criterion was that a child could not be on medication to improve attention span.

The children were recruited from 24 elementary schools within 2 school districts in the greater Boston area. Thirty boys and 15 girls whose parents consented to participate were included. Their ages ranged from 6 years, 2 months to 7 years, 11 months (M = 6 years, 11 months, SD = 5 months). One child was dismissed during the study because of extensive school absences, and another child was recruited for replacement.

Treatment Protocols

Kinesthetic training group. The two training tasks were presented in a counterbalanced order over a 6-day training period. The number of six training sessions was justified by the findings from Harris and Livesey's (1992) study in which children showed improvement in handwriting after six training sessions of the same kinesthetic intervention as this study. Each training session lasted 30 min. A small sticker was given at the end of each session after both tasks were completed to help maintain the children's interest in the training tasks.

In each session of the *runway task training,* the child was asked to differentiate with vision occluded the height of his or her arms on two tabletop runways. The runways were the same as those used for kinesthetic acuity testing, but the differences between the runways were different. The first difference in angle between the runways was set at 20°. The difference was reduced to 16°, 12°, 8°, and 4° in succeeding trials. Children progressed to the next step only if they gave the correct answer for four out of five trials at each difference in angle. The positions of the hands (which hand was to be higher) were randomly assigned for the training trials. Verbal feedback of whether the child gave the correct answer for each trial was provided. Visual feedback was also provided if the child gave two consecutive incorrect answers by allowing the child to see his or her hand position. Encouragement and positive rein-

forcement were provided throughout the sessions. Training time for this task was 15 min per session.

In each session of the *pattern task training,* the child was asked to reorient one of six stencil patterns presented in order of the least to the most complex. The patterns were different from those used for kinesthetic perception and memory testing. The child held a stylus, which was guided by the trainer through the cutout on a stencil pattern while the child's vision was blocked. The trainer then rotated the pattern and asked the child to look at the pattern and rotate it back to its original position. The child moved to the next, more difficult stencil only after he or she made no more than a 15° error for a particular pattern. The degrees of original positions, direction of rotation (clockwise, counterclockwise), and rotation degrees were randomly presented during the training session. Visual feedback was given by showing the correct original position after the child finished reorienting the pattern for each trial. Training time for this task was 15 min per session.

Handwriting practice group. For each child, six training sessions comparable in time and attention to the kinesthetic training group were conducted. The child was given letters, words, and sentences to copy. The handwriting tasks were presented from the least to the most complex (letters, shorter words, longer words, shorter sentences, longer sentences, paragraphs) to ensure the same features as the approach used in the kinesthetic training tasks. The handwriting practice books used one of the three different alphabet systems—Zaner–Bloser, palmer, and D'Nealian—to maintain ecological validity of the practice in relation to the children's actual handwriting in the classroom. Verbal and visual feedback were provided for letter size, alignment, and spacing. The training time for this task was 30 min. A small sticker was provided at the end of each training session to help maintain the children's interest in the training tasks.

No-treatment group. The children in this group continued to participate in their usual academic activities in the classroom. They were pulled out of the classroom only for pretesting and posttesting on a timeline similar to the children in the other groups.

Procedure

The children were randomly assigned to one of the three groups in blocks of three on the basis of order of entrance into the study. Treatments began within 1 week after pretest on the KST, the ETCH, and the teacher questionnaire. Kinesthetic training or handwriting practice was provided 30 min daily for 6 consecutive school days. In the cases where consecutive treatment sessions were not possible due to either the child's absence from school or a school closure on any particular day, the six treatment sessions were provided within a span of 2 weeks.

The children were reevaluated on the KST, the ETCH, and the teacher questionnaire within 1 week after the treatment period. Children in the no-treatment group were evaluated for their posttest performance approximately 2 weeks after the pretest. At follow-up (4 weeks after the posttest), only the teacher questionnaire was used.

A single scorer was used to score the ETCH. The scorer was blind both to the children's identities and to whether a particular handwriting sample was from pretest or posttest. Before the scoring began, the scorer was required to pass two quizzes provided in the test manual. The scorer's competence was maintained throughout the scoring period by retaking the same quizzes every 9 to 10 scorings.

Data Analyses

Each outcome variable was analyzed with a two-way (group × time) repeated-measures analysis of variance (ANOVA). The results that pertain to the hypothesis are the time main effect (indi-cates whether a significant change occurred from pretest to posttest) and the group × time inter-action effect (indicates whether the change was different among the groups). Only those statistics are reported here.

Results

Group Compatibility at Pretest

Using one-way ANOVA, no significant differences at pretest among the three groups for KST, ETCH total word legibility, ETCH total letter legibility, ETCH total numeral legibility, or level of handwriting legibility as judged by their teachers were found. Additionally, when each component of KST scores was examined separately, no significant difference was found among the groups for either the Runway task or the Pattern task. Therefore, the groups were acceptably comparable at the beginning of the study (see Table 24.1).

Effect of Kinesthetic Training on Kinesthesis

The KST score, which is a sum of the Runway and Pattern task Z scores and represents a general level of kinesthetic sensitivity of each child, was used for analysis. In addition, the Runway and Pattern task scores were analyzed separately to examine the pattern of change for each aspect of kinesthesis after kinesthetic training. Only 44 observations were available for the analyses because of one missing set of data of the posttest KST scores in the handwriting practice group.

Significant improvement of KST scores occurred over time, $F(1, 41) = 12.24$, $p = .001$; however, this improvement was not significantly different among the groups, $F(2, 41) = .78$, $p = .47$. When the Runway and Pattern task scores were analyzed separately, no significant improvement occurred in Runway task over time, $F(1, 41) = 2.06$, $p = .16$. The group × time interaction also was

Table 24.1. Scores of Outcome Variables at Pretest, Posttest, and Follow-Up Evaluations for the Three Groups

Group	KST[a] M (SD)	Runway Task[a] M (SD)	Pattern Task[a] M (SD)	ETCH–W[b] M (SD)	ETCH–L[b] M (SD)	ETCH–N[b] M (SD)	Teacher Questionnaire[c] M (SD)	Writing Time[d] M (SD)
KT								
Pretest	−2.09 (1.20)	−1.01 (0.65)	−1.08 (1.11)	50.30 (31.42)	61.77 (16.92)	69.37 (22.15)	−1.93 (0.88)	143.20 (41.73)
Posttest	−0.80 (1.78)	−0.63 (1.47)	−0.17 (0.86)	45.83 (34.41)	65.57 (30.67)	78.78 (12.74)	−1.07 (0.96)	150.73 (59.06)
Follow-up	—	—	—	—	—	—	−0.67 (1.23)	—
HP								
Pretest	−1.52 (0.89)	−0.57 (0.99)	−0.95 (0.68)	48.77 (19.34)	63.54 (9.95)	72.89 (10.61)	−2.20 (0.56)	163.80 (121.92)
Posttest	−0.90 (1.49)	−0.38 (1.13)	−0.52 (1.14)	49.51 (17.61)	63.07 (9.66)	71.72 (15.28)	−1.13 (0.99)	131.40 (46.27)
Follow-up	—	—	—	−1.00 (1.13)	—	—	—	—
NT								
Pretest	−1.73 (0.68)	−0.59 (0.96)	−1.14 (0.58)	54.24 (25.66)	71.45 (10.81)	74.85 (19.19)	−1.67 (0.62)	162.47 (58.63)
Posttest	−1.09 (1.61)	−0.44 (0.90)	−0.64 (1.28)	58.45 (27.04)	71.91 (14.68)	76.03 (16.42)	−0.67 (0.98)	130.40 (45.39)
Follow-up	—	—	—	—	—	—	−0.60 (1.05)	—

Note. KST = Kinesthetic Sensitivity Test; ETCH = Evaluation Tool of Children's Handwriting; ETCH–W = total word legibility; ETCH–L = total letter legibility; ETCH–N = total numeral legibility; KT = kinesthetic training; HP = handwriting practice; NT = no treatment.
[a]Unit in Z score.
[b]Unit in percentage.
[c]Unit in scale score (0 = average, −1 = one scaled score below average, −2 = two scaled scores below average).
[d]Unit in seconds.

not significant, $F(2, 41) = .14$, $p = .87$. For Pattern task scores, a significant improvement of Pattern task from pretest to posttest was found, $F(1, 41) = 8.06$, $p = .007$, although the improvement in Pattern task scores was not significantly different among the three groups, $F(2, 41) = .60$, $p = .55$.

Effect of Kinesthetic Training on Handwriting Legibility

Objective measurement (ETCH). ETCH scores for total word legibility, total letter legibility, and total numeral legibility were analyzed separately. These scores were not combined because they overlap. That is, the total letter and numeral scores are smaller unit scores that contribute to the level of total word scores (although not 100%). Therefore, the scores were highly correlated and not considered appropriate to combine or average to obtain a "total" score.

For the ETCH total word legibility scores, no significant difference was found between pretest and posttest, $F(1, 42) = .003$, $p = .96$. The group × time interaction also was not significant, $F(2, 42) = .63$, $p = .54$.

For the ETCH total letter legibility scores, no significant change occurred over time, $F(1, 42) = .63$, $p = .43$, and changes from pretest to posttest were not significantly different among the groups, $F(2, 42) = .66$, $p = .52$.

For the ETCH total numeral legibility scores, no significant difference was found from pretest to posttest, $F(1, 42) = 1.30$, $p = .26$. The group × time interaction also was not significant, $F(2, 42) = 1.36$, $p = .27$.

Because it is arguable that the lack of improvement in the total ETCH scores could be influenced by other factors, such as ability to recall (as in alphabet and numeral writing tasks), auditory processing (dictation), and spelling (sentence composition), the near-point copying and far-point copying tasks of the ETCH, which did not require these abilities, were further examined separately. No significant change was found from pretest to posttest of any score category in any of the groups: near-point word legibility, $F(1, 42) = .72$, $p = .40$; near-point letter legibility, $F(1, 42) = .00$, $p = .99$; far-point word legibility, $F(1, 42) = .64$, $p = .43$; and far-point letter legibility, $F(1, 42) = .04$, $p =$

.84. The group × time interactions were not significant: near-point word legibility, $F(2, 42) = .02$, $p = .98$; near-point letter legibility, $F(2, 42) = 1.48$, $p = .24$; far-point word legibility, $F(2, 42) = 1.03$, $p = .37$; and far-point letter legibility, $F(2, 42) = .08$, $p = .92$.

Subjective measurement (teacher questionnaire). Significant improvement of teacher questionnaire scores was found from pretest to posttest, $F(1, 42) = 52.12$, $p = .0001$. However, the amount of improvement was not significantly different among the groups, $F(2, 42) = .19$, $p = .83$. When the teacher questionnaire scores from posttest to follow-up were examined, a significant improvement was found, $F(1, 42) = 4.14$, $p = .048$. The improvement was, however, not significantly different among the three groups, $F(2, 42) = 1.07$, $p = .35$.

Effect of kinesthetic training on handwriting speed. The combined writing time for near-point copying and far-point copying tasks was used to represent handwriting speed because of the relatively few intervening factors that could affect the writing time. This time represented typical writing time because children were instructed to write at their usual pace during ETCH testing. No significant change in writing time was found from pretest to posttest, $F(1, 42) = 2.5$, $p = .12$. The group × time interaction also was not significant, $F(2, 42) = 1.22$, $p = .31$.

Discussion

Significant improvements of kinesthesis and handwriting legibility were found as judged by the teachers in all groups, whereas no significant improvement of handwriting legibility was found as measured by the standardized measurement tool or handwriting speed in any of the groups. These findings are different from those of past studies. The hypothesis that children who received kinesthetic training would improve significantly more in both kinesthesis and handwriting performance than children who received either handwriting practice or no treatment was not supported. Kinesthetic training was not any more effective than either handwriting practice or no treatment. The outcome of this study puts the theory proposed by Laszlo and Bairstow (1985b), on which the intervention is based, into question.

Three possible explanations need to be examined when attempting to interpret this outcome. First, kinesthetic and handwriting improvement (as judged by teachers) are related. Second, kinesthetic and handwriting improvement (as judged by teachers) have no direct relationship to each other. Third, the improvements seen may not represent a valid change of skills but rather a result of some uncontrolled measurement artifacts.

Improvement in Kinesthesis and Handwriting Are Related

Under this interpretation, the most likely explanation for kinesthetic improvement in all three groups is the exposure to the KST at pretest. Possibly being exposed to the KST had made the children more aware of their own movements. Consequently, their kinesthetic ability improved and led to improvement in their judged handwriting ability. This speculation, however, cannot be confirmed because of the lack of a non-pretest control group in the present study and lack of sufficient evidence from past research. A future study using the Solomon design (Campbell & Stanley, 1963) to control the exposure to pretest will help to answer the question of the influence of pretest exposure.

Subsequently, an explanation is needed about why teachers indicated improvement but the ETCH did not. On examination of the ETCH scoring criteria, certain aspects of handwriting, such as the ability to write on line, letter size, alignment, and the consistency of letter size and alignment within a sentence, would not be reflected by the ETCH scores, which reflect only global legibility (i.e., overall readability of letters, words, and numbers regardless of their appearances). It is conceivable that, if the children showed improvements in those aspects, their written work would have looked tidier and neater in the teachers' eyes, although those improvements would not have earned higher scores on the ETCH unless they changed the readability level of letters, words, and sentences. For future intervention studies, another tool that captures the other handwriting features as described should be considered in addition to measurement of global legibility.

Improvement in Kinesthesis and Handwriting Are Not Related

In the case that improvement in kinesthesis is not related to improvement in handwriting, natural development is the most likely explanation for the outcome. At the time of this study (which was later in the school year), the children had already received a substantial amount of handwriting education. Therefore, this period may already be a crucial one where gain would be expected even without additional interventions. Nonetheless, it seems extraordinary that the majority of the children would make significant gain in both kinesthesis and handwriting within a period of approximately 10 days. The explanation for the discrepancy between the improvement indicated by teachers and the ETCH score mentioned earlier also applies here.

Existing longitudinal developmental studies of handwriting have examined only the developmental pattern of cursive handwriting of children in 2nd grade and up (Blöte & Hamstra-Bletz, 1991; Hamstra-Bletz & Blöte, 1993; Smits-Engelsman & Van Galen, 1997) and over a long interval of at least 1 year. The lack of evidence for developmental progression of kinesthesis also makes it impossible to confirm the speculation for natural development of kinesthesis. For future research, multiple baseline measurements of these two variables before treatment will help identify children's develop-

mental patterns, which can be compared with the pattern during the training period.

Improvements in KST and Teacher Questionnaire Scores Are Due to Artifacts

When extreme scores are used, a tendency exists for the phenomenon of regression toward the mean even if no real change occurs (Campbell & Stanley, 1963), especially for a measurement instrument with low test–retest reliability such as the KST. In the present study, the pretest scores of all children were on the extreme low end (at or below the 25th percentile); therefore, the scores at posttest, according to Campbell and Stanley (1963), were likely to be higher even if no real improvement occurred. In support of this explanation, the significant improvement in KST scores was mainly the result of the improvement in Pattern task scores, which have very low test–retest reliability (.38 for 6-year-olds, .16 for 7-year olds), whereas the Runway task scores, which have higher test–retest reliability (.69 for 6-year-olds, .52 for 7-year-olds) did not show significant improvement.

To minimize the effect of regression toward the mean in future studies, a more reliable tool is needed for kinesthesis measurement. Changes may be needed in the testing procedure or the equipment structure. It has been shown that young children are capable of producing consistent responses (test–retest reliability of $r = .896$) when a different test of kinesthesis is used (Livesey & Coleman, 1997). Therefore, an acceptable test–retest reliability of a test designed to measure kinesthesis is possible to achieve and is needed for a more reliable score. Although it has an acceptable test–retest reliability, the test developed by Livesey and Coleman (1997) was not appropriate for measuring the outcome of the kinesthetic intervention used in the present study because no evidence exists that it measures the same aspects of kinesthesis as those targeted by the Laszlo and Bairstow kinesthetic intervention.

Another possibility is that the KST scores increased because of practice effect. This increase does not represent the improvement in kinesthesis but, rather, represents improvement in test-taking skills because of repeated test taking. The finding that the KST scores increased in all groups, with the largest increase seen in the kinesthetic training group, seems to support this explanation. It is logical that children in the kinesthetic training group would be expected to show the largest increase in the KST scores because they had the most practice. Again, taking multiple baselines before the treatment period as well as using a no-pretest control group in a future study would help to clarify the practice effect issue.

The increase in teacher questionnaire scores could have been a result of the teachers' expectations. No teachers were aware of group assignments, as they indicated in the posttest questionnaire, even for children who were in the no-treatment group. The children who received no-treatment were taken out of the classroom four times for testing (the teachers were not aware of that purpose), and the teachers could have thought that those children received some type of treatment during those times. The teachers' thought that all children received treatment may provide an alternative explanation from what was stated earlier about why the teacher questionnaire, which is a subjective judgment, showed improvement in handwriting, whereas the ETCH, which is an objective measurement, did not.

Limitations

The first limitation of this study is that the kinesthetic intervention proposed by Laszlo and Bairstow (1983) may not represent kinesthetic intervention presently used by occupational therapy practitioners in the United States. However, interpretation of these results can be the first step to questioning and examining theories that support the use of kinesthesis in treatment regimens that assume a direct relationship exists between kinesthesis and motor performance in children.

The second limitation is that the results can be generalized only to children who have similar characteristics to those who participated in this study. The effect of kinesthetic training on handwriting performance may be different in other groups of children.

Conclusion

The prediction that improvement in kinesthesis after kinesthetic training would lead to improvement in motor performance on the basis of the feedback control theory was not upheld. Effectiveness of the kinesthetic intervention on handwriting performance was not demonstrated in this study. Based on these results, not enough evidence supports the use of this intervention in clinics or school settings for the purpose of handwriting remediation at this time, at least for children with similar characteristics to those who participated in this study.

Acknowledgments

We thank the administrators, staff, and students of the Malden and Medford school districts of the greater Boston area for their generous help, accommodations, and commitment during the study. This study was partially funded by the Dudley Allen Sargent Research Fund of Sargent College of Health and Rehabilitation Sciences, Boston University, and the National Center for Medical Rehabilitation Research of the National Institutes of Health (National Institute of Child Health and Development), Grant 5T32HD07462. This study is based on the first author's dissertation.

References

Alston, J., & Taylor, J. (1987). *Handwriting: Theory, research, and practice.* New York: Nichols.

Amundson, S. J. (1992). Handwriting: Evaluation and intervention in school settings. In J. Case-Smith & C. Pehoski (Eds.), *Development of hand skills in the child* (pp. 63–78). Bethesda, MD: American Occupational Therapy Association.

Amundson, S. J. (1995). *Evaluation Tool of Children's Handwriting.* Homer, AK: OT KIDS.

Bairstow, P. J., & Laszlo, J. I. (1981). Kinaesthetic sensitivity to passive movements and its relationship to motor development and motor control. *Developmental Medicine and Child Neurology, 23,* 606–616.

Blöte, A. W., & Hamstra-Bletz, L. (1991). A longitudinal study on the structure of handwriting. *Perceptual and Motor Skills, 72,* 983–994.

Campbell, D. T., & Stanley, J. C. (1963). *Experimental and quasi-experimental designs for research.* Chicago: Rand McNally.

Cohen, J. (1988). *Statistical power analysis for the behavioral sciences* (2nd ed.). Hillsdale, NJ: Erlbaum.

Diekema, S. M., Deitz, J., & Amundson, S. J. (1998). Test–retest reliability of the Evaluation Tool of Children's Handwriting–Manuscript. *American Journal of Occupational Therapy, 52,* 248–254.

Escribano, M. C. (1991). *The effect of kinesthetic perception and memory practice on children's handwriting ability.* Unpublished bachelor's thesis, University of Sydney, Australia.

Hamstra-Bletz, L., & Blöte, A. W. (1993). A longitudinal study on dysgraphic handwriting in primary school. *Journal of Learning Disabilities, 26,* 689–699.

Harris, S. J., & Livesey, D. J. (1992). Improving handwriting through kinaesthetic sensitivity practice. *Australian Occupational Therapy Journal, 39,* 23–27.

Laszlo, J. I., & Bairstow, P. J. (1983). Kinesthesis: Its measurement, training, and relationship to motor control. *Quarterly Journal of Experimental Psychology, 35,* 411–421.

Laszlo, J. I., & Bairstow, P. J. (1984). Handwriting difficulties and possible solutions. *School Psychology International, 5,* 207–213.

Laszlo, J. I., & Bairstow, P. J. (1985a). *The Kinesthetic Sensitivity Test.* Subiaco, Australia: Senkit.

Laszlo, J. I., & Bairstow, P. J. (1985b). *Perceptual–motor behaviour: Developmental assessment and therapy.* New York: Praeger.

Levine, M. D. (1987). *Developmental variation and learning disorders.* Cambridge, MA: Educators.

Livesey, D. J., & Coleman, R. (1997). The development of kinesthesis and its relationship to motor ability in preschool children. In J. P. Piek (Ed.), *Motor behavior and human skill: A multidisciplinary approach* (pp. 253–265). Champaign, IL: Human Kinetics.

Livesey, D. J., & Intili, D. (1996). A gender difference in visual–spatial ability in 4-year-old children: Effects on performance of a kinesthetic acuity task. *Journal of Experimental Child Psychology, 63,* 436–446.

McClosky, D. I. (1978). Kinesthetic sensibility. *Physiological Review, 58,* 763–820.

McHale, K., & Cermak, S. A. (1992). Fine motor activities in elementary school: Preliminary findings and provisional implications for children with fine motor problems. *American Journal of Occupational Therapy, 46,* 898–903.

Mojet, J. (1991). Characteristics of the developing handwriting skill in elementary education. In J. Wann, A. M. Wing, & N. Sovik (Eds.), *Development of graphic skills: Research perspectives and educational implications* (pp. 53–75). London: Academic Press.

Rubin, N., & Henderson, S. E. (1982). Two sides of the same coin: Variations in teaching methods and failure to learn to write. *Special Education Trends, 9*(4), 17–24.

Sims, K., Henderson, S. E., Hulme, C., & Morton, J. (1996). The remediation of clumsiness. I: An evaluation of Laszlo kinesthetic approach. *Developmental Medicine and Child Neurology, 38,* 976–987.

Sims, K., Henderson, S. E., Morton, J., & Hulme, C. (1996). The remediation of clumsiness. II: Is kinesthesis the answer? *Developmental Medicine and Child Neurology, 38,* 988–997.

Smits-Engelsman, B. C. M., & Van Galen, G. P. (1997). Dysgraphia in children: Lasting psychomotor deficiency or transient developmental delay. *Journal of Experimental Child Psychology, 67,* 164–184.

CHAPTER 25

The Use of a Weighted Vest to Increase On-Task Behavior in Children With Attention Difficulties

Nancy L. VandenBerg

Nancy L. VandenBerg, MS, OTR, *is occupational therapist, Plainwell Community Schools, Plainwell, MI. At the time of this study, she was student, Master of Science in Occupational Therapy, Western Michigan University, Kalamazoo. Mailing address: 707 S. Woodhams, Plainwell, MI 49080; vanden4@aol.com.*

Children described as having attention deficit hyperactivity disorder (ADHD) show "a persistent pattern of inattention and/or hyperactivity–impulsivity that is more frequent and severe than is typically observed in individuals at a comparable level of development" (American Psychiatric Association, 1994, p. 78). These children often exhibit sensory-processing problems such as being easily distracted by irrelevant stimuli that is ignored by others, frequently shifting from one uncompleted activity to another, having difficulty remaining seated when expected to do so, performing messy written work, making noises or talking excessively, and grabbing objects or touching things excessively.

Children with ADHD who exhibit sensory-processing problems usually cannot function effectively within the regular classroom setting without accommodation and special education interventions (Ayres, 1979). Such children may be in constant motion or fatigue easily and have an activity level that is unusually high or unusually low. Behaviorally, these children are often impulsive and easily distractible and exhibit a lack of planning ability. They often cannot participate in seated activities, particularly fine motor activities, long enough to complete tasks. Theoretically, these children have sensory systems that are immature and work improperly, so abnormal neural signals are being sent to the brain cortex that interfere with "normal," organizing brain activity (Kranowitz, 1998). The brain, in turn, becomes overstimulated, making it difficult for the child to organize his or her behavior and to concentrate (Hatch-Rasmussen, 1995). This neural sequence often results in negative emotional responses or outbursts, so the child with ADHD is seen as a behavior problem (Hallowell & Ratey, 1994; Kranowitz, 1998).

Traditionally, the treatment of choice for children with ADHD has often been medication. Medications used to treat ADHD symptoms are believed to act on the ascending reticular activating system to help dampen some of the activating stimuli that cause hyperactivity; medications accomplish this by

Originally published 2001 in *American Journal of Occupational Therapy, 55*, 621–628.

increasing the neurotransmitters (dopamine, nor-epinephrine) that are suspected of being deficient (Silver, 1993; Taylor, 1994). Serotonin levels also have been found to be abnormally low in children with hyperactivity and attention deficits (Gainetdinov et al., 1999). Medication most likely affects the symptomology of ADHD by restoring balance among the brain chemicals.

Children with attention problems are often referred to occupational therapists for concerns regarding poor fine motor skills as well as other adaptive problems such as concentration difficulties, increased levels of purposeless activity, and inability to interact successfully within the classroom environment (Royeen & Lane, 1991). *Sensory modulation disorder* is a descriptive term that occupational therapists use to describe a person who "over responds, under responds, or fluctuates in response to sensory input in a manner disproportional to that input" (Koomar & Bundy, 1991, p. 268). A therapeutic activity program geared toward helping children learn to modulate their arousal levels effectively, referred to as *sensory integration treatment*, is often used in occupational therapy treatment for children with problems resulting from ADHD (Fisher, Murray, & Bundy, 1991).

School-based therapists increasingly are using weighted vests as an intervention strategy for children with conditions that affect sensory modulation and attention span, such as autism and ADHD (Joe, 1998; Maslow & Olson, 1999). Weighted vests are used as a means of applying deep pressure, which is believed to decrease purposeless hyperactivity and increase functional attention to purposeful activity (Miller, Moncayo, Treadwell, & Olson, 1999).

Farber (1982) supported a beneficial response to the application of deep pressure, suggesting that maintained pressure is calming as it facilitates an increase in parasympathetic or relaxed tone. In describing her own autism, Temple

Grandin related her experience of severe anxiety and how deep pressure ultimately helped her reduce the anxiety's debilitating effects by reducing overall arousal and facilitating attention and awareness (Grandin & Scariano, 1986). In studies done with children with autism, deep pressure has been found to have a calming effect (Edelson, Edelson, Kerr, & Grandin, 1999; Krauss, 1987; McClure & Holtz-Yotz, 1991; Miller et al., 1999; Zissermann, 1992). No published studies on the effects of deep pressure with children with ADHD were found.

Proprioception and deep touch–pressure are types of sensory information that can produce a calming effect (Ayres, 1972; Farber, 1982; Knickerbocker, 1980). Both are carried by the dorsal column system to higher levels in the thalamus and the reticular formation and then up to sensory areas in the parietal lobe of the cerebral cortex. According to Royeen and Lane (1991), "Since the reticular formation mediates arousal, the reticular projections of the dorsal column pathway may be related to the efficacy of these inputs in decreasing arousal and producing calming" (p. 115). The dorsal column system also has some connections with the limbic system via the hypothalamus and the anterolateral system. This functional redundancy in the nervous system may play a role in the efficacy of sensory integration intervention (Fisher et al., 1991).

An example of the nervous system's functional redundancy is seen in the registration of deep pressure. Deep pressure is registered in the limbic system, hippocampus, and reticular activating system and may stimulate production of neurotransmitters to modulate arousal levels, similar to the effects of medications. The action of the neurotransmitters norepinephrine, epinephrine, and serotonin is associated with the limbic structures and components of the reticular system, hypothalamus, and cortex (Ashton, 1987). Medications allow more of these neurotransmitters to be available to the brain, influencing the level of arousal in the nervous system of a child and thereby controlling hyperactivity and helping to increase the child's ability to attend (Cohen, 1998; Hallowell & Ratey, 1994). The reticular system is aroused to varying degrees of alertness by sensory stimuli (Ayres, 1972), and touch–pressure appears to be particularly effective in dampening overly activating stimuli.

Deep pressure also sends sensory information into the Purkinje cells in the cerebellum, which then work to dampen stimulation entering the reticular formation through brain chemistry or neurotransmitters (Hanschu, 1998; Reeves, 1998). Purkinje cells are rich in serotonin and are responsible for inhibition of motor activity (Edelson, 1995). Children with ADHD have been found to have high levels of hyperactivity related to lower levels of serotonin in their blood (Gainetdinov et al., 1999; Taylor, 1994). Deep pressure may stimulate the increase in serotonin, as well as other neurotransmitters, to create a natural calming on the central nervous system in the child with ADHD.

Weighted vests can provide deep, sustained pressure. Current school-based occupational therapy practice in the United States often incorporates the use of weighted vests to increase children's attention to school-based tasks (Joe, 1998; Maslow & Olson, 1999). The vests can be constructed inexpensively from materials that are attractive and do not stand out as a "therapeutic garment" so that the child does not look different from his or her peers. Vests can be administered by teachers (under the guidance of an occupational therapist) without removing the child from the classroom setting. They can be worn during purposeful activity within the child's learning environment, and children can even don the vests themselves. According to Hanschu (1998), "The right sensation, in the right amount, at the right time, can profoundly influence arousal,

alertness, attention, and how ably a person makes adaptive responses all day long" (p. 1). As Farber (1982) pointed out, however, when using maintained pressure on any part of the body, deciding how long and how often to apply the pressure is difficult. A more rigorous analysis is needed to measure the clinical effects of using a weighted vest to apply deep pressure for the purpose of increasing on-task behavior. Such analysis would help in determining the overall effectiveness of using such a vest to increase attention to purposeful activity and would contribute to evidence-based practice (Abreu, Peloquin, & Ottenbacher, 1998). The purpose of this study was to measure on-task behavior in children with attention difficulties while wearing a weighted vest calibrated at 5% of each child's body weight for a 15-min period while engaged in classroom fine motor activities.

Method

Sample

A convenience sample of four children receiving school-based occupational therapy services was selected for the study. The children had been diagnosed as having ADHD by a physician or scored in the high/problems range on the hyperactivity and attention scales of the Conners' Teacher Rating Scales (CTRS–39; Conners, 1989). The CTRS–39 requires that the teacher rate a student on 39 behavioral items from observations in multiple settings (playground, classroom, lunch) from which standard methods are used to derive *T* scores for the student. A *T* score of 65 or more indicates a high-problem area. The scales were scored by the school social worker and made available for the parents to share with their physician to help in making a determination of ADHD.

The four children selected for the study attended school in a Midwestern rural school district. Their ages ranged from 5 years, 9 months to 6 years, 10 months. During the previous academic year, all these students had attended special education or at-risk preschool programs in which developing school-readiness skills had been the primary goal. Students 1 and 2 were girls and eligible for special education services as speech and language impaired. Students 3 and 4 were boys and eligible for special education services as physically or otherwise health impaired due to ADHD as diagnosed by a physician. Before as well as during the study, Student 3 received medication as prescribed by his physician.

All four students received school occupational therapy services. The occupational therapist described each child as having a sensory modulation problem exhibited by excessive movement (constant playing with hair or clothing, picking at body parts such as nails, reaching or playing with objects excessively, unnecessarily getting in and out of the seat, rolling on the floor), overreaction to extraneous stimuli, and inability to complete an activity successfully. According to the occupational therapy clinical evaluation and as observed within the classroom, all four students had considerable difficulty writing their first names within the spaces of 1-in. ruled paper and had difficulty writing letters so that they rested on a line. When coloring, all four students did not stay within boundaries of simple shapes, and cutting did not remain on the lines of simple shapes.

The children were timed for on-task behavior while engaged in classroom fine motor activities, and data were recorded in the baseline phase and intervention phase. Varied activities such as coloring pictures, cutting shapes and gluing them onto paper, writing letters of the alphabet within squares on paper, counting out small objects according to a designated number, and stringing beads were typical tabletop activities performed during the timed observations.

Instruments

Weighted vests. Denim vests that buttoned down the front were purchased inexpensively from a thrift shop. Pockets from old jeans were removed and sewn into the inside of the vests so that weights could be placed into the pockets and would be evenly distributed. The pockets were positioned high enough on the chest anteriorly to prevent the weights from resting on the child's hips or legs when seated. A pocket was positioned posteriorly between the scapulae just below the scapular borders to ensure that the weight was supported from the shoulder girdle. The placement of the weights higher up on the shoulder girdle rather than predominantly below chest level has been used successfully by other therapists (Hanschu, 1999). Weights were purchased in 1/2-lb, 3/4-lb, and 1-lb fabric pouches and placed into the interior pockets so that they were evenly distributed front and back, with a total weight as close to 5% of the child's body weight as possible.

Stopwatches. Two dependable stopwatches and a timer set at 15 min were used.

Recording sheets. The total time a child spent on task during an activity was recorded to the hundredth of a second. The student number, date, and activity the class was instructed to perform for each observation were recorded.

Consent forms. Written permission to carry out the study was obtained from the special education supervisor of the school district. Parents signed consent forms authorizing their children to participate in the study after the purpose of the research was explained to them.

Procedure

The study was a quasi-experimental, single-system, AB design (Bloom, Fischer, & Orme, 1995; Ottenbacher & York, 1984). All prescribed medications and special education services that the students were eligible to receive, such as occupational therapy and speech–language services, continued as normally scheduled during the baseline and intervention phases. The study was initiated after the beginning of the second school semester so that the children would be familiar with classroom activities, procedures, and expectations.

Two observers were used in the study. One observer was the author, who was also the occupational therapist for the students at the study site. The other observer was an occupational therapy fieldwork student. Before beginning the study, the two observers randomly selected 11 nonparticipant students and practiced timing them performing the same types of classroom fine motor tasks as those timed in the baseline and intervention phases of the study. On-task behavior was defined as engagement in those processes that were necessary to complete the activity assigned by the teacher and were a part of the expected process. A child was timed as being on task while visually focused on the activity and engaging in the processes to complete the activity, such as reaching for required materials (e.g., scissors, crayons) as needed. Handling or reaching for materials no longer needed was timed as off task. Dropping something on the floor was allowed once but was timed as off task if more frequent. Talking to other children, unless continuing to work, was timed as off task. Interater agreement was defined as the observers being within 10 sec of one another in their timed observation of a child's on-task behavior. Practice timings with the 11 nonparticipant children were completed, with the last 6 consecutive timings being within 10 sec of one another.

The occupational therapist–observer showed the vests to each child on a day before observations began. The therapist fit the vest to each child, weighing the child so that the weights could be calibrated to 5% of his or her weight as closely as possible and ensured no distress to the shoulder girdle or posture. The children were asked whether the vest felt comfortable and whether they would wear it in the classroom when the teacher asked them to wear it along with some other children. They were not told the purpose of the vest nor that they would be timed while wearing it. Another volunteering child was given an unweighted vest to wear at the same time in the classroom so that the children in the study would not feel singled out. The children were also given the vest to wear at times other than during the observation periods so that they would not learn that putting on the vest meant that they would be observed or to "try" and be especially on task.

The observers spent time within the two study classrooms before beginning the baseline phase so that the children would not be distracted by their presence. The baseline phase spanned 6 different days within a 15-day period during which on-task behavior (dependent variable) was measured in seconds during a 15-min activity, totaling six observations for each child. The children were observed at different assigned times in accordance with their schedule of attendance (morning or afternoon kindergarten, preprimary). Each child's scheduled observation time was maintained throughout the study during the six baseline and six intervention observations.

Timings began after the teacher had given instructions to the class. Observations were recorded during a tabletop activity while the child was engaged in organizing materials, drawing, coloring, writing, pasting, or cutting as the teacher had instructed. One observer timed each child's on-task behavior during the baseline phase, and the other observer timed each child's on-task behavior during the intervention phase without knowledge of the baseline outcomes. The total time on task during each 15-min period was recorded as well as the name of the activity assigned that particular day.

The intervention phase followed in which observations were also completed within 15 days.

During the intervention phase, the four students wore a weighted vest and were timed by the other observer for six 15-min periods as described in the baseline phase. Each child's vest was put on 5 min before the beginning of the timing and removed after the completion of the 20-min to 30-min activity in which they were involved. Informal interviews with the classroom teachers and aides also were conducted to provide additional qualitative information regarding the outcomes of using the vest.

Results

Behavioral Data

Two methods of data analysis were used in this study to combine the strengths of several methods while avoiding some of their limitations (Bloom et al., 1995). The 2–standard deviation band approach (Bloom et al., 1995; Gottman & Leiblum, 1974; Ottenbacher & York, 1984) was chosen as a good fit because it is most useful with a relatively small number of baseline observations and the same number of intervention observations with some fluctuation in the baseline data but with no stable pattern present (Bloom et al., 1995). Because the study involved fewer than seven baseline observations, however, it was safer to assume that the data were autocorrelated (Bloom et al., 1995), as there could be some growth expected in attention over time due to practice or maturity (in spite of design precautions). Furthermore, transformation of data to remove autocorrelation, if present, could result in loss of data. Thus, to take into account the possibility that the data might be autocorrelated and not independent as assumed in the 2–standard deviation method, the celeration line approach was used to determine statistical significance because it is a better fit when autocorrelation of data is present (Bloom et al., 1995). The celeration line also takes any trends in the baseline into account.

Figure 25.1 represents the results of the data collected during the baseline phase and the intervention phase when the students were wearing the weighted vests while performing fine motor activities within the classroom. A mean number of minutes that each child was on task was computed for the baseline. The values associated with 2 standard deviations above the baseline mean were determined, with a horizontal line drawn on the scatterplot of each child's data representing this value. The lines are extended into the intervention phase to determine whether at least two consecutive observations (data points) during the intervention phase fell above the 2–standard deviation line (+2SD) (Gottman & Leiblum, 1974). Using the 2–standard deviation band method of analysis, all students except Student 2 demonstrate 2 consecutive data points above +2SD, indicating that a significant change ($p < .05$) occurred from the baseline phase to the intervention phase for Students 1, 3, and 4.

Additionally, a celeration line was also computed using median scores in the baseline (Gingerich & Feyerherm, 1979) and extended into the intervention phase; the extension predicts what course the students' on-task behavior would take in the absence of any intervention. Statistically, a significant change has occurred in the intervention phase if the required proportion of data points above the celeration line in that phase is sufficiently different from the number above the celeration line in the baseline phase. To represent a significant increase at the .05 level (Bloom et al., 1995), Students 1 and 2 needed 6 data points to be above the celeration line, Student 3 needed 5, and Student 4 needed 4. As seen in Figure 25.1 for all 4 students, the criteria of the necessary number of data points falling above the celeration line to indicate a significant change in the intervention phase at the .05 level was met.

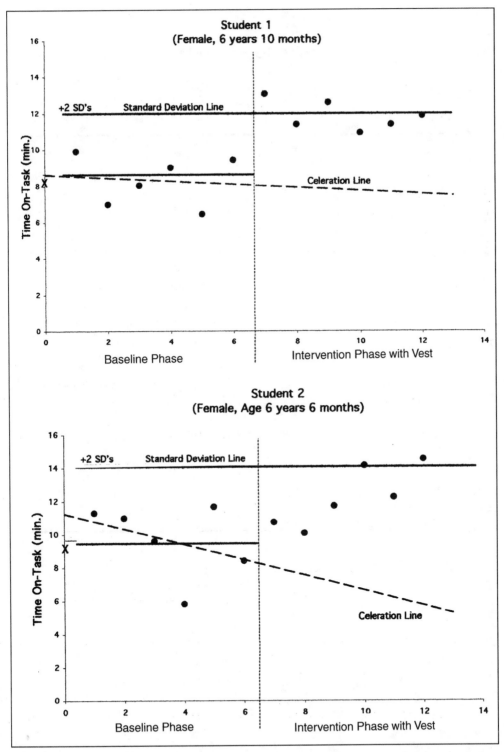

Figure 25.1. The 2–standard deviation band method is used to evaluate changes in minutes spent on task during a fine motor activity from the baseline phase to the intervention phase during which a weighted vest was worn. Two consecutive data points above the +2SD band during the intervention phase indicates a change at the .05 level. The celeration line method requires (for *p* < .05 level change) 6 data points above the celeration line during the intervention phase for Students 1 and 2, 5 data points for Student 3, and 4 data points for Student 4. *(continued)*

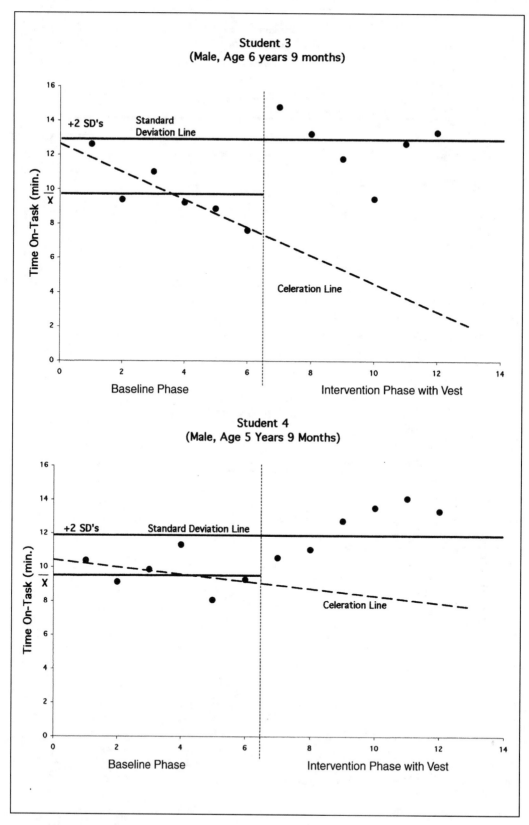

Figure 25.1. *(Continued)*

Ottenbacher and York (1984) cautioned that statistical analysis of data from single-system designs should be interpreted as an adjunct to visual analysis because the presence of serial dependency or unusual trends may compromise results. Although serial dependency and the presence of trends have been taken into consideration by using both the celeration line and 2–standard deviation band methods of analysis, visual analysis further supports the results that a significant change in on-task behavior occurred during the intervention phase. All four students showed a regressing trend line in Figure 25.1, but Students 2 and 3 appeared to be getting significantly worse over time, as illustrated by the steeper downward slope of the trend line. Only during the intervention phase with the use of the vest did any on-task behaviors measure more than 2 standard deviations above the mean, showing an upward trend.

The change from the baseline phase to the intervention phase with Student 1 indicates a 25% mean increase in the amount of time that this student was on task while wearing the vest (see Figure 25.2). The change from the baseline phase to the intervention phase with Students 2, 3, and 4 indicates a mean increase of 17% to 18% in on-task behavior while wearing the vests. Student 1's (girl, no medication) mean time spent on task during the baseline phase was only 54% and increased to a mean of 79% while wearing the weighted vest. Student 2 (girl, no medication) demonstrated a mean on-task behavior of 63% during the baseline, with an increase to 81% while wearing the vest. Student 3 (boy, receiving medication at the same scheduled time during both phases) demonstrated a mean of 64% for on-task behavior during the baseline phase, increasing to 82% while wearing the vest. Student 4 (boy, no medication) showed a baseline mean of 64%, with an increase to a mean of 81% for on-task behavior while wearing the vest.

Qualitative Information

Perhaps the most revealing questions to raise are those that are hard to answer with quantitative research methods. However, these questions give us a view of the child's reality and the meaning the intervention has for the child. Yerxa (1987) suggested that "the research subject might be one of the most important sources of information" (p. 417). The teachers reported that 3 of the 4 students (1, 3, 4) asked to wear the vest at times other than during the timed observations and wanted to put the vest on themselves. Student 3 asked to wear the vest during an occupational therapy treatment session (after completion of the study). The vest that was fitted to him for the study was not available in the occupational therapy room, so the therapist gave him another vest with less weight in it. He responded that this vest "did not have the same amount of weight in it," appearing to be aware of the difference in a 1/2 lb of pressure on his body. When asked why he wanted to wear the vest, Student 3 responded, "I like to wear the vest. It's comfortable." Student 4 wanted to keep the vest on after one observation was completed, and he had been wearing it for 20 min. He told the observer that the vest "made him feel good." Student 1 asked to wear the vest every day when she came into the kindergarten class, and the teacher believed that the student would have liked to have worn it all day. This child was observed to be the most hyperactive of the study group and demonstrated the greatest increase in on-task behavior while wearing the vest.

Yerxa (1987) also suggested that we "need to ask questions about how children relate to their peers, the nature of their play, and how satisfied they are with what they do" (p. 416). The classroom staff members for Students 1, 2, and 3 commented to the occupational therapist–observer that they noticed a visible difference in all three students, especially in Student 1. One support staff

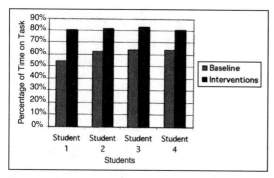

Figure 25.2. The mean percentage of time on task during the baseline phase (without the weighted vest) and the intervention phase (with the weighted vest).

member commented that "the vests really help the kids during centers [seated, fine motor activities]" and that "the vest especially kept [Student 1] in her seat." A staff member from the after-kindergarten school program asked to use the vest with Student 3, commenting that it seemed to help him organize himself on the playground and not run around so purposelessly; he seemed to be "slowing down more and stopping to think" when wearing the vest and to be interacting with other children more appropriately. She observed that, without the vest, Student 3 "was just all over the room."

Discussion

Yerxa (1991) stressed that, in occupational therapy, a need exists "to emphasize the skills and capabilities of the whole person and include the experience of engagement in occupation" (p. 201). This study attempted to measure the level of engagement in occupation of four students 5 to 6 years of age with attention difficulties by measuring on-task behavior while performing fine motor activities within their natural environment—the classroom. Weighted vests were used to apply deep-pressure sensory input and measure whether it changed on-task behavior.

Although a small sample size was used, the behavioral results indicate a clinically significant increase in on-task behavior in all 4 students while wearing a vest containing weights totaling 5% of their individual body weight. All 4 students demonstrated significant changes at the .05 level in on-task behavior while wearing the weighted vests according to the celeration line method of analysis. Students 1, 3, and 4 showed a significant change at the .05 level according to the 2–standard deviation band method of analysis.

These findings strongly suggest the need for further inquiry. Videotaping, as suggested by Miller et al. (1999), was not used so as not to distract the children or make them feel self-conscious. It is very important to watch the entire observation period rather than intervals. Observing the entire activity allows the observer to determine quickly whether the child's actions are on task as part of the activity or are purposeless, off-task behaviors that might be misinterpreted as on task if the sequence of the activity is not carefully observed in its entirety.

The AB design was used instead of the ABA design because of ethical concerns with discontinuing the vests, which appeared to be an effective intervention. Hence, the design limits this study's generalizability. Use of an ABA or alternating treatment design would further add to the power of a follow-up study and strengthen the validity of results by decreasing the effects of variables such as maturation or practice. Another limitation of this study is the small sample size. Future research using a larger sample size would increase generalizability, and an increase in age range would increase the generalizability of the findings to other age groups. Future studies can help to determine how different amounts of weight affect on-task behavior by using the 2–standard deviation method.

Conclusion

The use of a weighted vest as a means of applying deep-pressure sensory input is practical and convenient for classroom use. It is low cost and easily transported to therapy sessions with occupational therapists and speech–language therapists and for use in other learning environments where optimal on-task behavior is required for maximal learning.

This study supports the efficacy of using weighted vests on children with attention difficulties to increase on-task behavior. A significant increase ($p < .05$) in on-task behavior was demonstrated in four students when the weighted vests, calibrated at 5% of their individual body weight, were used during the intervention phase.

Acknowledgments

I thank Debra Lindstrom-Hazel, PhD, OTR, for her assistance throughout the project and Richard G. Cooper, EdD, OTR, for his comments on earlier drafts of this chapter. I also thank the students' teachers MaryBeth Ramm and Mary Warner, Plainwell Community Schools, for their cooperation in the research and Sheryl Lee (former occupational therapy student at Western Michigan University), who participated as an observer in this study. This research was completed as partial fulfillment of a master's degree in occupational therapy at Western Michigan University.

References

Abreu, B., Peloquin, S. M., & Ottenbacher, K. (1998). Competence in scientific inquiry and research. *American Journal of Occupational Therapy, 52,* 751–759.

American Psychiatric Association. (1994). *Diagnostic and statistical manual of mental disorders* (4th ed.). Washington, DC: Author.

Ashton, J. (1987). *Brain disorders and psychotropic drugs.* New York: Oxford University Press.

Ayres, A. J. (1972). *Sensory integration and learning disorders.* Los Angeles: Western Psychological Services.

Ayres, A. J. (1979). *Sensory integration and the child.* Los Angeles: Western Psychological Services.

Bloom, M., Fischer, J., & Orme, J. (1995). *Evaluating practice: Guidelines for the accountable professional.* Boston: Allyn & Bacon.

Cohen, C. W. (1998). *The attention zone: A parent's guide to attention deficit/hyperactivity disorder.* Washington, DC: Taylor & Francis.

Conners, C. K. (1989). *Conners' Teacher Rating Scales.* New York: Multi-Health Systems.

Edelson, S. M. (1995). *Self-injurious behavior.* Salem, OR: Center for the Study of Autism. Retrieved July 10, 1998, from http://www.autism.org/sib.html

Edelson, S. M., Edelson, M. G., Kerr, D. C. R., & Grandin, T. (1999). Behavioral and physiological effects of deep pressure on children with autism: A pilot study evaluating the efficacy of Grandin's hug machine. *American Journal of Occupational Therapy, 53,* 145–152.

Farber, S. D. (1982). *Neurorehabilitation: A multisensory approach.* Philadelphia: Saunders.

Fisher, A. G., Murray, E. A., & Bundy, A. C. (Eds.). (1991). *Sensory integration: Theory and practice.* Philadelphia: F. A. Davis.

Gainetdinov, R. R., Wetsel, W. C., Jones, S. R., Levin, E. D., Jaber, M., & Caron, M. G. (1999, January 15). Role of serotonin in the paradoxical calming effect of psychostimulants on hyperactivity. *Science, 283,* pp. 397–401.

Gingerich, W., & Feyerherm, W. (1979). The celeration line technique for assessing client change. *Journal of Social Service Research, 3*(1), 99–113.

Gottman, J. M., & Leiblum, S. R. (1974). *How to do psychotherapy and how to evaluate it.* New York: Holt, Rinehart, & Winston.

Grandin, T., & Scariano, M. M. (1986). *Emergence: Labeled autistic.* Novato, CA: Arena Press.

Hallowell, E. M., & Ratey, J. J. (1994). *Driven to distraction.* New York: Random House.

Hanschu, B. (1998, March). *Creating sensory diets.* Course and paper presented at the Spring Conference for the Michigan Alliance of School Physical and Occupational Therapists, Lansing.

Hanschu, B. (1999, April). *Sensory issues in autism.* Course presented at the Spring Conference for the Michigan Alliance of School Physical and Occupational Therapists, East Lansing.

Hatch-Rasmussen, C. (1995). *Sensory integration.* Salem, OR: Center for the Study of Autism. Retrieved July 10, 1998, from http://www.autism. org/si.html

Joe, B. E. (1998, May 21). Are weighted vests worth their weight? *OT Week, 12,* pp. 12–13.

Knickerbocker, B. M. (1980). *A holistic approach to learning disabilities.* Thorofare, NJ: Slack.

Koomar, J. A., & Bundy, A. C. (1991). Tactile processing and sensory defensiveness. In A. G. Fisher, E. A. Murray, & A. C. Bundy (Eds.), *Sensory integration: Theory and practice* (pp. 251–314). Philadelphia: F. A. Davis.

Kranowitz, C. S. (1998). *The out-of-sync child: Recognizing and coping with sensory integration dysfunction.* New York: Skylight Press.

Krauss, K. E. (1987). The effects of deep pressure touch on anxiety. *American Journal of Occupational Therapy, 41,* 366–373.

Maslow, B., & Olson, L, (1999, April). *Findings of a nationwide survey about occupational therapy practice with weighted vests.* Paper presented at the American Occupational Therapy Association Annual Conference and Exposition, Indianapolis, IN.

McClure, M. K., & Holtz-Yotz, M. (1991). Case Report—The effects of sensory stimulatory treatment on an autistic child. *American Journal of Occupational Therapy, 45,* 1138–1142.

Miller, A., Moncayo, Z., Treadwell, D., & Olson, L. (1999, April). *Children with autism using weighted vests: Two single-subject studies.* Paper presented at the American Occupational Therapy Association Annual Conference and Exposition, Indianapolis, IN.

Ottenbacher, K., & York, J. (1984). Strategies for evaluating clinical change: Implications for practice and research. *American Journal of Occupational Therapy, 38,* 647–659.

Reeves, G. D. (1998, October). *Brain gain: Prenatal and postnatal neural development.* Course presented at the Full Conference for the Michigan Alliance of School Physical and Occupational Therapists, Lansing.

Royeen, C. B., & Lane, S. J. (1991). Tactile processing and sensory defensiveness. In A. G. Fisher, E. A. Murray, & A. C. Bundy (Eds.), *Sensory integration: Theory and practice* (pp. 108–136). Philadelphia: F.A. Davis.

Silver, L. B. (1993). *Dr. Larry Silver's advice to parents on attention-deficit hyperactivity disorder.* Washington, DC: American Psychiatric Press.

Taylor, J. F. (1994). *Helping your hyperactive/attention deficit child.* Rocklin, CA: Prima.

Yerxa, E. J. (1987). Nationally Speaking—Research: The key to the development of occupational therapy as an academic discipline. *American Journal of Occupational Therapy, 41,* 415–419.

Yerxa, E. J. (1991). Nationally Speaking—Seeking a relevant, ethical, and realistic way of knowing for occupational therapy. *American Journal of Occupational Therapy, 45,* 199–204.

Zissermann, L. (1992). Case Report—The effects of deep pressure on self-stimulating behaviors in a child with autism and other disabilities. *American Journal of Occupational Therapy, 46,* 547–551.

CHAPTER 26

Outcomes of an Occupational Therapy Program for Mothers of Children With Disabilities

Impact on Satisfaction With Time Use and Occupational Performance

Betsy VanLeit and Terry K. Crowe

Betsy VanLeit, PhD, OTR/L, *is lecturer II, Occupational Therapy Program, Department of Orthopaedics, University of New Mexico, Health Sciences and Services Building, Room 215, Albuquerque, NM 87131-5641; bvanleit@salud.unm.edu.*

Terry K. Crowe, PhD, OTR/L, FAOTA, *is director and professor, Occupational Therapy Program, Department of Orthopaedics, University of New Mexico, Albuquerque.*

Originally published 2002 in *American Journal of Occupational Therapy, 56,* 402–410.

Maternal work is time and energy intensive, and the demands are particularly great if the child has a disability (Barnett & Boyce, 1995; Breslau, 1988; Eisner, 1993). Mothers caring for children with disabilities spend more time engaged in child care activities than mothers of children without disabilities (Crowe, 1993; Harris & McHale, 1989; Johnson & Deitz, 1985), and they often are prevented from doing other discretionary occupations (Breslau, Salkever, & Staruch, 1982; Cant, 1993; Crowe, 1993; Crowe, VanLeit, Berghmans, & Mann, 1997; Widerstrom & Goodwin, 1987).

In addition, mothers of children with disabilities often are expected to include atypical caregiving activities in the maternal role, such as developmental interventionist (Allen & Hudd, 1987; Odom & Chandler, 1990) and "culture broker" between the medical culture and the family world (Brinker, 1992; Lawlor & Mattingly, 1998). These additional occupational dimensions of the caregiving role may undermine the parent–child relationship (Bazyk, 1989) and place difficult expectations on parents (Case-Smith & Nastro, 1993; Hinojosa, 1990).

A number of authors have pointed out the unique worries, hassles, challenges, and recurring grief that may be associated with raising a child with a disability (Crnic, Friedrick, & Greenberg, 1983; Hobbs, Perrin, & Ireys, 1986; Pearlin, Mullan, Semple, & Skaff, 1990; Schilling, Schinke, & Kirkham, 1988; Schultz & Schultz, 1997; Shapiro, 1989). Women may be particularly vulnerable because they are usually the primary caregivers (Crowe, VanLeit, & Berghmans, 2000; Eisner, 1993; Smith, Innocenti, Boyce, & Smith, 1993; Traustadottir, 1993).

The concept of working with families of children with disabilities in family-centered care is well established, but occupational therapists and occupational therapy assistants have tended to view attention to parental concerns as peripheral to the needs of the children (Lawlor & Mattingly, 1998). Lawlor and

Mattingly (1998) explored in some depth the tendency of practitioners to view the child with the disability as the client and treatment of the child as the "real" work of therapy.

To address the needs of mothers of children with disabilities within this context, it is necessary to identify time use and occupational strategies that facilitate effective mothering. Occupational therapists are just now beginning to study the complexities of maternal work (Larson, 2000a). Potential strategies include careful orchestration of daily occupations, time use strategies of enfolding and unfolding occupations, and ecocultural accommodations.

Larson (2000b) described how mothers of children with disabilities "orchestrate" their daily occupations through the processes of planning, organizing, balancing, interpreting, anticipating, forecasting, perspective shifting, and meaning making. These processes appear to help mothers make sense of the past and plan more effectively for the future. Effective orchestration of daily occupations may be important to subjective well-being (Primeau, Clark, & Pierce, 1990) but requires more study (Larson, 2000b).

Segal (2000) studied time use strategies of mothers of children with attention deficit hyperactivity disorder and identified three adaptive approaches: (a) enfolding occupations (performing more than one at a time), (b) unfolding occupations by changing the time sequence, and (c) unfolding occupations by having someone else perform certain occupations. Effective use of these strategies depended on family financial and human resources.

Ecocultural theorists suggest that families actively attempt to establish daily routines that are sustainable, personally satisfying, and responsive to the needs of family members (Gallimore, Weisner, Kaufman, & Bernheimer, 1989). Families respond to ecological variables and cultural influences by accommodating or adjusting

their daily routines. Ten domains in which accommodation may occur were identified as (a) family subsistence, (b) services, (c) home and neighborhood safety and convenience, (d) domestic workload, (e) child care tasks, (f) child peer groups, (g) marital roles, (h) emotional support, (i) partner role, and (j) parent information (Gallimore, Weisner, Bernheimer, Guthrie, & Nihira, 1993). For example, choosing to cut back on paid employment is an example of an accommodation in the family subsistence domain. Building on an ecocultural model, Kellegrew (2000) studied the daily routines of mothers of children with disabilities and noted that participants identified lack of time as an important ecological constraint.

To address the needs of mothers of children with disabilities, an occupational therapy intervention program called Project Bien Estar (meaning "well-being" in Spanish) was developed, implemented, and evaluated. This chapter documents the outcomes of the program. The intent was to increase mothers' satisfaction with their time use and occupational performance, thereby positively affecting maternal and family well-being.

Method

Participants

A sample consisted of 38 mothers of children with disabilities who were randomly assigned to either the treatment or the control group (19 in each). The participants each had school-age children between 3 and 13 years of age with significant functional disabilities. A checklist rating functional concerns of the children with disabilities was developed by the researchers and used to assess inclusion criteria for study participation. Women met the inclusion criteria if they reported that their child required significant assistance in at least three of five functional domains (mobility, eating, toileting, communication, play). For purposes of this study, it was proposed that functional limitations were more important than the children's specific conditions, which included autism, neuromuscular conditions, developmental delay, and multiple disabilities.

Descriptive statistics for several factors believed to have the potential to affect perceptions of time use, occupational performance, and occupational satisfaction were compared for the participants in each group. Variables were participant's years of education (M = 16 years, range = 12–22 years), participant's age (M = 37 years, range = 26–47 years), number of children in the household, number of adults in the household, and weekly hours of paid employment (range = 0–40 hours/week). Unpaired, two-tailed t tests were conducted for these variables because they consisted of interval-level data (Rosenthal & Rosnow, 1991), and no significant differences were found between the groups.

Other demographics could not be compared with t tests because the data could not be ranked (e.g., ethnicity) or were not numerically continuous with equal intervals between categories (e.g., income level). Ethnicity for the two groups was compared with Fisher's exact test (Rosenthal & Rosnow, 1991), which is appropriate for nominal data and can be used more accurately with small samples than the chi-square test. More Hispanic women participated in the control group, and more Anglo women participated in the treatment group; however, these differences were not statistically significant. Level of income for the two groups was examined using the Wilcoxon rank-sum test (Monroe, 1997) as appropriate for data that are ordinal. No significant differences emerged between control and treatment groups for income. English was the first language for all participants.

Procedure

Participants were recruited from the greater metropolitan area of a city in the southwestern United States. Representatives from interested organizations and programs helped to identify mothers of children with disabilities, provided the mothers with written materials about the project, and encouraged them to contact the researchers for more information. In addition, some women learned about the program from other participants. Organizations that referred women to the study included parent advocacy groups, pediatric hospitals, private therapy practices, and public schools. Once a referral was made, the researchers completed the functional checklist with each potential participant by phone to determine whether the qualifying child criteria were met. Recruitment followed the University of New Mexico College of Education Human Research Review Committee guidelines, and all participants signed a Human Subjects Consent Form.

After 10 women were recruited who met the inclusion criteria, 5 were assigned randomly (using an SAS computerized randomization list) to participate in the intervention program. The other 5 were assigned to the control group. Intervention was offered to the control group after the posttest data collection phase. The process of recruiting 10 women occurred four times over 2 years. Participants who completed all phases of the study received a $50 stipend. Students enrolled in an accredited occupational therapy program provided free child care during the group sessions. The study did not take place during the summer because of a concern that the participants' time use might be different when their children were out of school.

Pretest data collection phase. After recruiting 10 mothers into the study, data were collected during a 90-min home visit to each participant in both the treatment and the control groups. Pretest data consisted of several self-administered questionnaires and administration of the Canadian Occupational Performance Measure (COPM; Law et al., 1998). The data collector was either an occupational therapist (the second author) or one of two other occupational therapy students. The second author systematically trained the data collectors in the administration of the research protocol. Before collecting data, the data collectors had to obtain at least a 95% agreement on interpretation of COPM problem identification. To ensure consistency of data collection, collectors had to obtain 95% agreement on procedural protocol administration. Three checks were conducted with each data collector during the pretest and posttest phases. During these phases, both data collectors were in 100% agreement with the problem identification on the COPM when compared with the second author. Procedural agreement was 100% for both data collectors during the data collection phases.

Ultimately, 42 women were recruited into the study. Four (two each in the treatment and control groups) dropped out of the study because they left the area or because their work schedules changed, making it impossible for them to participate in all phases of the study. An effort was made to collect pretest data for each cohort of 10 participants within 2 weeks. However, because of some participants' busy schedules, data collection occasionally took 3 weeks.

Treatment group intervention phase. Intervention strategies were based on a collaborative relationship between the first author (an occupational therapist with extensive experience conducting group interventions) and the 5 participants in each small treatment group. The intervention was client centered (Corring & Cook, 1999; Fearing, Law, & Clark, 1997; VanLeit & Crowe, 2000), with an emphasis on respect for and partnership with the study participants. The purpose of the intervention

was to increase participants' satisfaction with their time use and occupations. The intervention program began with an initial 60-min individual session at the participant's home so that the occupational therapist (first author) could become familiar with her particular interests and concerns. Use of participant occupational narrative and story making (Clark, 1993) was an essential feature of the intervention process, and occupational storytelling was used to help participants reflect on themselves as occupational beings (Kellegrew, 2000).

The initial individual intervention sessions occurred within 2 to 3 weeks of pretest data collection and focused on exploration of perceived time use and occupational performance and satisfaction. Occupations were framed from an occupational science perspective as the "chunks of activity within the ongoing stream of human behavior which are named in the lexicon of a culture" (Yerxa et al., 1989). Daily routines were defined as consistent temporal patterns of sequenced occupations (Clark, 2000). Actual discussions of "occupations" and "routines" typically included paraphrased descriptions. Participants were asked to reflect on their occupational routines, strengths, needs, and concerns. Exploration of occupational performance emphasized attention to the interaction of personal, environmental, and occupational factors as described by the Person–Environment–Occupation Model (Strong, Stewart, Law, Letts, & Cooper, 1999) and the COPM (Canadian Association of Occupational Therapists [CAOT], 1997). Participants were encouraged to identify and develop occupational goals for change. Many needed reminders to focus on their own feelings and wishes. They were so accustomed to explaining their child's needs to professionals that sometimes they naturally tended to talk about their children and excluded discussion about themselves.

After the initial individual intervention sessions, the five participants were brought together in a group format to capitalize on synergistic opportunities for group problem solving and support. The occupational therapist (first author) was the group facilitator and ensured that each participant had an opportunity to participate in the group discussions. The occupational therapist did not choose the specific topics for the six group sessions or serve as the "expert" in the group. However, she did encourage participants to reflect on their current and desired future involvement in occupations within the group setting. In addition, she occasionally asked questions, summarized central discussion points, and reinforced ideas or suggestions that seemed particularly useful.

As in the individual sessions, the group sessions revolved around discussion of occupational routines and concerns. Generally, participants spent the majority of group time (a) engaged in discussions identified to increase self-awareness of their current perceived occupational performance and satisfaction, (b) problem solving creatively individual time use and occupational dilemmas, (c) examining strategies to communicate needs more effectively to others, (d) providing social support to each other and exploring ways to increase support in everyday life, and (e) discussing ways to expand involvement in discretionary occupations (e.g., hobbies) that currently did not fit into their extremely busy daily routines. (For a more detailed description of the group process and content, refer to VanLeit & Crowe, 2000.)

After completing the six group intervention sessions, each participant once again met individually with the occupational therapist (first author) for a final 60-min intervention session. An effort was made to complete the individual sessions within 2 weeks of the last group session. Each participant examined her group participation and reflected on perceptual and behavioral accom-plishments achieved since the beginning of the intervention sessions.

Posttest data collection phase. All 38 participants completed the same outcome measures, including self-administered questionnaires and the COPM, to examine the immediate effects of the intervention program. The posttest home visit took about 60 min and was completed approximately 2 weeks after the end of the group sessions.

Instruments

A demographic questionnaire was developed by the researchers and used to gather the basic demographic information reported earlier. The full demographic questionnaire was administered during the pretest data collection phase. A shortened version was used in the posttest data collection phase to identify important demographic changes (e.g., a change in the number of adults in the household).

Outcome measures that addressed satisfaction with time use, perceptions of occupational performance, and occupational satisfaction examined program effectiveness. These measures are described in the following paragraphs.

Time Perception Inventory (TPI). The TPI (Canfield, 1987) is a self-administered, one-page questionnaire that evaluates the way in which individuals view their time use. Such questions as "How often do you get the feeling that you should probably be spending your time doing something other than what you are doing at the time?" and "How often does your day end up being less productive than you had planned?" are answered with a 4-point scale (*rarely, occasionally, frequently, a great deal*). The TPI is a succinct, objective measurement that can be easily quantified and compared across groups. Percentile norms were developed from a sample of more than 2,000 students (Canfield, 1987); however, reliability and validity are not reported in the test manual and have not been determined to date.

Time Use Analyzer (TUA). The main purpose of the TUA (Canfield, 1990) is to clarify current time use and satisfaction in eight areas: work, sleep, personal hygiene, personal and family business, community and church, family and home, education and development, and recreation and hobbies. For each area, the person is asked to select the response that best reflects his or her perspective from the following choices: I would like to spend *a lot less time* (1), *a little less time* (2), *no more or no less time* (3), *a little more time* (4), or *a lot more time* (5). The scores from the TUA provide information about another dimension of time use to add to the data collected with the TPI. Normative data for the TUA have been collected (Canfield, 1990); however, reliability and validity studies are not reported in the test manual.

COPM. The COPM (CAOT, 1997) detects changes in a person's self-perception of occupational performance and satisfaction over time (Law et al., 1998). It is administered in interview format and is semistructured. Individuals are asked to list concerns in the areas of self-care, productivity (work), and leisure; rate the concerns in terms of importance; identify the five most important concerns; and evaluate performance and satisfaction relative to those five performance areas on a 10-point scale. For example, a woman might identify a concern with gardening, which she recognizes as an important leisure task. She is then asked to rate how well she gardens and how satisfied she is with her gardening performance. The COPM gives the researcher important information about which daily tasks the study participants would like to perform more effectively. In addition, the COPM is sensitive to changes in perceptions of satisfaction with performance over time (Law et al., 1998). Bosch (1995) found test–retest reliability to be

.89 for performance scores and .89 for satisfaction scores. Evidence for content and construct validity also has been found in a number of studies (Law et al., 1998).

As part of the posttest data collection phase, descriptive program evaluation data were collected about the participants' perceptions of the usefulness of the program. Treatment group participants also were asked verbally what they liked and disliked about the program during the posttest home visit.

Data Analysis

Differences in satisfaction with time use between participants in the treatment and control groups were tested with the TPI and TUA outcome measures. Perceptions of occupational performance and satisfaction changes were tested with the COPM. Baseline pretesting and posttesting allowed for comparisons within groups over time as well as for comparisons between groups both before and after the treatment group completed the intervention program. For the TPI and TUA, a score *decrease* from Time 1 to Time 2 is favorable, representing an improvement in perceptions of time use satisfaction. For the COPM, a score *increase* from Time 1 to Time 2 is favorable, representing improvement in perceptions of occupational performance and satisfaction. The alpha level of significance was set at the conventional .05 for all analyses. Two-tailed tests were used because no previous studies could be used to rationalize the use of one-tailed tests.

It was important to measure within-group changes because of the concern that asking women to complete the pretest measures might have sensitized them to time use issues that could potentially lead to score changes in the control group as well as the treatment group. Within-group changes were analyzed with paired, two-tailed t tests because the TPI, TUA, and COPM provide data that are both ranked and continuous. The TUA results were calculated as absolute scores. Changes from extreme scores (a score of either 1 or 5) were calculated identically because they were equally distant from the most satisfied score of 3 for each question.

Results and Discussion

Table 26.1 describes pretest and posttest TPI, TUA, and COPM scores for both participant groups. In addition, *p* values were calculated for *within-group* changes from Time 1 (pretest) to Time 2 (posttest). Table 26.2 highlights *between-group* comparisons for both COPM outcome measures (occupational performance, occupational satisfaction) using unpaired, two-tailed *t*-test analyses.

The TPI scores improved significantly for both control and treatment groups, suggesting that the instrument had a notable sensitizing effect. Asking such questions as "How often does your day end up being less productive than you had planned?" and "How often do you find yourself complaining about your lack of time to get things done?" perhaps heightened awareness of time use and planted the idea for all the participants to make efforts to improve their per-

ceptions of control over time. The treatment group demonstrated greater pretest to posttest score changes than the control group, but not significantly so. This finding may suggest that a larger sample size was required to have enough power to detect a treatment effect.

It is possible that the TPI is too global in scope to measure specific changes resulting from treatment. A participant may have improved her perceptions of time use in discrete ways that were not addressed by the particular questions. For example, a woman who was pleased that she was now exercising regularly as a result of involvement in the program might still believe that she could use more hours in the day. In this case, her TPI score would probably not reflect her satisfaction with having increased time devoted to exercise. In addition, the questionnaire may be sensitive to situational factors so that if a participant had a good (or bad) day on the posttest date, her responses to the questions could obscure the actual treatment effect.

The TUA scores did not change significantly for either the treatment or the control groups between pretest and posttest. In both groups, scores decreased (more so for the treatment than for the control group), but no significant differ-

Table 26.1. Within-Group Outcome Measure Perception Shifts Over Time

Measure and Condition	Pretest M (SD)	Posttest M (SD)	Change M (SD)	t (2-tailed)	p (2-tailed)
Time Perception Inventory					
Control	25.4 (7.9)	22.9 (7.3)	2.5 (3.8)	2.89	.01*
Treatment	25.6 (6.6)	22.4 (6.1)	3.2 (4.5)	3.10	.01*
Time Use Analyzer					
Control	7.6 (3.0)	7.2 (3.0)	0.4 (2.7)	0.67	ns
Treatment	7.1 (2.5)	6.3 (2.6)	0.8 (1.8)	2.00	ns
COPM–Performance					
Control	3.4 (1.2)	4.2 (1.7)	0.8 (1.7)	2.07	.05
Treatment	3.6 (1.0)	5.3 (1.4)	1.7 (1.3)	5.70	.0001**
COPM–Satisfaction					
Control	2.7 (1.5)	4.3 (2.0)	1.6 (2.0)	2.96	.01*
Treatment	2.7 (1.0)	5.7 (1.6)	3.0 (1.8)	7.07	.0001*

Note. n = 19 for both the control and the treatment groups. COPM = Canadian Occupational Performance Measure; ns = nonsignificant.
*Significant at *p* < .05. **Significant at *p* < .001.

Table 26.2. Between-Group Comparisons of Occupational Performance and Satisfaction Perceptions

Measure	Control Change M (SEM)	Treatment Change M (SEM)	t (2-tailed)	p (2-tailed)
COPM–Performance	0.8 (0.4)	1.7 (0.3)	1.85	.07
COPM–Satisfaction	1.6 (0.5)	3.0 (0.4)	2.09	.04*

Note. n = 19 for both the control and the treatment groups. COPM = Canadian Occupational Performance Measure.
*Significant at $p < .05$.

ences between the groups were found. One possible explanation addresses the nature of the questionnaire itself. The TUA asks about satisfaction with time use for eight categories (see "Method" section), making it quite comprehensive in scope. Potentially, a participant could desire more time in *all* categories, which is clearly impossible to accomplish within a 24-hr day. In fact, a time increase in one category is likely to require a lessening of time in another category. This time shift could result in increased satisfaction in some time use categories coupled with decreased satisfaction in other time use categories. In such a scenario, the overall score would reflect very little change from pretest to posttest, and no treatment effect would be measured, even if the participant had made positive changes in the categories that she identified as the highest priorities.

The COPM measures perceptions of performance and satisfaction for specific occupations, and a number of significant changes were detected. Both groups demonstrated positive changes in perceptions of occupational performance and satisfaction between Time 1 and Time 2. Similar to the TUA, the COPM seems to have a substantial sensitizing effect. Verbalizing the intention to improve performance and satisfaction in an individualized occupation (anything from spending more time with friends to finding better child care) seemed to lead to perceptual and behavioral changes reflected in improved posttest scores for both participant groups. However, the treatment group reported statistically greater gains in COPM satisfaction scores (also greater

gains in performance scores that were not statistically significant), suggesting a treatment effect related to satisfaction.

Although the intervention took place in a group context, it was individualized. Participants were asked to consider their own particular needs and to apply a problem-solving approach to their own everyday experiences. This approach may account for the changes in perceptions reflected on the COPM Performance and Satisfaction subscales. Participant perceptions of performance did not change as much as perceptions of satisfaction. This finding suggests that, although participants did not necessarily change their task performance as measured in the study, their level of satisfaction with the performance did change. For example, several participants discussed their initial dissatisfaction with their housecleaning performance and level of satisfaction. With encouragement from other group participants and the facilitator, they eventually may have been able to conclude that it is acceptable to maintain a home in a less-than-spotless condition. Thus, housecleaning performance may have been perceived to remain unchanged, but satisfaction with performance improved.

Implications for Professionals Working With Families

The fact that participants in the control group made significant gains in some of their test scores between the pretest and posttest suggests that exposure to questions about satisfaction with time use and occupations is stimulus enough to lead to some type of change (perceptual, attitudinal, or behavioral). This finding suggests that even a single yet meaningful opportunity to reflect on daily occupational routines may sometimes be enough to lead to positive changes. If so, then professionals working with women who have children with disabilities may be able to assist mothers by giving them a chance to discuss how they are feeling about their time use and occupations. This discussion process reflects the occupational storytelling described by Clark (1993).

The participants in the treatment group commented very favorably about their involvement in the program on an open-ended questionnaire provided during the posttest data collection phase. In addition, many spontaneously talked about how useful they found the program during the final group session and in the final individual intervention session (Helitzer, Sabo-Cunningham, VanLeit, & Crowe, in press). These descriptive data were not analyzed statistically but were overwhelmingly positive in nature. Participants placed great value on having a supportive opportunity to discuss their feelings and thoughts in a setting that was nonjudgmental and comfortable. The emphasis placed on exploring adult needs (as opposed to children's needs) was important to them, and several participants stated that their usual experience was that professionals focused exclusively on the child while de-emphasizing the mother. Their comments highlight the importance of being family centered (Lawlor & Mattingly, 1998) and attending to the needs of other family members in addition to the child with the disability. Many of the participants spoke of becoming better advocates for themselves and their families. The experience of reflection and group sharing seemed to allow them to clarify their own strengths and needs and to identify occupational issues that they now felt more competent to address. From an ecocultural vantage point (Gallimore et al., 1989), the partici-

pants described how they were exploring possible accommodations in a variety of domains (e.g., family subsistence, emotional support) to address their own needs and the needs of other family members, including the child with a disability.

The participants also liked the fact that they were responsible for deciding what to discuss, and they commented frequently that the group facilitation was effective in that it provided a certain amount of structure without being directive or controlling. In fact, many participants discussed how professionals often are authoritarian and, as "experts," tend to minimize or ignore the parent's perspective. Such a phenomenon is consistent with findings from other studies (Case-Smith & Nastro, 1993; Lawlor & Mattingly, 1998). The participants described their frustration with professionals who may appear harsh and judgmental, and they stated that professional arrogance might contribute to parental stress and feelings of either inadequacy or anger.

Limitations

This research was an exploratory pilot study in which a sample of 38 women from a metropolitan area in the southwestern United States participated. As a group, the participants were college educated and in their mid-30s. Recruitment was one of the most difficult aspects of conducting this research project. Many women reported that, although they were interested in participating in the program, they could not make one more time commitment. On the other hand, some may not have chosen to participate because they believed that they were already coping adequately. Thus, the self-selected group of women who did participate in the study may differ in their perceptions of time and coping from those who did not. Caution must be used in any effort to generalize findings to the larger population of women who have children with disabilities.

The lack of reliability and validity studies for the TPI and TUA is of concern. It is possible that these measures do not accurately or reliably reflect the dimensions of time that they are purported to measure.

Conclusion

Many of the study participants said that they had not thought about their own needs in years. Assisting mothers of children with disabilities to increase their satisfaction with their time use and occupations is an area that traditionally has been ignored or neglected. This preliminary study suggests that attending to the time use and occupational concerns of mothers of children with disabilities can have a positive impact on their perceptions and satisfaction with time use and occupations. The COPM appears to have great promise as a tool for measuring changes in client perceptions of occupational performance and satisfaction and for opening discussion about occupations and daily routines with clients.

Acknowledgments

We thank the women who generously gave their time and taught us so much through the sharing of their life experiences. We also thank the many University of New Mexico occupational therapy students who assisted us, especially April Boardman, OTR/L, and Kim Wilson, OTR/L. We thank Nikki Love, OTR/L, for data entry and Clifford Qualls, PhD, for statistical consultation. Finally, we acknowledge the American Occupational Therapy Foundation and the General Clinical Research Program (NCRR-GCRC M01 RR00997) for funding this research. This work was based on a dissertation completed by the first author in partial fulfillment of a doctor of philosophy degree in health, physical education, and recreation at the University of New Mexico.

References

Allen, D., & Hudd, S. (1987). Are we professionalizing parents? Weighing the benefits and the pitfalls. *Mental Retardation, 25,* 133–139.

Barnett, W. S., & Boyce, G. C. (1995). Effects of children with Down syndrome on parents' activities. *American Journal on Mental Retardation, 100,* 115–127.

Bazyk, S. (1989). Changes in attitudes and beliefs regarding parent participation and home therapy programs: An update. *American Journal of Occupational Therapy, 43,* 723–728.

Bosch, J. (1995). *The reliability and validity of the Canadian Occupational Performance Measure.* Unpublished master's thesis, McMaster University, Hamilton, Ontario.

Breslau, N. (1988). Childhood disabilities: Economic and psychological effects. *Perspectives on Behavioral Medicine, 3,* 143–168.

Breslau, N., Salkever, D. S., & Staruch, K. S. (1982). Women's labor force activity and responsibilities for disabled dependents: A study of families with disabled children. *Journal of Health and Social Behavior, 23,* 169–182.

Brinker, R. P. (1992). Family involvement in early intervention: Accepting the unchangeable, changing the changeable, and knowing the difference. *Topics in Early Childhood Special Education, 12,* 307–332.

Canadian Association of Occupational Therapists. (1997). *Enabling occupation: An occupational therapy perspective.* Ottawa, ON: CAOT Publications.

Canfield, A. (1987). *Time Perception Inventory* (rev. ed.). Los Angeles: Western Psychological Services.

Canfield, A. (1990). *Time Use Analyzer manual.* Los Angeles: Western Psychological Services.

Cant, R. (1993). Constraints on social activities of care-givers: A sociological perspective. *Australian Occupational Therapy Journal, 40,* 113–122.

Case-Smith, J., & Nastro, M. A. (1993). The effect of occupational therapy intervention on mothers of children with cerebral palsy. *American Journal of Occupational Therapy, 47,* 811–817.

Clark, F. (1993). Occupation embedded in a real life: Interweaving occupational science and occupational therapy [1993 Eleanor Clarke Slagle lecture]. *American Journal of Occupational Therapy, 47,* 1067–1078.

Clark, F. (2000). The concepts of habit and routine: A preliminary theoretical synthesis. *Occupational Therapy Journal of Research, 20*(Suppl. 1), 123S–137S.

Corring, D., & Cook, J. (1999). Client-centered care means that I am a valued human being. *Canadian Journal of Occupational Therapy, 66,* 71–82.

Crnic, K. A., Friedrick, W. N., & Greenberg, M. T. (1983). Adaptation of families with mentally retarded children: A model of stress, coping and family ecology. *American Journal of Mental Deficiency, 88,* 125–138.

Crowe, T. K. (1993). Time use of mothers with young children: The impact of a child's disability. *Developmental Medicine and Child Neurology, 35,* 621–630.

Crowe, T. K., VanLeit, B., & Berghmans, K. K. (2000). Mothers' perceptions of child care assistance: The impact of a child's disability. *American Journal of Occupational Therapy, 54,* 52–58.

Crowe, T. K., VanLeit, B., Berghmans, K. K., & Mann, P. (1997). Role perceptions of mothers with young children: The impact of a child's disability. *American Journal of Occupational Therapy, 51,* 651–661.

Eisner, C. (1993). *Growing up with a chronic disease: The impact on children and their families.* London: Jessica Kingsley.

Fearing, V. G., Law, M., & Clark, J. (1997). An occupational performance process model: Fostering client and therapist alliances. *Canadian Journal of Occupational Therapy, 64,* 7–15.

Gallimore, R., Weisner, T. S., Bernheimer, L. P., Guthrie, D., & Nihira, K. (1993). Family responses to young children with developmental delays: Accommodation activity in ecological and cultural context. *American Journal on Mental Retardation, 98,* 185–206.

Gallimore, R., Weisner, T. S., Kaufman, S. Z., & Bernheimer, L. P. (1989). The social construction of ecocultural niches: Family accommodation of developmentally delayed children. *American Journal on Mental Retardation, 94,* 216–230.

Harris, V. S., & McHale, S. M. (1989). Family life problems, daily caregiving activities, and the psychological well-being of mothers of mentally retarded children. *American Journal on Mental Retardation, 94,* 231–239.

Helitzer, D. L., Sabo-Cunningham, L. D., VanLeit, B., & Crowe, T. K. (in press). Perceived changes in self-image and coping strategies of mothers of children with disabilities. *Occupational Therapy Journal of Research.*

Hinojosa, J. (1990). How mothers of preschool children with cerebral palsy perceive occupational and physical therapists and their influence on daily life. *Occupational Therapy Journal of Research, 10,* 144–162.

Hobbs, N., Perrin, A., & Ireys, S. (1986). *Chronically ill children and their family.* San Francisco: Jossey-Bass.

Johnson, C. B., & Deitz, J. C. (1985). Time use of mothers with preschool children: A pilot study. *American Journal of Occupational Therapy, 39,* 578–583.

Kellegrew, D. H. (2000). Constructing daily routines: A qualitative examination of mothers with young children with disabilities. *American Journal of Occupational Therapy, 54,* 252–259.

Larson, E. A. (2000a). Mothering: Letting go of the past ideal and valuing the real. *American Journal of Occupational Therapy, 54,* 249–251.

Larson, E. A. (2000b). The orchestration of occupation: The dance of mothers. *American Journal of Occupational Therapy, 54,* 269–280.

Law, M., Baptiste, S., Carswell, A., McColl, M. A., Polatajko, H., & Pollock, N. (1998). *Canadian Occupational Performance Measure* (3rd ed.). Ottawa, ON: CAOT Publications.

Lawlor, M. C., & Mattingly, C. F. (1998). The complexities embedded in family-centered care. *American Journal of Occupational Therapy, 52,* 259–267.

Monroe, B. H. (1997). *Statistical method for health care research.* Philadelphia: Lippincott.

Odom, S. L., & Chandler, L. (1990). Transition to parenthood for parents of technology-assisted infants. *Topics in Early Childhood Special Education, 9,* 43–54.

Pearlin, L. I., Mullan, J. T., Semple, S. J., & Skaff, M. M. (1990). Caregiving and the stress process: An overview of concepts and their measures. *Gerontologist, 30,* 584–594.

Primeau, L., Clark, C., & Pierce, D. (1990). Occupational therapy alone has looked upon occupation: Future applications of occupational science to pediatric occupational therapy.

Occupational Therapy in Health Care, 6(4), 19–31.

Rosenthal, R., & Rosnow, R. L. (1991). *Essentials of behavioral research: Methods and data analysis* (2nd ed.). New York: McGraw-Hill.

Schilling, R. F., Schinke, S. P., & Kirkham, M. A. (1988). The impact of developmental disabilities and other learning deficits on families. In C. S. Chilman, E. W. Nunally, & F. W. Cox (Eds.), *Chronic illness and disability* (pp. 156–170). Beverly Hills, CA: Sage.

Schultz, N. C., & Schultz, C. L. (1997). *Care for caring parents leader's manual: A programme for parents of children with special needs.* Melbourne, Australia: Australian Council for Educational Research.

Segal, R. (2000). Adaptive strategies of mothers with children with attention deficit hyperactivity disorder: Enfolding and unfolding occupations. *American Journal of Occupational Therapy, 54,* 300–306.

Shapiro, J. (1989). Stress, depression, and support group participation in mothers of developmentally delayed children. *Family Relations, 38,* 169–173.

Smith, T. B., Innocenti, M. S., Boyce, G. C., & Smith, C. S. (1993). Depressive symptomatology and interaction behaviors of mothers having a child with disabilities. *Psychological Reports, 73,* 1184–1186.

Strong, S., Stewart, D., Law, M., Letts, L., & Cooper, B. (1999). Application of the person–environment–occupation model: A practical tool. *Canadian Journal of Occupational Therapy, 66,* 122–133.

Traustadottir, R. (1993). Mothers who care: Gender, disability and family life. In M. Nagler (Ed.), *Perspectives on disability* (pp. 173–184). Palo Alto, CA: Health Markets Research.

VanLeit, B., & Crowe, T. K. (2000, June 19). Promoting well-being in mothers of children with disabilities. *OT Practice,* pp. 26–31.

Widerstrom, S. H., & Goodwin, L. D. (1987). Effects of an infant stimulation program on the child and the family. *Journal of the Division for Early Childhood, 11,* 143–153.

Yerxa, E. J., Clark, F., Frank, G., Jackson, J., Parham, D., Pierce, D., et al. (1989). An introduction to occupational science: A foundation for occupational therapy in the 21st century. *Occupational Therapy in Health Care, 6*(4), 1–17.

V

Scholarship of Discovery:

New Information
for Application
to Practice

CHAPTER 27

Sensory-Processing Correlates of Occupational Performance in Children With Fragile X Syndrome

Preliminary Findings

Grace T. Baranek, PhD, OTR/L, *is assistant professor, Division of Occupational Science, Department of Allied Health Sciences, CB7120, University of North Carolina at Chapel Hill, Chapel Hill, NC 27599-7120; gbaranek@med.unc.edu.*

Yuki H. Chin, MS, OTR, *is occupational therapist, Greater Anaheim SELPA, Anaheim, CA.*

Laura M. Greiss Hess, MS, OTR, *is occupational therapist, San Joaquin County Office of Education, Stockton, CA.*

Jann G. Yankee, MS, OTR/L, *is occupational therapist, University of North Carolina Hospitals, Chapel Hill.*

Deborah D. Hatton, PhD, *is research investigator, Frank Porter Graham Child Development Center, University of North Carolina at Chapel Hill.*

Stephen R. Hooper, PhD, *is associate professor, Department of Psychiatry, and psychology section head, Center for Development and Learning, University of North Carolina at Chapel Hill.*

Originally published 2002 in *American Journal of Occupational Therapy,* 56, 538–546.

Grace T. Baranek, Yuki H. Chin, Laura M. Greiss Hess,
Jann G. Yankee, Deborah D. Hatton, and Stephen R. Hooper

Fragile X syndrome (FXS) is an X-linked disorder that is the most common inherited cause of mental retardation. It affects persons of all races and ethnic groups, with an estimated frequency at 1 in 4,000 males and 1 in 8,000 females (Crawford et al., 1999; Turner, Webb, Wake, & Robinson, 1996). The gene FMR-1 (Fragile X Mental Retardation-1) is located on the X chromosome, and a mutation in this gene causes FXS. The genetic code for this gene normally contains between 5 and 50 repetitions of CGG (cytosine–guanine–guanine) sequences, the average being around 30 (Bailey, 1997). Some persons may have an expansion of 50 to 200 CGG repeats and are referred to as *premutation carriers*. Although many persons with the premutation may show no effects of the disorder (Mazzocco & Holden, 1996), mounting evidence shows that others are affected (Hagerman, 1996). Persons with *full-mutation* FXS are those having 200 or more CGG repeats. In most cases, an expansion of this size results in decreased production of the FMR protein assumed to be essential for normal brain functioning.

A variety of unusual behaviors (e.g., tactile defensiveness, gaze aversion, hyperactivity, hyperarousal, hand flapping) thought to reflect difficulties in sensory processing are observed clinically in children with FXS (Scharfenaker et al., 1996; Shopmeyer & Lowe, 1992; Stackhouse, 1994). Occupational therapists often receive referrals for children with FXS to mitigate sensory-processing difficulties and help families cope more effectively. Anecdotal reports based on expert clinical observations add to our understanding of the potential impact of sensory-processing difficulties on occupational performance; however, empirical evidence is lacking.

Within the field of occupational therapy, one study (Baranek, Hooper, Hatton, & Bailey, 2002) documented the nature of sensory-processing disruptions in boys with FXS and its association with behavioral problems. Miller et al. (1999) and Miller and McIntosh (1998) found that children with FXS manifested the most severe sensory-processing disorders of all the clinical groups they studied (e.g., autism, attention deficit hyperactivity disorder). Researchers from fields outside of occupational therapy have provided the bulk of the scientific literature about FXS (e.g., Bailey, Hatton, & Skinner, 1998; Belser & Sudhalter, 1995; Boccia & Roberts, 2000; Cohen, 1995; Hatton, Bailey, Hargett-Beck, Skinner, & Clark, 1999; Warren & Nelson, 1994). These important studies document physical and behavioral features, genotypic and phenotypic correlates, developmental profiles, or consequences of physiological hyperarousal. Unusual sensory responses are described occasionally as aspects of temperament (Bailey, Hatton, Mesibov, Ament, & Skinner, 2000) or a consequence of physiological hyperarousal (Cohen, 1995) but are not targeted for study specifically.

Occupational performance of persons with FXS has not been investigated directly. A few studies that address the consequences of FXS on adaptive behavior (Dykens et al., 1996; Freund, Peebles, Aylward, & Reiss, 1995) focus on developmental changes, noting that age correlates significantly with increases in adaptive skills during the preschool years and that adaptive skills often surpass cognitive performance on standardized tests as boys with FXS approach adulthood. None of these studies specifically relates sensory processing to individual differences in occupational performance.

Few conceptual models guide interventions in this area. Assumptions of linear causality are evident in some practices (i.e., remediation of sensory-processing deficits), whereby impairments in one subsystem (sensory processes) are thought to directly affect occupational performance and guide the therapist's treatment accordingly. However, newer theories using dynamical systems perspectives (Thelen, 1989; Thelen & Smith, 1994) highlight interactions among various intrinsic

capacities and stress the importance of self-organizing functions that partially depend on performance in contextually relevant tasks. Thus, a less direct relationship between components (i.e., sensory processing) and occupational performance is implied in the newer perspective. This perspective offers insights into alternate interventions, such as providing task and environmental modifications to support engagement in occupation.

The purpose of this preliminary study was to investigate whether sensory-processing functions are associated with occupational performance in children with FXS. Based on our review of the literature, we hypothesized that children with higher levels of sensory-processing vulnerabilities would present with greater challenges in occupational performance across areas of school function, self-care, and play. Findings generated from this study will be used to guide further research and evidence-based practice.

Method

This study used a correlational design to measure the association between sensory processing and occupational performance. Descriptive methods also were used.

Participants

Fifteen boys with full-mutation FXS, ranging in age from 53 to 126 months (M = 93 months, SD = 22), participated in this study. The boys were recruited through a large, multistate research project studying the developmental trajectories of children with FXS. Genetic testing (blood samples) confirmed full mutation for each child. Only boys were recruited for this study because boys are typically more severely affected than girls. Informed consent was obtained from the all the children's parents. The children received a toy; their parents received financial remuneration, including travel expenses.

Race or socioeconomic status was not restricted for this study. Thirteen (87%) children were Caucasian, and 2 (13%) were African American. Two families received public assistance. Educational levels of the primary caregivers (mothers) were reported. Three (20%) mothers were high school graduates; 7 (47%) attended some college courses; and 5 (33%) were college graduates. Data on the fathers were not collected because in some cases fathers were not caregivers or providers.

The children had a mean Brief IQ Composite Score in the mild range of mental retardation ($M = 60$, $SD = 14.29$) on the Leiter International Performance Scale–Revised (Roid & Miller, 1997), a nonverbal measure of cognitive skills. Considerable variability existed in cognitive performance (score range = 42–93). Seven children were functioning 3 to 4 standard deviations below the normative mean of the Leiter standardization sample. Three children's scores fell 2 to 3 standard deviations below the normative mean. Only 1 child was functioning within the average range on this standardized test. (One child was untestable.) As a group, the four subtests from the Visualization and Reasoning Battery comprising the Brief IQ reflected little variation, with child scores averaging about 2 standard deviations below the normative mean for all four subtests.

Measures

Assessment of sensory-processing components. Few well-standardized tools exist to measure sensory-processing functions in a population of children with mental retardation. Furthermore, different formats (parent reports, standardized behavioral tests, naturalistic observations) yield contrasting information about sensory-processing abilities (Baranek, Foster, & Berkson, 1997). Thus, we opted to use a comprehensive, multimodal assessment process.

To tap these functions, we used one parent-report measure (Sensory Profile [Dunn, 1999]) and two observational measures (Tactile Defensiveness and Discrimination Test–Revised [TDDT–R; Baranek, 1997] and Sensory Approach–Avoidance Rating).

The Sensory Profile is a 125-item parent questionnaire that inquires about a child's responses to sensory events in his or her daily environment (e.g., Is your child bothered by loud noises?). It has been validated for use with school-age children but does not provide norms for children with FXS, specifically. The items are scored on a 5-point Likert scale ranging from *always* (1) to *never* (5). Lower scores on this assessment indicate greater problems in processing sensory information. We used two scores in our analyses: (a) total score for the Short Sensory Profile (SSP; 38 items) and (b) total score of Group 1 items (auditory, visual, vestibular, touch, multisensory, and oral sensory-processing categories [total of 65 items]) from the original research version of the Sensory Profile. The SSP provides published cut-off scores. Scores at or above 155 points are considered "typical"; scores from 154 through 142 are reported as a "probable difference" (1 *SD* below the mean for the typical reference sample); and scores at or below 141 are reported as a "definite difference" (2 *SD*s below the mean for the typical reference sample). Reliability (Cronbach's alpha) of the SSP total score ranges from .90 to .95 for published reference samples (Dunn, 1999).

The TDDT–R is a standardized behavioral assessment measuring tactile processing that has been validated previously for use with children with developmental disabilities between the ages of 3 and 12 years (Baranek & Berkson, 1994; Baranek et al., 1997). The tool has been used reliably in these studies to discriminate levels of sensitivity (aversive responses) to tactile stimuli, an indication of construct validity. Total scores are derived for each of two scales: *externally controlled* tactile experiences (responses to stimuli such as stickers or a finger puppet applied by the examiner) and *internally controlled* tactile experiences (responses during child-initiated exploration of tactile media, such as lotion, dried noodles, or sand). Higher scores on the TDDT–R reflect greater difficulties with tolerating tactile experiences. Interrater reliability was reassessed and is reported later within this section.

The Sensory Approach–Avoidance Rating was developed for this study as an observational measure of sensory defensiveness in a more naturalistic context of interaction with novel toys. Item selection was based on current conceptual models of sensory processing (Baranek, Reinhartsen, & Wannamaker, 2000; Dunn, 1997) and evidence from a review of the empirical and clinical literature indicating that children with sensory defensiveness are less tolerant of sensory experiences across modalities and less likely to engage with materials that encompass such properties (Ayres, 1979; Dunn, 1997; Kimball, 1993; Kinnealey, Oliver, & Wilbarger, 1995). Toys were chosen for their novelty as well as for their inherent multisensory properties with which the child could interact spontaneously. These methods provided preliminary construct and face validity for use of such a measure in this study.

For the Sensory Approach–Avoidance Rating, the children were presented with nine novel multisensory toys to explore individually. The specific toys were a water log, porcupine fish, neon-colored molding sand, rain stick, switch-activated fan, car with sound–light activation, kaleidoscope, spinning board, and large blue ball. Although the research team classified the toys on the basis of their sensory properties for descriptive purposes, it should be emphasized that we were interested in the multisensory nature of the experiences. In fact, all children's toys available commercially inherently exhibit some level of tactile and visual prop-

erties, and it is impossible to isolate sensory features of toys in naturalistic observations.

All toys contained a minimum of three interactive sensory features. For example, the water log provided a smooth and slippery tactile experience and contained bright-blue water and glitter that reflected the light and attracted visual inspection. When squeezed, the toy elicited an audible sound. The classifications for the sensory properties were derived by research team consensus (100% agreement across independent raters for the most salient sensory properties of the toy). The primary features of the toys were three tactile, three auditory, one visual, and two vestibular. The secondary sensory features were six visual, two tactile, and one auditory. The tertiary sensory features were four auditory, three tactile, and two visual. A variety of sensory properties were represented in this task, and all toys contained a minimum of three sensory features. Gustatory-olfactory features were not included in this study because they rarely occur in toys designed for school-age children. The child's level of approach or avoidance for each toy was observed and rated on a 3-point scale (0 = *engages–approaches*, 1 = *approach–avoidance behavior*, 2 = *avoids engagement–aversion*) for each toy. The sum total across all novel sensory toys was used for analysis. Interrater reliability is reported later within this section. This measure differs from the TDDT–R in that it measures level of engagement during free-play exploration of novel multisensory toys rather than level of discrete responses to structured tactile stimuli. Like the TDDT–R, higher scores indicate greater problems tolerating sensory experiences.

Assessment of occupational performance. Three domains were selected to assess occupational performance: self-care, school function, and play. Measures included the Vineland Adaptive Behavior Scales–Daily Living Skills

(VABS; Sparrow, Balla, & Cicchetti, 1984), the School Function Assessment (SFA; Coster, Deeney, Haltiwanger, & Haley, 1998), and a measure of play duration with the toys.

The VABS is an interview-based survey administered to the parents of children birth through 18 years of age. It assesses the child's proficiency and independence in performing various daily activities across several domains (social, daily living, communication, motor). Only the Daily Living Skills section was used in this study because the occupational performance domain of interest was self-care and not overall adaptive functioning. Standard scores were used in the analyses. Reliability of the VABS is reported to be .93 to .99 (Sparrow et al., 1984).

The SFA is a questionnaire that obtains reports of a child's functional performance on school-related activities compared with his or her same-age peers. The classroom teacher was used as the informant for the children in this study. We derived three quantitative measures of "school functioning": (a) the sum score of Part I: Participation (the level of the child's participation summed across 6 school settings: classroom, playground, transportation, bathroom, transition, meals); (b) the sum score of all criterion scores in Part III: Activity Performance–Physical Tasks (12 physical tasks, such as maintaining and changing positions, using materials, eating and drinking, and going up and down stairs); and (c) the sum score of all criterion scores in Part III: Activity Performance–Cognitive/Behavioral Tasks (9 tasks such as functional communication, following social conventions, task behavior and completion, and behavioral regulation). Internal consistency reliability is reported as .92 to .98; test–retest coefficients ranged from .82 to .98 for the reference samples (Coster et al., 1998).

The third occupational performance category—play duration—was a measure of the amount of time the child engaged (i.e., physically interacted) with the novel sensory toys provided during the seminaturalistic play assessment in our laboratory. The total time playing was calculated in whole seconds (to a maximum of 5 min) for each toy and then summed across all multisensory toys for use in the analyses. This measure is not meant as a comprehensive or generalizable measure of play but, rather, as a snapshot of one play context with novel toys. Amount of time attending to or interacting with materials has been documented as an important component of engagement and participation (McWilliam, Trivette, & Dunst, 1985); such measures have been used previously with children with developmental disabilities (Case-Smith & Bryan, 1999; McWilliam & Bailey, 1995; Stone, Lemanek, Fishel, Fernandez, & Altemeier, 1990). The importance of physical exploration of toys as a basis for development of higher level play skills (Belsky & Most, 1981) and participation in joint interactions with caregivers (Bakeman & Adamson, 1984) also is well documented.

Interrater Reliability

Interrater reliability estimates for the TDDT–R, Sensory Approach–Avoidance Rating, and play duration were established by two independent raters from videotaped observations of three children (20% of sample). On the TDDT–R, above 90% agreement was obtained. Agreement was 98% for the Sensory Approach–Avoidance Rating and play duration measures.

Procedure

These measures were administered as part of a larger research protocol that included a full 2-hr occupational therapy evaluation and a cognitive assessment. The occupational therapy and psychological evaluations were conducted in a counterbalanced order to minimize fatigue effects across measures. All sessions were videotaped for later coding on the following measures:

TDDT–R, Sensory Approach–Avoidance Rating, and play duration. Assessment was done either on site (a small carpeted clinic room at the university) or in a small room in the child's school or home. Unnecessary distractions were minimized across environments. Families brought the child's favorite toys to ease the transition and increase comfort in a new environment. Parents or a familiar adult were present during the initial free play until the child was comfortable with the examiner. When the child's comfort level seemed appropriate, the caregiver left the room, and the child remained with one examiner and one videographer. Breaks and access to caregivers were provided as needed.

One parent (in most cases, mother) for each child filled out the Sensory Profile and was interviewed about self-help skills on the VABS by a trained examiner (psychologist or educational specialist). The SFA was completed by the child's classroom teacher. Because teachers usually were not present on the day of the child assessments, the SFA forms were completed and returned to the research team for scoring and interpretation within a few weeks of the other assessments.

Data Analysis

Descriptive statistics were used to report participant profiles on the measures. Summaries of group performance were reported, and the percentages of children below age expectations were calculated. Partial correlations, adjusting for age and IQ (see Licht, 1995), tested associations between sensory-processing variables and occupational performance using the Statistical Package for the Social Sciences, version 10.0 (SPSS, 1999).

Results

Demographic Correlates

Table 27.1 presents demographic information about the cognitive levels (standardized IQ

Table 27.1. Correlations Between All Measures and IQ and Age

Variable	IQ	Age
Sensory-processing component		
Short Sensory Profile	.12	.65*
Sensory Profile–Group 1 items	−.07	.65*
TDDT–R (external score)	−.23	−.03
TDDT–R (internal score)	.23	.13
Sensory Approach–Avoidance Rating	−.49	.21
Occupational performance		
Self-care (VABS)		
Daily living skills	.59*	.18
School function (SFA)		
Part I: Total participation	.06	.64*
Part III: Total physical tasks	.19	.83**
Part III: Total cognitive–behavioral tasks	.56	.78**
Play duration with novel toys	.44	−.01

Note. N = 15. SFA = School Function Assessment; TDDT–R = Tactile Defensiveness and Discrimination Test–Revised; VABS = Vineland Adaptive Behavior Scales.
*p < .05. **p < .01.

scores) and ages of the children in our study as well as the intercorrelations between these demographics and the various measures used in the study. The scores on the VABS were positively correlated with IQ; SFA scores and Sensory Profile scores were positively correlated with age. Thus, these two demographic variables (age in months, IQ) were statistically controlled using partial correlations in the final analyses to remove potentially confounding influences of maturational factors and general cognitive ability on performance for those measures that were correlated (Licht, 1995).

Correlations Among Sensory Measures

Pearson correlation coefficients were calculated to see the relationships among the sensory-processing measures used. We found that the TDDT–R external-control score and the Sensory Approach–Avoidance Rating were not related (r = −.11, p > .05); however, the TDDT–R internal-control score was correlated with the Sensory Approach–Avoidance Rating (r = .62, p < .05). The SSP was not correlated with either the TDDT–R (external-control score, $r = .29$, $p > .05$; internal-control score, $r = .20$, $p > .05$) or the Sensory Approach–Avoidance Rating ($r = .09$, $p > .05$), indicating that these measures perhaps were tapping different aspects of sensory processing. These findings are not surprising given that the Sensory Profile includes both hyporesponsiveness and hyperresponsiveness patterns, whereas the other measures represent only hyperresponsiveness patterns.

Descriptive Findings

Descriptive analyses provide details of the range of individual differences present in our sample. Several commonalities among the children were noted; however, not all were found to have significant sensory-processing problems despite the fact that all 15 had full-mutation FXS. For example, on the SSP, the average score was more than 2 standard deviations below the mean of the typical reference sample (see Table 27.2). The majority of boys ($n = 11$) had scores that indeed fell more than 2 standard deviations below the norm. However, 2 obtained scores in the typical ranges, and 2 had scores that fell between 1 and 2 standard deviations from the norm.

Although reference norms are not available for children developing typically on either the TDDT–R or the Sensory Approach–Avoidance Rating, our observations from previous pilot work indicated that sensory-defensive behaviors are quite unusual for school-age children who are typically developing and without sensory modulation disorders; scores for children developing typically tend to show floor effects (total scores near 0) on both scales. In our FXS sample, we found that 2 boys had scores that fell at or near 0 on the TDDT–R; 3 showed low scores (few concerns) on the Sensory Approach–Avoidance Rating. The remainder had scores demonstrating varying levels of sensory difficulties, with 4 showing very high levels of aversion–avoidance on at least one of the two scales.

The range of performance across occupational domains of play, self-care, and school function also varied among the children, although both the SFA criterion scores and VABS standard scores were generally much

Table 27.2. Descriptive Statistics for All Measures for Boys With Fragile X Syndrome

Variable	Range of Scores Possible	Fragile X Syndrome Sample		
		Range	*M*	*SD*
Sensory processing				
Short Sensory Profile	38–190	75–164	131	26
Sensory Profile–Group 1 items	65–325	143–281	226	37
TDDT–R (total external score)	0–48	0–40	20	12
TDDT–R (total internal score)	0–33	0–14	7	4
Sensory Approach–Avoidance Rating	0–18	0–8	5	3
Occupational performance				
Self-care (VABS) *M* = 100 (*SD* = 15)[a]	28–71	56	14	
School function (SFA criterion scores)				
Part I: Participation	0–100	45–100	73	20
Part III: Sum physical tasks	0–1200	488–1062	840	174
Part III: Sum cognitive–behavioral tasks	0–900	243–767	545	158
Play duration with novel toys (in sec)	0–1800	163–622	356	157

Note. N = 15. SFA = School Function Assessment; TDDT–R = Tactile Defensiveness and Discrimination Test–Revised; VABS = Vineland Adaptive Behavior Scales.

[a]The VABS is a standardized, norm-referenced test; thus, the exact mean and standard deviation are presented for the normative sample.

below the range of typical performance in the reference samples. Reference scores are not available for the measure of play duration. On the VABS, the mean standard (composite) score was 56.4 (SD = 13.5), falling near the cut-off between the mildly to moderately delayed range of performance. Compared with the norms for samples of children who are typically developing, all but 1 boy fell more than 2 standard deviations below the mean; 4 boys' scores fell more than 3 standard deviations below the mean.

We note that the SFA uses criterion scores that reflect the teacher's perceptions of the child's functioning levels compared with their same-aged peers in the same classroom; thus, the scores are not intended as a measure of normative performance. However, for descriptive purposes, full participation on the SFA Part I would be indicated by criterion scores near 100. In our sample, 3 boys received a full participation score of 100 on Part I of the SFA, and 1 additional boy received a score of 93, indicating that these 4 boys were participating in school functional activities at or near the level of their classroom peers. The remainder of the sample showed relatively low participation in school tasks compared with peers.

Correlational Findings: Sensory Processing and Occupational Performance Areas

Pearson partial correlations were used to examine relationships between each of the sensory-processing variables and each of the occupational performance measures, controlling for effects of age and IQ for those measures that were correlated with these demographic variables. Both conventional ($p < .05$) and conservative ($p < .01$) significance levels are reported (see Table 27.3).

Sensory processing and daily living skills. Results revealed a significant negative relationship between the TDDT–R internal-control score and the VABS score ($r = -.63$, $p = .02$), suggesting that the boys who demonstrated a lower level of self-initiated approach (more aversive–avoidance reactions) with tactile media were less independent in daily living skills.

Sensory processing and school function. The Sensory Approach–Avoidance Rating was significantly negatively correlated with all three of the SFA variables, indicating that children who demonstrated more aversive–avoidance behaviors (less engagement) while exploring sensory toys had relatively lower scores in school function. A moderately strong but nonsignificant correlation was noted for the

Table 27.3. Correlations Between Measures of Sensory Processing and Occupational Performance

Occupational Performance	Sensory Processing				
	Sensory Profile		TDDT–R		
	Short Form	Total Group 1	External	Internal	Sensory Approach–Avoidance Rating
Self-care (VABS)					
Daily living skills	.01	.09	.40	−.63*	−.39
School function (SFA)					
Part I: Total participation	.25	.33	.53	−.34	−.76**
Part III: Total physical tasks	.28	.29	.31	−.09	−.79**
Part III: Total cognitive–behavioral tasks	.49	.55	.52	.12	−.86**
Play duration with novel toys	−.04	.07	.11	−.38	−.56*

Note. N = 15. SFA = School Function Assessment; TDDT–R = Tactile Defensiveness and Discrimination Test–Revised; VABS = Vineland Adaptive Behavior Scales.
*$p < .05$. **$p < .01$.

Sensory Profile with SFA cognitive–behavioral tasks. Although we predicted negative correlations, we found positive correlations of moderate effect sizes (nonsignificant) between the TDDT–R external-control score and the three SFA measures.

Sensory processing and play. As expected, Sensory Approach–Avoidance Rating scores were significantly negatively correlated with play duration ($r = -.56$, $p = .05$)—the children who demonstrated more aversive–avoidance behaviors toward sensory properties of toys also spent less time engaging in play with novel toys. A moderately strong negative correlation (not significant) was noted for the TDDT–R internal-control score and play duration.

Discussion

Overall group findings indicated that these 15 boys with FXS were found to perform at ranges much below "typical" levels on sensory-processing functions and "criterion" cutoffs for occupational performance relative to classroom peers. However, significant individual differences were noted despite the fact that all of the boys had the full-mutation FXS and significant developmental delays. Surprisingly, 3 boys (20%) performed within normal ranges on at least one of the measures of interest.

This study supports our hypotheses that controlling for age and IQ, some measures of sensory processing are associated with measures of occupational performance; however, these associations were not always in the direction predicted, and not all measures were equally associated. These empirical findings support existing clinical literature (e.g., Hagerman, 1996; Stackhouse, 1994) and further clarify the nature of individual differences.

Specifically, those children with greater *internally controlled* aversion (avoidance) to sensory features of toys, as measured by either the TDDT–R or the Sensory Approach–Avoidance Rating, had lower levels of participation and performance in school activities, were less independent in self-care at home, and engaged for shorter durations of play with novel toys. These avoidance responses appear to be a coping strategy used to deal with high levels of arousal, defensiveness, or fear of new sensory experiences, characteristics known to be prevalent in FXS (Belser & Sudhalter, 1995; Boccia & Roberts, 2000; Cohen, 1995). Dunn (1997) also described a pattern of "sensation avoiding" for persons attempting to counteract low neurological thresholds to stimulation. Many learning experiences inherently require approach and engagement in novel tasks; however, for some boys with FXS, low sensory tolerance may add challenges to their self-regulation and coping abilities and, ultimately, to their participation in daily occupations.

Our findings can be further elucidated through the lens of dynamical systems theory (Kamm, Thelen, & Jensen, 1990; Thelen, 1989), demonstrating how a developing system chooses the most stable, comfortable, or "efficient" pattern or solution given a specific context and developmental time point. For children with FXS, avoidance of sensory features may be one such stable pattern; however, if the pattern is not flexible enough to accommodate new challenges, exploration, adaptation, and occupational performance may be affected.

Considerable variability was evident across the children in our study, and intercorrelations were not uniformly strong across the measures. The Sensory Profile indicated that 11 of the 15 boys (73% of our sample) had definite sensory modulation differences, but this measure was not significantly associated with occupational performance. These scores, however, were significantly related to age such that the younger boys had greater levels of sensory symptoms than the older boys. Given that the Sensory Profile merges hyporesponsive and hyperresponsive patterns into one total score, this measure may obscure some potential relationships between sensory processing and occupational performance in a population prone to hyperresponsiveness. Use of the factor scores on the Sensory Profile may be indicated in future work.

Our results demonstrated outcomes in both positive and negative directions; these findings suggest that perhaps there is not a direct (causal) relationship between sensory-processing vulnerabilities and occupational performance. Rather, these variables may have a dynamic interrelationship mediated by other factors producing an array of individual performance outcomes. That is, sensory-processing components, however "deficient" in children with FXS, are likely not a sufficient explanation for difficulties in occupational performance. Deficits in participation likely arise from a transaction of multiple factors, including the context, that may or may not support a child's intrinsic vulnerabilities.

As an example, we found that high levels of aversion to touch from unpredictable external sources (that the child cannot easily avoid) indicated a tendency toward increased independence in self-care and greater participation in school activities in some children with FXS studied. Although these results seemed potentially incongruent with our other findings and previous speculations in the occupational therapy literature (Kimball, 1993; Kinnealey et al., 1995), it appears that sensory-processing vulnerabilities per se did not translate automatically into decreased occupational performance. The relationship between these variables appears more dynamic than linear, consistent with dynamical systems theory (Law et al., 1994). Furthermore, it is possible that, in some cases, these sensory-processing vulnerabilities may actually facilitate other adaptive coping

or self-regulation strategies ("I'll do it myself") if, for example, protective factors (high intellectual abilities) or appropriate environmental supports (calm atmosphere) are available to an individual child. These findings speak to the importance of using dynamic, occupation-centered interventions that incorporate the child's strengths and facilitate effective coping strategies that mitigate a constrained sensory-processing system, perhaps bypassing the need to remediate some "deficits" altogether.

Conclusion

These preliminary findings clarify some complex issues surrounding sensory processing in a special-needs population. Independent of general maturational and cognitive factors, avoidance of self-controlled sensory experiences significantly correlated with decreased occupational performance in the areas of self-care, school function, and play in this sample of boys with FXS. However, tremendous individual differences were noted—some children with high levels of aversive responses to sensory experiences do quite well participating within supportive environments or in situations in which they exert adaptive self-regulatory strategies, such as performing tasks more independently. These findings provide insight into understanding the dynamic nature of self-organizing systems and the variables potentially mediating the relationship between sensory-processing components and complex occupational behaviors.

Replication studies with larger samples of children with FXS, as well as children with other developmental disorders, are needed to determine the generalizability of these findings. Further research also needs to address the limitations inherent in some measures developed for this study. For example, better-validated assessments of play across multiple contexts would be useful. Additionally, given that many of the significant findings depended on the validity of the Sensory Approach–Avoidance Rating, clinical interpretations warrant caution until further validation and replication studies are conducted.

Acknowledgments

We thank the families who participated in this study. We acknowledge the Carolina Fragile X Project and the Center for Development and Learning for their support. Special thanks to Lorin McGuire, Don Bailey, Jennifer Roberts, Jane Roberts, Renee Clark, Michelle Ozgen, and Ruth Humphry for their contributions and to Winnie Dunn and Wendy Coster for allowing us to use research versions of their respective assessments.

Partial funding for this study was provided by the U.S. Department of Education, Office of Special Education Programs (Grant H023C950034-98).

This study was conducted in partial fulfillment of the master of science degree in occupational therapy at the University of North Carolina at Chapel Hill for the second, third, and fourth authors.

References

Ayres, A. J. (1979). *Sensory integration and the child.* Los Angeles: Western Psychological Services.

Bailey, D. B. (1997). Genetic issues in mental retardation: A report on the Arc's human genome education project. *The Arc, 2*(2), 1–4.

Bailey, D. B., Hatton, D. D., Mesibov, G., Ament, N., & Skinner, M. (2000). Early development, temperament, and functional impairment in autism and fragile X syndrome. *Journal of Autism and Developmental Disorders, 30,* 557–567.

Bailey, D. B., Hatton, D. D., & Skinner, M. (1998). Early developmental trajectories of males with fragile X syndrome. *American Journal on Mental Retardation, 103*(1), 29–39.

Bakeman, R., & Adamson, L. (1984). Coordinating attention to people and objects in mother–infant and peer–infant interaction. *Child Development, 55,* 1278–1289.

Baranek, G. T. (1997). *Tactile Defensiveness and Discrimination Test–Revised.* Unpublished manuscript, University of North Carolina at Chapel Hill.

Baranek, G. T., & Berkson, G. (1994). Tactile defensiveness in children with developmental disabilities: Responsiveness and habituation. *Journal of Autism and Developmental Disorders, 24,* 457–471.

Baranek, G. T., Foster, L. G., & Berkson, G. (1997). Tactile defensiveness and stereotyped behaviors. *American Journal of Occupational Therapy, 51,* 91–95.

Baranek, G. T., Hooper, S., Hatton, D. D., & Bailey, D. B. (2002). *Sensory processing correlates of cognitive and social–behavioral functioning in boys with fragile X syndrome.* Manuscript submitted for publication.

Baranek, G. T., Reinhartsen, D. B., & Wannamaker, S. W. (2000). Play: Engaging children with autism. In R. Heubner (Ed.), *Sensorimotor interventions in autism* (pp. 311–351). Philadelphia: F. A. Davis.

Belser, R. C., & Sudhalter, V. (1995). Arousal difficulties in males with fragile X syndrome: A preliminary study. *Developmental Brain Dysfunction, 8,* 270–279.

Belsky, J., & Most, R. K. (1981). From exploration to play: A cross-sectional study of infant free play behavior. *Developmental Psychology, 17,* 630–639.

Boccia, M. L., & Roberts, J. E. (2000). Behavior and autonomic nervous system function assessed via heart period measures: The case of hyperarousal in boys with fragile X syndrome. *Behavior Research Methods, Instruments, and Computers, 32*(1), 5–10.

Case-Smith, J., & Bryan, T. (1999). The effects of occupational therapy with sensory integration emphasis on preschool-age children with autism. *American Journal of Occupational Therapy, 53,* 489–497.

Cohen, I. L. (1995). A theoretical analysis of the role of hyperarousal in the learning and behavior of fragile X males. *Mental Retardation and Developmental Disabilities Research Reviews, 1,* 286–291.

Coster, W. J., Deeney, T. A., Haltiwanger, J. T., & Haley, S. M. (1998). *School Function Assessment.* San Antonio, TX: Psychological Corporation/ Therapy SkillBuilders.

Crawford, D. C., Meadows, K. L., Newman, J. L., Taft, L. F., Pettay, D. L., Gold, L. B., et al. (1999). Prevalence and phenotype consequence of FRAXA and FRAXE alleles in a large, ethnically diverse, special education-needs population. *American Journal of Human Genetics, 64,* 495–507.

Dunn, W. (1997). The impact of sensory processing abilities on the daily lives of young children and their families: A conceptual model. *Infants and Young Children, 9*(4), 23–35.

Dunn, W. (1999). *Sensory Profile.* San Antonio, TX: Psychological Corporation.

Dykens, E., Ort, S., Cohen, I., Finucane, B., Spiridigliozzi, G., Lachiewicz, A., et al. (1996). Trajectories and profiles of adaptive behavior in males with fragile X syndrome: Multicenter studies. *Journal of Autism and Developmental Disorders, 26,* 287–300.

Freund, L. S., Peebles, C. D., Aylward, E., & Reiss, A. L. (1995). Preliminary report on cognitive and adaptive behaviors of preschool-aged males with fragile X. *Developmental Brain Dysfunction, 8,* 242–251.

Hagerman, R. J. (1996). Physical and behavioral phenotypes. In R. J. Hagerman & A. Cronister (Eds.), *Fragile X syndrome: Diagnosis, treatment, and research* (2nd ed., pp. 3–87). Baltimore: Johns Hopkins University Press.

Hatton, D. D., Bailey, D. B., Hargett-Beck, M. Q., Skinner, M., & Clark, R. D. (1999). Behavioral style of young boys with fragile X syndrome. *Developmental Medicine and Child Neurology, 41*(9), 1–8.

Kamm, K., Thelen, E., & Jensen, J. L. (1990). A dynamical systems approach to motor development. *Physical Therapy, 70,* 763–775.

Kimball, J. G. (1993). Sensory integrative frame of reference. In P. Kramer & J. Hinojosa (Eds.), *Frames of reference for pediatric occupational therapy* (pp. 87–175). Baltimore: Williams & Wilkins.

Kinnealey, M., Oliver, B., & Wilbarger, P. (1995). A phenomenological study of sensory defensiveness in adults. *American Journal of Occupational Therapy, 49,* 444–451.

Law, M., Cooper, B., Letts, L., Rigby, P., Stewart, S., & Strong, S. (1994). *A model of person–environment interactions: Application to occupational therapy.* Hamilton, ON: McMaster University.

Licht, M. H. (1995). Multiple regression and correlation. In L. G. Grimm & P. R. Yarnold (Eds.), *Reading and understanding multivariate statistics* (pp. 19–64). Washington, DC: American Psychological Association.

Mazzocco, M. M., & Holden, J. J. (1996). Neuropsychological profiles of three sisters homozygous for the fragile X premutation. *American Journal of Medical Genetics, 2,* 323–328.

McWilliam, R. A., & Bailey, D. B. (1995). Effects of classroom social structure and disability on engagement. *Topics in Early Childhood Special Education, 15*(2), 123–147.

McWilliam, R. A., Trivette, C. M., & Dunst, C. J. (1985). Behavior engagement as a measure of the efficacy of early intervention. *Analysis and Intervention in Developmental Disabilities, 5*(1–2), 59–71.

Miller, L. J., & McIntosh, D. N. (1998, March). The diagnosis, treatment, and etiology of sensory modulation disorder. *Sensory Integration Special Interest Section Quarterly,* pp. 1–4.

Miller, L. J., McIntosh, D. N., McGrath, J., Shyu, V., Lampe, M., Taylor, A., et al. (1999). Electrodermal responses to sensory stimuli in individuals with fragile X syndrome: A preliminary report. *American Journal of Medical Genetics, 83,* 268–279.

Roid, D., & Miller, L. (1997). *Leiter International Performance Scale–Revised.* Wood Dale, IL: Stoelting.

Scharfenaker, S., O'Connor, R., Stackhouse, T., Braden, M., Hickman, L., & Gray, K. (1996). An integrated approach to intervention. In R. J. Hagerman & A. Cronister (Eds.), *Fragile X syndrome: Diagnosis, treatment, and research* (2nd ed., pp. 349–411). Baltimore: Johns Hopkins University Press.

Shopmeyer, B., & Lowe, F. (1992). *The fragile X child.* San Diego, CA: Singular.

Sparrow, S., Balla, D., & Cicchetti, D. (1984). *Vineland Adaptive Behavior Scales.* Circle Pines, MN: American Guidance Services.

SPSS, Inc. (1999). Statistical Package for Social Sciences for Windows 10.0 [Computer software]. Chicago: Author.

Stackhouse, T. M. (1994, March). Sensory integration concepts and fragile X syndrome. *Sensory Integration Special Interest Section Newsletter*, pp. 2–6.

Stone, W. L., Lemanek, K. L., Fishel, P. T., Fernandez, M. C., & Altemeier, W. A. (1990). Play and imitation skills in the diagnosis of autism in young children. *Pediatrics, 86*, 267–272.

Thelen, E. (1989). The (re)discovery of motor development: Learning new things from an old field. *Developmental Psychology, 25*, 946–949.

Thelen, E., & Smith, L. (1994). *A dynamic systems approach to the development of cognition and action.* Cambridge, MA: MIT Press.

Turner, G., Webb, T., Wake, S., & Robinson, H. (1996). Prevalence of the fragile X syndrome. *American Journal of Medical Genetics, 64,* 196–197.

Warren, S. T., & Nelson, D. L. (1994). Advances in molecular analysis of fragile X syndrome. *Journal of the American Medical Association, 271,* 536–542.

CHAPTER 28

Toddlers' Persistence in the Emerging Occupations of Functional Play and Self-Feeding

Sally J. Bober, Ruth Humphry,

Heather West Carswell, and Amanda J. Core

Sally J. Bober, MS, OTR/L, *is project STIR coordinator, Clinical Center for the Study of Development and Learning, CB 7255, University of North Carolina at Chapel Hill, Chapel Hill, NC 27599-7255; sally.bober@cdl.unc.edu.*

Ruth Humphry, PhD, OTR/L, *is professor, Division of Occupational Science, University of North Carolina at Chapel Hill.*

Heather West Carswell, MS, OTR/L, *is occupational therapist, Frye Regional Medical Center, Hickory, NC.*

Amanda J. Core, MS, OTR/L, *is occupational therapist, Backus Children's Hospital, Memorial Health University Medical Center, Savannah, GA.*

Originally published 2001 in *American Journal of Occupational Therapy, 55,* 369–376.

Occupations are purposeful, intrinsically motivating, and socially valued (Yerxa, 1993). Two occupations acquired in the toddler period are the ability to play with objects in a functional manner and to self-feed with a utensil (Belsky & Most, 1981; Gessell & Ilg, 1943). The development of occupations among toddlers is influenced by the interaction of the child, the task at hand, and the environment (Gray, Kennedy, & Zemke, 1996; Thelen, 1995). Thus, dynamic systems theory (DST), which reflects this interconnectedness, serves as a lens through which to view occupations and development. DST conceptualizes humans as complex, multifaceted beings who change and evolve over time (Kamm, Thelen, & Jensen, 1990). Furthermore, a small change in the function of a body system can disturb the preferred pattern of an activity, leading to re-organization of how the activity is performed (Thelen, 1995). Thus, the emergent nature of occupational performance results in constant skill refinement in play and self-feeding during early childhood. In addition, DST recognizes the individual as open to the influences of the environment. A toddler's most immediate influences, as recognized by an ecological view of development, are experiences within the family (Bronfenbrenner, 1979). In addition to the family-created social context, the interaction of the subsystems in the toddler's development, such as cognition and motor skills, influence emerging skills. Therefore, the framework we used to investigate development of occupations is a blend of DST and the ecological view of development.

Within the sensorimotor learning process, satisfactory occupational performance is achieved by resolving issues of *what needs to be done* and *how* (Gentile, 1998). Thus, as the people or events in the environment present novel food textures, toys, or playmates, the young child must reorganize and adapt his or her behavior while repeatedly responding to *how*. Therefore, a critical issue in understanding skill development is to further appreciate the child's motivation to make repeated attempts, or persist, in a challenging task.

Literature Review

Mastery motivation has been defined as "a psychological force that stimulates an individual to attempt independently, in a focused and persistent manner, to solve a problem or master a skill or task which is at least moderately challenging" (Morgan, Harmon, & Maslin-Cole, 1990, p. 319). *Persistence* is typically measured as "the percentage of time in which the child was engaged in task-directed behaviors" (Yarrow, Morgan, Jennings, Harmon, & Gaiter, 1982, p. 134). In addition, moderately challenging tasks have been proposed as ideal situations in which to elicit mastery motivation (Redding, Morgan, & Harmon, 1988). A moderately challenging task for young children without disabilities is one in which part but not all of the task is solved within 2 minutes (MacTurk, Morgan, & Jennings, 1995).

The concept of mastery motivation, rooted in psychology, includes the general domains of social, object, and gross motor mastery and posits that persistence results from the child's inner drive to be competent (Wachs & Combs, 1995). This perspective suggests that the urge for competence originates from the need to challenge some inner-body systems. For example, a child's goal may be to conquer dexterity challenges, and two occupations with similar fine motor challenges might tap the same intrinsic urge.

In studying occupations, however, the meaning of an activity as experienced by the person is important in understanding his or her motivation for doing the activity (Christiansen, 1994; Clark, Wood, & Larson, 1998). For toddlers, interacting with others, particularly family members, shapes what young children experience as important (Bronfenbrenner, 1979; Vygotsky, 1978). Occupational meaning and purpose must be inferred, as the developmental status of the toddler's subsystems and unique experiences with family members determine the internal perspective. If occupational meaning for the child goes beyond developing competence in intrinsic abilities, such as dexterity, two occupations that share commonly observed characteristics could emerge from uniquely different motivations.

Occupational therapy has applied to intervention the perspective of developmental psychology's grand theories (Coster, 1995). Consistent with a Piagetian framework, some researchers suggest that specific fine motor abilities and means–end understanding are prerequisites for performance of complex play and self-care tasks (Case-Smith, 1995; Exner, 1996; Henderson, 1995). Guided by the presumed link of fine motor skills and occupational performance, Case-Smith (1996) conducted a descriptive, correlational study of weekly intervention for 26 preschool-age children (mean age = 4.7 years) with mild to moderate fine motor delays. At the beginning and end of the school year, she measured the accuracy and speed of the preschooler's in-hand manipulation, tool use, eye–hand coordination, and grasping strength. Case-Smith used the Pediatric Evaluation of Disability Inventory (PEDI; Haley, Coster, Ludlow, Haltiwanger, & Andrellos, 1992) to measure functional performance in self-care, mobility, and social function. Her findings suggested a moderate association at the end of the year between increased dexterity in tool use and motor accuracy and self-care abilities ($r = .44–.61$). She proposed that opportunities to practice fine motor skills in therapy and the classroom generalized to better performance of self-care activities at home.

An alternative explanation for Case-Smith's (1996) findings is that supportive experiences with challenging therapeutic activities and success in these activities positively affected an underlying inclination to work harder at a variety of difficult activities. The result would be that both effort on testing activities and self-help skills would increase as the child perceives himself or herself as more competent and tries harder in general. Another alternative explanation is that the children showing the greatest change in both areas experienced a developmental transition in their awareness of the cultural criteria related to occupational performance and organized their behavior to meet newly perceived expectations for performance in both testing conditions and self-care. In either case, change relates to the *experience* of mastering occupations rather than the inner drive to master fine motor abilities.

Functional object play replaces mouthing and simple visually guided manipulation in the second half of the first year of life (Belsky & Most, 1981; Bornstein, Haynes, Pascual, Painter, & Galperin, 1999). Barrett and Morgan (1995) proposed that this transition to functional play reflects children's increasing awareness of what objects can do and that goal-oriented behavior is a prerequisite for mastery motivation. An example of functional object play is intentionally sliding a door on a busy box. Functional–relational play follows as the child brings together two objects in a manner consistent with a toy's purpose, for example, putting pegs in a pegboard (Belsky & Most, 1981). By selecting toys and engaging children in functional play in a certain manner, parents instill meaning to play and influence what is perceived as successful performance (Uzgiris & Raeff, 1995). Compared with other cultures that may put greater stress on social play, North American parents especially encourage functional play (Bornstein et al., 1999), which likely increases the meaningfulness of this form of play.

Learning to use utensils for self-feeding reflects a child's response to culturally determined expectations of performance in self-care (Henderson, 1995). Although Gessell and Ilg (1943) described the emergent and changing behaviors of self-feeding decades ago, little attention has been paid to *how* children come to acquire

skilled abilities to use utensils. Connolly and Dalgleish (1989) initially purported that the acquisition of spoonfeeding abilities, as influenced by the neuromaturational process, occurs in a fairly universal developmental sequence for children who are typically developing. In a second study on the emergence of tool-using skills, Connolly and Dalgleish (1993) concluded that there are distinct individual differences consistent with a more dynamic system perspective of learning tool use.

The ecological view of development recognizes the social context, specifically experiences in the family, as a source of individual differences in young children (Bronfenbrenner, 1979). This influence is not accidental; rather, parents actively create an ecocultural niche based on interconnected values, expectations, and meanings (Gallimore, Weisner, Kaufman, & Bernheimer, 1989). Two strategies are used to capture variations in parenting. Direct observations of adults' behaviors can reveal how parents support toddlers' activities and communicate meaning (Drucker, Hammer, Agras, & Bryson, 1999; Rogoff, Mosier, Mistry, & Goncu, 1993). Alternatively, parental value systems are affected by ethnic background and educational levels that offer an indirect measure of the ecocultural niche parents create (Humphry & Thigpen-Beck, 1997). In addition to parenting practices, siblings can play an important role in young children's experiences (Lamb, 1988; Teti, Bond, & Gibbs, 1988). Therefore, describing parents' background and family structure reflects the social contexts of toddlers.

This study assumes that the meaning that parents and children ascribe to the performance of occupations in addition to an inherent drive to overcome a perceptual–motor challenge contribute to the child's persistence. The issue of motivation is made relevant because persistence toward a goal ensures practice and potentially affects the child's emerging quality of performance in play and self-care. Therefore, the goal of this study was to expand our understanding of how two different occupations are associated with the persistence demonstrated by toddlers who are typically developing. We used a descriptive, correlational design to capture the relationships among several variables that cannot be manipulated experimentally (Isaac & Michael, 1995). The questions specifically addressed in this study are as follows:

- Is there a correlation between persistence in object manipulation during functional play and in self-feeding with a utensil among toddlers?
- What is the size of the association between the standardized measure of fine motor skills and persistence in functional play and self-feeding with a utensil?
- What is the association between measures of social contexts and the toddler's persistence with challenging occupations?

Method

Participants

Thirty-five children who were typically developing participated in this study. Videotapes from 2 children could not be scored due to lack of cooperation with the methodology. Of the 33 remaining toddlers, 18 (55%) were boys. The average age of the children was 15.7 months (*SD* = 2.0, range = 12–19 months).

Most of the children (88%) came from two-parent families, and 13 (41%) had older siblings. The average age of the participants' mothers was 33 years (*SD* = 4.9), and the fathers' average age was 35.8 years (*SD* = 5.8). The participants' parents were generally well educated. Mothers completed an average of 17.36 years (*SD* = 1.71) of school, and the fathers completed an average of 17.51 years (*SD* = 2.56) of school.

Toddlers and their families were recruited from the community. Parents were informed of the study through announcements placed in the newspaper; fliers at play groups, day care centers, and housing areas; and word of mouth. When a family indicated interest in the study, a screening call was made to ensure the child's fit with the participation criteria, which were the following: (a) chronological age between 12 and 19 months, (b) no known developmental delay, (c) parental report of some experience with utensils but not proficiency, and (d) at least one English-speaking parent. The age range was selected as a period of emerging spoon use based on norms from the PEDI (Haley et al., 1992).

Data Collection

Three data collection procedures were used: The child was administered the fine motor portion of the Peabody Developmental Motor Scales (PDMS; Folio & Fewell, 1983), a videotape was made of the child during functional play, and another videotape was made of the self-feeding session. Two of the researchers with at least 4 years' experience with pediatric standardized assessments administered the PDMS. Initially, they co-scored four PDMS evaluations and compared age equivalence scores, which were the same in all conditions. It was believed that this level of agreement reflected sufficient interrater reliability of the PDMS.

The four researchers formed two separate coding teams of two persons each for viewing the videotapes of functional play and self-feeding with a utensil. Thus, each team was blind to the toddlers' percentage of time spent persisting in a moderate challenge in the other mastery situation. For data coding, the coding team watched a videotaped session and identified the moderately challenging situations. Each coder then individually timed with a stopwatch and documented the total amount of time the child was presented with moderate challenges as well as the amount of time the child was on task during the moderate challenges. The coders discussed their total and on-task times and negotiated concordance. If a greater than 5-sec discrepancy existed on a videotape, observation and timing were repeated until agreement was reached.

For the functional play session, functional and functional–relational play were considered on-task behaviors. Off-task behavior consisted of engaging in any of the following behaviors for more than 5 sec: visual inspection; mouthing, banging, patting, or shaking the toy; or looking away. In the play session, unanticipated interruptions did not occur. In the self-feeding session, children were considered to be off-task if they engaged in any of the following behaviors for more than 5 sec: finger feeding, banging or setting down the utensil, playing with the food, or looking away. Unlike the uninterrupted play sessions, distractions occurred during the self-feeding sessions (e.g., father walked into the room). In these situations, the time during the distraction was not coded as part of the overall session.

At the end of observing the self-feeding videotape, the coders rated the parent's behavior on a scale of 1 to 5 regarding how much prompting the toddler was given to use the utensil (i.e., 1 = *none or only a few prompts to use the utensil*, 3 = *5–7 prompts*, 5 = > *10 prompts*). The ratings for amount of prompting were coded independently, and differences were negotiated between coders.

Procedure

A home visit was scheduled for a time when the parent anticipated the child would become hungry. At the beginning of the home visit, an interview with the parents was completed to obtain informed consent, demographic information, and details about the child's typical mealtimes. When possible, the PDMS was completed before the feeding session. At times, the feeding session was videotaped first if the parent believed that the child was hungry.

For the functional play session, toys were selected by the researcher to present varying levels of fine motor challenge. Many of the toys included a cause-and-effect element (e.g., pop-up figures busy box, shape sorter with sound). Three levels of difficulty were selected to represent a 12-month to 13-month level of challenge, a 14-month to 16-month level of challenge, or a 17-month to 19-month level of challenge. For example, round shapes for the one-hole shape sorter represented the lowest level, whereas the four-shape sorter represented the highest level.

Parents were asked to identify one parent to sit on the floor near the child during the play session, and siblings were asked not to participate with or distract the participant. Frequently, parents selected times when someone else would be available to watch older children; otherwise, the second researcher would engage the sibling somewhere else in the room. Parents were asked to minimize interactions with their child during videotaping. A warm-up period with toys not used in the study allowed the child to become comfortable with the researcher who presented the child with the toys. Videotaping began as the child was presented with a toy the parent reported as novel and at the level of difficulty thought to be moderately challenging on the basis of the age equivalence score from the PDMS. However, if the child was able to complete the entire task within 2 min, he or she was considered competent, and an alternative toy was introduced. The opportunity to play with a toy was terminated if the child demonstrated competence, refused the toy, or was off-task for more than 20 sec. Although times varied, effort was made to videotape 10 min of play with moderately challenging toys.

For the feeding session, the child was seated in his or her usual mealtime location and used the utensil reported to be typical for his or her meals. The food consistency selection was based on earlier parental interview. The children were thought to experience a moderate challenge if they spilled food from the utensil in the first two bites. To ensure a moderate challenge, the food consistency or utensils were altered if the child was initially proficient. The range of food consistencies used to ensure a challenge included pudding or yogurt at the easy level, applesauce at the moderate level, and small cooked vegetables or cereal in milk at the difficult level. Some older toddlers demonstrated remarkable proficiency with a spoon, so novel utensils, such as an adult-sized teaspoon, mother care spoon, or fork, were introduced to create a challenging self-feeding condition. Although the criteria for a challenging feeding condition was the same across participants, parental preferences and input were considered in making any modifications; therefore, standardizing food among the children was not possible. During videotaping, the parent was asked to hand the toddler the utensil and give one verbal cue as each new food was presented or when the child dropped the utensil or began to finger feed but to avoid other feedback. The length of videotape for the self-feeding sessions varied on the basis of the toddler's appetite and amount of food consumed, although effort was made to videotape 10 min of moderate challenge.

Data Analysis

Data were analyzed using the SAS statistical solution (SAS Institute, 1999). Pearson product-moment correlations were used to investigate the relationships between persistence in the two observational situations and to address the questions related to possible factors affecting how long children continued with moderately challenging activities. A *t* test was used to compare persistence between children grouped according to sibling status. The correlations between gender and

chronological age and the children's persistence did not reveal significant associations.

Results

Because each child varied slightly in the length of time in the functional play and self-feeding situations, a means of finding a comparable unit of measure was important. Persistence in each occupation was calculated as the percentage of time the child was on task while presented with moderate challenges. The sample of functional play ranged from 5 min to 10 min of moderately challenging tasks. Average persistence was 84% ($SD = 11$) of the time. The range of time children were presented with moderately challenging self-feeding tasks was 1 min to 10 min. On average, they persisted in feeding themselves with a utensil 50% ($SD = 22$) of the time.

The relationship between persistence in functional play with a challenging toy and persistence in self-feeding with a utensil was examined first. A modest but significant correlation was found between the observed percentage of on-task time across the two occupations ($r = .44, p < .01$). This finding suggests an underlying variable affecting persistence in both activities to a modest degree.

The association between maturity of fine motor abilities and persistence was explored using the age equivalence scores from the PDMS fine motor scale. Although no significant association was found between chronological age and persistence in either condition, the PDMS age equivalence score was significantly associated with the percentage of on-task time during moderately challenging functional play ($r = .39, p < .03$). No significant association was found between the PDMS fine motor score and persistence in self-feeding with a utensil ($r = .15, p < .40$).

Finally, the relationships between the two measures of persistence and features of social contexts, as defined by demographic characteristics of parents, presence of older siblings, and frequency of verbal prompts to use the utensil, were explored. No association was found between the age or educational background of either parent and the child's persistence in either activity. In comparing participants with siblings to those without siblings, a significant difference was found in percentage of time persisting in functional play and having or not having an older sibling, $t(32) = 3.02$, $p = .005$. On average, toddlers with older siblings persisted 90% of the time when confronted with moderately challenging functional play compared with toddlers without siblings, who persisted 79% of the time. No significant difference was found in persistence in self-feeding with a utensil when comparing toddlers with or without a sibling.

Immediate social context was examined by using the rating of how often the parent urged the child to use the utensil. No significant association was found between how often the parent encouraged utensil use and actual percentage of time using the utensil to self-feed ($r = -.28$, $p < .15$).

Discussion

The results of this initial descriptive study of typically developing toddlers' persistence in two challenging occupations, if supported in future research with larger samples of children with or without disabilities, suggest implications for occupational therapy practice. Therefore, after a discussion of these results, potential application to therapy will be covered.

The first purpose of this study was to examine the association between persistence in object manipulation during two challenging situations—functional object play and use of a utensil for self-feeding. The findings revealed a moderate, positive correlation between percentage of time persisting in functional play and self-feeding with a utensil. The activities were selected because they

shared similar object manipulation characteristics. Thus, an explanation for the finding of a significant correlation is that, regardless of the differences in the activities, motivation to master fine motor challenges in any task may organize children's behavior. This explanation is consistent with literature suggesting that mastery motivation is organized in general domains, such as object manipulation (Wachs & Combs, 1995). However, because the size of the correlation was modest, other sources may contribute to persistence. We propose that occupational meaning may contribute to persistence in occupations because, presumably, toddlers would not demonstrate focused effort and remain on task if an activity has no meaning for them.

The next question was whether the level of maturity of a child's fine motor abilities related to persistence. Redding et al. (1988) found that children tend to persist longer with moderate rather than very difficult tasks. In the current study, each activity was tailored to provide a moderate challenge. Therefore, the status of fine motor skills should not have been a factor in the children's persistence. No association between maturation of fine motor skills and how long the toddlers tried to use utensils in self-feeding was found, but a positive correlation between the PDMS age equivalence scores and persistence during functional play was found. Direction or cause of the association cannot be determined in correlational analyses. It may be that, despite efforts to match toys with emerging abilities, the protocol was not completely successful, and children with more fine motor abilities worked harder to master the toys. Alternatively, because none of the PDMS fine motor items for this age group are timed, the individual differences in these toddlers' persistence in object manipulation was captured in the fine motor scores. That is, children inclined to work longer with objects in general were more likely to eventually answer the *how* question of motor learning (Gentile, 1998) and succeed in test items, thus earning higher age-equivalent scores.

The final question, which asked how social context is associated with persistence in challenging occupations, explored factors thought to contribute to meaning of functional play and self-feeding. The lack of association of parents' age or education is inconclusive because the convenience sample of participants came from a fairly homogeneous group of families.

Other findings, though, reinforce the importance of exploring the possible impact of social context on motivation for an occupation. The presence of an older sibling in the family was positively related to persistence with toys. Older siblings did not participate in the functional play session, thus suggesting an indirect influence of having a playmate. Lamb (1988) found that older siblings tend to lead play interactions with their younger siblings; the younger siblings subsequently imitate their older siblings' behaviors. Having a model to share the activity not only enables the child to refine abilities but also enriches the meaning of the activity (Bandura, 1986).

An association between persistence in self-feeding with a utensil and having siblings was not found. All children typically ate some meals with family members. Adults who may not engage in as much functional play may be equally as effective as siblings in communicating meaning of utensil use in self-feeding.

Social encouragement to use a spoon or fork, on the other hand, did not affect the child's persistence in the self-feeding situation. Conversely, Drucker et al. (1999) found that mothers' frequencies of eating prompts significantly correlated with the amount their 3.5-year-old children ate. Barrett and Morgan (1995) suggested that mastery motivation to meet social criteria for performance emerges around 2 years of age. Thus,

the lack of association between verbal encouragement and persistence in the current study may be explained by the participants' ages (< 2 years). Toddlers seemed to be motivated by the desire to use utensils to eat like others rather than to please their parents.

Implications for Occupational Therapy Practice

Findings from this study raise questions about a traditional assumption that enhancement of underlying capacities, such as fine motor abilities, leads to improved occupational performance. This linear assumption leads to evaluation and intervention at the fine motor level when children experience delays in daily life activities. Interventions designed to enhance fine motor ability focus on how to provide the just-right challenge in such areas as in-hand manipulation, tactile processing, or grip. If challenges to a toddler's hand skills are the major factors organizing persistence and enhancing learning, then one-on-one sessions in which the therapist creates and modifies activities according to the sensorimotor challenge may be most effective. However, the current study suggests only modest overlap in the amount of organized effort in two occupations requiring manipulation of objects. Therefore, it appears that what captures interest and relates to persistence is more than challenging hand skills. More recently, therapists have been encouraged to move away from contrived activities as therapeutic means and provide interventions where meaningful occupations in natural context serve as both means and ends (Fisher, 1998; Gray, 1998). In occupational therapy practice, enhanced meaning of the occupation (e.g., realizing other children do the activity) may increase the likelihood that the child will try something challenging and persist to gain greater proficiency. Most specifically, the finding that older siblings are associated with the child's level of persistence in functional play supports the use of siblings or peers as ways to enrich meaning and, thus, effort.

The association between PDMS age equivalence scores and persistence in functional play warrants further consideration. Until further study is completed, therapists may want to consider when using this assessment that, in addition to fine motor abilities, test scores may also capture individual differences in intrinsic desire to master manipulation of objects.

Limitations

Several limitations make these findings tentative. First, research procedures create artificial conditions for the children by having strangers (researchers) in their home and asking parents to limit social interactions. Furthermore, this is the first study to address persistence in self-feeding, so credibility of actually capturing mastery motivation is not as well established as with functional play, and other factors such as hunger could organize efforts or distract from the child's utensil use for self-feeding.

Collecting even more information on the toddlers' social contexts is recommended for future studies. For example, the ages of siblings would be useful in determining whether the association between siblings and persistence in functional play differed for various ages. In addition, knowing which toddlers are in day care would be useful in looking further at any associations between young children's experiences around age-mates and persistence in functional play or self-feeding. Because occupational meaning is constructed in a social context, socioeconomic status and ethnicity of parents in a more heterogeneous group need further investigation to determine their associations with toddlers' persistence.

Differences existed between toddlers in test situations. In some situations, the child was already familiar with some of the research toys, and consequently, those toys were not used with

that particular child. In addition, parents' or toddlers' preferences for food meant that complete standardization of procedures was impossible.

Another limitation is that the same researchers conducted the PDMS evaluations, observed the play and self-feeding sessions, and served on the videotape coding teams. Although the PDMS scoring and the videotape coding typically took place weeks apart, bias could have been introduced. In addition, the videotapes were coded only once, so consistency in application of criteria for observations was not checked.

Finally, many methods of statistical analysis are linear and limited in their ability to investigate the interrelationships in a dynamic system. Sample size limited the use of multivariate analyses. The correlational method of analysis, however, was beneficial for this initial exploration into the degree to which mastery motivation is present in two occupations requiring object manipulation.

Conclusion

Data from this study revealed a significant but moderate correlation between percentage of time toddlers persist in functional play and self-feeding with a utensil. This finding of a modest correlation suggests that what organizes young children's efforts can only partially be explained by an intrinsic drive to master manipulation challenges. We believe that the individually experienced meaning of these occupations emerges from social context and that many dynamic factors determine a child's persistence. Our findings suggest a special role for siblings to serve as models and enrich the meaning of some activities, contributing to the toddlers' organized efforts in challenging occupations, especially during functional play. If consistent with future work, the results provide evidence that occupational therapists may be most effective in supporting sensorimotor learning by using actual, not contrived, occupations within a peer-rich environment as the means of affecting occupations (Fisher, 1998; Gray, 1998). Additionally, adults should not expect that verbally instructing the toddler to do an activity in a certain way will lead to persistent effort that refines skill. Rather than coaching the child in an activity, finding ways to enhance meaning may lead to greater persistence and greater learning.

Acknowledgments

We thank the 35 families who participated in this study. This study was a research project completed in partial fulfillment of master's degree requirements from the University of North Carolina at Chapel Hill.

References

Bandura, A. (1986). *Social foundations of thought and action: A social–cognitive theory.* Englewood Cliffs, NJ: Prentice-Hall.

Barrett, K. C., & Morgan, G. A. (1995). Continuities and discontinuities in mastery motivation during infancy and toddlerhood: A conceptualization and review. In R. H. MacTurk & G. A. Morgan (Eds.), *Mastery motivation: Origins, conceptualizations, and applications* (pp. 57–93). Norwood, NJ: Ablex.

Belsky, J., & Most, R. K. (1981). From exploration to play: A cross-sectional study of infant free play behavior. *Developmental Psychology, 17,* 630–639.

Bornstein, M. H., Haynes, O. M., Pascual, L., Painter, K. M., & Galperin, C. (1999). Play in two societies: Pervasiveness of process, specificity of structure. *Child Development, 70,* 317–331.

Bronfenbrenner, U. (1979). *The ecology of human development.* Cambridge, MA: Harvard University Press.

Case-Smith, J. (1995). Grasp, release, and bimanual skills in the first two years of life. In A. Henderson & C. Pehoski (Eds.), *Hand function in the child: Foundations for remediation* (pp. 113–135). St. Louis, MO: Mosby.

Case-Smith, J. (1996). Fine motor outcomes in preschool children who receive occupational therapy services. *American Journal of Occupational Therapy, 50,* 52–61.

Christiansen, C. (1994). Classification and study in occupation: A review and discussion of taxonomies. *Journal of Occupational Science: Australia, 1*(3), 3–21.

Clark, F., Wood, W., & Larson, E. A. (1998). Occupational science: Occupational therapy's legacy for the 21st century. In M. E. Neistadt & E. B. Crepeau (Eds.), *Willard and Spackman's occupational therapy* (9th ed., pp. 13–21). Philadelphia: Lippincott.

Connolly, K., & Dalgleish, M. (1989). The emergence of a tool-using skill in infancy. *Developmental Psychology, 25,* 894–912.

Connolly, K., & Dalgleish, M. (1993). Individual patterns of tool use by infants. In A. F. Kalverboer, B. Hopkins, & R. Geuze (Eds.), *Motor development in early and later childhood: Longitudinal approaches* (pp. 174–204). Cambridge, MA: Cambridge University Press.

Coster, W. (1995). Developmental aspects of occupation. In C. B. Royeen (Ed.), *Self-Study Series: Lesson 10. The practice of the future: Putting occupation back into therapy.* Bethesda, MD: American Occupational Therapy Association.

Drucker, R. R., Hammer, L. D., Agras, W. S., & Bryson, S. (1999). Can mothers influence their child's eating behavior? *Developmental and Behavioral Pediatrics, 20,* 88–92.

Exner, C. E. (1996). Development of hand skills. In J. Case-Smith, A. S. Allen, & P. N. Pratt (Eds.), *Occupational therapy for children* (3rd ed., pp. 268–306). St. Louis, MO: Mosby.

Fisher, A. G. (1998). Uniting practice and theory in an occupational therapy framework [1998 Eleanor Clarke Slagle Lecture]. *American Journal of Occupational Therapy, 52,* 509–522.

Folio, R. M., & Fewell, R. (1983). *Peabody Developmental Motor Scales.* Chicago: Riverside.

Gallimore, R., Weisner, T. S., Kaufman, S. Z., & Bernheimer, L. P. (1989). The social construction of ecocultural niches: Family accommodation of developmentally delayed children. *American Journal on Mental Retardation, 94,* 216–230.

Gentile, A. M. (1998). Implicit and explicit processes during acquisition of functional skills.

Scandinavian Journal of Occupational Therapy, 5, 7–16.

Gessell, A., & Ilg, F. L. (1943). *Infant and child in the culture of today: The guidance of development in home and nursery school.* New York: Harper & Brothers.

Gray, J. M. (1998). Putting occupation into practice: Occupation as ends, occupation as means. *American Journal of Occupational Therapy, 52,* 354–364.

Gray, J. M., Kennedy, B. L., & Zemke, R. (1996). Application of dynamic systems theory to occupation. In R. Zemke & F. Clark (Eds.), *Occupational science: The evolving discipline* (pp. 309–324). Philadelphia: F. A. Davis.

Haley, S. M., Coster, W. J., Ludlow, L. H., Haltiwanger, J. T., & Andrellos, P. J. (1992). *Pediatric Evaluation of Disability Inventory: Development, standardization and administration manual.* Boston: New England Medical Center Hospitals.

Henderson, A. (1995). Self-care and hand skill. In A. Henderson & C. Pehoski (Eds.), *Hand function in the child: Foundations for remediation* (pp. 164–283). St. Louis, MO: Mosby.

Humphry, R., & Thigpen-Beck, B. (1997). Caregiver role: Ideas about feeding infants and toddlers. *Occupational Therapy Journal of Research, 17,* 237–264.

Isaac, S., & Michael, W. B. (1995). *Handbook in research and evaluation* (3rd ed.). San Diego, CA: Edits.

Kamm, K., Thelen, E., & Jensen, J. L. (1990). A dynamical systems approach to motor development. *Physical Therapy, 70,* 763–775.

Lamb, M. E. (1988). Social and emotional development in infancy. In M. H. Bornstein & M. E. Lamb (Eds.), *Developmental psychology: An advanced textbook* (2nd ed.). Hillsdale, NJ: Erlbaum.

MacTurk, R. H., Morgan, G. A., & Jennings, K. D. (1995). The assessment of mastery motivation in infants and young children. In R. H. MacTurk & G. A. Morgan (Eds.), *Mastery motivation: Origins, conceptualizations, and applications* (pp. 19–56). Norwood, NJ: Ablex.

Morgan, G. A., Harmon, R. J., & Maslin-Cole, C. A. (1990). Mastery motivation: Definition and measurement. *Early Education and Development, 1,* 318–339.

Redding, R. E., Morgan, G. A., & Harmon, R. J. (1988). Mastery motivation in infants and toddlers: Is it greatest when tasks are moderately challenging? *Infant Behavior and Development, 11,* 419–430.

Rogoff, B., Mosier, C., Mistry, J., & Goncu, A. (1993). Toddlers' guided participation with their caregivers in cultural activity. In E. A. Forman, N. Minick, & C. A. Stone (Eds.), *Context for learning: Sociocultural dynamics in children's development* (pp. 230–253). New York: Oxford University Press.

SAS Institute. (1999). SAS Institute statistical solution [Computer software]. Cary, NC: Author.

Teti, D. M., Bond, L. A., & Gibbs, E. D. (1988). Mothers, fathers, and siblings: A comparison of play styles and their influence upon infant cognitive level. *International Journal of Behavioral Development, 11,* 415–432.

Thelen, E. (1995). Motor development: A new synthesis. *American Psychologist, 50,* 79–95.

Uzgiris, I. C., & Raeff, C. (1995). Play in parent–child interactions. In M. H. Bornstein (Ed.), *Handbook of parenting* (Vol. 4, pp. 353–376). Mahwah, NJ: Erlbaum.

Vygotsky, L. S. (1978). *Mind in society: The development of higher psychological processes.* Cambridge, MA: Harvard University Press.

Wachs, T. D., & Combs, T. T. (1995). The domains of infant mastery motivation. In R. H. MacTurk & G. A. Morgan (Eds.), *Mastery motivation: Origins, conceptualizations, and applications* (pp. 147–164). Norwood, NJ: Ablex.

Yarrow, L. J., Morgan, G. A., Jennings, K. D., Harmon, R. J., & Gaiter, J. L. (1982). Infants' persistence at tasks: Relationships to cognitive functioning and early experience. *Infant and Behavior Development, 5,* 131–141.

Yerxa, E. J. (1993). Occupational science: A new source of power for participants in occupational therapy. *Occupational Science: Australia, 1,* 3–10.

CHAPTER 29

Pencil Grasp and Children's Handwriting Legibility During Different-Length Writing Tasks

Julie L. Dennis and Yvonne Swinth

Julie L. Dennis, MOTR/L, *is occupational therapist, Highline Community Hospital Specialty Center, 12844 Military Road South, Tukwila, WA 98168; jldennis74@hotmail.com.*

Yvonne Swinth, PhD, OTR/L, *is assistant professor, School of Occupational Therapy, University of Puget Sound, Tacoma, WA.*

Throughout their educational careers, students use writing to record, express, and communicate ideas (Tseng & Cermak, 1993). Students who struggle to acquire and master handwriting skills may experience frustration and anxiety, which in turn may negatively affect overall school performance (Bonney, 1992). Many students with handwriting difficulties are referred to occupational therapy either as the primary reason for referral or in conjunction with other issues (Bonney, 1992; Weil & Amundson, 1994). Occupational therapists who practice in the school setting need to understand what factors influence writing performance so that they are better able to help children improve these skills.

Several researchers have investigated the effects of pencil grasp, amount of pressure on pencil, perceptual–motor abilities, and kinesthetic sensitivity on handwriting speed, accuracy, and legibility (Bailey, 1988; Harris & Livesey, 1992; Schneck, 1991; Weil & Amundson, 1994; Ziviani & Elkins, 1986). Only a limited number of studies, however, have examined how these factors influence handwriting endurance, or the ability to maintain consistent performance over longer periods. Students frequently use writing to record notes and complete exams, particularly in higher grades. As students progress through school, they are generally expected to be able to write for longer periods. The handwriting grasps that may affect performance during these longer writing tasks have usually been established by the end of elementary school and may be difficult to change as the child matures. Teachers and therapists who work with elementary-age children need more concrete evidence regarding the relationship between pencil grasp and endurance to provide effective instruction and treatment in this area.

Background

Originally published 2001 in *American Journal of Occupational Therapy, 55,* 175–183.

Children typically develop their preferred pencil grasp at a young age (Erhardt, 1994; Rosenbloom & Horton, 1971). Erhardt (1994) outlined a normal progression from immature to mature grasp patterns that occurs from 1 year to 6 years of age. Between 1 year and 2 years of age, children usually grasp their pencils or crayons in a palmar-supinate pattern (see Figure 29.1). The hand is fisted around the pencil, with the ulnar side toward the pencil tip, and the arm moves as a whole unit from the shoulder. Next, around 2 years to 3 years of age, the digital pronate grasp emerges. The thumb and index finger lie closest to the pencil tip, with the other digits curling around the upper shaft and the end of the pencil extending beyond the ulnar side of the hand. A static tripod grasp emerges around 3 years to 4 years of age. In this grasp, the pencil is held against the radial side of the middle finger, with the pad of the index finger on top of the shaft, and the pad of the thumb in opposition to the index finger. The arm is still moving as a unit, with some mobility at the wrist and elbow. As the child's fine motor control improves, the dynamic tripod grasp emerges, usually between 4 years and 6 years of age. The position of the pencil in the fingers is identical to the static tripod, but the proximal arm joints are stable, and the writing movement is controlled by the intrinsic hand muscles.

Because of this distal control, the dynamic tripod grasp is generally considered by both occupational therapists and teachers to be the optimal grasp for handwriting performance (Amundson & Weil, 1996; Bonney, 1992; Tseng & Cermak, 1993). This grasp, however, is not the only one used by persons without handwriting difficulties. Grasp patterns in addition to those just out-

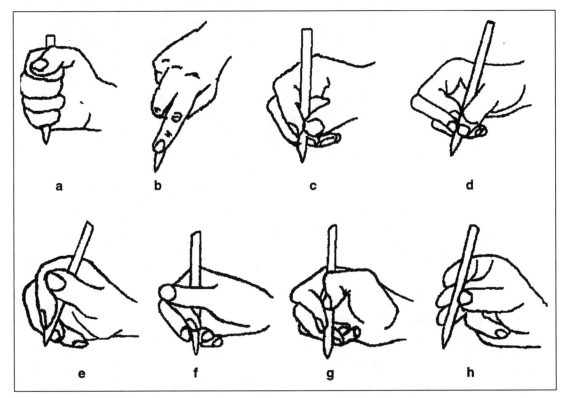

Figure 29.1. Typical developmental progression of pencil grasp: (a) palmar supinate grasp, (b) digital pronate grasp, (c) static or dynamic tripod grasp. Atypical pencil grasps: (d) quadropod grasp, (e) lateral tripod grasp, (f) lateral quadropod grasp, (g) tripod grasp without web space, (h) four finger with tips only grasp.

lined have been described by other researchers. Bergmann (1990) conducted a descriptive study of pencil grasps with occupational therapy students, medical students, and voters. Of the 447 right-handed adults studied, 64 (14.3%) used grasps other than the dynamic tripod grasp while signing their name. The most common atypical grasp was the lateral tripod in which the thumb lies adducted against the lateral aspect of the index finger rather than in opposition as in the dynamic tripod (see Figure 29.1). Bergmann noted that most of the participants with atypical grasps still displayed mature grasp patterns, characterized by the use of intrinsic hand musculature, dynamic wrist control, and distal finger control of the writing tool. This finding suggested that perhaps emphasis should be on immature versus mature grasp patterns rather than on the specific type of grasp.

Another descriptive study of pencil grasp focused on children who were typically developing, ranging in age from 3 years to 6 years, 11 months (Schneck & Henderson, 1990). The 320 children were observed during drawing and writing tasks, and the data on pencil grasp were separated according to 6-month age groups. The dynamic tripod grasp was the most common across all age groups. Some children used the lateral tripod grasp as well, particularly the older children. Approximately 25% of the children between 5 years and 6 years, 11 months of age used the lateral tripod grasp. The authors classified only the dynamic tripod and lateral tripod grasps as being mature grasps. It is not clear, however, whether the researchers classified the grasps on the basis of hand and wrist movement patterns, as in Bergmann's study, or whether the grasps were listed as mature simply because they were seen more frequently in the older children.

The distributions of pencil grasps in these two descriptive studies were similar. In both cases, most participants used the dynamic tripod,

although a substantial minority used the lateral tripod grasp. This similarity suggests that many people establish their preferred pencil grasp at an early age. In fact, other authors have noted that therapists or teachers who wish to attempt to change a student's grasp pattern should do so by the second grade (Amundson & Weil, 1996).

Researchers have not found a clear relationship, however, between pencil grasp and handwriting performance. Ziviani and Elkins (1986) examined four components of grasp for 282 children between 7 years and 14 years of age who were typically developing: degree of index finger flexion, degree of forearm pronation and supination, number of fingers used on the pencil shaft, and opposition of the thumb and fingers. They found that neither speed nor legibility was affected by atypical grasp patterns and concluded that grasp patterns may not significantly affect overall handwriting performance. A similar study also investigated the relationship between pencil grasp and handwriting speed with children who were normally developing (Sassoon, Nimmo-Smith, & Wing, 1986). The 294 participants, 7 years to 16 years of age, were grouped according to their grasp, and writing speeds were compared. As in Ziviani and Elkins's study, the researchers did not find a relationship between type of pencil grasp and speed of writing.

In contrast, Schneck (1991) found differences in grasp between children with good and poor handwriting, as rated by classroom teachers. The first graders' pencil grasps were scored according to a 5-point scale on the basis of a drawing task. The scale, devised previously by the author, assigned a rank to specific grasps on the basis of the age at which each grasp was seen in young children. Then the children were rated on legibility and accuracy of letter formation after printing the alphabet in lowercase letters and copying a sentence. The participants were also evaluated for proprioceptive finger awareness.

Results indicated that students with poor hand-writing received lower grasp scores. In addition, the children with lower grasp scores displayed decreased proprioceptive awareness, indicating a possible relationship between decreased proprio-ception and lower grasp scores on the scale used in this study.

In all these studies, the tasks used to evaluate the relationship between pencil grasp and hand-writing performance were short writing samples consisting of only one or two sentences. Some authors have suggested that performance during longer tasks, or endurance, could be affected by grasp patterns (Bailey, 1988; Bonney, 1992; Tseng & Cermak, 1993). One study of 40 adult participants examined the influence of pencil grasp on fatigue, legibility, and speed after writ-ing three paragraphs (Jaffe, 1987). No significant differences were found on any of the dependent variables between participants using the dynamic tripod grasp and those using other grasp patterns. The author noted, however, that the writing samples used in the study may not have been long enough to reveal differences in fatigue for adults.

Because endurance during handwriting tasks has not been given much attention in school-age populations, the current study focused on the rela-tionship between pencil grasp and performance on short and long writing tasks in elementary school children. Legibility was chosen as the measure of handwriting performance because legible writing is crucial for successful written communication, although other important factors also exist. From previous research, it is unclear whether the use of specific pencil grasps, such as the dynamic tripod, might affect students' abilities to write legibly dur-ing longer tasks. Thus, the purpose of this study was to examine the influence of pencil grasp on handwriting legibility during both short and long writing tasks in fourth-grade students who were typically developing.

Method

Design

A quasi-experimental, mixed repeated-measures design, as described in Portney and Watkins (1993), was used in this study, with one indepen-dent factor and one repeated factor. The inde-pendent, or between-subjects, variable was grasp pattern (atypical vs. dynamic tripod), and the repeated, or within-subjects, variable was length of writing task (short vs. long). The dependent variables were letter legibility and word legibility. Matched samples were used to control for vari-ability due to age, gender, hand dominance, and classroom. This design enabled the researchers to compare the performance of students with atypi-cal grasps on short tasks with their performance on long tasks as well as to compare their perfor-mance on both tasks to that of their peers who used the dynamic tripod grasp. The mixed design also allowed the researchers to examine the inter-action between the two independent variables.

Participants

Students in the fourth grade were thought to be appropriate participants because instruction in cursive handwriting has usually been completed at this point and the amount of writing expected from students has increased (Cornhill & Case-Smith, 1996). In addition, in Washington State, the Commission on Student Learning (1997) provided standards for several academic subjects, including writing, and the first set of standards was developed for the fourth-grade level. A con-venience sample of 46 fourth-grade students from two western Washington school districts partici-pated in the current study. In the first district, 20 students attended two classrooms in the same elementary school, whereas 4 more students attended another school in the same district. The remaining 22 students attended two class-rooms in the same school in the second district.

Both districts used the D'Nealian curriculum for handwriting instruction (Hillandale Elementary School, 1999). Participants with an atypical grasp were first identified by the primary researcher after observation in the five different fourth-grade classrooms. These participants were then matched with the participants with a dynamic tripod grasp on the basis of gender, age, hand dominance, and classroom. None of the students was receiving occupational therapy treatment or any other support services related to motor or cognitive development.

Instrument

The writing tasks used in this study were the participants' regular class assignments so that the level of difficulty would be appropriate for fourth-grade students. In the first district, 14 participants (two classrooms) performed creative writing tasks. The teachers asked the participants to write about the topics "What I Do at Recess" and "The Things That Bother Me." The remaining 10 participants (one classroom) performed copying tasks. The teacher selected passages about the history of St. Patrick's Day and the original 13 colonies, which were relevant to the current classwork. In the second district, the primary researcher assisted the teachers in creating the passages for the participants to copy to lessen the burden on the teachers at a busy time of year. Both passages (short and long) were about Washington State government because both classes were currently learning about that topic. The teachers read over the text to check for level of difficulty.

For all classrooms, the shorter samples consisted of 2 to 4 sentences, with approximately 5 to 10 words per sentence. Longer samples consisted of at least 8 sentences. The participants wrote in either manuscript or cursive, depending on the teacher's instructions, although the teachers were asked to try to give the same instructions for both short and long tasks. Decisions about specific instructions were left up to each teacher so that the tasks would reflect the participants' typical performance based on the usual practices in each class. Legibility of the samples was scored according to the letter and word legibility criteria used in the Evaluation Tool of Children's Handwriting (ETCH) scale (Amundson, 1995).

For short samples, the entire sample was scored. On longer samples, the first, middle, and last 5 words were scored. For example, if the sample consisted of 100 words, then words 1 through 5, 48 through 52, and 95 through 100 were scored. For all samples, each letter and word was determined to be either legible or illegible. The number of legible items was divided by the total number of items to produce letter and word percentage legibility scores for the total sample. Letter legibility scores were also calculated for each subsection of the longer writing samples. Word legibility for the longer samples was calculated only for the total score because each subsection contained only 5 words.

The ETCH manual provided a set of specific criteria for determining legibility of cursive or manuscript writing for children in grades 1 through 6 (United States). Although the manual provided several examples of legible and illegible letters and words, the test author clarified that raters must still use their own clinical judgment in determining whether a given letter met the criteria for legibility. Because the words in the current samples differed from the words used when administering the ETCH, scoring decisions for word legibility were based on the general written criteria. For total letter legibility, the ETCH manual reported intraclass correlation coefficients for interrater reliability of .84 on the manuscript scale and .89 on the cursive scale, and .48 on the manuscript scale and .94 on the cursive scale for total word legibility. Because the ETCH scale was published while still under construction, normative data have not been compiled to provide an expected range of performance for students.

The ETCH manual provided two practice tests for test administrators or researchers to establish proficiency in administering the scale. Before the study, the researchers achieved a reliability of .90 with the practice tests, the level required by the test author. The primary researcher scored all of the samples, and every fifth writing sample was also scored by the secondary researcher to check for rater drift. Both point-by-point reliability and percentage of agreement on total legibility scores were calculated for interrater reliability.

Procedure

Before any contact with the participants, this study was approved by the Institutional Review Board at the University of Puget Sound and by the participating school districts. The parents or guardians of all children in the five classrooms were contacted in writing to explain the purpose and procedure of the study and to obtain consent. Participants were given an opportunity to ask questions about the study and to give their consent, and they were reassured that their performance during the study would have no bearing on their academic evaluations. Permission forms were sent out for all 118 students, and permission was obtained for 51. When possible, the primary researcher spent at least 30 minutes observing in the classroom before data collection began to allow the participants to become accustomed to the researcher's presence. Each teacher introduced the researcher and the purpose of the study.

The participants who used an atypical grasp (n = 23) were identified first by the primary researcher. Then each participant who used the dynamic tripod grasp (n = 23) was selected at random from a pool of the remaining students who matched on gender, hand dominance, classroom, and age (i.e., within 6 months of age of each participant with an atypical grasp). Any students who were receiving support services for cognitive or motor development were not included. The primary researcher then coordinated with the teacher to observe both the short and long writing tasks, which were completed on the same day in each classroom. Field notes were recorded regarding the structure of the classroom and the reactions of the participants to the assignments, such as signs of muscle fatigue, as well as the prevalence of atypical grasps in each class. These qualitative data were taken to check the validity of the quantitative data. Photocopies were made of the writing samples, and the originals were returned to the teacher. The copies were kept in a secure location to which only the researchers had access. The researchers then scored the letter and word legibility of each sample. Information regarding each participant's grasp pattern was kept separate from the writing samples so that the researchers were blind to grasp type while scoring.

Data Analysis

The legibility scores were grouped according to type of grasp and length of writing task. The letter legibility scores for each subsection of the long task (first, middle, last) were also included in the analysis for a total of five data sets for letter legibility (short task, long task, three subsections of the long task). As stated previously, for word legibility, only the total scores for each sample were analyzed because each section of the long task only contained 5 words. Means and standard deviations were calculated for each set of scores, and the means were compared using a two-way analysis of variance (ANOVA) with one repeated measure (Portney & Watkins, 1993). The ANOVA for the letter legibility scores was conducted separately from the ANOVA for the word legibility scores. An F ratio was calculated for each main effect of grasp or writing task and for the interaction between grasp and writing task. For letter legibility, post hoc tests were also conducted between the mean for the short task and the mean for the total long task as well as between each of the means for the three sections of the long task. A separate comparison between the mean for the total long task and the means for the three sections was not conducted because the total scores were averages of the three subscores. An alpha level of .05 was used to determine significance of all statistical comparisons.

Results

The 18 boys and 28 girls who participated in this study ranged in age from 9.3 years to 10.9 years (M = 10.2 years, SD = .40). Four participants were left-hand dominant, and 42 were right-hand dominant. Half used the dynamic tripod grasp during writing, whereas the other half used an atypical grasp (one other than dynamic tripod). Of those who used an atypical grasp, the quadropod (four-finger) grasp was the most common (n = 13). The next most common grasp was a combination of the lateral tripod and quadropod grasps, referred to as the lateral quadropod grasp (n = 4), followed by the lateral tripod grasp (n = 2), a tripod grasp without web space between the thumb and index finger (n = 2), the static tripod grasp (n = 1), and a quadropod grasp where only the tips of the fingers were used (n = 1). All atypical grasps are illustrated in Figure 29.1.

Letter Legibility

The ANOVA data for letter legibility are summarized in Table 29.1. No significant main effect was found for grasp pattern, $F(1, 44)$ = 3.90, p = .054, nor was a significant interaction effect for grasp by task length found, $F(4, 176)$ = 1.75, p = .142. A significant main effect was found, however, for task length, $F(4, 176)$ = 12.42, p = .000. Because the repeated-measures ANOVA is sensitive to violations of the assumption of homogeneity of variance (Portney & Watkins, 1993), the variables

were tested for homogeneity of variance. Unequal variances can lead to an increased risk of Type I errors, or an increased risk of finding significant differences when none exist. The variances for the scores of the third section of the long task were found to be unequal, so correction factors (epsilons) were generated and used to calculate new p values (Portney & Watkins, 1993). Even with these correction factors, the main effect for task length was still significant (see Table 29.1).

Post hoc testing using Tukey's honestly significant difference revealed an overall significant difference between the short task and the long task, with participants scoring higher on the short task than on the long task. Within the long task, significant differences were found between the first section and the middle section and between the first section and the last section but not between the middle and last sections. The scores on the first section were higher than those on the second and last sections. Thus, participants' letter legibility was greater on the short task than on the long task and greater at the beginning of the long task than at the middle or end of the long task.

Word Legibility

The ANOVA summary data for word legibility scores are presented in Table 29.2. No significant main effects were found for grasp pattern,

Table 29.1. Comparison of Letter Legibility Scores by Grasp Pattern and Task Length

Source of Variance	df	F	p	G–G[a]	H–F[b]
Between subjects					
Grasp (A)	1	3.90	.054	NA	NA
Error	44	(132.9)			
Within subjects					
Task (B)	4	12.42	.000	.000	.000
Grasp × task (A × B)	4	1.75	.142	.171	.167
Error	176	(18.41)			

Note. Values in parentheses represent mean square errors. G–G = Greenhouse–Geisser corrected p values; H–F = Huynh–Feldt corrected p values.
[a]G–G epsilon = .614.
[b]H–F epsilon = .668.

Table 29.2. Comparison of Word Legibility Scores by Grasp Pattern and Task Length

Source of Variance	df	F
Between subjects		
Grasp (A)	1	0.48
Error	44	(119.6)
Within subjects		
Task (B)	1	3.86
Grasp × Task (A × B)	1	0.16
Error	44	(29.23)

Note. Values in parentheses represent mean square errors.

$F(1, 44) = .48$, $p = .492$, or task length, $F(1, 44) = 3.86$, $p = .056$, nor was any significant interaction effect for grasp by task length found, $F(1, 44) = .16$, $p = .689$. Because none of the comparisons yielded significant differences, correction factors were not generated. Additionally, because each independent variable contained only two levels, no post hoc comparisons were calculated.

Other Analyses

Interrater reliability on every fifth writing sample ranged from 89.0% to 98.7% for letter legibility and from 86.7% to 100% for word legibility using the point-by-point agreement method. Total percentage of agreement ranged from 96.9% to 99.4% for letter legibility and from 86.7% to 100% for word legibility.

The field notes collected during the writing tasks revealed several interesting patterns. First, the participants in one classroom that used creative writing assignments were allowed to move about the room, retrieving dictionaries and washing hands. Because spelling was not scored on the creative writing samples, the teacher discouraged the dictionary use by telling the participants to write as if it were a first draft. Second, one of the participants in that same class who used an atypical grasp (quadropod) was observed shaking out her hand once during the longer writing task. After the legibility scoring was completed, this participant's scores were found to be at or above the mean for each subsection of the long task.

In one classroom in the second district, many of the participants shook their hands several times and took breaks during the long task. They also made comments about the length of the task. These participants required at least 15 additional minutes to complete the task compared with the other class in the same school. After the assignments were completed, their teacher mentioned that the writing sample was longer than what she usually required during a typical writing assignment. The other class in the same school did not display similar reactions to the identical task. Averages of the legibility scores for these two classrooms were almost identical.

Not all students who used atypical grasps were included in this study. This was because their parent or guardian did not grant permission for their participation, they did not meet the inclusion criteria, or they were absent during administration of one of the writing tasks. All of the atypical grasp patterns noted previously were seen in these students as well. On the basis of the primary researcher's observations, between 25% and 48% of the students in the five classrooms used atypical grasp patterns.

Discussion

The results of this study support previous findings that pencil grasp does not have a significant effect on handwriting legibility (Sassoon et al., 1986; Ziviani & Elkins, 1986). The significant main effect for task length indicated that endurance may have influenced legibility for the participants, regardless of pencil grasp. According to the field notes, several other issues arose regarding the variables examined.

Grasp Pattern

All of the atypical grasps were more mature, developmentally; that is, no participants displayed a primitive grasp, such as the palmar-supinate or digital pronate grasp. This finding was expected because the study focused on upper elementary students with typical motor development. Any student who still used immature grasp patterns likely would have been referred to an occupational therapist or other special education service provider and, thus, would have been exempt from the study.

The atypical grasps observed in this study were not consistent with the distributions or descriptions reported in previous literature (Bergmann, 1990; Erhardt, 1994; Rosenbloom & Horton, 1971; Schneck & Henderson, 1990). Instead of the lateral tripod, the quadropod grasp was the most common atypical grasp. Two grasp patterns were also observed that had not been described in previous studies. These grasps were labeled by the first author as the lateral quadropod grasp and the tripod grasp without web space. These two grasps were possibly included in the lateral tripod groups of previous studies because they are similar, yet neither one fits the descriptions provided in earlier research.

Although the main effect for grasp was not significant, the difference in the means was close to achieving significance ($p = .054$), and the mean for the participants who used an atypical grasp (95.14% legibility) was higher than the mean for the dynamic tripod grasp (92.87% legibility). This finding could simply be random variation, or error, in the legibility scores. Another possible explanation is that, among participants with poorer handwriting, those who use an atypical grasp may be referred for intervention in fine motor skills more frequently than those who use a dynamic tripod grasp. Teachers may see the use of an atypical grasp as further evidence of fine motor deficits. Therefore, students with poor legibility who use an atypical grasp would have been underrepresented in this study because students receiving support services were excluded. The development of the atypical grasps may also

be an effective adaptation for these students. Other aspects of a student's pencil use, besides just the grasp pattern, need to be examined if handwriting problems are present. For students who do not have handwriting difficulties, the use of an atypical grasp may not be a sufficient reason to provide intervention.

On the other hand, all of the atypical grasps that were observed, except the static tripod grasp and the four finger with tips grasp, seemed to allow greater surface area of contact between the fingers and the pencil shaft. This may reflect a need for more stabilization of the pencil and may result in less use of intrinsic hand musculature during writing. The long-term biomechanical effects of these grasps on the soft tissue structures of the hand are not known. By allowing greater contact with the pencil shaft, these grasps could also allow greater pressure to be placed on the pencil. Writing with too much pressure on the pencil, regardless of grasp pattern, can cause greater muscle fatigue (Tseng & Cermak, 1993).

Legibility Scores

Although the ETCH scale was useful for providing specific guidelines for legibility, decisions about individual letters were still based on the researchers' opinions and interpretations of those guidelines. The procedure outlined in the manual requires raters to examine each word or letter out of context, which is difficult because so much of reading depends on context. The situation also arises where individual letters may be illegible when considered alone, but the whole word is legible. The reverse can also be true, where all the letters may be legible, but the word is scored as illegible because of poor erasures or inadequate spacing between words (see Figure 29.2). Any test for handwriting legibility is likely to encounter the same problems because it must be specific enough to produce reliable scores yet flexible enough to be useful in clinical settings.

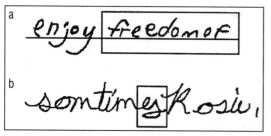

Figure 29.2. Sample legibility scoring: (a) "Freedom" and "of" are illegible because of inadequate spacing; (b) the final "s" is illegible when examined out of context, but the word "sometimes" is legible.

Related to the need for interpretation in scoring, the raters found it more difficult to achieve reliability using a point-by-point reliability, where agreement is checked letter by letter or word by word. Agreement on overall legibility scores, however, was easier to achieve. The difference may be partly because the actual ETCH tool was not administered; rather, the ETCH criteria were used on different writing tasks. Because the Washington State standards provide only a general guideline for legibility (Washington State Commission on Student Learning, 1997), a more global score, such as total word or letter legibility, may be more appropriate. Additionally, the ETCH manual notes that the interrater reliabilities for the total legibility scores are generally greater than the reliabilities for the individual tasks (Amundson, 1995). Because other states may have established writing standards that address legibility differently than Washington, therapists who frequently work with handwriting issues may want to review the specific standards for their state.

Strengths and Limitations

By matching the participants in the two grasp pattern groups on several demographic variables, some of the error variability in the scores was reduced. The two research groups contained equal distributions of students on gender, age, classroom, and hand dominance. Another strength of the study was the use of classroom assignments for the writing samples. By using these samples, the data reflected real-life performance of students in their natural environment. Although the participants did not all perform the same tasks, this was also a realistic situation because teachers make decisions about a student's handwriting performance that are based on comparisons with peers who may not be completing an identical task.

The classroom differences in tasks introduced more error variability in the legibility scoring, which was a limitation. The variety of writing samples made group differences more difficult to identify particularly because some participants produced creative writing samples rather than copied samples. A school-based practitioner with experience in handwriting intervention noted that she has observed students reverting to immature or atypical grasps when presented with a more challenging task, such as creative writing (S. J. Amundson, personal communication, June 25, 1999). This did not appear to be a factor in this study because the classrooms that performed creative tasks had 36% of participants using atypical grasps, whereas the classrooms that performed copying tasks ranged from 25% to 48% of students using atypical grasps. The results of this study also have limited generalizability due to the small sample size and the narrow age range from which the sample was drawn. Using copies of the students' work, rather than original writing samples, presented another limitation; edges of words were occasionally cut off, and the writing was not always as dark on the copy as on the original because pencil marks do not copy well.

Directions for Future Research

A replication of the design of this study is needed to investigate the validity of the results for other school districts in other states. Future studies should also be expanded to include a greater range of grade levels to examine the relationship between grasp and handwriting performance throughout a student's academic career. Once a clearer picture of this relationship is established for students who are typically developing, researchers then need to conduct studies with students with disabilities. The use of an atypical grasp may affect the performance of a student with a particular disability in a different way than the use of the same grasp would affect the performance of a child without that disability. Occupational therapists could then use the results of these studies to determine when and whether any intervention to change a student's grasp pattern is appropriate. Future researchers using a similar design as the current study may also wish to use only copying tasks, which would allow them to examine writing speed or efficiency as another measure of writing performance because the students would not have to pause during writing to create the text.

Other suggestions for future research arose from the observations made in this study. The percentages of students in the classrooms who used an atypical grasp were higher than reported in previous studies. This difference indicates that the prevalence of atypical grasps may have increased since those previous studies were conducted. Further descriptive studies that document the distributions of types of pencil grasps would give teachers and therapists current information regarding the prevalence of atypical grasps. Researchers could then also follow students who use atypical grasps in a longitudinal study. Given that the atypical grasps seen in this study may allow students to exert greater pressure on the pencil, longitudinal studies could address whether long-term use of such grasps results in biomechanical changes to the soft tissue structures of the hand. In addition, investigators could compare the grasps that students use during creative tasks with the grasps used during copying tasks to

determine whether students revert to more primitive grasps or to atypical grasps during creative writing tasks.

Another issue raised by this and previous research is how to consistently critique legibility of handwriting. The Washington State criteria for writing specify only that students should demonstrate "correct cursive letter formation and legible handwriting" (Washington State Commission on Student Learning, 1997, p. 32), leaving interpretation of what is legible up to individual teachers and therapists. Legibility is certainly a crucial component of written communication but can be quite difficult to define. An in-depth qualitative evaluation of how legibility is defined by practitioners would determine whether teachers and therapists across school districts and states have a consistent method for grading legibility. A further component of such research could focus on establishing norms for students' handwriting legibility on the ETCH or other assessments.

Summary

This study examined the effects of pencil grasp and length of writing task on fourth-grade students' handwriting legibility. A significant difference was found between the letter legibility scores on the short task and the letter legibility scores on the long task. Participants' handwriting was more legible on the short task than on the long task across both grasp conditions. No significant difference was found in scores between participants who used dynamic tripod grasps and those who used atypical grasps, nor was there a significant interaction between grasp and task length. No significant differences were found between word legibility scores by grasp or by task length. Because of the limited sample size in this study, the results should be interpreted with caution. The results do indicate that, although endurance was a factor in handwriting performance, the type of pencil grasp the students used was not, suggesting that changing a student's grasp to "improve" legibility may not always be appropriate. More research in handwriting performance and pencil grasp, particularly related to endurance and legibility standards, is necessary to establish clear expectations and treatment strategies for students.

Acknowledgment

We thank Katherine B. Stewart, MS, OTR/L, and Martins Linauts, PhD, PT, for serving as thesis committee members and providing editorial assistance; George Tomlin, PhD, OTR/L, for statistical support; and Sandi Koch, OTR/L, for serving as a liaison between the researchers and participating teachers.

This chapter is based on research conducted in partial completion of a master of occupational therapy degree at the University of Puget Sound.

References

Amundson, S. J. (1995). *Evaluation tool of children's handwriting.* Homer, AK: OT KIDS.

Amundson, S. J., & Weil, M. (1996). Prewriting and handwriting skills. In J. Case-Smith, A. S. Allen, & P. N. Pratt (Eds.), *Occupational therapy for children* (3rd ed., pp. 524–544). St. Louis, MO: Mosby.

Bailey, C. A. (1988). Handwriting: Ergonomics, assessment, and instruction [Research Supplement]. *British Journal of Special Education, 15*(2), 65–71.

Bergmann, K. P. (1990). Incidence of atypical pencil grasps among nondysfunctional adults. *American Journal of Occupational Therapy, 44,* 736–740.

Bonney, M. (1992). Understanding and assessing handwriting difficulty: Perspectives from the literature. *Australian Occupational Therapy Journal, 39*(3), 7–15.

Cornhill, H., & Case-Smith, J. (1996). Factors that relate to good and poor handwriting. *American Journal of Occupational Therapy, 50,* 732–739.

Erhardt, R. P. (1994). *Developmental hand dysfunction: Theory, assessment, and treatment* (2nd ed.). Tucson, AZ: Therapy SkillBuilders.

Harris, S. J., & Livesey, D. J. (1992). Improving handwriting through kinaesthetic sensitivity practice. *Australian Occupational Therapy Journal, 39*(1), 23–27.

Hillandale Elementary School. (1999). *The D'Nealian™ Handwriting Method.* Available from www.hillandale.org/dnealian.htm

Jaffe, L. (1987). *Influence of grip on legibility, speed, and fatigue in adult handwriting.* Unpublished manuscript, Boston University.

Portney, L. G., & Watkins, M. P. (1993). *Foundations of clinical research: Applications to practice.* Norwalk, CT: Appleton & Lange.

Rosenbloom, L., & Horton, M. E. (1971). The maturation of fine prehension in young children. *Developmental Medicine and Child Neurology, 13,* 3–8.

Sassoon, R., Nimmo-Smith, I., & Wing, A. M. (1986). An analysis of children's penholds. In H. S. R. Kao, G. P. van Galen, & R. Hoosain (Eds.), *Graphonomics: Contemporary research in handwriting* (pp. 93–106). New York: North Holland.

Schneck, C. M. (1991). Comparison of pencil-grip patterns in first graders with good and poor writing skills. *American Journal of Occupational Therapy, 45,* 701–706.

Schneck, C. M., & Henderson, A. (1990). Descriptive analysis of the developmental progression of grip position for pencil and crayon control in nondysfunctional children. *American Journal of Occupational Therapy, 44,* 893–900.

Tseng, M. H., & Cermak, S. A. (1993). The influence of ergonomic factors and perceptual–motor abilities on handwriting performance. *American Journal of Occupational Therapy, 47,* 919–926.

Washington State Commission on Student Learning. (1997). *Essential academic learning requirements: Technical manual.* Olympia: Author.

Weil, M. J., & Amundson, S. J. C. (1994). Relationship between visuomotor and handwriting skills of children in kindergarten. *American Journal of Occupational Therapy, 48,* 982–988.

Ziviani, J., & Elkins, J. (1986). Effects of pencil grip on handwriting speed and legibility. *Education Review, 38,* 247–257.

CHAPTER 30

Sensory-Processing Issues Associated With Asperger Syndrome
A Preliminary Investigation

Winnie Dunn, Brenda Smith Myles, and Stephany Orr

Winnie Dunn, PhD, OTR, FAOTA, *is professor and chair, Department of Occupational Therapy Education, University of Kansas, 3033 Robinson, 3901 Rainbow Boulevard, Kansas City, KS 66160-7602.*

Brenda Smith Myles, PhD, *is professor, Department of Special Education, University of Kansas, Kansas City.*

Stephany Orr, MSEd, *is director of children's ministries, United Methodist Church of the Resurrection, Leawood, KS.*

Individuals with Asperger syndrome, their parents, and professionals have debated whether sensory-processing issues are a salient part of Asperger syndrome (Attwood, 1998; Fling, 2000; Myles & Simpson, 1998; Myles & Southwick, 1999; Stagnitti, Raison, & Ryan, 1999; Willey, 1999), despite original assumptions that sensory issues were integral to the syndrome. Psychiatrist Hans Asperger (1944) first described a syndrome that he referred to as a social disability. In a study of four children, he observed a unique group of characteristics that set these children apart from any he had studied (Frith, 1991; Wing, 1991). Although each child was unique, Asperger noted the following traits common among the children: (a) social isolation and awkwardness, (b) self-stimulatory responses, (c) insistence on environmental sameness, (d) normal intellectual development, and (e) normal communication development.

The children in Asperger's (1944) study displayed a range of hyposensitivities and hypersensitivities to taste, tactile, and auditory stimuli. In taste, he found them to have very specific likes and dislikes. For example, many preferred very sour or strongly spiced foods. Similarly, the children had a strong dislike for certain fabrics or an aversion to specific daily life activities containing strong tactile sensory input, such as cutting fingernails. The children displayed extreme levels of noise sensitivity; at times, they were hypersensitive to noise in certain environments and appeared to be hyposensitive to the same noises in other environments. Further, the children manifested a lack of respect or understanding for other people and their space. Asperger reported that they leaned on total strangers or touched them as if they were pieces of furniture.

However, these impressions about sensory-processing challenges are not directly reflected in current diagnostic criteria for Asperger syndrome. Currently, the fourth edition of the American Psychiatric Association's (APA's) *Diagnostic and Statistical Manual of Mental Disorders* (DSM-IV; APA, 1994) is the source containing the most widely used diagnostic criteria for identifying Asperger

Originally published 2002 in *American Journal of Occupational Therapy, 56,* 97–102.

syndrome. DSM-IV places Asperger syndrome under the category of pervasive developmental disorders (PDD). According to these criteria, Asperger syndrome can be recognized by three behavioral criteria and three exclusion criteria. Behavioral criteria are (a) qualitative social impairment, (b) repetitive and restrictive stereotyped patterns of behavior, and (c) significantly decreased social function. Exclusion criteria are (a) language delays; (b) cognitive delays; and (c) other significant conditions, including schizophrenia or autism.

Further criteria are specified. For example, under "qualitative social interaction impairment" (APA, 1994, p. 65), the DSM-IV describes (a) significant impairment in nonverbal communication skills, (b) inability to establish appropriate peer relationships, (c) inability to initiate interactions with others, and (d) difficulty reciprocating socially or emotionally in ways social interaction might be impaired. The specific criteria listed under "repetitive and restricted stereotyped patterns of behavior, activities, and interests" (p. 65) are (a) abnormal preoccupation with stereotyped, specific areas of interest; (b) inflexible adherence to nonfunctional routines or rituals; (c) high repetition of nonfunctional motor movements; and (d) preoccupation with parts of an object. Some authors view these patterns as reflections of poor sensory processing (Huebner, 2000; Zero to Three, 1994), but sensory processing has not been incorporated into formally accepted definitions (Frith, 1991; Gillberg, 1992).

Scholars have reported about the relationships between sensory processing and functions in daily life, including learning, play, work, and socialization (e.g., Anderson & Emmons, 1996; Ayres, 1972, 1979; Cook & Dunn, 1998; Fisher, Murray, & Bundy, 1991). No empirical evidence exists, however, regarding whether children with Asperger syndrome tend to have difficulties with sensory processing. Thus, the purpose of this study was to provide initial evidence about the sensory-processing patterns of children and youths with Asperger syndrome.

Method

Design

This study used a group comparison design to identify possible differences in sensory processing between children with and without Asperger syndrome on the Sensory Profile. The Sensory Profile is a standardized parent-reporting measure of sensory processing.

Sample

Parents of 42 children (39 boys, 3 girls) with Asperger syndrome ranging in age from 8 to 14 years ($M = 11.33$ years) completed the Sensory Profile. All the children attended public school; a licensed professional diagnosed these children as having Asperger syndrome consistent with criteria in the DSM-IV (APA, 1994).

Using the random selection function of the Statistical Package for the Social Sciences (SPSS), version 9.0 computer program (SPSS, 2001), we selected a random sample of 42 children without disabilities between 8 and 14 years of age ($M = 9.6$ years) from the Sensory Profile standardization sample to serve as a comparison group (Dunn, 1999). Although this group is somewhat younger, all previous studies indicate that virtually no differences exist in scores on the Sensory Profile from preschool-age to school-age children (Dunn, 1999).

Instrument

The Sensory Profile (Dunn, 1999) is a 125-item questionnaire that describe responses to sensory events in daily life. The caregiver reports on a 5-point Likert scale how frequently the child uses that response to particular sensory events (i.e., *always, frequently, occasionally, seldom, never*).

This Sensory Profile was normed on more than 1,000 children without disabilities and 150 children with disabilities (Dunn, 1999). Reliability includes internal consistency estimates (range = .47–.91) and standard error of measurement (range = 1.0–2.8). Dunn (1999) also reported on content (three types established) and construct validity (i.e., convergent, discriminant). The validity findings indicate that the Sensory Profile has higher correlations with measures of sensory perception and behavioral regulation and lower correlations with particular skill demands.

The Sensory Profile measures the degree to which children exhibit problems in (a) sensory processing, (b) modulation, (c) behavioral and emotional responses, and (d) responsiveness to sensory events (i.e., hyporesponsive, hyperresponsive). The instrument evaluates the possible contributions of sensory processing to a child's individual performance patterns, provides information about the child's responses to stimuli, and identifies systems that contribute to or create barriers to functional performance. For this study, we used the children's raw summary scores for section and factor clusters as specified in the manual (Dunn, 1999). To make it easier for family members to understand scores, lower scores reflect poorer performance (i.e., a higher rate of behavior, because items are written to reflect potential difficulty with the sensory experience). Hence, if a child never engages in the behavior, he or she obtains a raw score of 5, whereas if the child always engages in the behavior, he or she yields a raw score of 1.

Procedure

The researchers mailed packets containing several questionnaires, including the Sensory Profile, to families who indicated an interest in being part of a comprehensive research study on Asperger syndrome being conducted by a large midwestern university. In most cases, the parent completed the Sensory Profile at home; some completed the instrument at a clinic while their child was being tested as part of the larger study.

Data Analysis

The researchers conducted two multivariate analyses of variance (MANOVAs) to identify differences between the groups. The first MANOVA addressed comparisons between groups on the Sensory Profile section scores (i.e., sensory processing, modulation, behavioral responses), and the second addressed comparisons between groups on the factor scores (Dunn, 1999; Dunn & Brown, 1997). We used SPSS 9.0 to conduct the analyses.

Results

This study was designed to determine the sensory-processing characteristics of children with Asperger syndrome. Specifically, we sought to determine the (a) sensory processing, (b) modulation, (c) behavioral and emotional responses, and (d) responsiveness as characterized in the factor scores that might be characteristic of children with Asperger syndrome as tested by the Sensory Profile.

Tables 30.1 and 30.2 contain the results of the MANOVAs. We had a sufficient sample size to identify real differences (i.e., all power estimates were .997–1.00), and effect sizes were large (i.e., η^2 = .310–.692), suggesting that differences would be clinically meaningful. (See Green, Salkind, and Akey [1997] for interpretation of η^2 calculation used in SPSS and Cohen [1992] for a conceptual discussion of effect size.) Of the 23 possible statistical comparisons, 22 were significantly different ($p < .05$), with the children

Table 30.1. MANOVA Results for Section Scores on the Sensory Profile

Section	F	p	Effect Size (h^2)	Power
Auditory processing	112.22	< .001	.63	1.00
Visual processing	41.18	< .001	.39	1.00
Vestibular processing	47.70	< .001	.42	1.00
Touch processing	130.10	< .001	.67	1.00
Multisensory processing	104.11	< .001	.61	1.00
Oral sensory processing	42.17	< .001	.39	1.00
Sensory processing related to endurance/tone	59.67	< .001	.48	1.00
Modulation related to body position and movement	45.79	< .001	.41	1.00
Modulation of movement affecting activity level	70.68	< .001	.52	1.00
Modulation of sensory input affecting emotional responses and activity level	108.60	< .001	.62	1.00
Modulation of visual input affecting emotional responses and activity level	0.05	.82	.00	0.05
Emotional/social responses	129.19	< .001	.69	1.00
Behavioral outcomes of sensory processing	175.10	< .001	.73	1.00
Items indicating thresholds for response	23.26	< .001	.26	0.99

Note. MANOVA = multivariate analysis of variance.

having Asperger syndrome reported as performing more poorly than the children without disabilities in each case.

Tables 30.3 and 30.4 contain the means, standard deviations, and 95% confidence intervals for the two groups on each comparison. Evident from these tables is that the 95% confidence interval raw score ranges for the two groups are quite separate from each other.

Discussion

Beginning with Asperger (as translated by Frith, 1991), researchers have reported that behaviors of children with Asperger syndrome suggest diffi-

culty with sensory processing (Attwood, 1998; Bettison, 1996; Fling, 2000; Iwanaga, Kawasaki, & Tsuchida, 2000; Myles & Simpson, 1998; Myles & Southwick, 1999; Stagnitti et al., 1999; Willey, 1999). Others have reported on the link between sensory processing and the ability to conduct daily life successfully (e.g., Ayres, 1979; Cook & Dunn, 1998; Dunn, 1997, 1999; Fisher et al., 1991). In this study, we report about the performance of children with Asperger syndrome on the Sensory Profile, a validated measure of sensory processing in daily life.

Interpretation of Specific Findings

Group performance (raw) scores reveal that the confidence intervals for the two groups are quite separate from each other, making differentiation between performance of children with and without Asperger syndrome clear (see Tables 30.3 and 30.4). That is, children with Asperger syndrome consistently have lower scores (i.e., *always displays the behavior* = 1) than children without disabilities. For example, when considering the scores on auditory processing (see Table 30.3), the lower boundary of the confidence interval for the children without disabilities was 33.03, whereas the upper

Table 30.2. MANOVA Results for Factor Scores

Factor	F	p	Effect Size (h^2)	Power
Sensation seeking	44.93	< .001	.37	1.00
Emotionally reactive	168.24	< .001	.69	1.00
Low endurance/tone	75.05	< .001	.50	1.00
Oral sensory sensitivity	31.30	< .001	.29	1.00
Inattention/distractibility	79.32	< .001	.51	1.00
Poor registration	64.86	< .001	.46	1.00
Sensory sensitivity	33.68	< .001	.31	1.00
Sedentary	43.98	< .001	.37	1.00
Fine motor/perceptual	71.76	< .001	.48	1.00

Note. MANOVA = multivariate analysis of variance.

Table 30.3. Means, Standard Deviations, and 95% Confidence Intervals for Groups on Each Section

Section	Typical M (SD)	Asperger M (SD)	Typical CI	Asperger CI
Auditory processing	34.28 (0.63)	23.73 (0.78)	33.03–35.52	22.18–25.28
Visual processing	38.80 (0.71)	31.50 (0.89)	37.37–40.23	29.73–33.27
Vestibular processing	52.53 (0.73)	44.54 (0.90)	51.08–53.98	42.74–46.34
Touch processing	83.50 (1.22)	61.31 (1.52)	81.06–85.94	58.28–64.33
Multisensory processing	30.88 (0.50)	22.81 (0.62)	29.88–31.87	21.58–24.04
Oral sensory processing	54.85 (1.18)	42.65 (1.46)	52.50–57.21	39.73–45.58
Sensory processing related to endurance/tone	42.28 (0.89)	31.27 (1.11)	40.49–44.06	29.05–33.49
Modulation related to body position and movement	46.48 (0.70)	38.92 (0.87)	45.08–47.87	37.19–40.66
Modulation of movement affecting activity level	27.45 (0.56)	20.00 (0.69)	26.34–28.56	18.62–21.38
Modulation of sensory input affecting emotional responses and activity level	18.43 (0.36)	12.46 (0.45)	17.71–19.14	11.57–13.35
Modulation of visual input affecting emotional responses and activity level	17.45 (2.21)	16.65 (2.74)	13.04–21.86	11.19–22.12
Emotional/social responses	72.03 (1.23)	49.81 (1.52)	69.57–74.48	46.68–52.85
Behavioral outcomes of sensory processing	26.13 (0.48)	16.12 (0.59)	25.18–27.07	14.94–17.29
Items indicating thresholds for response	13.53 (0.32)	11.08 (0.40)	12.89–14.16	10.29–11.87

Note. CI = 95% confidence interval. Lower scores indicate poorer performance; that is, the children engage in the difficult behaviors more often (*always* = 1, *never* = 5). Children without disabilities (typical) have a low rate of the behaviors on the Sensory Profile; fewer behaviors yield a higher score.

boundary was only 25.28 for the children with Asperger syndrome. Therefore, it is highly likely that children with Asperger syndrome will have poor auditory processing on the basis of the Sensory Profile. These findings are consistent with other reports that children with Asperger syndrome have difficulty with auditory processing. Bettison (1996) reported specific sensitivity to sounds that led to distress. Bettison then provided an auditory intervention, and participants demon-strated significantly improved behavior over a 12-month period in conditions of auditory train-ing or listening to music, suggesting that interventions addressing sensory-processing differences may be fruitful once a pattern of sensory process-ing is identified.

In the current study, children with Asperger syndrome were the same as the children without disabilities on modulation of visual input affect-ing emotional responses and activity level. Reports

Table 30.4. Means, Standard Deviations, and 95% Confidence Intervals for Groups on Each Factor

Factor	Typical M (SD)	Asperger M (SD)	Typical CI	Asperger CI
Sensation seeking	74.83 (1.32)	60.38 (1.70)	72.20–77.47	56.99–63.77
Emotionally reactive	66.35 (1.17)	41.72 (1.50)	64.03–68.68	38.74–44.71
Low endurance/tone	42.19 (0.77)	31.38 (0.99)	40.66–43.71	29.42–33.34
Oral sensory sensitivity	40.02 (1.02)	30.72 (1.31)	37.99–42.05	28.11–33.34
Inattention/distractibility	28.71 (0.62)	19.72 (0.80)	27.48–29.94	18.14–21.31
Poor registration	36.73 (0.58)	29.17 (0.74)	35.58–37.88	27.70–30.65
Sensory sensitivity	18.94 (0.37)	15.41 (0.48)	18.20–19.68	14.46–16.37
Sedentary	15.06 (0.50)	9.66 (0.64)	14.07–16.06	8.37–10.94
Fine motor/perceptual	13.67 (0.32)	9.24 (0.41)	13.03–14.31	8.42–10.06

Note. CI = 95% confidence interval. Lower scores indicate poorer performance; that is, the children engage in the difficult behaviors more often (*always* = 1, *never* = 5). Children without disabilities (typical) have a low rate of the behaviors on the Sensory Profile; fewer behaviors yield a higher score.

in the literature suggest that children with Asperger syndrome have strengths in visual–perceptual skills (Miller & Ozonoff, 2000; Quill, 1995, 1997, 1998). This section of the Sensory Profile addresses a child's way of using visual information to keep track of the context (e.g., watches everyone as they move around the room). However, the children with Asperger syndrome had a significantly lower score on visual processing. This section contains items related to basic responsivity (e.g., How does the child respond to particular visual stimuli? Prefers to be in the dark or bothered by bright lights). These data suggest that children with Asperger syndrome can process visual–perceptual information in context and, perhaps, can orient to social situations using their visual systems in a similar manner to other children, even though other behavioral responses might be different. Quill (1995, 1997, 1998) suggested that children with Asperger syndrome are visual learners and described visually cued instruction as a method to support them in instructional situations and communication. By providing direct cuing related to the visual environment, perhaps professionals and parents can link contextual cues, which the child notices, to expected behavioral patterns, which the child may not know how to select or use appropriately. The role of visual processing in the performance of children with Asperger syndrome, particularly in social contexts, will be important to study further.

On examination of the factor scores (see Table 30.4), it is interesting that the children with Asperger syndrome had difficulty with factors associated with both hyporesponsiveness and hyperresponsiveness. Low endurance/tone and poor registration are associated with hyporesponsiveness (i.e., the children do not notice stimuli that others notice), whereas emotionally reactive and sensory sensitivity are associated with hyperresponsiveness (i.e., the children notice stimuli more readily than others) (Dunn & Brown,

1997). These score patterns suggest that the children with Asperger syndrome in this study may have poor modulation (i.e., poor ability to regulate responses) rather than one way of responding. When children have poor modulation, their responses can vary dramatically from one situation to another, and predicting how the child will behave can be difficult (Dunn, 1999; Fisher et al., 1991; Huebner, 2000). The resulting behavioral repertoire may reflect a vulnerability to input rather than erratic performance per se.

Implications for Diagnostic Criteria for Asperger Syndrome

As reported by the parents, the children with Asperger syndrome demonstrated a significantly different pattern of sensory-processing from their peers without disabilities according to the Sensory Profile, suggesting a sensory-processing correlate in Asperger syndrome that needs to be included in the diagnosis. Bagnato and Neisworth (1999) described methods for early identification of regulatory disorders as described in the Zero to Three (1994) diagnostic classification system; this classification contains a predominance of items reflecting poor ability to process sensory information and is associated with early identification of autism spectrum disorders (Greenspan, Wieder, & Simons, 1998). Revisiting the diagnostic criteria to consider the contributions of sensory processing to Asperger syndrome may be useful.

For example, socialization challenges are criteria of the Asperger syndrome diagnosis (APA, 1994). Some evidence suggests that difficulties with socialization can be linked to poor sensory-processing. Persons with Asperger syndrome have reported on the relationships among sensory-processing functions in daily life, including learning, play, work, and socialization (Grandin, 1995; Shore, 2001; Willey, 1999). Shore (2001), an adult with Asperger syndrome, reported that as a toddler he would not kiss his father because the smell of coffee on his father's breath and the scratchiness of his moustache were too much to tolerate. As an adult, Shore stated that he was unable to work in companies that had traditional wardrobe requirements. He found suits and ties to be uncomfortable to the point that he could not perform his job.

However, these relationships do not reveal which problem leads to the other; people might exhibit poor sensory processing because they have not been able to engage in their environment to gather appropriate experiences or may not be able to engage because they have poor sensory processing. Researchers have attempted to uncover the nature of these relationships with intervention studies. For example, in intervention studies using sensory-processing approaches with children who have PDD, researchers have reported improvements in play schemas and social engagement with decreases in disruptive social behaviors (Case-Smith & Bryan, 1999; Linderman & Stewart, 1999), suggesting that poor sensory processing underlies the child's ability to engage in the complexities of social situations and communication.

The current diagnostic criteria for Asperger syndrome also address unusual patterns of behavior (i.e., repetitive and restricted patterns of stereotyped behavior). Some researchers hypothesized a "sensory-generating" function in repetitive and stereotypic behaviors (see Huebner & Dunn, 2000). Willemsen-Swinkels, Buitelaar, Dekker, and van-Engeland (1998) created a subtyping structure for stereotypic behaviors, and four of the five subtypes related to sensory intensity of the behavior. Our findings indicate that children with Asperger syndrome have difficulty with sensory modulation; perhaps the stereotypic behaviors serve an organizing function in that their repetitiveness provides a method for equalizing the tendency for hyporesponsiveness and hyperresponsiveness. If so, including sensory-processing status in diagnostic criteria might be warranted.

Limitations and Directions for Future Research

It must be noted that this study used a convenience sample of children with Asperger syndrome and selected a comparison group from the standardization data of the Sensory Profile. A larger sample reflecting broader geographic representation would verify the findings of this initial study about sensory processing in children with Asperger syndrome. The dramatic differences found between the two groups suggest that further study about the nature of sensory processing challenges for children with Asperger syndrome would be useful for the field.

We also did not evaluate the impact of these sensory-processing differences on the children's and their families' daily routines. A person's sensory-processing patterns are only important to evaluate if we link their patterns to successes and challenges in daily life. People with all types of sensory-processing patterns are living satisfying lives; it is only when a particular pattern of sensory processing interferes with life choices that this information becomes relevant to quality of life. In future studies, researchers need to study the relationship between the differences we found here and performance in daily life.

Further studies about the sensory-processing aspects of performance in children with Asperger syndrome are needed to validate the observations that professionals and families make about the children's behaviors and responses during daily life. If we can understand this aspect of their performance more clearly, we can design more refined interventions to support adaptive responses to the demands of development and learning.

References

American Psychiatric Association. (1994). *Diagnostic and statistical manual of mental disorders* (4th ed., rev.). Washington, DC: Author.

Anderson, E., & Emmons, P. (1996). *Unlocking the mysteries of sensory dysfunction.* Arlington, TX: Future Horizons.

Asperger, H. (1944). Die ëAutistischen Psychopathení im Kindesalter. *Archiv fur Psychiatrie und Nervenkrankheiten, 117,* 76–136.

Attwood, T. (1998). *Asperger's syndrome.* London: Jessica Kingsley.

Ayres, A. J. (1972). *Sensory integration and learning disorders.* Los Angeles: Western Psychological Services.

Ayres, A. J. (1979). *Sensory integration and the child.* Austin, TX: PRO-ED.

Bagnato, S. J., & Neisworth, J. T. (1999). Collaboration and teamwork in assessment for early intervention. *Child and Adolescent Psychiatric Clinics of North America, 8,* 347–363.

Bettison, S. (1996). The long-term effects of auditory training on children with autism. *Journal of Autism and Developmental Disorders, 26,* 361–374.

Case-Smith, J., & Bryan, T. (1999). The effects of occupational therapy with sensory integration emphasis on preschool-age children with autism. *American Journal of Occupational Therapy, 53,* 489–497.

Cohen, J. (1992). A power primer. *Psychological Bulletin, 112,* 155–159.

Cook, D. G., & Dunn, W. (1998). Sensory integration for students with autism. In R. L. Simpson & B. S. Myles (Eds.), *Educating children and youth with autism: Strategies for effective practice* (pp. 191–229). Austin, TX: PRO-ED.

Dunn, W. (1997). The impact of sensory processing abilities on the daily lives of young children and their families: A conceptual model. *Infants and Young Children, 9*(4), 23–35.

Dunn, W. (1999). *Sensory Profile.* San Antonio, TX: Psychological Corporation.

Dunn, W., & Brown, C. (1997). Factor analysis on the Sensory Profile from a national sample of children without disabilities. *American Journal of Occupational Therapy, 51,* 490–495.

Fisher, A., Murray, E., & Bundy, A. (Eds.). (1991). *Sensory integration: Theory and practice.* Philadelphia: F. A. Davis.

Fling, E. (2000). *Eating an artichoke: A mother's perspective on Asperger syndrome.* London: Jessica Kingsley.

Frith, U. (1991). Asperger and his syndrome. In U. Frith (Ed.), *Autism and Asperger syndrome* (pp. 1–36). London: Cambridge University Press.

Gillberg, C. L. (1992). Autism and autistic-like conditions: Subclasses among disorders of empathy. *Journal of Child Psychology and Psychiatry, 33,* 813–842.

Grandin, T. (1995). How people with autism think. In E. Schopler & G. Mesibov (Eds.), *Learning and cognition in autism: Current issues in autism* (pp. 137–156). New York: Plenum.

Green, S. B., Salkind, N. J., & Akey, T. M. (1997). *Using SPSS for Windows: Analyzing and understanding data.* Upper Saddle River, NJ: Prentice Hall.

Greenspan, S., Wieder, S., & Simons, R. (1998). *The child with special needs: Encouraging intellectual and emotional growth.* Reading, MA: Addison Wesley Longman.

Huebner, R. (Ed.). (2000). *Autism and related disorders: A sensorimotor approach to management.* Gaithersburg, MD: Aspen.

Huebner, R., & Dunn, W. (2000). Introduction and basic concepts of sensorimotor approaches to autism and related disorders. In R. Huebner (Ed.), *Autism and related disorders: A sensorimotor approach to management* (pp. 3–40). Gaithersburg, MD: Aspen.

Iwanaga, R., Kawasaki, C., & Tsuchida, R. (2000). Brief report: Comparison of sensory–motor and cognitive function between autism and Asperger syndrome in preschool children. *Journal of Autism and Developmental Disorders, 30,* 169–174.

Linderman, T. M., & Stewart, K. B. (1999). Sensory integrative–based occupational therapy and functional outcomes in young children with pervasive developmental disorders: A single-subject design. *American Journal of Occupational Therapy, 53,* 207–213.

Miller, J. N., & Ozonoff, S. (2000). The external validity of Asperger disorder: Lack of evidence from the domain of neuropsychology. *Journal of Abnormal Psychology, 109,* 227–238.

Myles, B. S., & Simpson, R. L. (1998). *Asperger syndrome: A guide for educators and parents.* Austin, TX: PRO-ED.

Myles, B. S., & Southwick, J. (1999). *Asperger syndrome and difficult moments: Practical solutions for tantrums, rage, and meltdowns.* Shawnee Mission, KS: Autism Asperger Publishing.

Quill, K. A. (1995). Visually cued instruction for children with autism and pervasive developmental disorders. *Focus on Autistic Behavior, 10*(3), 10–20.

Quill, K. A. (1997). Instructional considerations for young children with autism: The rationale for visually cued instruction. *Journal of Autism and Developmental Disorders, 27,* 697–714.

Quill, K. A. (1998). Environmental supports to enhance social communication. *Seminars in Speech and Language, 19,* 407–424.

Shore, S. (2001). *Beyond the wall: Experiences in autism and Asperger syndrome.* Shawnee Mission, KS: Autism Asperger Publishing.

Stagnitti, K., Raison, P., & Ryan, P. (1999). Sensory defensiveness syndrome: A paediatric perspective and case study. *Australian Occupational Therapy Journal, 46,* 175–187.

Willemsen-Swinkels, S. H., Buitelaar, J. K., Dekker, M., & van-Engeland, H. (1998). Subtyping stereotypic behavior in children: The association between stereotypic behavior, mood, and heart rate. *Journal of Autism and Developmental Disorders, 28,* 547–557.

Willey, L. H. (1999). *Pretending to be normal: Living with Asperger's syndrome.* London: Jessica Kingsley.

Wing, L. (1991). The relationship between Asperger's syndrome and Kanner's autism. In U. Frith (Ed.), *Autism and Asperger syndrome* (pp. 93–121). London: Cambridge University Press.

Zero to Three. (1994). *Diagnostic classification of mental health and developmental disorders of infancy and early childhood.* Baltimore: Author.

CHAPTER 31

Time Use and Leisure Occupations of Young Offenders

Louise Farnworth

Louise Farnworth, OT, MA, PhD, *is lecturer, School of Occupational Therapy, La Trobe University, Bundoora, Victoria, Australia, 3083; l.farnworth@latrobe.edu.au.*

The assumption that a relationship exists between balanced, purposeful, and varied use of time and a person's health and well-being has formed the basis for occupational therapy practice since its formation (Meyer, 1922/1977). In the founding years of the profession, Meyer identified four areas, or categories, of daily occupations—work, play, rest, and sleep—that, he argued, in interaction determined the overall adaptation of the person to the requirements of daily life. His views suggested that, by providing opportunities for engagement in these daily occupations, especially work, a person should be able to fulfill personal interests and meet needs for physical and psychological well-being. In practice, occupational therapy has helped persons to develop ways to use their time in balanced and meaningful ways.

There is empirical support for the assumption that humans need a balance of daily occupations. Time budget studies, completed by social scientists in industrialized nations, have consistently found that humans have a natural temporal order to their daily living that is organized around the occupations of self-maintenance, work, and leisure (Castles, 1993; Robinson, 1996; Robinson, Andreyenkov, & Patrushev, 1988; Statistics Canada, 1986; Szalai, 1977).

Studies of the time use of adolescents also indicate consistency of findings across different countries. Csikszentmihalyi and Larson (1984) completed a comprehensive study of the ecology of the daily lives of adolescents in the United States. Their study, on which the study described here was modeled, used a stratified random sample, including male and female students from four high school grades and two contrasting residential zones. Using a research methodology that allows on-the-spot sampling of time use, the Experience Sampling Method, these researchers collected 2,734 self-reports on the daily occupations of 75 students. They found that 29% of the main occupations engaged in by the group during their wakeful hours were what the researchers described as productive occupations, primarily those relating to school. An additional 31% of their time

Originally published 2000 in *American Journal of Occupational Therapy, 54,* 315–325.

use was spent in various self-maintenance occupations such as eating, bathing, and dressing. The rest of the time (40%) was spent engaged in occupations that could be described as leisure, for example, talking, playing sports, and reading. Sixteen percent of this leisure time was spent socializing and 7% watching television. These percentages closely resemble the findings of the Australian Bureau of Statistics (ABS, 1993) of the time use of 15- to 18-year-olds in a national time use survey.

Bruno (1996), using a time allocation preference survey with 494 adolescents attending school in the United States, found that girls were far more likely to allocate their time in directed occupations than were boys. However, those students of both genders who were considered by their teachers to have at-risk behaviors, such as being absent from school, had the least preference for occupations that involved external rules and the most preference for nondirected occupations such as entertainment and just passing time. Bruno's study indicated that the use of time may be important in understanding adaptation and, in particular, at-risk behaviors. The study further suggests that the occupational challenges for some adolescents may be greater and may predispose them to engaging in risk-taking behaviors.

There has been some empirical research in occupational therapy literature on humans' use of time (e.g., Hayes & Halford, 1996; Lo, 1996; Lo & Zemke, 1997; Ludwig, 1997, 1998; McKinnon, 1992; Neville, 1980; Passmore, 1998a; Suto & Frank, 1994; Wilcock et al., 1997; Yerxa & Locker, 1990). Although Passmore (1998a) explored the leisure occupations of adolescents and Lederer, Kielhofner, and Watts (1985) compared the values, personal causation, and skills of offenders and nonoffenders, no one has studied the time use of young offenders. Recently, several theoretical papers written by scholars in occupational science have stated the

need for further research on the relationship between time use and adaptation to the demands of living (Christiansen, 1994, 1996; Clark et al., 1991; Farnworth, 1990; Parham, 1996; Pettifer, 1993; Primeau, 1996a, 1996b). In response to this call, the present study sought to understand the time use and, in particular, the leisure occupations of young offenders.

Adolescent Leisure Occupations and Health

Csikszentmihalyi and Larson (1984) found that the 75 adolescents in their study engaged in 51 different activities that they reported as being most enjoyable, most of which were leisure occupations. The most intrinsically rewarding leisure occupations in their study were those that were highly structured and highly organized and in which adolescents could use their skills. These included such pursuits as art, hobbies, music, and sports. All involved external rules and challenges.

Interest in participating in leisure occupations arises from a variety of sources. One source is a natural proclivity to find enjoyment within particular occupations that do not need external support (Kielhofner, 1995). However, for interests to be developed and maintained, opportunities for engagement generally need to be available as well as cultural instructions for appreciation of the experience. For example, a person first must appreciate that regular practice of a musical instrument is required before the pleasure of competent performance can be achieved.

According to Passmore (1998b), young people from families having higher socioeconomic status have the financial capacity to explore and gain satisfaction from a larger range of leisure occupations. Leisure occupations such as music, ballet, or tennis lessons may be beyond the finances available in many family budgets as well as resources for transportation to and from such lessons. The more exposure a person has to a range of potential leisure occupations, the more likely it is that he or she will also be able to make realistic choices based on preferences (Kielhofner, 1995). Garton and Pratt (1991) also found that leisure occupations are determined by the availability of suitable resources. Yet, according to Passmore (1998b), those engaged in a wide range of leisure occupations, in addition to being from economically better-off families, are usually the higher academic achievers in school. The directionality of these factors is unclear. However, not only is it likely that young persons who are exposed to a range of leisure occupations will be advantaged academically over persons who have fewer choices, but also it is more likely that they will be able to engage in those occupations for which they have a greater preference.

There is some agreement that engagement in play and leisure occupations can facilitate cognitive, physical, and social skills as well as develop self-esteem and identity (Hendry, 1983; Parham & Primeau, 1997; Wood, 1996). Passmore (1998b), who studied the leisure experiences of nearly 1,200 Australian adolescents 12 to 18 years of age, found that some forms of leisure contribute positively to personal growth and development and to maintenance and enhancement of mental health and well-being, whereas others may lead to negative mental health outcomes. She identified three typologies of leisure occupations: achievement, social, and time-out leisure.

According to Passmore (1998b), achievement leisure occupations are those that provide challenge, are demanding, and require commitment, such as sports and music performances. She found that engaging in achievement leisure occupations influenced participants' self-efficacy beliefs and competencies and had a direct relationship with self-esteem. Passmore's social leisure occupations are those that exist primarily for the purpose of being with others. This form of leisure occupation

also supported the development of competencies, particularly in the areas of relationships and social acceptance, which positively, albeit indirectly, influenced self-esteem. Time-out leisure, according to Passmore, is for relaxation. However, this type of leisure occupation supported neither competence nor self-esteem enhancement and was found to be negatively related to mental health outcomes. Time-out leisure occupations included watching television and reflecting or listening to music, activities that tended to be socially isolating, less demanding, and frequently passive.

Time Use of Young Offenders

Juvenile crime has enormous human and economic costs and, as such, needs to be understood further. Surprisingly little is known, however, about how young offenders occupy their time, including time in leisure occupations. A young offender is one who is arrested and processed through the Children's Court (juvenile court) for committing an illegal act. Research findings indicate that young offenders spend their time with friends in public places, such as shopping centers and street corners, where most of their illegal behavior occurs (Felson, 1994; White & Sutton, 1995). However, this criminological research has not studied why young offenders choose these social and physical contexts in which to spend their time. In one study, Hagell and Newburn (1996) briefly mentioned the time use of young offenders. They interviewed 74 British, predominantly male, repeat criminal offenders about their family and social contexts. As a peripheral issue, they found that most of the young offenders reported that they were either unemployed (50%) or not engaged in studying or work training. Most were, in effect, doing "nothing" (p. 13). However, data in this study did not include any in-depth information about what this nothing meant or why they perceived themselves as doing nothing.

Criminological studies indicate that many young persons who come to the formal attention of the legal system are those who are truant from school and who often engage in activities that result in suspension or expulsion from school (Carrington, 1990; Galloway, 1985; Knight, 1997). One consequence of leaving school is that they become more vulnerable to long-term unemployment (Alder, 1986; Braithwaite & Chappell, 1994; Sullivan, 1989). Increasingly high levels of youth unemployment in Australia have further exacerbated the problems for young offenders. According to Commonwealth of Australia (1998) figures, the average unemployment rate for 15- to 19-year-olds seeking full-time employment in Victoria, where this study was completed, was more than 30% during 1998. The figure for the United States during the same period was 14.6% (U.S. Department of Labor, 1999).

From these studies, it appears that young offenders may differ in their time use from their peers who are nonoffenders. Occupations, such as paid employment and attending school, help to structure time and develop routines and habits for independent living (Allen & Steffensmeier, 1989; Csikszentmihalyi & Larson, 1984; Jahoda, 1981). However, the time use of young offenders is largely unknown.

Purpose of Study

Occupational science and occupational therapy literature indicates that humans need a balance of daily occupations to maintain their health and well-being. This assumption is supported, in part, by empirical data from time use surveys. Occupational science literature also suggests that some occupations may have more positive mental health outcomes than others. Although much has been written about delinquency, there is little empirically generated information about the time use of young offenders. The current study sought to redress this gap in the literature by exploring the time use occupations and, in particular, the leisure time use occupations of young offenders in Melbourne, Australia. Understanding the relationship between occupation and health is of central concern to occupational therapists. Hence, the findings from this study also may expand the profession's knowledge of human occupation. In particular, findings may help us to understand the relationships among use of time, leisure occupations, and social well-being—specifically those of young offenders. Additionally, this study may potentially inform current and future occupational therapy practices with young offenders.

Method

This study used a combination of research methodologies—Experience Sampling Method, a methodology developed by Larson and Csikszentmihalyi (1983) and Csikszentmihalyi and Csikszentmihalyi (1988), and qualitative interviewing. The Experience Sampling Method yields both quantitative and qualitative data (Farnworth, Mostert, Harrison, & Worrell, 1996) and involves each participant carrying a pager and a pad of experience sampling forms (ESFs). At random intervals during the day, a signal is sent to the pager, alerting the participant to complete a questionnaire (the ESF) about what he or she is doing, the social and physical environment, and various subjective experiences at that moment.

Participants

Thirty-seven offenders, 13 to 18 years of age and literate, were recruited for this study. Participants lived in an outer industrialized suburb of Melbourne, a city of 4 million people, in the state of Victoria, Australia. Eligibility for inclusion in the study was based on having appeared before the Children's Court for committing an illegal act. In Victoria, the age of criminal responsibility under the jurisdiction of the juvenile court system is 10 to 17 years. In Australia, just 4% of the total population of 10- to 17-year-olds are processed by police caution, panel hearing, or court appearance.

All participants were on probation and lived in the community with relative freedom to choose the structure of their daily occupations. Thirty-one participants were referred by probation officers and youth workers. Five additional offenders were referred by other participants. The 16 girls and 21 boys ranged in age from 13 to 18 years ($M = 16$ years).

Whereas 12 lived with a family member and 10 lived in accommodations arranged by government and nongovernment agencies, 7 were homeless (see Table 31.1). Seventeen participants had been expelled or suspended from school, and 10 had left school voluntarily ($M = 7.7$ years achieved). Ten were still enrolled in school. However, only 4 of these 10 regularly attended school while in the study. Three participants were currently employed in casual and shift work. Although 26 were at least second-generation Australians, 11 were first-generation Australians or had been born overseas. This cultural mix was typical of the population living in the district.

The offenses for which the participants were on probation included shoplifting, assault, and drug trafficking (see Table 31.2), which were representative of offenses committed by juveniles in Victoria. Twenty-one participants reported using alcohol, marijuana, speed, heroin, or methadone.

Table 31.1. Living Situation of Participants

Living Situation	Number
Government or nongovernment agency	10
Living with family member	12
Living with boyfriend or girlfriend	7
Itinerant or homeless	7
Living alone	1

Table 31.2. Most Serious Offense Committed by Participants

Offense	Number
Crime against person	
Sexual or indecent assault	4
Assault and robbery	2
Assault (indictable; i.e, serious)	3
Assault (summary; i.e., less serious)	3
Crime against property	
Theft (of goods)	6
Burglary	7
Theft of motor vehicle	2
Handle stolen goods	1
Criminal damage	1
Other crime	
Drug trafficking	4

Four reported being under the influence of mind-altering substances more than half of the times they were beeped.

Instrument

A modified version of an ESF originally developed by Csikszentmihalyi and Larson (1984) was used. Each ESF contained the open-ended question, "What was the main activity that you were doing?" to record the occupation that the person was engaged in at the moment that he or she was paged. The ESF also contained open-ended questions related to the social and physical contexts of the occupations, including, "Who are you with?" and "Where are you?" An additional question—"What are you thinking about?"—was included. Two cognitive questions directly related to the main activity when paged were, "What are the challenges of the activity?" and "What are your skills in the activity?" These cognitive questions had Likert response categories; participants indicated their response on a scale ranging from 1 to 7 where 1 corresponded to *low* and 7 to *high*. Although the ESF contained 22 additional items on motivation, cognitive efficiency, activation, and affect, only the questions about the occupation, social and physical contexts, thoughts, challenges, and skills are discussed in this chapter.

Data Collection

Data were gathered between 1995 and 1997, and a total of 1,535 ESFs were completed. Each participant responded to 12 to 60 ESFs when paged, with a mean response rate of 43/60 (72%). Seventy-eight percent of the beeper signals were responded to within 5 min, 87% within 10 min, and 92% within 20 min. These response rates compare favorably with other Experience Sampling Method studies with nonoffender populations of young persons attending educational institutions (e.g., Clarke & Haworth, 1994; Csikszentmihalyi & Larson, 1984). Each participant was paid for his or her participation in the study, which may, in part, explain the high response rate. No ESFs or participants were excluded from the data analysis, except one participant who lost her booklet. Therefore, the Experience Sampling Method data analysis was carried out using data from 36 participants only.

Procedure

Informed consent was gained from each participant or his or her guardian. As a condition of ethical approval for the study, participants were warned that they did not need to make comments that may have been incriminating or that constituted a breach of their probation. I met with each participant in a location of his or her choice. Each participant was introduced to the study and received instructions on the use of the pager and how to fill out the questions on a pad of 30 double-sided self-report forms (ESFs). I asked participants to fill out a practice ESF and then gave them a pager and pad to carry for 7 consecutive days.

Experience Sampling Method procedure. In this study, a standard method of paging was applied. Each participant was asked about his or her normal sleep–wake pattern so that a beeping schedule could be arranged around wakeful hours. At one random moment within approximately every 2-hour period, a signal was sent to the pager, causing it to beep or vibrate. Each participant was paged 60 times during the week. At the time of the beep, the participant answered questions on the ESF, a process that took approximately 2 min. At the completion of the 7 days, I met with each participant for debriefing and collected the pager and the pad of ESFs.

Interview procedure. Participants were interviewed twice. Interviews in conjunction with the Experience Sampling Method have been used in other studies (Hurlburt, Happe, & Frith, 1994; Hurlburt & Melancon, 1987; Kimiecik & Stein, 1992; Mokros, 1993; Voelkl & Nicholson, 1992) to check the validity and authenticity of findings and their interpretation. Using a semi-structured interview schedule, I interviewed each participant during the week of the Experience Sampling Method study to develop rapport and to gather background information about their engagement in illegal activities and their past and current occupations, including questions about their schooling and leisure occupations. This first interview process involved an informal conversational style that lasted from .5 hr to 1.5 hr. The interview was tape-recorded and transcribed fully.

After I studied the initial interview transcript and analyzed the data from the ESFs (approximately 2 weeks after collecting the pager and ESFs), I again met with each participant for another interview. I gave the young person a copy of the transcript to read and discussed information from the first interview and ESFs that required further clarification. This procedure included checking with the participant about how he or she would interpret ambiguous categories in the open-ended items. The findings from the Experience Sampling Method were also shared with each participant. This second interview also was tape-recorded and transcribed.

I kept field notes and an analytical log throughout the research data collection (Minichiello, Aroni, Timewell, & Alexander, 1990). Field notes included additional information about each participant that arose during the data collection, such as my description of the participants' living situations, their appearance, or their relationship with me. The analytical log was a record of daily schedules and logistics, a personal diary about my impressions, and a methodological log about questions that presented themselves and changes in thinking about the research process as it was evolving.

Data Analysis

All ESF data were coded and entered into the data analysis program Statistical Package for the Social Sciences[1] (V6 for Macintosh computers). Categories from the ABS survey on *How Australians Use Their Time* were used for coding occupations (Castles, 1993). The 10 broad functional categories were labor force occupations, domestic occupations, child care, purchasing goods and services, personal care, educational occupations, voluntary work and community participation, social life and entertainment, active leisure occupations, and passive leisure occupations. Because illegal activities are an important category for this study, they were coded separately. The frequency and mean percentage of completed ESFs for each participant, and for the total group's engagement in each occupation, were computed. Time diaries and the Experience Sampling Method have the potential to produce almost identical values of time allocation for different daily occupations (Csikszentmihalyi & Larson, 1984, 1987); therefore, the ABS time use data were used as a basis for comparison with the Experience Sampling Method data.

An individual synthesis was constructed for each participant that integrated the nonnumerical ESF data, field notes, and textual data into a comprehensive whole for each participant. In collecting and analyzing the qualitative data, a comparative method was followed (Bogdan & Biklen, 1992; Strauss & Corbin, 1990). This type of analysis is an iterative process of observing, recording, coding, and comparing data and emerging interpretations of the data (Glaser & Strauss, 1967; Polkinghorne, 1986). Data related to daily routines and leisure occupations are presented in this chapter. A computer program, NUD*IST (Richards & Richards, 1997), was used to aid in handling the nonnumerical and unstructured data and in supporting processes of coding data in an index system. All participants' names are pseudonyms.

Results

Reported Beep Times Engaged in Main Occupation

Table 31.3 summarizes the 1,421 responses to the question "What was the main thing you were doing?" Passive leisure occupations included watching television, talking, thinking, and listen-

Table 31.3. Percentage of Beep Times Engaged in Main Occupation of Sample Compared With Australian Bureau of Statistics (ABS, 1993) for 15- to 18-Year-Olds[a]

Occupational Category	Main Occupation Sample (% of Time)	ABS 15- to 18-Year-Olds (% of Time)
Passive leisure	48.8	18.2
Personal care	21.2	16.4
Household	9.3	9.1
Active leisure	6.7	8.6
Education	6.3	22.1
Labor force	3.3	11.1
Legal related	3.0	
Social leisure	1.4	14.0

[a]Not including sleep.

[1]SPSS Inc., 233 Wacker Drive, 11th Floor, Chicago, IL 60606-6307.

ing to music; personal care occupations included smoking, drinking, eating, or resting; household occupations included domestic, child care, and purchasing goods and services (e.g., selecting a video); active leisure occupations included playing computer games, sport, hobbies, and having sex; education occupations included both school-based occupations and homework; labor force occupations included voluntary work; legal-related occupations included shoplifting, purchasing and using illegal substances, and police-related matters; and social leisure occupations included attending social events (e.g., going to the movies).

Nearly 80% of the reported beep times of the group was spent engaged in leisure, particularly passive leisure (49%), or personal care occupations. Conversely, when beeped, few participants reported being engaged in education or labor force occupations, although there were wide individual variations in this time use. The percentage of reported beep times engaged in legal-related activities, such as shoplifting and use of illegal substances, is small (3%), and because recording it had the potential to incriminate, this figure probably underestimates participants' engagement in these activities.

For a comparison with the time use of a larger population of adolescents, Table 31.3 presents the 1992 ABS Time Use Study percentage of time engaged in main occupations for boys and girls 15 to 18 years of age (not including sleep). When the occupations of the two groups are compared, the most obvious differences are that the young offender group spent the most time in passive leisure occupations (30% higher than the ABS population) and 3% engaged in legal-related activities. Time engaged in educational occupations was 16% higher (almost three times as much) in the ABS sample. Engagement in labor force occupations was 7% higher (almost three times as much) in the ABS sample, and social leisure occupations were almost nonexistent in

the young offender population. The percentage of time reported in personal care and household occupations are similar for both groups. In considering participants' engagement in active leisure occupations, only 39 (2.5%) of the ESFs contained reports of engagement in occupations such as kicking a football or skateboarding. Thirty-two of these occupations were reported by the four participants who were still regularly attending school. Just 11 (0.7%) ESFs reported participants engaged in hobby-related leisure occupations, such as drawing.

These time use findings strongly suggest that young offenders do not spend their time in the same way as their peers who are nonoffenders. Passive leisure occupations appear to dominate their lives, whereas nonoffenders use more time engaged in productive occupations such as education and labor force occupations and social leisure.

Leisure Occupations

All participants were asked about their current leisure occupations. Although it is usual for adolescents to engage in a range of structured leisure occupations (Castles, 1993; Csikszentmihalyi & Larson, 1984) or, using Passmore's (1998b) typology, achievement leisure occupations (e.g., music, sports), surprisingly few participants could mention any achievement leisure occupations in which they currently engaged. Their time use was dominated by passive, or time-out, leisure occupations. The reason for this was explored further through questioning.

Loss of Active Leisure Occupations After Leaving School

Most participants talked about leisure occupations that they had developed in the past, in the context of the school environment. These may have included active sports, such as athletics or team sports, or artistic pursuits. Of the five participants who more regularly engaged in sporting occupations during the study, four were still attending school. Ten participants reported that they had ceased their engagement in achievement leisure occupations as a direct consequence of leaving school.

Chung, 17 years of age, explained that he was expelled from school because he took too much time off to attend to his girlfriend's problematic pregnancy. He was one of those who had stopped engaging in sporting occupations. He had subsequently become immersed in an illicit drug culture and was currently on probation for heroin dealing. In discussing activities he enjoyed, I (L. F.) asked him whether he had ever played sports, to which he replied,

> *Chung:* Yeah. I played volleyball for [a state team] and we came fifth.
> *L.F.:* This is at school?
> *Chung:* Yeah. Through school. Yeah, at high school.
> *L.F.:* So, do you still play volleyball?
> *Chung:* No, I quit for 2 years, 3 years. Yeah, as soon as I left school.

Similarly, John, 16 years of age, also stopped his athletics when he left school. He had originally received an athletic scholarship in a private school. However, his expulsion from school also coincided with drug taking and engagement in other illegal activities. At the time of the study, he was on probation for a series of burglaries that were committed to finance his drug addiction. According to John,

John: I represented Victoria and stuff. I was a sprinter. I've got, like, a big newspaper article and medals and stuff. I went to the Pan Pacific games and stuff like that. Got sponsorship by Nike.
L.F.: Do you do any sports now?
John: Oh, not really, not much time. I was training every day and stuff. I am going to get back into it soon. Get fit again.

John acknowledged, "I smoke [marijuana—bongs] all the time," in part because "normally after a smoke it motivates me in a way." He was under the influence of drugs 45% of the times he was beeped and engaged in passive leisure occupations 52% of the times. These occupations included listening to music, watching television, and smoking marijuana. His only active leisure occupation was having sex. The Saturday described in Table 31.4 is an example of his routine daily occupations. Although he began the day by trying to mend the lawnmower so that he could mow his girlfriend's mother's lawn, by midday he was smoking bongs. He then ran out of drugs and needed to "score" (purchase more marijuana). Under the influence of these drugs, he began cleaning at 9:49 p.m. before going to bed by 1:19 a.m. For a young man who had previously won a scholarship to a private school for his athletic prowess, his routine, as indicated by this Saturday, would not support his resumption of athletic activities. His most challenging activities for this day are scoring drugs at the local shopping mall and smoking them at home.

Table 31.4. John's Experience Sampling Form (Saturday)

Time	Thoughts	Where	Occupation	With Whom	Challenge	Skill
10:29 a.m.	Lawn mowers	Garage	Talking	[not answered]	4	7
12:35 p.m.	Smoking bongs	Bedroom	Smoking	Girlfriend	2	7
3:06 p.m.	Scoring	[Local shopping mall]	Walking		7	7
4:44 p.m.	Bongs	Home	Smoking a bong	Girlfriend	2	7
7:29 p.m.	Bongs	Home	Having a bong	Girlfriend and friend	2	7
9:49 p.m.	Cleaning	Home	Cleaning	Girlfriend	2	7
1:19 a.m.	Sleep	Bed	Sleeping	Girlfriend	1	7

Loss of Capacities

Other participants had also experienced prior successful participation in achievement leisure occupations. Sue, on probation for two assault charges, had won prizes for her drawings. Drawing was important to her because it was the only activity she had engaged in that had gained her external praise. She explained,

> Sketching. That's all I've been good at. And that's all I know I've been good at because I always won awards since I was little, and I won the [local] show, first prize. It was so exact. But the thing about me is I only draw right, but if I'm actually supposed to do something, I can't concentrate.

Sue, 16 years of age, had stopped attending school at 14 when the demands of attending to her boyfriend's needs had become too much for her to keep up with her schoolwork. At that time, however, she had demonstrated some artistic talent. Although this skill could have been developed further, without the structure and routine provided by school, she now found it difficult to draw because she lacked the required concentration skills. In the week of the study, Sue was engaged in passive leisure 74% of the times she responded to the beeper, in household occupations 13% of the time, in personal care 10% of the time, and in purchasing goods from the local milk bar 3% of the time (see Table 31.5). The

drawing that she enjoyed, and in which she had some skill, was not practiced, nor did she engage in any other activities in which she was likely to develop further skills. Even attending to a noisy washing machine became a highly challenging activity—the highest challenge, but her lowest perceived skill—in the week that Sue participated in the study.

Lack of Resources to Pursue Leisure Occupations

Not having money to pay for leisure occupations was raised by several participants. For example, Martin said that, apart from signing on at the local police station every day,

> *Martin:* [I] sit down and do nothing. Sometimes I drink, sometimes I just smoke cigarettes all day. Read the newspaper or do puzzles in a magazine. And that's it.
> *L.F.:* Would you rather be doing something else?
> *Martin:* Yeah, but I haven't got the money.

Martin was living (illegally) in an accommodation provided through a Youth Support scheme with four other persons. None of them had enough money to even buy a television. Although Martin suggested that he might have to steal one, he was trying to get through his probation without further charges. His $240 biweekly allowance did not allow him to buy extras apart from food and rent. Previously, Martin had been able to use

Table 31.5. Sue's Experience Sampling Form (Tuesday)

Time	Thoughts	Where	Occupation	With Whom	Challenge	Skill
12:25 p.m.	Nothing	In car	Listening to music	Brother	1	7
2:00 p.m.	Friend's house	Friend's house	Looking around friend's house	Friends	1	7
4:45 p.m.	Nothing	Friends	Talking	Friends	1	7
6:15 p.m.	Turning the noisy thing [the washing machine] off	Home	Washing clothes	Family	7	1
8:21 p.m.	The Golden [listening to music]	In car	Sitting in the car	Friends	1	7
11:25 p.m.	Going home	Friend's house	Thinking	Friends	1	7

a barter system to pay for some of his entertainment. For example, he had worked at his local "[pinball]-parlor" mopping floors and cleaning up pool tables "just to get a few credits." But as a condition of his probation, he was no longer allowed to go to the suburb, so he lacked both the opportunity and financial resources to pursue this leisure occupation.

Lost Leisure Occupation Opportunities

Some facilities that provided care for young offenders appeared to lack opportunities for realistic leisure occupations. I met both Laura and Linda through a safe house that provided supported accommodation for young female offenders who also had been victims of sexual assault. The program had an excellent reputation for the care and support offered to these young women. By coincidence, I was party to an ongoing saga about four bicycles.

Linda, now 16 years of age, had previously been a keen bike rider. She explained,

> I used to do it when I was a child, that was my escape. Sort of piss off and ride for hours and get [as] far away as possible, and then since I went out on the streets and all that sort of bisso [business], I sort of didn't get the chance to even get my hands on a bike to ride, or do anything I liked.

Linda—who had had a baby when she was 11 years old, earned a living through prostitution, had been addicted to heroin, and attempted suicide—now was staying in her first stable, supported accommodation facility in 5 years. The facility had four bicycles; however, all of them required minor repairs. Linda had asked whether the bikes could be fixed, and one of the workers had purchased some repair equipment, but none were repaired before Linda moved out. When I asked about the repair equipment, no one could find it.

Laura had different reasons for wanting to use the bikes. She had been raised in a rural town and, after escaping an abusive home situation, had fled to the city. She responded well to open, natural environments. For example, at one time when beeped during the study, she was walking in a park with her youth worker while the worker walked her two dogs. Laura's affect at that beep was her highest during a traumatic week of periodic suicidal thoughts. She feared walking alone into the local parks but would have been happy to go by herself with a bike if one had been repaired. Had the bikes been repaired, both Linda and Laura might have learned that leisure occupations can be enjoyed regularly, with little cost, and from within their regular living environment.

Discussion

The lives of many of these young offenders were dominated by passive leisure with few achievement leisure occupations, time use that differs greatly from their peers who were nonoffenders. This finding is important because it identifies a problematic area of concern: That is, young offenders engage in passive leisure occupations at the expense of engagement in achievement leisure or productive occupations. Hoge, Andrews, and Leschied's (1996) research indicated that effective use of leisure time is one factor that protects young offenders from engaging in criminal activities. The clear predominance of passive leisure reported by the participants in the study indicates that these young offenders were not using their leisure time effectively. These findings strongly suggest that occupation-based interventions with young offenders should reflect the need for these clients to develop effective use of leisure time.

Many of the participants had fragmented family lives and experienced financial and emotional deprivation. One consequence of this is that they potentially had fewer opportunities to engage in a range of achievement leisure occupations than did adolescents from more secure families. For those participants who had developed achievement leisure occupations at school, accessibility to these was lost once they left school. In consequence, not only did they lose the time structure and routine of attending school (as evidenced through the descriptions of their daily routines), but they also lost the potential health benefits of engaging in achievement leisure occupations. For several participants, leaving school coincided with their initial or deepening immersion in the use of drugs that also had an impact on their physical and psychological ability to engage in achievement leisure occupations.

Passmore's (1998a) research indicated that passive time-out leisure is likely to negatively affect mental health, competence, and self-esteem; one might, therefore, assume that this pattern of time use was unlikely to encourage the mental health of the participants in this study. That is, the time use of young offenders not engaged in work, school, or achievement leisure occupations potentially may have negative health implications.

From findings presented here, relationships, if any, between this pattern of time use and young offenders' engagement in criminal activities are not explained. Greater understanding of this relationship is likely to be found by further studying their experiences while engaged in occupations. Although the experience of boredom is cited as coexisting with engagement in criminal activities (Csikszentmihalyi & Larson, 1978; Farnworth, 1998; Glassner & Loughlin, 1987; Hirsch, 1969), the relationship between boredom and different occupations, such as passive and achievement leisure, needs further exploration. The use of the Experience Sampling Method to identify any such relationships is strongly recommended.

Passmore (1998a) also found that achievement leisure occupations not only are more likely to lead to improved mental health but also are more likely to lead to the development of values and skills necessary for work settings, such as commitment, personal control, and learning to work with others. Additionally, social leisure is about forming interpersonal relationships, developing a sense of belonging, and resolving differences. Hence, both achievement and social leisure occupations are conducive to developing skills for the workplace; however, these are the very leisure occupations least likely to have been engaged in by young offenders. In support of this, Hong, Milgram, and Whiston (1993) found in an 18-year follow-up study that adolescent leisure activities predicted subsequent employment choices. As has been suggested by Passmore (1998a), achievement and social leisure occupations may lay the foundations for supporting a range of occupational roles, including the worker role. It is likely that the young offenders in this study may be disadvantaged by their lack of engagement in achievement and social leisure pursuits not only in the present but also in the future.

Occupational Repetition

As Clark et al. (1991) postulated, occupations and routines facilitate or limit a person's ability to successfully adapt to and meet environmental demands. Hence, understanding one's daily routines may give us insight into the person's occupational adaptation. According to Carlson (1996), people tend to repeat engagement in the same or similar occupations, or to engage in occupational repetition, producing a sequential pattern of occupations with little variability. So, for example, if a young woman watches television at the exclusion of other occupations, she may lose interest in seeking alternative daily occupations. Occupational repetition sets in. She may come to define her social identity in relationship to her regular pattern of television watching. In this way, the young woman's use of time not only affects her self-perception but also leads to acceptance of this use of time as normal, resulting in little personal investment to change. As Carlson explained, occupational repetition would be an implicit and positive requirement of achievement leisure occupations, such as sports, that demand repeated practice over time. However, repetition of less fulfilling, passive occupations, such as watching television, may indirectly lead to wasted talent and personal mediocrity.

The long-term consequences of occupational repetition may potentially affect all levels of cognitive, physical, and emotional growth and development from adolescence to adulthood. To this end, the use of time by young offenders as described in this study—dominated by passive leisure and few achievement leisure occupations—might lead, without intervention, to similar patterns of occupations in adulthood. Future research on the use of time of young offenders, therefore, should concentrate further on the occupational history of a larger group of young offenders and, in particular, their development of leisure interests from childhood to the present. Additionally, to further understand the relationships between different forms of leisure occupations in adolescence and future occupational roles, longitudinal studies of young offenders are necessary.

Conclusion

The overall goal of this study was to explore the time use and, in particular, the leisure occupations of young offenders. Findings indicate that these young offenders do not use their time in the same way as their peers who are nonoffenders. Their lives are dominated by passive leisure and self-care occupations, and they engage in few productive occupations such as labor force or education

occupations. The findings also suggest that these young offenders engage in few achievement leisure occupations, that is, those that may contribute to their mental health and well-being and that could lay the foundation for supporting a range of productive occupational roles. The pattern of time use found in this study may negatively affect the young offenders' future development of skills for independent living.

This research has also contributed to the study of occupation by furthering our knowledge on human use of time and its relationship to health and well-being. Many young offenders in this study who experienced problems at home and who left school subsequently lost achievement leisure occupations. Their current use of time, therefore, was a consequence of a problematic occupational history.

As has been indicated, data from this study also revealed that those working with young offenders do not always appreciate the benefits of engaging young people in ordinary everyday occupations that may have health benefits. Expert knowledge on human occupation is the domain of occupational therapists. Hence, findings from this study help us to understand the use of time—particularly, the leisure occupations—of young offenders and will help to inform current and future occupational therapy practices with such groups.

Acknowledgments

This study was supported by faculty research grants from the Faculty of Health Sciences, La Trobe University, and OT National: Australian Association of Occupational Therapists, Victorian Branch. This chapter is based on material submitted in partial fulfillment of the requirement for a doctorate of philosophy in occupational science at the University of Southern California, Los Angeles.

References

Alder, C. (1986). Unemployed women have got it heaps worse: Exploring the implications of female youth unemployment. *Australian and New Zealand Journal of Criminology, 19*, 210–224.

Allen, E., & Steffensmeier, D. (1989). Youth, under-employment, and property crime: Differential effects of job availability and job quality on juvenile and young adult arrest rates. *American Sociological Review, 54*, 107–123.

Australian Bureau of Statistics. (1993). 1992 *time use survey* (Cat. No. 4150.0). Canberra: Author.

Bogdan, R., & Biklen, S. (1992). *Qualitative research for education: An introduction to theory and methods.* Needham Heights, MA: Allyn & Bacon.

Braithwaite, J., & Chappell, D. (1994). The job compact and crime: Submission to the Committee on Employment Opportunities. *Current Issues in Criminal Justice, 5*, 295–300.

Bruno, J. (1996). Time perceptions and time allocation preferences among adolescent boys and girls. *Adolescence, 31*, 109–126.

Carlson, M. (1996). The self-perpetuation of occupations. In R. Zemke & F. Clark (Eds.), *Occupational science: The evolving discipline* (pp. 143–157). Philadelphia: F. A. Davis.

Carrington, K. (1990). Truancy, schooling and juvenile justice: "She says she hates school." *Australian and New Zealand Journal of Criminology, 23*, 259–268.

Castles, I. (1993). *How Australians use their time* (ABS Cat. No. 4153.0). Canberra: Australian Bureau of Statistics.

Christiansen, C. (1994). Classification and study in occupation: A review and discussion of taxonomies. *Occupational Science: Australia, 1*(3), 3–21.

Christiansen, C. (1996). Three perspectives on balance in occupation. In R. Zemke & F. Clark (Eds.), *Occupational science: The evolving discipline* (pp. 431–451). Philadelphia: F. A. Davis.

Clark, F., Parham, D., Carlson, M., Frank, G., Jackson, J., Pierce, D., et al. (1991). Occupational science: Academic innovation in the service of occupational therapy's future. *American Journal of Occupational Therapy, 45*, 300–310.

Clarke, S., & Haworth, J. (1994). "Flow" experience in the daily lives of sixth-form college students. *British Journal of Psychiatry, 85*, 511–523.

Commonwealth of Australia. (1998). *Labour market review–Victoria–October 1998.* Canberra: Labour Economics Office. (Available from www.dewrsb.gov.au)

Csikszentmihalyi, M., & Csikszentmihalyi, I. (1988). *Optimal experience: Psychological studies of flow in consciousness.* New York: Cambridge University Press.

Csikszentmihalyi, M., & Larson, R. (1978). Intrinsic rewards in school crime. *Crime and Delinquency, 24*, 322–335.

Csikszentmihalyi, M., & Larson, R. (1984). *Being adolescent: Conflict and growth in the teenage years.* New York: Basic.

Csikszentmihalyi, M., & Larson, R. (1987). Validity and reliability of the Experience Sampling Method. *Journal of Nervous and Mental Disease, 175*, 526–536.

Farnworth, L. (1990). *Understanding work, self-care, and leisure in human occupation.* Paper presented at the 10th International Congress of the World Federation of Occupational Therapists, Melbourne, Australia.

Farnworth, L. (1998). Doing, being, and boredom. *Journal of Occupational Science, 5*(3), 140–146.

Farnworth, L., Mostert, E., Harrison, S., & Worrell, D. (1996). The Experience Sampling Method: Its potential use in occupational therapy research. *Occupational Therapy International, 3*(1), 1–17.

Felson, M. (1994). *Crime and everyday life: Insight and implications for society.* Thousand Oaks, CA: Pine Forge.

Galloway, D. (1985). *Schools and persistent absentees.* Oxford, UK: Pergamon.

Garton, A., & Pratt, C. (1991). Leisure activities of adolescent school students: Predictors of participation and interest. *Journal of Adolescence, 14*, 305–321.

Glaser, A., & Strauss, B. (1967). *The discovery of grounded theory.* New York: Aldine.

Glassner, B., & Loughlin, J. (1987). *Drugs in adolescent worlds: Burnouts to straights.* New York: St. Martin's Press.

Hagell, A., & Newburn, T. (1996). Family and social contexts of adolescent re-offenders. *Journal of Adolescence, 19*, 5–18.

Hayes, R., & Halford, K. (1996). Time use of un-employed and employed single male schizophrenia subjects. *Schizophrenia Bulletin, 22,* 659–669.

Hendry, L. (1983). *Growing up and going out: Adolescents and leisure.* Aberdeen, UK: Aberdeen University Press.

Hirsch, T. (1969). *Causes of delinquency.* Berkeley: University of California Press.

Hoge, R., Andrews, D., & Leschied, A. (1996). An investigation of risk and protective factors in a sample of youthful offenders. *Journal of Child Psychology and Psychiatry, 37,* 419–424.

Hong, E., Milgram, R., & Whiston, S. (1993). Leisure activities in adolescents as a predictor of occupational choice in young adults: A longitudinal study. *Journal of Career Development, 19,* 221–229.

Hurlburt, R., Happe, F., & Frith, U. (1994). Sampling the form of inner experience in three adults with Asperger syndrome. *Psychological Medicine, 24,* 385–395.

Hurlburt, R., & Melancon, S. (1987). Goofed-up images: Thought sampling with a schizophrenic woman. *Journal of Nervous and Mental Disease, 175,* 575–578.

Jahoda, M. (1981). Work, employment, and unemployment: Values, theories, and approaches in social research. *American Psychologist, 36,* 184–191.

Kielhofner, G. (1995). *A model of human occupation: Theory and application* (2nd ed.). Baltimore: Williams & Wilkins.

Kimiecik, J., & Stein, G. (1992). Examining flow experiences in sport contexts: Conceptual issues and methodological concerns. *Journal of Applied Sport Psychology, 4*(2), 144–160.

Knight, T. (1997). Schools, delinquency, and youth culture. In A. Borowski & I. O'Connor (Eds.), *Juvenile crime, justice, and corrections* (pp. 79–97). Melbourne, Australia: Longman.

Larson, R., & Csikszentmihalyi, M. (1983). The Experience Sampling Method. In H. Reis (Ed.), *Naturalistic approaches to studying social interaction: New directions for methodology of social and behavioral science* (Vol. 15, pp. 41–56). San Francisco: Jossey-Bass.

Lederer, J., Kielhofner, G., & Watts, J. (1985). Values, personal causation, and skills of delinquents and nondelinquents. *Occupational Theory in Mental Health, 5*(2), 59–77.

Lo, J. L. (1996). The relationship between daily occupational affective experiences and subjective well-being. *Occupational Therapy International, 3*(3), 190–203.

Lo, J. L., & Zemke, R. (1997). The relationship between affective experiences during daily occupations and subjective well-being measures: A pilot study. *Occupational Therapy in Mental Health, 13*(3), 1–21.

Ludwig, F. M. (1997). How routine facilitates well-being in older women. *Occupational Therapy International, 4,* 213–228.

Ludwig, F. M. (1998). The unpackaging of routine in older women. *American Journal of Occupational Therapy, 52,* 168–178.

McKinnon, A. (1992). Time use for self care, productivity, and leisure among elderly Canadians. *Canadian Journal of Occupational Therapy, 59,* 102–110.

Meyer, A. (1977). The philosophy of occupation therapy. *American Journal of Occupational Therapy, 3,* 639–642. (Original work published 1922)

Minichiello, V., Aroni, R., Timewell, E., & Alexander, L. (1990). *In-depth interviewing.* Melbourne, Australia: Longman Cheshire.

Mokros, H. (1993). Communication and psychiatric diagnosis: Tales of depressive moods from two contexts. *Health Communication, 5,* 113–127.

Neville, A. (1980). Temporal adaptation: Application with short-term psychiatric patients. *American Journal of Occupational Therapy, 34,* 328–331.

Parham, D. (1996). Perspectives on play. In R. Zemke & F. Clark (Eds.), *Occupational science: The evolving discipline* (pp. 71–80). Philadelphia: F. A. Davis.

Parham, D., & Primeau, L. (1997). Play and occupational therapy. In L. D. Parham & L. S. Fazio (Eds.), *Play in occupational therapy for children* (pp. 2–21). St. Louis, MO: Mosby.

Passmore, A. (1998a). Does leisure have an association with creating cultural patterns of work? *Journal of Occupational Science, 5,* 161–165.

Passmore, A. (1998b). *The relationship between leisure and mental health in adolescents.* Unpublished doctoral dissertation, University of Western Australia, Perth.

Pettifer, S. (1993). Leisure as compensation for unemployment and unfulfilling work: Reality or pipe dream? *Journal of Occupational Science: Australia, 1*(2), 20–26.

Polkinghorne, D. (1986). *Methodology for the human sciences systems of inquiry.* Albany: State University of New York Press.

Primeau, L. (1996a). Work and leisure: Transcending the dichotomy. *American Journal of Occupational Therapy, 50,* 569–577.

Primeau, L. (1996b). Work versus nonwork: The case of household work. In R. Zemke & F. Clark (Eds.), *Occupational science: The evolving discipline* (pp. 57–70). Philadelphia: F. A. Davis.

Richards, L., & Richards, T. (1997). NUD*IST (Version 4) [for Apple Macintosh]. Melbourne, Australia: Qualitative Solutions and Research.

Robinson, J. (1996). Time, housework, and the rest of life. *Journal of Family and Economic Issues, 17,* 213–229.

Robinson, J., Andreyenkov, V., & Patrushev, V. (1988). *The rhythm of everyday life: How Soviet and American citizens use time.* San Francisco: Westview.

Statistics Canada. (1986). *General social survey* (Public use microdata file documentation and user's guide). Ottawa: Author.

Strauss, A., & Corbin, J. (1990). *Basics of qualitative research: Grounded theory procedures and techniques.* Newbury Park, CA: Sage.

Sullivan, M. (1989). *Getting paid: Youth crime and work in the inner city.* New York: Cornell University Press.

Suto, M., & Frank, G. (1994). Future time perspective and daily occupations of persons with chronic schizophrenia in a board and care home. *American Journal of Occupational Therapy, 48,* 7–18.

Szalai, A. (1977). *Cross-national comparative survey research: Theory and practice.* New York: Pergamon.

U.S. Department of Labor. (1999). *Comparative labor force statistics in ten countries, 1959–1998.* Washington, DC: Bureau of Labor Statistics. (Available from: http://ststs.bls.gov/flsdata.htm)

Voelkl, J., & Nicholson, L. (1992). Perceptions of daily life among residents of a long-term-care facility. *Activities, Adaptation, and Aging, 16,* 99–114.

White, R., & Sutton, A. (1995). Crime prevention, urban space, and social exclusion. *Australian and New Zealand Journal of Sociology, 31,* 82–99.

Wilcock, A., Chelin, M., Hamley, N., Morison, B., Scrivener, L., Townsend, M., et al. (1997). The relationship between occupational balance and health: A pilot study. *Occupational Therapy International, 4,* 17–30.

Wood, W. (1996). The value of studying occupation: An example with primate play. *American Journal of Occupational Therapy, 50,* 327–337.

Yerxa, E., & Locker, S. (1990). Quality of time use by adults with spinal cord injuries. *American Journal of Occupational Therapy, 44,* 318–326.

CHAPTER 32

Effects of Billing Medicaid for Occupational Therapy Services in the Schools

A Pilot Study

Charlotte Brasic Royeen, PhD, OTR, FAOTA, *is associate dean for research and professor in occupational therapy, School of Pharmacy and Allied Health Professions, Creighton University, 2500 California Plaza, Omaha, NE 68178; croyeen@creighton.edu.*

Maureen Duncan, OTD, OTR, *is assistant professor in occupational therapy, Program in Occupational Therapy, School of Pharmacy and Allied Health Professions, Creighton University, Omaha, NE.*

Jeffrey Crabtree, OTD, FAOTA, *is program director in occupational therapy, University of Texas at El Paso, El Paso.*

Jeannette Richards, OTD, OTR, *is instructor, School of Allied Health Professions, Louisiana State University Medical Center, Shreveport.*

Gloria Frolek Clark, MS, OTR/L, FAOTA, *is school occupational therapist, Heartland Area Education Agency, Adel, IA.*

Originally published 2000 in *American Journal of Occupational Therapy, 54,* 429–433.

Charlotte Brasic Royeen, Maureen Duncan, Jeffrey Crabtree, Jeannette Richards, and Gloria Frolek Clark

Many local education agencies across the United States have implemented a billing structure for school-based occupational therapy services that accesses Medicaid dollars. This structure was made possible through a series of amendments to the Medicaid Program: (1) Title XIX of the Social Security Act (P.L. 89–97), (2) Medicare Catastrophic Coverage Act of 1988 (P.L. 100–360), and (3) the Omnibus Budget Reconciliation Act of 1987 (P.L. 100–203). These amendments gave school administrators the authority to bill Medicaid for "related services" provided to schoolchildren with disabilities who met financial eligibility. Related services, as defined in the Education for All Handicapped Children Act of 1975 (EHA; P.L. 94–142), are those services, such as occupational therapy and physical therapy, provided to students with disabilities that permit them to benefit from special education within the least restrictive education environment.

The intent of the Title XIX amendment was to allow expensive equipment, such as technologically advanced wheelchairs that would help special education students function within the education setting, to be funded through Medicaid. In actuality, however, Medicaid began to be billed not only for technology equipment for students, a medically related service, but also for all school-based occupational therapy services, regardless of whether the service was educationally or medically related.

There is a difference between medically and educationally related occupational therapy services. Medically related services focus primarily on the individual student, whereas educationally related services focus on parent and teacher concerns and student interactions within the specific education setting. When using the medical model, evaluation of a student relies on standardized tests to identify underlying physical problems, which may or may not be related to the student's educational performance in the classroom. When using the education model, evaluation focuses on the student's educational performance within the classroom or education setting, using expert observation (American Occupational Therapy Association [AOTA], 1997). Other distinctions between these two types of related services are shown in Table 32.1.

The need to distinguish educationally related occupational therapy services from medically related occupational therapy services was an outcome of the EHA and its stress on an educational context for the delivery of related services. The EHA was amended by the Individuals With Disabilities Education Act of 1990 (IDEA; P.L. 101–476) and reauthorized in 1997 (P.L. 105–17). This reauthorization continues to ensure that children and young adults with disabilities, 3 to 21 years of age, are entitled to a free, appropriate public education. This legislation also continues to ensure the place of occupational therapy as a related service in special education.

The practice of billing Medicaid for occupational therapy services in the school is required by EHA. Because Medicaid, now a major reimburser for school-based services, is predicated on a medical model that is not in accord with providing the educationally related services mandated by the IDEA, we were concerned that occupational therapists may be making decisions about services that are driven by resources rather than by the student's needs. Therefore, we conducted a pilot study of the effects on practice of billing Medicaid for school-based occupational therapy services.

Understanding the influence of a payment system on practice will help us to assure quality of services. Understanding the influence of a payment system that embraces a medically related practice model will help us to meet the challenge of maintaining educationally related occupational therapy in the public school setting per IDEA and the *Standards of Practice for Occupational Therapy* (AOTA, 1998). Finally, understanding the influence of a payment system has implications for how services for children are provided overall (Diekema, 1996).

Method

A nine-item questionnaire was developed for this pilot study and reviewed by members of the

Table 32.1. Medically Related Versus Educationally Related Occupational Therapy Services

Medically Related	Educationally Related
Assumes an underlying cause with diagnosis based on symptomatology.	Assumes no underlying cause. Focus in on what behavior or functional need is to be accomplished.
Evaluation to reveal underlying problems.	Evaluation to determine what functional problem needs resolution (i.e., targeted behavioral outcome).
Dysfunction is within the student.	Dysfunction is a mismatch between student's abilities and what is being demanded or asked.
Intervention focuses on "curing" the cause and tends to be long term because underlying causes are often never able to be fully cured.	Interventions focus on function and are more short term.
Treatment is usually one to one and occurs in a setting outside of the classroom.	Treatment is group oriented and can be in classroom or other school settings.
Provider uses medical terms that are not generally understood by parents and teachers.	Provider uses everyday language that is understood by parents and teachers.

Note. From Ottenbacher (1991) and Royeen (1991, 1992).

School System Special Interest Section and the AOTA Practice department for completeness, readability, and accuracy. Respondents were to answer "yes" or "no" to seven of the nine questions and to further explain (open-ended responses) their answers to seven of the questions (see Table 32.2).

The questionnaire, published in the January 16, 1997, issue of *OT Week*, invited practitioners who were employed by or worked in the public schools to complete the survey. From this mailing to 40,000 subscribers, a self-selected sample of 200 occupational therapy practitioners completed the survey (see Table 32.3). Frequency counts of the yes and no responses were tabulated, and the respondents' written comments were categorized according to five of the six principles of the

Occupational Therapy Code of Ethics (AOTA, 1994) by three separate reviewers.

Results

Respondents reported little concern regarding billing of Medicaid for occupational therapy services in the schools (see Table 32.2). The majority did bill Medicaid for services and reported that this did not affect which students received services. Most continued to provide services that had been regularly provided before implementing Medicaid billing. Seventy-nine reported that billing Medicaid affected documentation, 29 agreed that administrative problems with billing Medicaid hampered services, and 15 reported

Table 32.2. Questions and Responses

	Response				
Question	Yes	No	N/A	No Response	Provided Comments
1. Do you or your employer bill Medicaid for OT services in the public school setting?	170	50	—	—	—
2. Has billing for Medicaid for OT services affected or changed how you provide services? If yes, please explain.	34	186	—	—	34
3. Has billing for Medicaid services affected which students receive OT services? If yes, please explain.	4	216	—	—	2
4. Are you aware of any services you regularly provide that you are no longer able to provide under Medicaid requirements? If yes, please explain.	10	210	—	—	12
5. Has billing Medicaid affected your documentation? Please specify.	79	113	—	28	112
6. Have administrative problems hampered delivery of services? If yes, please explain.	29	191	—	—	24
7. Has billing Medicaid had significant effects on the use of OTAs in the schools? Please explain.	15	80	109	16	25
8. How is Medicaid funding used within your state?					
Flows into general education	21	—	—	—	—
Flows to district	75	—	—	—	—
Flows to noneducation state funds	12	—	—	—	—
Don't know	85	—	—	—	—
Other	26	—	—	—	—
No response	22	—	—	—	—
9. Comment on areas of concern or benefits from Medicaid billing that you have witnessed regarding OT services in the public school setting.	—	—	—	—	119

Note. OT = occupational therapy; OTA = occupational therapy assistant.

Table 32.3. Geographic Distribution of Respondents by State

State	OT	OTA	State	OT	OTA
Alabama	1	—	Nebraska	1	—
Alaska	1	—	New Hampshire	4	—
California	2	1	New Jersey	6	—
Colorado	1	0	New Mexico	3	4
Delaware	2	—	New York	13	—
Florida	8	1	North Carolina	2	1
Georgia	3	—	North Dakota	3	—
Hawaii	1	—	Ohio	17	1
Illinois	16	3	Oregon	1	—
Indiana	3	—	Pennsylvania	9	—
Kansas	2	1	Rhode Island	5	—
Kentucky	2	—	South Carolina	2	1
Louisiana	2	—	Tennessee	2	—
Maine	2	—	Texas	17	2
Maryland	10	1	Virginia	1	—
Massachusetts	1	—	Washington	11	—
Michigan	21	—	West Virginia	2	—
Minnesota	1	—	Wyoming	4	—
Montana	1	—	Unknown	7	—

Note. OT = occupational therapist; OTA = occupational therapy assistant.

that occupational therapy assistants had been affected by this billing.

Written comments explaining responses yielded a different picture. Respondents' comments were categorized into the following eight areas of concern:

1. Paperwork and billing requirements for reimbursement take away from time previously spent in direct care and in collaboration with students, parents, and teachers.
2. Smaller school districts cannot afford to participate in such billing because of increased administrative costs and record keeping.
3. Medicaid funds may become "tapped out" and unavailable once a student reaches adulthood.
4. There are potential ethical issues in billing Medicaid such that some practitioners have thought of resigning.
5. Medicaid supervision regulations for occupational therapy assistants may be different

from those of state and professional license boards and, thereby, cause legal and ethical problems. Occupational therapists were being asked to sign off for unsupervised occupational therapy assistants.

6. Children who receive educationally related services may be denied services if they lose their Medicaid benefits. Medicaid enrollment status may encourage or discourage identification and placement.
7. Special education service providers are forced to follow a medical model approach to school-based practice to ensure that services are reimbursed.
8. Billing agencies are editing occupational therapy documentation records to meet Medicaid reimbursement requirements.

Discussion

Respondents' concerns reveal potential ethical dilemmas for school-based occupational therapy practitioners posed by the Medicaid billing structure (see Table 32.4). *Principle 1* of the *Code of Ethics* relates to beneficence, or the "obligation to help others further their important and legitimate interests" (Beauchamp & Childress, 1989). Respondents wondered whether a reimbursement system that pays for medically necessary services will benefit only children who are eligible for Medicaid and thus compromise the quality of educationally related services.

Principle 3 pertains to the professional duty to attain and maintain competence, to use appropriate procedures, and to ensure that services provided are commensurate with qualifications and experience. Within a system that encourages the use of medically related contract services, respondents were concerned that therapy expectations might shift away from educationally relevant services to the more limited medically necessary services. They were concerned that this system will encourage the inappropriate use of occupational therapy assistants as direct service providers without the supervision by occupational therapists, which is mandated by our practice standards.

Principle 4 places responsibilities on therapists to, among other things, abide by all local, state, and federal laws; the *Standards of Practice* (AOTA, 1998); and institutional rules. Respondents commented that the Medicaid billing structure might contribute to "double dipping"—the payment of services already paid for by other sources—which violates the therapist's obligation to abide by the law. Although this principle does not deal expressly with distributive justice, such as balancing the needs of one person against the needs of the community, respondents were concerned that this system could unfairly divert funds away from needy populations other than special education students and deplete the total allowed monies for Medicaid per individual, resulting in "using up" lifetime benefits.

Principle 5 dictates that occupational therapists provide truthful and accurate information about their services. Respondents expressed concern that providing Medicaid services without some consensus or understanding among school therapists and administrators about the differences between medical versus educational occupational therapy services could create an ethical dilemma for the provider. Many respondents were confused about the difference between medical versus educational occupational therapy services and wondered whether the blending of educationally based and medically based services might result in misrepresentation of services or lack of accountability to families.

Principle 6 pertains to treating colleagues and other professionals fairly and truthfully. Several respondents believed that providing Medicaid services in the school setting contradicted the therapist's legal mandate regarding educationally relevant services. They wondered whether these two types of services should be segregated by billing mechanisms. They expressed concern that meeting the school's needs for Medicaid-reimbursable service was at the expense of the student's need for educational services to benefit from special education.

The resolution of these potential ethical dilemmas has relevance to schools, the children and families whom therapists serve, and the occupational therapy profession. Currently, thousands of students in special education receive services from at least 7,183 occupational therapists and occupational therapy assistants (U.S. Department of Education, 1998). Implementation of billing Medicaid for school-based occupational therapy services has led to related ethical issues such as those addressing parental consent, student privacy, the legality of billing Medicaid for educational services, institutions where schools aggressively push medically necessary services, and the possible harm done to

Table 32.4. Principles of the *Occupational Therapy Code of Ethics* and Respondents' Major Concerns[a]

Principle	Respondent Concerns
Principle 1. Occupational therapy personnel shall demonstrate a concern for the well-being of recipients of their services (beneficence).	• "My greatest concern is that a possible future 'cap' may leave the disabled without resources in the future." (017) • "Concerned about the depletion of Medicaid funds in general. In the event that a student requires a wheelchair or operation down the road, will that be restricted or denied as the level of funding for those categories has been previously shifted elsewhere." (040) • "Money does not come back to the students." (062) • "Billing may reduce the lifetime benefits for the children we work with." (065) • "Concerned about impact of managed care and of lifetime quota for students followed in clinical private sector." (220)
Principle 3. Occupational therapy personnel shall achieve and continually maintain high standards of competence (duty).	• "How long will Medicaid pay students who make little or no change?" (071) • "Am uncomfortable with charging Medicaid because it is so clinically oriented. We believe that this will have a negative impact on school therapy services and what they can entail." (188)
Principle 4. Occupational therapy personnel shall comply with laws and Association policies guiding the profession of occupational therapy (justice).	• "Confusion exists between educationally relevant and medically relevant services. Multiple agencies might be tapping Medicaid for OT services." (015) • "It seems like 'double dipping.'" (015) (85) (142) (149) • "Seems like we are charging the state for services already paid by tax bases." (101) • "Services provided by a school district are supposed to be educationally relevant...Medicaid was designed to cover expenses based on medical needs. Therefore, by definition the two systems are incompatible." (123) • "It is my understanding that Medicaid funds are used for medical services, not educational. I provide educationally related services." (168) • "What is Medicaid doing reimbursing educational needs?" (190) • "This seems to add another layer of cost in funding—it all comes from taxpayers in the end." (194)
Principle 5. Occupational therapy personnel shall provide accurate information about occupational therapy services (veracity).	• "I am concerned about the misrepresentation to families and accountability of reimbursement funds." (088) • "We are billing for medically related OT services yet providing educationally related services." (152)
Principle 6. Occupational therapy personnel shall treat colleagues and other professionals with fairness, discretion, and integrity (fidelity, veracity).	• "We've worked hard to explain educationally related therapy, and Medicaid billing contradicts our efforts." (012) • "There is more pressure to provide 'medical' therapy in school." (037) • "Billing Medicaid for educationally related services could begin to change our practice—a discouraging thought since we worked so hard to achieve educationally related therapy." (103) • "I am uncomfortable with use of medical funding for school services. I spent many years developing educational relevance in my school-based OT programs." (114) • "What started out to be a simple issue ended up with the replacement of an entire OT department of seven therapists (with a combined total of 120 years of experience) by foreign therapists (with a total of less than 10 years of experience), a loss of consistent services to the students, a loss of continuity in their treatment, a loss to the students of working New Mexican role models who were familiar with their Hispanic culture, and a financial loss to this community and state." (175)

Note. OT = occupational therapy.

[a]Representative respondent statements organized according to five of the six ethical principles of the *Occupational Therapy Code of Ethics* (American Occupational Therapy Association, 1994).

children who do not receive occupational therapy because they do not qualify for Medicaid.

Many of these concerns are similar to those reported by Ahearn (1993) in a larger scale study of Medicaid billing in the public school setting. Ahearn reported the following concerns: (a) conflicting interpretations about what constitutes a Medicaid-reimbursable service, (b) school difficulty in hiring qualified personnel who meet Medicaid regulations for provider prerequisites, (c) potential school difficulty in planning and managing services to ensure nonduplication of services (need for intra-agency collaboration), (d) changes in family income that may result in inconsistency in eligibility for Medicaid benefits, and (e) substantial loss of education dollars to support a rapidly growing Medicaid budget. The fact that two studies yielded similar concerns warrants serious consideration.

Limitations

The current study was based on a convenience sample. The findings are not based on calculation of statistical probabilities but identify issues for continued research. The number of written responses by participants for questions 2 through 9 (see Table 32.2) do not align with only those who responded yes because many who answered no responded anyway, and some who answered yes provided no explanation.

Conclusion

The effects of billing Medicaid for occupational therapy services in the schools warrant further study. This is especially true because reauthorization of IDEA requires that Medicaid be billed for occupational therapy services provided in the school setting. Because this billing structure may put school-based therapists in the position of violating principles of the *Occupational Therapy Code of Ethics,* we recommend that practitioners be well versed with the code as well as with the billing mechanism in the settings where they work.

Acknowledgments

We thank Leslie Jackson, Med, OT/L, federal affairs representative, Federal Affairs department, American Occupational Therapy Association, and Gail Jensen, PhD, PT, associate, Center for the Study of Ethics and Health Policy, Creighton University, for expert consultation. Partial funding for this study was provided by the Center for the Study of Children's Issues, Creighton University.

References

Ahearn, E. M. (1993). *Medicaid as a resource for students with disabilities: Project FORUM.* Alexandria, VA: National Association of State Directors of Special Education. (ERIC Document Reproduction Service No. ED 366 127)

American Occupational Therapy Association. (1994). Occupational therapy code of ethics. *American Journal of Occupational Therapy, 48,* 1037–1038.

American Occupational Therapy Association. (1997). *Occupational therapy services for children and youth under the Individuals With Disabilities Education Act.* Bethesda, MD: American Occupational Therapy Association.

American Occupational Therapy Association. (1998). Standards of practice for occupational therapy. *American Journal of Occupational Therapy, 52,* 866–869.

Beauchamp, T. L., & Childress, J. F. (1989). *Principles of biomedical ethics* (3rd ed.). New York: Oxford University Press.

Diekema, D. S. (1996). Children first: The need to reform financing of health care services for children. *Journal of Health Care for the Poor and Underserved, 7*(1), 3–14.

Individuals With Disabilities Education Act (1990). Pub. L. 101–476, 20 U.S.C., Ch 33.

Omnibus Budget Reconciliation Act. (1987). Pub. L. 100–203, 42 U.S.C. § 4211.

Ottenbacher, K. (1991). Conflicting views: Who knows best? In C. B. Royeen (Ed.), *School-based practice for related services (Lesson 2)*. Rockville, MD: American Occupational Therapy Association.

Reauthorization of the Individuals With Disabilities Education Act. (1997). Pub. L. 105-17.

Royeen, C. B. (Ed.). (1991). *School-based practice for related services*. Bethesda, MD: American Occupational Therapy Association.

Royeen, C. B. (Ed.). (1992). *Classroom applications for school-based practice*. Rockville, MD: American Occupational Therapy Association.

U.S. Department of Education. (1998). *20th annual report to Congress on the implementation of Individuals With Disabilities Education Act*. Washington, DC: U.S. Government Printing Office.

CHAPTER 33

Relationships Between Handwriting and Keyboarding Performance of Sixth-Grade Students

Janet Rogers and Jane Case-Smith

Janet Rogers, MS, OTR/L, BCP, *is in private practice, Pickerington, OH.*

Jane Case-Smith, EdD, OTR/L, BCP, FAOTA, *is associate professor, School of Allied Medical Professions, Ohio State University, 1583 Perry Street, Columbus, OH 43210; case-smith.1@osu.edu.*

Occupational therapists working in school-based settings have become increasingly involved in the remediation of children's illegible handwriting (Amundson, 2001). An estimated 12% to 21% of school-age children struggle with handwriting skills (Alston, 1985; Rubin & Henderson, 1982). Many children continue to demonstrate difficulty with handwriting despite months of intervention. Written communication allows the child to express what he or she knows. When a child struggles with the process of writing, the actual expression of knowledge can be compromised (Rubin & Henderson, 1982). As a result, children with poor handwriting often are given poorer grades on the content of their written work than good handwriters (Briggs, 1980). Relationships also have been shown between poor handwriting and difficulties in many other areas of academic learning (e.g., spelling, writing composition, grammar) (Berninger, Mizokawa, & Bragg, 1991; Campbell, 1973). With the increasing numbers of computers available in elementary and secondary schools, word processing is a viable option for students who struggle with handwriting.

Use of Computer-Based Word Processing in Schools

As early as 1926 in first-grade classrooms at the Horace Mann School at Columbia University, educators considered the value of using typewriters within the educational curriculum (Sinks & Thurston, 1972). Early studies in the United States demonstrated that the use of a typewriter in the elementary classroom had a positive effect on academic learning (Conard, 1935; Rowe, 1959; Tate, 1942; Wood & Freeman, 1932). This initial enthusiasm for typing as a tool for enhancing academic learning subsided with the realization of the cost and effort required to incorporate it effectively into the elementary classroom (Balajthy, 1988).

Originally published 2002 in *American Journal of Occupational Therapy,* 56, 34–39.

In the mid-1980s, computers began to appear in public school programs (Cochran-Smith, 1991). In the 1990s, the number of computers in schools and homes increased substantially. It was recently estimated that one in three American homes has a personal computer (Belsie, 1995) and that 75% of the public schools have computers, with one computer available for every nine students (Brown, 1995). This accessibility to computers has added new learning options for students in a variety of academic areas.

The use of word processors for written communication is an emerging academic area in the public school curriculum that has recently received considerable attention by educators and school administrators. Many public school systems have recognized these benefits and have mandated keyboarding (i.e., word processing using a computer keyboard) instruction in elementary schools (Balajthy, 1988; Nieman, 1996).

Comparison of Keyboarding and Handwriting

Findings from a number of studies have demonstrated the functional benefits of keyboarding in the development of writing and reading skills in elementary school children who are typically developing and children with disabilities (Campbell, 1973; Dybdahl & Shaw, 1989; MacArthur & Graham, 1987; Sinks & Thurston, 1972). Cochran-Smith (1991) reported that students' composing skills improve when they use word processors. Students reportedly made a greater number of revisions, although these were usually surface-level rather than meaning-level revisions. Students also tended to write longer and more error-free texts as well as wrote for longer periods.

Word processing appears to have a number of distinct advantages when compared with handwriting (Cochran-Smith, 1991). The advantages include increasing the ease of editing, increasing content quality and quantity of written work, and increasing the legibility of written work. Surveyed elementary school students reported a preference for keyboarding because pushing a button was easier than writing a letter (Kahn & Freyd, 1990). By simplifying text production, children appear to concentrate on the content and meaning of composing.

For keyboarding to be considered a possible alternative to handwriting, a certain level of keyboarding performance is necessary. According to Balajthy (1988), "For touch typing to be useful, the process must be automatic and students must reach a typing speed at least equivalent to their handwriting speed" (p. 41). Dunn and Reay (1989) demonstrated this concept in a study of 52 12-year-old and 13-year-old students identified by their teachers as having difficulty in writing composition. They examined the relationship of handwriting and typing transcription rates and found that students whose typing speed equaled or exceeded their handwriting speed showed greater competence in the content of narrative writing when using a word processor than when handwriting. Conversely, when students' typing speed was less than their handwriting speed, they demonstrated less competency in the content of the narrative writing when using the word processor than when handwriting.

Studies have found that handwriting speed correlates with keyboarding speed: Those students who write quickly also tend to be relatively strong initial keyboarders (Kahn & Freyd, 1990). Pisha (1993) found that students who wrote quickly tended to develop keyboarding skills more quickly than students who wrote slowly. Handwriting speed typically never approached the same levels as keyboarding. Freeman (1954) reported that the average adult can handwrite legibly 130 letters per minute (or approximately 26 words per minute [WPM]). For advanced typists, however, typing speed can reach and exceed 100 WPM (West, 1969).

Occupational therapy practitioners seem to agree about the importance of keyboarding as an alternative form of written communication for students who struggle with handwriting (Amundson, 2001; Penson, 1990). Few guidelines, however, are provided to therapists to determine when a student should use keyboarding as an alternative to handwriting. Being able to identify a child who can benefit from computer word processing and initiating early keyboarding instruction may help that child to avoid the compositional writing disabilities often associated with dysgraphia (Berninger et al., 1991).

The purpose of this study was to investigate the relationship between handwriting and keyboarding performance in sixth-grade children who had received a standard instructional program in keyboarding. Specifically,

1. Does handwriting speed and legibility relate to keyboarding speed and accuracy?
2. Can handwriting speed and legibility correctly categorize students as slow or fast in keyboarding?

Method

Participants

The sample of convenience consisted of sixth-grade students from a central Ohio elementary school. All students participated in the school's computer keyboarding classes, which were taught by one keyboarding instructor. Students with sensory, motor, cognitive, or social–emotional impairments were excluded from the sample. Of the 98 children who met these criteria, 41 returned the consent form to participate in the study. Of these, 1 student was unable to complete the

testing. Table 33.1 provides comparative demographic data about the 40 study participants.

Instrument

Handwriting legibility was assessed by scoring a timed handwriting sample using the Test of Legible Handwriting (TOLH; Larsen & Hammill, 1989). This test was designed to measure the holistic legibility of students' handwriting in grades 2 to 12. Writing samples can be taken in any number of ways, including samples from verbal prompts, from picture prompts, or from the child's previous written work. The sample is compared with one of three scoring guides for a rating score of 1 to 9. In the current study, the scored handwriting samples were taken during the handwriting speed test as described in the next section.

Handwriting and keyboarding speed were assessed using 2-min samples of each. To assess handwriting speed, participants were asked to copy a poem in their "usual cursive handwriting" until told to stop. The poem was a modified version of "Twinkle Twinkle Little Star." The participants were told not to erase or mark out words. If they paused before the 2-min period ended, they were encouraged by verbal prompts to continue writing. To derive a WPM score, a score for letters per minute was first computed and then

Table 33.1. Participant Demographics (*N* = 40)

Characteristic	*n*
Gender	
Male	20
Female	20
Ethnicity	
Caucasian	36
African-American	3
Asian	1
Hand dominance	
Right	36
Left	4
Has a home computer	
Yes	34
No	6

divided by 5 (i.e., this method assumes that the average length of a word is 5 letters).

Keyboarding speed was measured using the same model as that used in the handwriting speed test. The participants were instructed to type a modified version of the poem "Twinkle Twinkle Little Star" using a printed model. They were instructed to type the poem in their "usual way" until told to stop. The number of keystrokes per minute was computed and divided by 5 to calculate the WPM score. Keyboarding errors were calculated on the basis of omitted key strikes (letters, punctuation marks, spaces), additional key strikes (letters, punctuation, spaces, shifting to capitalize), or incorrect key strikes (misspelled words). Each omitted key strike counted as one error. Completely skipped lines of text were not penalized.

Procedure

Students in the sample participated in the keyboarding instruction class required by the school for 12 weeks. The class met for 30 sessions (40 min per session), which were integrated into the language arts class. The formal class included group instruction using a textbook on keyboarding and word processing and a self-paced computer instructional program (Mavis Beacon Teaches Typing[1]). In the final 3 weeks of the keyboarding class, language arts assignments were integrated into the program. Students were tested in the final week of this class so that each would have a baseline of instructional background to keyboarding and would have achieved a basic level of competence.

Data Analysis

Means, ranges, and standard deviations were computed for all measures. Pearson product-moment correlations were used to determine the relationships among keyboarding speed, keyboarding errors, handwriting speed, and handwriting legibility. A discriminant analysis was done to determine the ability of the handwriting performance scores to identify correctly a student's group membership as either slow or fast in keyboarding.

Results

Means and standard deviations for the measures are presented in Table 33.2. Examination of mean scores revealed 2 participants who had keyboarding scores that were approximately 25 WPM higher than the mean scores. These 2 were considered outliers and were eliminated from the analyses. The correlations among measures are presented in Table 33.3.

Keyboarding speed correlated with handwriting legibility ($n = 38$, $r = .361$, $p = .026$) and handwriting speed ($n = 38$, $r = .342$, $p = .036$). These correlations indicate that legibility accounts for 13% and handwriting speed for 12% of the variability in keyboarding speed.

The participants were categorized as slow keyboarders if speed was less than 15 WPM or fast keyboarders if speed was 15 WPM or greater. Slow or fast keyboarding speed was predicted by handwriting legibility and handwriting speed ($\chi^2 = 7.7$, $df = 2$, $p = .021$). The standardized canonical discriminant function coefficient was .532 for handwriting speed and .661 for handwriting legibility. When combined, handwriting performance correctly classified 71.4% of the students

Table 32.2. Measures for Handwriting Legibility and Speed and Keyboarding Speed and Error Rate ($N = 38$)

Measure	M	SD
Handwriting speed (words/minute)	9.3	2.73
TOLH (raw scores)	11.55	3.72
Keyboarding errors	5.71	4.53
Keyboarding speed (words/minute)	14.9	6.35

Note. TOLH = Test of Legible Handwriting.

[1]Published by Mindscape, Inc., 88 Roland Way, Novato, CA 94945.

Table 33.3. Correlations Between Handwriting and Keyboarding Measures

Measure	TOLH r (p)	Handwriting Speed r (p)	Keyboarding Speed r (p)
Handwriting speed	.487** (.002)		
Keyboarding speed	.361* (.026)	.342* (.036)	
Keyboarding errors	.213 (.198)	.261 (.113)	.203 (.222)

Note. TOLH = Test of Legible Handwriting.
*p < .01. **p < .05.

in the slow keyboarding group and 70.6% of students in the fast keyboarding group. Overall, 71.1% of the original grouped cases were correctly classified.

Discussion

Handwriting Performance

The 38 participants exhibited a mean handwriting speed of 46.3 letters per minute (range = 17–81.5 letters per minute), or 9.3 WPM. The range of handwriting speeds of sixth-grade students across the studies reviewed (Groff, 1961; Hamstra-Bletz & Blote, 1990; Phelps, Stempel, & Speck, 1985; Ziviani & Elkins, 1984) was 46.1 to 66 letters per minute. The mean handwriting speed in these studies was 54.7 letters per minute, or 10.9 WPM. Variations in the methods used to obtain the handwriting samples most likely contributed to the wide range of handwriting speeds across these studies. In our study, the participants were asked to copy a poem in their "usual way" and were timed for 2 min. In other studies (e.g., Graham, Berninger, Weintraub, & Schafer, 1998; Sassoon, Nimmo-Smith, & Wing, 1986), students were asked to copy as fast as they could, possibly accounting for faster speeds.

Participants' handwriting legibility was assessed with the TOLH, obtaining a standard mean score of 11.58. This score was within the average range (8–12; Larsen & Hammill, 1989). Throughout the testing, several students com-

plained about writing in cursive and stated that manuscript was their preferred form of handwriting. Graham et al. (1998) found that, when given a choice of handwriting style in a copying test, 50% of sixth-grade students chose manuscript or a mixed style of primarily manuscript. Because students were required to use cursive in the present study, legibility scores and handwriting speeds may have been decreased.

Keyboarding Performance

The participants' mean keyboarding speed after a 30-session keyboarding instruction program was 14.9 WPM (more than 5 WPM more than handwriting), with a range of 6.2 to 33.9 WPM. These speeds are consistent with the mean keyboarding speeds of other sixth-grade students who received 12 to 15 sessions of keyboarding instruction (Sormunen, 1988). In studies by Sormunen (1988) and Kahn and Freyd (1990), the mean keyboarding speed was 13.90 WPM, or 1 word less than the mean handwriting speed for our participants.

Keyboarding errors were also considered in this study as a function of keyboarding performance. Overall, the errors were minimal. The participants demonstrated a mean keyboarding error rate of 5.71, with a range of 0 to 18. Errors consisted of reversed letters, omitted spaces, additional spaces, omitted letters, and additional letters.

Relationship of Handwriting and Keyboarding

Handwriting speed and legibility demonstrated low to moderate correlations with keyboarding speed. Although these relationships were significant, the handwriting variables accounted for less than 15% of the variance in keyboarding. This level of correlation suggests that the two skills not only have some common elements (e.g., motor performance) but also have many elements that differ, which may include differing levels of motor planning, perceptual–motor skill, visual–motor integration, visual memory, and cognitive processing. The low level of correlation suggests that some children with relatively poor handwriting legibility can be effective in keyboarding.

Handwriting performance as measured by legibility and speed demonstrated a moderate ability to predict whether a participant was a slow or fast keyboarder. Among children who are typically developing, a good handwriter will often demonstrate speed and competence in keyboarding. Five participants (29.4%) whose handwriting performance indicated that they should be slow in keyboarding were fast keyboarders, meaning that between one-quarter and one-third of the participants with low legibility and low handwriting speed became fast keyboarders (i.e., >15 WPM).

Pisha (1993) and Kahn and Freyd (1990) also found moderate correlations between handwriting speed and keyboarding speed. Combined, these results suggest that handwriting performance is a moderate predictor of keyboarding performance. In our study, 70% of the students produced more text using keyboarding versus handwriting. Of the 20 slowest handwriters, 75% achieved faster text production using keyboarding rather than handwriting. Because keyboarding is more legible than handwriting, students with illegible handwriting would almost certainly have more legible written production with keyboarding.

Limitations

This exploratory study examined the relationship of handwriting performance to keyboarding performance. A sample of convenience was used with limited diversity in ethnicity, socioeconomic status, and ability. A larger sample and broader range of participants may increase the expression of relationships and would produce results with greater generalizability.

Conclusion

The low to moderate association between handwriting legibility and speed and keyboarding speed and errors suggests that some children with difficulty in handwriting may nonetheless become proficient in using a keyboard to word process. Teaching children with poor handwriting to word process may simplify their text production. This simplification of text production may allow certain children to concentrate on content and meaning when composing and encourage them to engage in compositional writing. The low correlations also suggest that additional studies are needed to identify the variables that predict a child's ability to use a keyboard.

References

Alston, J. (1985). The handwriting of seven to nine year olds. *British Journal of Special Education, 12,* 68–72.

Amundson, S. (2001). Prewriting and handwriting. In J. Case-Smith (Ed.), *Occupational therapy for children* (4th ed., pp. 545–570). St. Louis, MO: Mosby.

Balajthy, E. (1988). Keyboarding, language arts, and the elementary school child. *Computing Teacher, 15*(5), 40–43.

Belsie, L. (1995). Computer industry sales brisk, but some blips ahead on screen. *Christian Science Monitor, 87*(244), 1–8.

Berninger, V., Mizokawa, D., & Bragg, R. (1991). Theory-based diagnosis and remediation of writing disabilities. *Journal of School Psychology, 29,* 57–79.

Briggs, D. (1980). A study of the influence of handwriting upon grades using examination scripts. *Educational Review, 32,* 185–193.

Brown, G. E. (1995). *Educational technology in the 21st century: Joint hearing before the Committee on Science and the Committee on Economic and Educational Opportunities, House of Representatives,* 104th Cong., 1st Sess. 23. (Eric Document Reproduction Service No. ED 392 400)

Campbell, D. D. (1973). Typewriting contrasted with handwriting: A circumvention study of learning disabled children. *Journal of Special Education, 7,* 155–168.

Cochran-Smith, M. (1991). Word processing and writing in elementary classrooms: A critical review of related literature. *Review of Educational Research, 61,* 107–155.

Conard, E. U. (1935). A study of the influence of manuscript writing and of typewriting on children's development. *Journal of Educational Research, 29,* 254–265.

Dunn, B., & Reay, D. (1989). Word processing and the keyboard: Comparative effects of transcription on achievement. *Journal of Educational Research, 84,* 237–245.

Dybdahl, C. S., & Shaw, D. G. (1989). Issues of interaction: Keyboarding, word processing, and composing. *Journal of Research on Computing in Education, 21,* 380–391.

Freeman, F. (1954). Teaching handwriting. *What Research Says to Teachers, 4,* 1–33.

Graham, S., Berninger, V., Weintraub, N., & Schafer, W. (1998). *The development of handwriting speed and legibility in Grades 1 through 9.* Manuscript submitted for publication.

Groff, P. J. (1961). New speeds of handwriting. *Elementary English, 38,* 564–565.

Hamstra-Bletz, L., & Blote, A. (1990). Development of handwriting in primary school: A longitudinal study. *Perceptual Motor Skills, 70,* 759–770.

Kahn, J., & Freyd, P. (1990). Touch typing for young children: Help or hindrance? *Educational Technology, 30*(2), 41–45.

Larsen, S. C., & Hammill, D. O. (1989). *Test of Legible Handwriting.* Austin, TX: PRO-ED.

MacArthur, C. A., & Graham, S. (1987). Learning disabled students' composing under three methods of text production: Handwriting, word processing, and dictation. *Journal of Special Education, 21*(3), 22–42.

Nieman, P. (1996). Introducing early keyboarding skills. *Business Education Forum, 51*(10), 27–30.

Penson, D. E. (1990). *Keyboard, graphic, and handwriting skills: Helping people with motor disabilities.* New York: Chapman & Hall.

Phelps, J., Stempel, L., & Speck, G. (1985). The Children's Handwriting Evaluation Scale: A new diagnostic tool. *Journal of Educational Research, 79,* 46–50.

Pisha, B. (1993). *Rates of development of keyboarding skills in elementary school-aged children with and without identified learning disabilities.* Unpublished doctoral dissertation. Harvard University, Boston.

Rowe, J. L. (1959). Readin', typin', and 'rithmatic. *Business Education World, 19*(5), 9–12.

Rubin, N., & Henderson, S. E. (1982). Two sides of the same coin: Variation in teaching methods and failure to learn to write. *Special Education: Forward Trends, 9*(4), 17–24.

Sassoon, R., Nimmo-Smith, I., & Wing, A. (1986). An analysis of children's penholds. In H. Kao, G. van Galen, & R. Hoosain (Eds.), *Graphonomics: Contemporary research in handwriting* (pp. 93–106). Amsterdam: Elsevier Science.

Sinks, T. A., & Thurston, J. F. (1972). Effect of typing on school achievement in elementary grades. *Educational Leadership, 29,* 344–348.

Sormunen, C. (1988). A comparison of speed achievement of students in Grades 3 to 6 who learn keyboarding on the microcomputer. *Delta Pi Epsilon Journal, 30*(2), 47–57.

Tate, M. W. (1942) Use of the typewriter in remedial reading and language. *Elementary School Journal, 43,* 481–485.

West, L. J. (1969). *Acquisition of typewriting skills: Methods and research in teaching typewriting.* New York: Pitman.

Wood, B. D., & Freeman, F. N. (1932). *An experimental study of the educational influences of the typewriter in the elementary classroom.* New York: Macmillan.

Ziviani, J., & Elkins, J. (1984). An evaluation of handwriting performance. *Educational Review, 36,* 249–261.

CHAPTER 34

The School as Social Context

Social Interaction Patterns of Children With Physical Disabilities

Pamela K. Richardson

Pamela K. Richardson, PhD, OTR, *is assistant professor, Department of Occupational Therapy, San Jose State University, One Washington Square, San Jose, CA 95192-0059; crichar007@aol.com.*

The relationship between physical disabilities and impaired social development in children has been well documented. Children with physical disabilities have been found to have a variety of social deficits, including limited participation in active and social play and increased dependence on others to make social arrangements (Brown & Gordon, 1987; Mulderij, 1996, 1997; Rubin, Fein, & Vandenberg, 1983), poor social skills (Philip & Duckworth, 1982), limited intrinsic motivation (Levitt & Cohen, 1977), lack of drive, and decreased concentration (Salomon, 1983; Sheridan, 1975). They have shown a significantly restricted ability to initiate and direct social interactions with siblings (Dallas, Stevenson, & McGurk, 1993a) and a tendency to engage in rigidly hierarchical relationships in which they assume the role of the younger child (Dallas, Stevenson, & McGurk, 1993b). At school, children with disabilities participate in less cooperative play, more solitary play, and more play with teachers than typically developing peers (Nabors & Badawi, 1997). Medical and therapeutic interventions during school hours can disrupt children's class and free play time, making them less accessible to peers for unstructured social interactions (Lightfoot, Wright, & Sloper, 1999).

The play deprivation caused by lack of environmental engagement can result in secondary social, emotional, and psychological disabilities that persist into adulthood (Missiuna & Pollock, 1991). These secondary disabilities can include isolation, poor self-esteem, poor social adjustment, and unemployment (Blum, Resnick, Nelson, & St. Germaine, 1991; Kokkonen, Saukkonen, Timmonen, Serlo, & Kinnunen, 1991; LaGreca, 1990; Law & Dunn, 1993; Stevens et al., 1996; Varni, Rubenfeld, Talbot, & Setoguchi, 1989; Wallander, Feldman, & Varni, 1989; Wallander & Varni, 1989; Yude & Goodman, 1999). Lack of mobility, overprotection by parents, and lack of opportunities for peer interaction have been cited as contributing factors to the poor social adjustment of many young adults with physical disabilities (Lightfoot et al., 1999; Stevens et al., 1996; Strax, 1991).

Originally published 2002 in *American Journal of Occupational Therapy, 56,* 296–304.

Contemporary theoretical and practice frameworks in occupational therapy support a focus on the interaction between the individual and the environment (Dunn, Brown, & McGuigan, 1994; Law et al., 1996; Yerxa et al., 1989). Additionally, current pediatric frameworks advocate a top–down approach to evaluation in which the quality of the child's participation in the environment is of primary concern (Coster, 1998). However, to apply these frameworks to the social functioning of children with physical disabilities, it is necessary to develop a better understanding of what specific factors in the social environment experienced by children with physical disabilities facilitate or inhibit social and occupational performance.

The school environment is an appropriate context in which to investigate children's socialization. The early school environment appears to be a critical point in children's social development at which they establish an attitude toward school and themselves that is closely related to the quality of peer relationships (Ladd, 1990). The limited amount of literature on how children with physical disabilities experience their school social environment suggests that these children experience physical, organizational, and interactional barriers to social participation (Lightfoot et al., 1999; Nabors & Badawi, 1997).

The concept of social networks frames investigation of how children's social environments affect their social development. A major function of social networks is to provide *support*, which is defined as "resources that are provided by other people and that arise in the context of interpersonal relationships [and] reach individuals through their social network connections" (Belle, 1989, p. 1). When well-functioning, social networks prepare children to become competent within the particular cultural or ecological context in which they live (Tietjen, 1989) and provide them with the skills to develop their own social

networks (Cochran & Brassard, 1979). Through interactions with members of the social network, children learn the essential skill of reciprocal exchanges, or the ability to offer support as well as to receive it. Children who do not engage in reciprocal exchanges will not acquire the ability to offer help and support and, consequently, will have difficulty establishing and maintaining relationships that facilitate the development of adaptive social networks (Cochran & Brassard, 1979).

In a longitudinal study of children's social networks, Feiring and Lewis (1989) found that the biggest change in the number of peers in children's networks occurred between 6 and 9 years of age, reflecting children's transition to school and increased exposure to peers. Lewis, Feiring, and Brooks-Gunn (1988) found that children with handicapping conditions had larger social networks than typically developing peers, but unlike their peers, the social networks of children with disabilities did not show an increase in the number of peers relative to the number of adults with increasing age. The authors concluded that children's developmental delays might have limited their ability to access peers for social interactions independently, consequently limiting the number of peers in their social networks.

The positive aspects of social networks for children with physical disabilities also have been documented. Perceived social support has been suggested as an important protective factor against psychological maladjustment for children with physical disabilities (Varni & Setoguchi, 1991). In a study of children with limb deficiencies and amputations, the most powerful predictor of depressive symptoms was lack of classmate social support (Varni et al., 1989), which was also found to be correlated with trait anxiety and general self-esteem (Varni, Setoguchi, Rappaport, & Talbot, 1992). Children who were able to develop early relationships with peers had higher self-esteem, better mental health, greater levels of independence, and better employment records as adults (Strain & Smith, 1996).

The data on social networks of children with physical disabilities suggest that differences in the composition of their social networks limit opportunities to engage with peers. However, children with physical disabilities value the peer support available in their social networks and have better psychosocial and functional outcomes when this support is present. Further investigation of the school social environment can provide occupational therapists with an understanding of the interactive processes that support or inhibit children's social interactions and, hence, a framework for intervention. Therefore, this study sought to answer the following questions:

1. What are the characteristics of the school social environment experienced by children with physical disabilities?
2. What are the social interactional characteristics of children with physical disabilities in the school environment?

Method

A qualitative approach was used to investigate the school social environment and interactional characteristics of children with physical disabilities. Data were collected through naturalistic observation as well as through semistructured and informal interviews of the child and adult participants.

Participants

I used purposive sampling to select three children with physical disabilities (pseudonyms Edgar, Rosa, and Richard) who were between 5 and 8 years of age and enrolled in age-appropriate regular education classrooms. I chose this age group to observe children in the process of making the transition from primarily family-centered to more peer-oriented social networks (Feiring & Lewis,

1989; Howes, 1988; Ladd, 1990). To limit the scope of the study to social issues related to physical disability, I selected participants who were at or near grade level academically and were free of significant cognitive, communication, or behavioral problems that could affect their ability to enter into age-appropriate social engagement with peers. The children attended three different school programs in the same California community. Adult participants included the classroom teachers, special education teachers and aides, and occupational therapists and physical therapists who worked with the children at each site. The participants and their school programs are described in Table 34.1.

Data Collection

I used naturalistic observation combined with participant interviews to collect data on social behaviors. I conducted classroom observations over an 8-week period in the last quarter of the school year. At each of the three sites, I observed 10 to 11 full school days, observing 1 or 2 school days at each site during any given week. Each teacher helped me to design the observation schedule for her classroom in advance, structuring it to include typical school days as well as occasional special events, such as assemblies, field days, or special projects. During the observations, I maintained field notes that described the interactions and experiences of each child throughout the entire scope of daily school activities, including classroom, recess, lunch, transitions, arrival and departure, and specialist times. This approach allowed me to observe children's interactions during times in the school day when varying levels of structure and varying amounts of adult and peer involvement were expected. When recording behaviors in field notes, I also recorded antecedent events and outcomes of the interactions.

I conducted individual, semistructured interviews with each child's classroom teacher, occu-

Table 34.1. Characteristics of Child Participants and Educational Programs

Child	Child Characteristics	Program Characteristics
Edgar	Eight-year-old third grader Spanish-speaking family: parents and infant sister Fluent in spoken English Myelomeningocele, independent in wheelchair Receives occupational therapy twice a week, daily reading tutor, and catheterization program at school. *Teacher quote:* "Good-natured, loving, and caring but lacking in self-confidence. He wants to reach out to other children and be part of the group but doesn't always know the appropriate way."	Open alternative program Multigraded classroom (grades 3–6); 24 students Full-time instructional assistant to help with lesson preparation and general classroom management Eight students receive resource room intervention and occasional occupational therapy consultation for learning or behavioral issues (Edgar is not one of them) Approximately 25% of class from Spanish-speaking or bilingual homes Almost all instruction done in English
Rosa	Six-year-old first grader Bilingual family: parents and two older sisters Fluent in spoken English Myelomeningocele, independent in wheelchair Receives 1.5 hr pull-out special education daily and occupational therapy and physical therapy after school twice a week *Teacher quote:* "Friendly, well-liked, and open but needing to be more assertive and more self-aware as to how she is perceived by others."	K–1 combination class; 25 students Special education teacher coteaches class 4 hr per day Three students fully included (Rosa and one student each with Down syndrome and developmental delay), one student with severe behavioral problems mainstreamed part-time Approximately 50% of class from Spanish-speaking or bilingual homes All instruction done in English
Richard	Five-year-old prekindergarten student English-speaking family: adoptive grandfather, aunt, and 5-year-old cousin Spastic diplegia, uses walker Receives occupational therapy and physical therapy after school twice a week *Teacher quote:* "He has great spirit and self-confidence and an ability to deal with whatever life presents to him."	Private child care and preschool Approximately 20 students per day in prekindergarten class (some part-time students) Four students fully included in class (Richard, two students with mild autism, and one student with behavioral problems) Full-time special education aide in class, consulting special education teacher present 1 to 2 days per week. Special education support was being withdrawn gradually to prepare Richard to enter kindergarten in fall with no support.

Note. All names are pseudonyms.

pational therapist, physical therapist, and special education teacher or classroom aide. Interviews focused on the adult's perceptions and observations of the child's social engagement and peer relationships at school. I also conducted informal interviews with all child and adult participants throughout the study to check findings with the participants (Lincoln & Guba, 1985). One adult participant from each site also reviewed the initial draft of this chapter to check the validity of the conclusions. An experienced qualitative researcher reviewed portions of the raw data, coded data, and thematic data analysis to check the credibility of the coding scheme and analysis as well as to check the assumptions and hypotheses developed during the data collection and analysis process.

Data Analysis

I coded the data from the field notes and interviews using constant comparative analysis (Glaser, 1965). Coding categories were developed through the process of examining and sorting the data. I identified 10 categories that described aspects of children's social interactions and social experiences through this process: solitary play (parallel play, playing alone), adversarial interactions (e.g., arguments, teasing, physical aggression), helper interactions (child takes the role of helper), helpee interactions (child is being helped by others), play/social (engagement in play or socialization with peers), unsuccessful interactions (attempts to initiate an interaction were unsuccessful), individual adult attention (any adult attention), special or different treatment (e.g., special teaching techniques, therapy intervention, physical assistance), on-task/independent activity (child was working independently at a task), and off-task (child was not attending to or participating in the task). When coding was complete, I prepared a data display for each coding category.

The 10 descriptive codes generated 4 pattern codes from which I identified interactive patterns between the children and the social environment (Miles & Huberman, 1984). The pattern codes were reciprocity, effects of adult involvement, characteristics of play interactions, and quality of occupational engagement.

Results

Reciprocity

The children in the study offered help frequently to both adults and peers. Helping efforts were often directed toward other children who had special needs. Relationships with these classmates seemed to provide important opportunities to engage in reciprocal interactions. All three children had a friend with special needs, and numerous instances of reciprocal helping were observed within these relationships. The most naturally animated, assertive, and caring behaviors observed occurred during these interactions. Other helping interactions suggested a strong desire to be a useful member of the class.

> The teacher asks for volunteers to harvest cilantro in the class garden. Edgar raises his hand and says, "Me, me!" The teacher calls on two other children, then comes over to Edgar and

tells him to help the two other children. He goes outside with a small trowel and digging fork. The cilantro is in the middle of a raised bed, and Edgar cannot reach it from his wheelchair. He sits at the edge of the bed and chops at the chard with his tools.

This type of "helping" experience was observed for all three children. Others appeared to not always take the children's offers of help seriously and, consequently, did not give them the chance to take a productive role in activities. The lack of opportunity to take on the role of helpers marginalized their participation and limited their ability to experience meaningful engagement in classroom occupations.

By contrast, a desire to help did not always extend to taking a role in classroom jobs, such as cleanup or group projects. Teachers were inconsistent in conveying their expectations that the children do their fair share, although they expressed frustration that the children did not take responsibility for being contributing class members. The response of their peers to the lack of cooperative effort ranged from resentment to an "I'll take care of it myself" attitude.

> The teacher announces cleanup for recess. The children start to pick up rapidly so that they can be dismissed. Rosa closes her journal, and her crayon falls to the floor. She wheels up to Iris, who is nearby at the sink washing her hands and asks her to pick up the crayon. Megan is busily straightening up the table. Iris finishes washing her hands and hurries back to the table to be dismissed. The crayon is still on the floor. Rosa goes directly outside, and Megan puts Rosa's journal away.

Not surprisingly, most of the help the children received involved physical assistance. Many peers, particularly those in the upper grades, had developed the ability to anticipate needs and offer help unobtrusively. These helping instances often served as a positive peer interaction opportunity.

Edgar in particular appeared to revel in these brief interactions.

> The kids head in from recess across the field. Tim struggles to push Edgar's wheelchair across the grass. Edgar drops a book (it looks like on purpose). Tim says, "I'll get that for you." Edgar laughs, almost a shriek, as Tim gives it to him.

This tendency to equate helping with socializing was seen on numerous occasions in this study. Peers and adults approached readily to help, resulting in an interaction that was usually positive as well as centered on the child's needs. These interactions seemed to encourage inappropriate bids for attention at other times, as the children in the study attempted to re-create the positive social experiences attained during helping interactions.

Although adults and other children appeared to be able to ascertain when help was truly needed, numerous instances of unsolicited and unneeded help offered to each child were observed.

> Rosa is in a group of children making spiders out of pipe cleaners and felt. The teacher asks each child to pick out four pipe cleaners to be the legs. Anna and Andrea immediately start helping Rosa get pipe cleaners. The teacher tells them, "You help her pick them out." Anna lays the legs out on the felt body of the spider. Rosa sits quietly and watches. The teacher explains how to glue the spiders, then gives everyone a glue bottle. Rosa starts to squeeze glue onto her spider. Anna says, "No, Rosa!" She takes Rosa's glue bottle and puts the glue on, then folds the felt over to make the body. Rosa raises her hands and says to the teacher, "We're done!"

The children rarely declined this type of unnecessary help. The value of the positive social interaction appeared to outweigh the value of performing the task independently.

Effects of Adult Involvement

All of the children in the study received substantial adult attention, which ranged from assistance with physical, self-care, and academic tasks to monitoring of academic and play activities. Adults were very present in the children's environment, even during inherently unstructured activities such as recess or lunch. At times, the children sought out adults as social partners. The adults were willing to adjust their interactive style to suit the children's needs, providing interaction experiences that were less challenging and more immediately rewarding.

> Richard sits down at the table at the play kitchen. He plays by himself for a few minutes, until the aide comes over. They talk and play for a couple of minutes until the aide leaves, then Richard plays by himself for a while. The aide is sitting nearby, and Richard initiates a conversation with her about a TV show. He approaches a nearby table where the teacher is sitting. He talks to her and plays around with her for a few minutes, doing a lot of giggling.

Adults may have approached the children in this study for interactions because they were less frequently engaged with peers and, therefore, more available for interactions with adults. Adults also were observed to interrupt children's play interactions by involving themselves in the play activities or offering assistance.

> Rosa is in a group of children playing word bingo. The special education teacher sits down to play with them. Rosa looks at her card and says "I got a Bingo." The teacher says "Not yet." The teacher compliments Rosa each time she marks a square correctly. She rarely does this with the other children.

Although at times the adult assistance facilitated the children's abilities to participate in activities, interaction with adults during recess and play times often served to remove them from the opportunity to be part of a peer interaction group and disrupted the flow of play activities. The time spent in one-to-one or small group activities with adults appeared to form the basis for a more social adult–child relationship.

> The special education teacher takes Rosa and two other children to the special education room. They stop in the office to visit. Rosa gets a kiss and hug from the speech therapist and resource room teacher in the office. The children stop to pet the office cat. They stop to count toy pigs in the window of the resource room.

Numerous incidents were observed where teachers and aides provided significant support for the children's classroom and social participation, and on balance the influence of adults on the children's social environment was positive. Richard's special education teacher commented, however, that one of her biggest dilemmas was how to provide enough support that the regular education teacher was willing to have her and her students in the class but not so much that the students became overly dependent on her presence. This statement illustrates the fine line between support that facilitates social inclusion and "support" that inhibits peer interactions.

Characteristics of Play Interactions

The children in the study were observed to have many unsuccessful attempts at initiating interactions with others. Causes appeared to be poor timing, interaction attempts that were interpreted by peers as inappropriate, and lack of interest on the part of the potential play partner. In addition, their difficulty with physically approaching children for play sometimes resulted in verbal compensations, such as shouting at children from a distance or, in some cases, tattling.

> Edgar watches three girls play jump rope. The recess supervisor tells him to move away from the girls so that the rope will not hit him. He laughs at the girls, who are starting to get silly with the jump rope rhymes. He moves closer to one of the girls who is turning the rope. She pushes his wheelchair away with her foot and says, "Move!" He moves back.

As this anecdote demonstrates, the children in the study were frequently onlookers rather than active participants in play. At times, this behavior was a result of their initiations being rebuffed. Other episodes of onlooking occurred because physical limitations precluded participation in the activity.

When unsuccessful in engaging their peers, the children often approached an adult to socialize, almost always receiving a positive response. Adults also approached them to offer assistance or socialize. Consequently, as stated earlier, many of their play and social interactions involved adults.

A second play characteristic observed in the children in the study was a lack of depth of engagement, or superficiality, of their social and play interactions. During recess and other free play times, the children moved freely between groups of peers. Episodes of extended one-on-one play interactions were infrequent. A "hit-and-run" quality to their socialization was observed. They engaged with many children but did not stay long with a specific individual or group. Many of their play and social interactions centered on themselves through helping interactions and conversations about their equipment.

> Rosa leaves the classroom with a group of girls to go out for recess and a snack. The girls cluster around Rosa, opening her yogurt and juice containers for her and getting out her cookies. Rosa and the others chatter away as they eat the snack. The girls leave after a few minutes, and another group of girls approaches Rosa to ask her about her wheelchair.

The children in the study did not engage in a large amount of solitary play, and when they did, it often was by default rather than by choice, usually because attempts at engaging others were unsuccessful. During solitary play, they were not fully engaged in their activities, often directing their attention to other children playing nearby.

> Richard plays with the cars on the car mat, watching as two other boys play with a marble game a foot or two away. He repeatedly makes overtures to the two boys that are barely acknowledged. The other boys continue to play together enthusiastically. Richard plays alone, occasionally looking over at the boys.

Quality of Occupational Engagement

The quality of engagement by the children in the study in academic and play occupations was inconsistent. Although at times all three demonstrated episodes of absorbed attention in activities, at other times they required adult attention to persist at ordinary tasks. They received adult supervision and encouragement during both play and classroom activities. When attention was not focused on them, they frequently sought attention from others nearby. When directed at other children, these interaction initiation attempts were most often rebuffed.

> The teacher is sitting on the floor with a group of children, introducing a counting activity. Rosa puts her arm around Megan and leans into her. Megan gently pushes her away. Rosa crawls off around the perimeter of the group. The teacher sees her and tells her to sit next to Iris. Rosa crawls up to Iris, who smiles and puts her arm around her. Rosa sits there for a moment, then crawls behind the teacher, telling her that she is going to sit in the circle because she cannot see her. The special education teacher looks over from her group and says "Rosa, quit messing around."

None of the children's teachers identified them as having attention deficits. Rather, the frequent pursuit of adult attention appeared to be more related to the experience of having adults constantly available for assistance and praise.

Edgar's teacher noted that although he was very capable academically, he seemed to require adult attention to complete even routine assignments. Even when engaged in an activity, he managed to find a way to attract attention to himself.

> During quiet seat work time, Edgar picks up a book he had chosen earlier and makes a couple of brief attempts to read. He takes the book back to his cubby, wheeling close to several children and peering over their shoulders. They each stop to look at him briefly and return to their work. Edgar goes back to his seat to write a poem. He lays his head on the table and sighs loudly as he writes.

Each of the children spent time away from classmates because of interventions such as therapy, catheterization, tutoring, and adaptive physical education. The missed classroom time sometimes disrupted the children's ability to be fully engaged in the classroom activities.

> Edgar returns to the room as the class is quietly listening to the teacher read a story. He pulls up next to the counter, plays briefly with the geosafari game, and then picks up a book. Edgar makes a show of holding the book up in front of his face. He is utterly uninvolved with the story.

Richard was more successful than the other two children at engaging in extended object-centered or make-believe play with other children. He was not as focused on obtaining adult attention, which allowed him to direct his own attention to his peers and the task.

> Richard is working a large alphabet floor puzzle. Two girls walk across the puzzle. Richard says to them "Don't walk on the rug!" He looks over at me and says "We're making a carpet. We take the letters out." I tell him I like the carpet. He says "You can't help us." Another boy comes and watches. He holds a letter L like a gun and pretends to shoot Richard, who continues to work diligently.

Richard's ability to immerse himself in play and to maintain his engagement in activities without the help of adults was commensurate with that of his peers. Consequently, he seemed more likely to be viewed as "just another kid," as a play partner rather than as someone who needed help. This ability to maintain occupational engagement seemed to facilitate his ability to engage in reciprocal play with peers.

Discussion

The importance of reciprocity in the peer relationships of children with disabilities has been emphasized in recent studies (Grenot-Scheyer, Staub, Peck, & Schwartz, 1998; Van der Klift & Kunc, 1994). Of primary importance is the opportunity for children with disabilities to develop a balance between providing and receiving help. In this study, each of the children had developed reciprocal relationships with other children in their class who had special needs. These relationships had evolved into friendships. However, classroom structures to support reciprocity were limited and inconsistently applied. Teachers seemed to have difficulty identifying situations in which the children with physical disabilities could offer authentic assistance to others.

Snell, Janney, and Colley (2000) argued that help should be provided on an as-needed basis, not on the basis of global perceptions of the individual as "able" or "not able." The children in this study appeared to be quite skilled at identifying situational needs for help. However, the fact that interactions with peers were more reliably positive when they were being helped than when they attempted to engage socially seemed to encourage them to seek or accept help when it was not truly necessary. This acceptance of helping interactions tended to reinforce the perception among children and adults that they were not able and, therefore, not truly a peer.

Meyer et al. (1998) discussed "friendship frames" that characterize the social relationships between adolescents with and without disabilities. The authors found that the "I'll help" frame was the most frequently observed social interaction pattern, and when children with disabilities were viewed within this frame, they were not viewed in the "just another kid" frame. Consequently, adults who supported helping behaviors of children without disabilities may have actually facilitated the development of unbalanced peer relationships, making it more difficult for the children with disabilities to be perceived as equals. Staub, Schwartz, Galluci, and Peck (1994) described helping relationships that evolved into friendships but emphasized that both parties had something to contribute, facilitating the reciprocity of the relationship.

The findings of the present study related to the effects of adult interaction support the findings of these previous studies. The adults were able to limit inappropriate helping by peers and actively encouraged the children with disabilities to be independent. However, they were less able to provide opportunities for the children with disabilities to help others, perhaps for several reasons. Time limitations and the need to manage the class as a whole were challenges for the classroom teachers. Teachers and aides did not appear to have a clear understanding of the children's physical disabilities, as evidenced by the many questions on this topic directed toward me. Consequently, it was often difficult for them to develop and communicate performance expectations confidently. The occupational and physical therapists were knowledgeable about the children's functional skills, but because they spent little time in the classroom, this knowledge was not conveyed consistently to the teachers. The aides were better acquainted with the children as social beings than the teachers because of the individual time spent with them. However, their duties as classroom helpers seemed to result in more helping and social interactions, which tended to draw the children away from peer interaction opportunities and did not nurture the children's roles as helpers.

The quality of the children's social and play interactions in this study suggested that they lacked skills in the initiation and maintenance of interactions. These deficits could be attributed to difficulty reading social cues, lack of knowledge of appropriate ways to engage others in interactions, and lack of real-life experience to draw on to enrich the social or play experience. The frequency with which they engaged in supported social interactions with adults may have detracted from their opportunities to engage in more developmentally appropriate interactions with peers. It also created expectations about the structure and theme of play and social interactions that could not always be met when interacting with peers.

The findings regarding the quality of the children's occupational engagement also appeared to relate to the adult involvement in their school and play activities. Interactions with adults were child-centered. The expectations developed during these interactions of being the center of attention seemed to result in attention seeking during other activities, which affected the children's abilities to experience meaningful engagement in occupations of play and schoolwork. Each classroom program offered many opportunities for active participation, but the children were not always able to take advantage of these opportunities because of their difficulty with fully immersing themselves in their daily occupations. These daily occupations are the basis for the development of friendships and social support networks (Cochran & Brassard, 1979; Hartup, 1979). Occupational engagement that is decreased in quality and quantity can potentially affect children's social relationships, adjustment, and life satisfaction (Ladd, 1990; Lightfoot et al., 1999; Strain & Smith, 1996).

Implications for Occupational Therapy Practice

The results of this study suggest several areas in which school-based occupational therapists can improve the social learning context for children with physical disabilities. The focus of intervention must expand beyond the child to include adults and peers in the school environment. Treatment frameworks that address the interaction between the child and the social environment as well as psychosocial components of function are essential (Cronin, 2000; Richardson, Florey, & Greene, 2001). Key areas for intervention include the following: developing strategies for children with physical disabilities to exploit fully opportunities to engage in daily school occupations, educating adults on ways to create opportunities for children to be actively engaged participants in daily occupations, and facilitating reciprocal interactions between children with and without disabilities that promote the development of friendships and supportive peer networks. The occupational therapist's knowledge of physical and psychosocial development and the effects of disabling conditions as well as the interaction between the individual and the performance context can be used to educate adults and children; to alter or adapt the social and physical environment; to provide consultation to other professionals; to develop programs; and to provide direct intervention to children in groups, classrooms, and individual contexts. This involvement requires a broader and more visible role for occupational therapists in school-based practice.

Directions for Future Research

Further study of the structure of the social networks of children with physical disabilities can elucidate how their play and socialization compare with typical peers and identify areas for further research and intervention. Analysis of the structure and theme of social interactions between children with and without physical disabilities can inform us of the relationship between helping and social interactions in peer relationships. Investigation into the role of childhood occupations in the play, socialization, and friendship of children with physical disabilities can yield important information on the relationship between the quality of occupational engagement and success in social interactions. Additionally, exploration into children's perceptions of helping, playing, and reciprocating may help us to understand how children with and without physical disabilities construct their social relationships and negotiate the roles of helper, helpee, and play companion. Finally, within the school environment, the relationship between adult involvement in children's socialization and children's social success with peers deserves further investigation. In the meantime, this study contributes a conceptual frame with which to observe the effects of the social environment on the ability of children with physical disabilities to engage in interactions that will support the development of social support networks.

Acknowledgments

I thank all the children and adults who participated in the study; Ilene Schwartz, PhD, Jean Dietz, PhD, OTR, FAOTA, Owen White, PhD, and Susan Nolen, PhD, for their expert guidance and oversight; research assistants Gina Matheney and Alyson Zuppero; and the occupational therapy writing group at San Jose State University. I especially thank Kay Schwartz, EdD, OTR, FAOTA, for her thoughtful critique and feedback.

This study was completed in partial fulfillment of the dissertation requirements for the author's doctor of philosophy degree at the University of Washington.

References

Belle, D. (1989). *Children's social networks and social supports.* New York: Wiley-Interscience.

Blum, R. W., Resnick, M. D., Nelson, R., & St. Germaine, A. (1991). Family and peer issues among adolescents with spina bifida and cerebral palsy. *Pediatrics, 88,* 280–285.

Brown, M., & Gordon, W. A. (1987). Impact of impairment on activity patterns of children. *Archives of Physical Medicine and Rehabilitation, 68,* 828–832.

Cochran, M. M., & Brassard, J. A. (1979). Child development and personal social networks. *Child Development, 50,* 601–616.

Coster, W. (1998). Occupation-centered assessment of children. *American Journal of Occupational Therapy, 52,* 337–344.

Cronin, A. F. (2000). Psychosocial and emotional domains. In J. Case-Smith (Ed.), *Occupational therapy for children* (pp. 413–452). St. Louis, MO: Mosby.

Dallas, E., Stevenson, J., & McGurk, H. (1993a). Cerebral-palsied children's interactions with siblings—I. Influence of severity of disability, age, and birth order. *Journal of Child Psychology and Psychiatry, 34,* 621–647.

Dallas, E., Stevenson, J., & McGurk, H. (1993b). Cerebral-palsied children's interactions with siblings—II. Interactional structure. *Journal of Child Psychology and Psychiatry, 34,* 649–671.

Dunn, W., Brown, C., & McGuigan, A. (1994). The ecology of human performance: A framework for considering the effect of context. *American Journal of Occupational Therapy, 48,* 595–607.

Feiring, C., & Lewis, M. (1989). The social networks of girls and boys from early through middle childhood. In D. Belle (Ed.), *Children's social networks and social supports* (pp. 119–150). New York: Wiley-Interscience.

Glaser, B. (1965). The constant comparative method of qualitative analysis. *Social Problems, 12,* 436–445.

Grenot-Scheyer, M., Staub, D., Peck, C. A., & Schwartz, I. S. (1998). Reciprocity and friendships: Listening to the voices of children and youth with and without disabilities. In L. H. Meyer, H. Park, M. Grenot-Scheyer, I. S. Schwartz, & B. Harry (Eds.), *Making friends: The influences of culture and development* (pp. 149–167). Baltimore: Brookes.

Hartup, W. W. (1979). The social worlds of childhood. *American Psychologist, 34,* 944–950.

Howes, C. (1988). Peer interaction of young children. *Monographs of the Society for Research in Child Development, 53*(1, Serial No. 217).

Kokkonen, J., Saukkonen, A. L., Timmonen, E., Serlo, W., & Kinnunen, P. (1991). Social outcome of handicapped children as adults. *Developmental Medicine and Child Neurology, 33,* 1095–1100.

Ladd, G. W. (1990). Having friends, keeping friends, making friends, and being liked by peers in the classroom: Predictors of children's early school adjustment? *Child Development, 61,* 1081–1100.

LaGreca, A. M. (1990). Social consequences of pediatric conditions: Fertile area for future investigation and intervention? *Journal of Pediatric Psychology, 15,* 285–307.

Law, M., Cooper, B., Strong, S., Stewart, D., Rigby, P., & Letts, L. (1996). The Person–Environment–Occupation model: A transactive approach to occupational performance. *Canadian Journal of Occupational Therapy, 63,* 9–23.

Law, M., & Dunn, W. (1993). Perspectives on understanding and changing the environments of children with disabilities. *Physical and Occupational Therapy in Pediatrics, 13*(3), 1–17.

Levitt, E., & Cohen, S. (1977). Parents as teachers: A rationale for involving parents in the education of their young handicapped children. In L. G. Katz (Ed.), *Current topics in early childhood education* (Vol. 1, pp. 165–178). Norwood, NJ: Ablex.

Lewis, M., Feiring, C., & Brooks-Gunn, J. (1988). Young children's social networks as a function of age and dysfunction. *Infant Mental Health Journal, 9,* 142–157.

Lightfoot, J., Wright, S., & Sloper, P. (1999). Supporting pupils in mainstream school with an illness or disability: Young people's views. *Child: Care, Health, and Development, 25,* 267–283.

Lincoln, Y. S., & Guba, E. G. (1985). *Naturalistic inquiry.* Beverly Hills, CA: Sage.

Meyer, L. H., Minondo, S., Fisher, M., Larson, M. J., Dunmore, S., Black, J. W., et al. (1998). Frames of friendship: Social relationships among adolescents with diverse abilities. In L. H. Meyer, H. Park, M. Grenot-Scheyer, I. S. Schwartz, &

B. Harry (Eds.), *Making friends: The influences of culture and development* (pp. 189–221). Baltimore: Brookes.

Miles, M. B., & Huberman, A. M. (1984). *Qualitative data analysis.* Newbury Park, CA: Sage.

Missiuna, C., & Pollock, N. (1991). Play deprivation in children with physical disabilities: The role of the occupational therapist in preventing secondary disability. *American Journal of Occupational Therapy, 45,* 882–888.

Mulderij, K. J. (1996). Research into the lifeworld of physically disabled children. *Child: Care, Health, and Development, 22,* 311–322.

Mulderij, K. J. (1997). Peer relations and friendship in physically disabled children. *Child: Care, Health, and Development, 23,* 379–389.

Nabors, L., & Badawi, M. (1997). Playground interactions for preschool-age children with special needs. *Physical and Occupational Therapy in Pediatrics, 17*(3), 21–31.

Philip, M., & Duckworth, D. (1982). *Children with disabilities and their families.* Windsor, UK: NFER-Nelson.

Richardson, P. K., Florey, L., & Greene, S. (2001). Facilitating social interactions in children with disabilities. *OT Practice, 6*(1), CE-1–CE-8.

Rubin, K. H., Fein, G. G., & Vandenberg, B. (1983). Play. In P. H. Mussen & E. M. Hetherington (Eds.), *Handbook of child psychology* (Vol. 4, pp. 693–774). New York: Wiley.

Salomon, M. K. (1983). Play therapy with the physically handicapped. In C. E. Schaeffer & K. J. O'Connor (Eds.), *Handbook of play therapy* (pp. 455–469). New York: Wiley.

Sheridan, M. D. (1975). The importance of spontaneous play in the fundamental learning of handicapped children. *Child: Care, Health, and Development, 1,* 3–17.

Snell, M. E., Janney, R., & Colley, K. M. (2000). Approaches for facilitating positive social relationships. In M. E. Snell & R. Janney (Eds.), *Social relationships and peer support* (pp. 35–77). Baltimore: Brookes.

Staub, D., Schwartz, I. S., Galluci, C., & Peck, C. A. (1994). Four portraits of friendship at an inclusive school. *Journal of the Association for Persons With Severe Disabilities, 19,* 314–325.

Stevens, S. E., Steele, C. A., Jutai, J. W., Kalnins, I. V., Bortolussi, J. A., & Biggar, W. D. (1996).

Adolescents with physical disabilities: Some psychosocial aspects of health. *Journal of Adolescent Health, 19*, 157–164.

Strain, P. S., & Smith, B. J. (1996). Developing social skills in young children with special needs. *Preventing School Failure, 41*, 24–27.

Strax, T. E. (1991). Psychological issues faced by adolescents and young adults with disabilities. *Pediatric Annals, 20*, 507–511.

Tietjen, A. M. (1989). The ecology of children's social support networks. In D. Belle (Ed.), *Children's social networks and social supports.* New York: Wiley-Interscience.

Van der Klift, E., & Kunc, N. (1994). Beyond benevolence: Friendship and the politics of help. In J. S. Thousand, R. A. Villa, & A. I. Nevin (Eds.), *Creativity and collaborative learning: A practical guide to empowering students and teachers* (pp. 391–401). Baltimore: Brookes.

Varni, J. W., Rubenfeld, L. A., Talbot, D., & Setoguchi, Y. (1989). Stress, social support, and depressive symptomatology in children with congenital/acquired limb deficiencies. *Journal of Behavioral Medicine, 15*(1), 31–44.

Varni, J. W., & Setoguchi, Y. (1991). Psychosocial factors in the management of children with limb deficiencies. *Physical Medicine and Rehabilitation Clinics of North America, 2*, 395–404.

Varni, J. W., Setoguchi, Y., Rappaport, L. R., & Talbot, D. (1992). Psychological adjustment and perceived social support in children with congenital/acquired limb deficiencies. *Journal of Behavioral Medicine, 15*, 31–44.

Wallander, J. L., Feldman, W. S., & Varni, J. W. (1989). Physical status and psychosocial adjustment in children with spina bifida. *Journal of Pediatric Psychology, 14*, 89–102.

Wallander, J. L., & Varni, J. W. (1989). Social support and adjustment in chronically ill and handicapped children. *American Journal of Community Psychology, 17*, 185–201.

Yerxa, E. J., Clark, F., Frank, G., Jackson, J., Parham, D., Pierce, D., et al. (1989). Occupational science: The foundation for new models of practice. *Occupational Therapy in Health Care, 6*(4), 1–17.

Yude, C., & Goodman, R. (1999). Peer problems of 9- to 11-year-old children with hemiplegia in mainstream schools: Can these be predicted? *Developmental Medicine and Child Neurology, 41*, 4–8.

CHAPTER 35

Perceptual–Motor Function of School-Age Children With Slow Handwriting Speed

Mei Hui Tseng and Susanna M. K. Chow

Mei Hui Tseng, ScD, OTR, *is associate professor, School of Occupational Therapy, College of Medicine, National Taiwan University, No. 7, Chung-Shan S. Road, Taipei, Taiwan 10016 ROC; mhtseng@ha.mc.ntu.edu.tw.*

Susanna M. K. Chow, BSc, MSc, MA, *is assistant professor, Department of Rehabilitation Sciences, Hong Kong Polytechnic University, Hong Kong.*

Proficiency in handwriting is essential if students are to accomplish an acceptable amount of work in the classroom and meet the standards of the teacher and the curriculum. Elementary school children typically spend up to 50% of the school day engaged in paper-and-pencil tasks (McHale & Cermak, 1992). Many of these tasks, including most tests and examination papers, are performed under time constraints (Amundson & Weil, 1996). Unfortunately, although a traditional instructional approach is sufficient for many children to become competent handwriters by 6 or 7 years of age, handwriting difficulties are common among children in both regular and special education classrooms (Bergman & McLaughlin, 1988). As a result, remediation of handwriting difficulties is one of the most important areas of school occupational therapy.

Handwriting, however, is a complex skill. It follows that, before more systematic ways of teaching children to write can be developed, the constellation of skills that are necessary for efficient writing will need to be better understood. Competent handwriting depends on the maturation and integration of cognitive, visual–perceptual, and fine motor skills (Maeland, 1992; Rubin & Henderson, 1982; Sovik, 1975; Tseng & Murray, 1994; Weil & Amundson, 1994; Ziviani, Hayes, & Chant, 1990). Handwriting requires finely graded manipulation of pencils to produce letter forms, in a fluent and ballistical manner, with a specific orientation and size, in a specific serial order, and in specific positions on a writing surface (van Galen, 1993). Further, according to Sovik and Arntzen (1991), fluent writing is produced by an integrated pattern of coordinated movements subject to visual monitoring and sensorimotor feedback. In support of this range of requirements, visual–motor integration was found to be the best predictor of legibility for both American and Norwegian children (Sovik, 1975) and for a group of Chinese school-age children (Tseng & Murray, 1994). Visual–perceptual skills, including visual–spatial perception, visual size discrimination, visual retrieval, and left–right orientation, enable children to distinguish visually

Originally published 2000 in *American Journal of Occupational Therapy, 54,* 83–88.

among graphic forms and to judge their correctness (Sovik, 1975; Thomassen & Teulings, 1983). Fine motor skills are also essential, because accurately formed letters can be produced only by the proper timing and force control of coordinated arm, hand, and finger movements (Alston & Taylor, 1987; Thomassen & Teulings, 1983).

Much also can be inferred from the various ways in which handwriters do not achieve functional competence. Handwriting can be deficient either in terms of legibility or in terms of speed. Common handwriting problems such as incorrect letter formation, poor alignment, reversals, uneven size of letters, irregular spacing between letters and words, and slow motor speed (Alston & Taylor, 1987; Johnson & Carlisle, 1996) do not necessarily arise from identical underlying mechanisms. Most studies to date, however, have focused primarily on the relationship between illegibility and various visual–perception skills, fine motor skills, and visual–motor integration (Alston & Taylor, 1987; Carlson & Cunningham, 1990; Cornhill & Case-Smith, 1996; Johnson & Carlisle, 1996; Maeland, 1992; Tseng & Murray, 1994). Illegible handwriting also has been investigated in connection with other functional deficiencies. For example, Levine, Oberklaid, and Meltzer (1981) not only found that 72% of 26 children with "developmental output failure" (low academic work output) had difficulty with fine motor tasks, they further postulated that these children's uncoordinated finger movements and diminished pencil control accounted for their "illegible and/or laborious, hesitant, and slow" (p. 20) handwriting.

Although slow handwriting speed often affects functional performance because it prevents students from meeting the time constraints involved in schoolwork (Amundson & Weil, 1996; Cermak, 1991; Levine et al., 1981; Oliver, 1990), few investigators have focused on this form of handwriting deficiency. Previous studies

include that of Berninger and Rutberg (1992), who contended that finger function is the best predictor of handwriting dysfunction in that fine motor skill accounted for 52.5% of the variance in handwriting speed. Sovik, Arntzen, and Teulings (1982) found that poor coordination in the form of poor dissociation (e.g., exaggerated wrist and thumb movement) was inversely correlated with writing speed. Curiously, although Hamstra-Bletz and Blote (1993) found no relationship between slow handwriting and dysgraphia, children with dyslexia were found to write more slowly than children without reading disabilities (Martlew, 1992). This suggests that visual–perception or cognitive skills might also affect handwriting speed.

In this chapter, we attempt to identify more clearly the factors associated with slow handwriting in the hope that this may help to elucidate the underlying mechanisms. Because inadequate attention span also has been clinically observed to impair handwriting proficiency (see also Levine et al., 1981, who found that 60% of their 26 low-productivity subjects also had serious difficulty concentrating), a vigilance test was included in the present study. We hypothesized that children with slow handwriting would obtain lower scores on a series of standard visual–perception, motor, visual–motor integration, and attention tests than did children with normal handwriting speeds.

Method

Participants

Teachers at two elementary schools in the greater Taipei area nominated 110 children from Grades 2 to 6 to participate in the study. On the basis of between 6 and 18 months of classroom observations, the teachers evaluated 71 children as slow handwriters and the other 39 as having normal handwriting speed.

To ensure the accuracy of these groupings, the 110 referrals were each given the Chinese Handwriting Speed Test (CHAST; Tseng & Hsueh, 1997). In this test, children copy a text in pencil from a previously studied Chinese textbook, and handwriting speed is expressed as the number of Chinese characters written per minute. Incompletely written characters (three or more strokes omitted) are not counted. Characters with added strokes are counted. The intraclass correlation coefficient (ICC) for retest reliability was .98 with a 1-week interval. In this study, the ICC for interrater reliability was .95.

Using one standard deviation below the norm as the cutoff point, the children who scored below the cutoff point for the CHAST were assigned to the slow handwriter group ($n = 34$), and the children who scored above the cutoff point were assigned to the normal-speed handwriting group ($n = 35$). Children whose teachers' evaluations of handwriting speed and CHAST scores were inconsistent ($n = 41$) did not take further part in the study.

All participants had been receiving handwriting instruction in Chinese characters since Grade 1 and had normal intellectual function according to their school reports. The age and handwriting speed of the two groups of children are shown in Table 35.1.

Instruments

Four measures, including three perceptual or motor tests and a vigilance test, were used in the present study. The Upper Limb Speed and Dexterity (ULSD) subtest of the Bruininks–Oseretsky Test of Motor Proficiency (BOTMP; Bruininks, 1978) was used to measure fine motor function. The BOTMP has been standardized on children ranging from 4.5 to 14.5 years of age. The ULSD subtest consists of eight items that involve placing pennies, sorting cards, stringing beads, displacing pegs, drawing vertical lines, and

Table 35.1. Age and Writing Speed of Slow Handwriters and Normal Speed Handwriters

Group	n	Mean Age (SD)	Mean Writing Speed (SD)
Slow handwriting			
Grade 2	4	84.8 (3.1)	3.6 (0.4)
Grade 3	8	101.3 (8.6)	4.5 (1.0)
Grade 4	12	109.1 (2.3)	8.9 (1.4)
Grade 5	5	125.4 (4.2)	9.0 (1.7)
Grade 6	5	135.6 (6.2)	9.3 (2.8)
Normal-speed handwriting			
Grade 2	7	87.4 (3.1)	7.6 (2.4)
Grade 3	9	103.9 (6.6)	13.3 (2.8)
Grade 4	8	113.6 (3.8)	15.2 (2.2)
Grade 5	5	120.4 (4.6)	18.7 (2.8)
Grade 6	6	133.2 (7.1)	22.0 (2.8)

Note. $N = 69$, where $n = 34$ for the slow handwriting group and $n = 35$ for the normal-speed handwriting group.

making dots. The test–retest reliability of the ULSD subtest was .89 for Grade 2 and .86 for Grade 6, with an interval of 7 to 12 days. The test–retest reliability ranged from .86 to .89, and the interrater reliability ranged from .79 to .97.

The Test of Visual–Perceptual Skills–Non-Motor (TVPS; Gardner, 1982), which measures nonmotor visual perception in children ranging from 4 years of age to 12 years, 11 months of age, was selected for the study because it covers a wide age range and examines various aspects of visual perception, including discrimination, memory, spatial relationships, form constancy, sequential memory, figure ground, and figure closure. It is also relatively easy to administer and score. The child is shown the test plates and is asked to point to the correct response from a series of choices. The TVPS has satisfactory internal consistency, with Cronbach's alpha ranging from .66 (visual discrimination) to .97 (visual closure).

The Developmental Test of Visual-Motor Integration (VMI; Beery, 1989), which consists of 24 geometric forms to be copied in sequence from a test booklet, was designed for children ranging from 2 to 15 years of age. The geometric forms become progressively more complex, and the points for each successive, correctly copied form are added to the child's score. Scores continue to accumulate either until all 24 forms have been copied or until three consecutive forms are copied incorrectly. The interrater reliability ranged from .58 to .99, and the test–retest reliability was .63 for an interval of 7 months and .92 for an interval of 2 weeks.

The Vigilance Task of the Gordon Diagnostic System (Gordon, 1991) was used to test the participant's ability to focus and maintain attention over time and in the absence of feedback. The task presents a series of digits at a rate of one per second. The child is told to press the response button whenever a "9" follows a "1." For the purpose of this study, the number of correct responses was totaled. Norms have been established on youngsters without hyperactivity who are 4 to 16 years of age ($n = 1,300$). Test–retest reliability was .68 to .85 with a 3-week interval.

Procedure

All children were tested one at a time in a separate, quiet room in the child's own school. The perceptual or motor tests and the Vigilance Task (Gordon, 1991) were administered consecutively, with a 3-min break between each. Testing took approximately 40 min to 50 min for each child.

Data Analysis

Because many of the tests or subtests used in the current study have not been normed on Chinese children, raw scores were used for analysis. A multivariate analysis of variance (MANOVA) was performed to compare the scores of the slow and normal-speed handwriting groups using the perceptual or motor measures and the Vigilance Task, and Pearson product-moment correlation was used to analyze the overall correlations. Stepwise regression analyses were performed to identify the best set of predictors, with handwrit-

ing speed entered as the dependent variable and the perceptual or motor measures and the Vigilance Task as predictor variables. Because the participants were drawn from Grades 2 to 6, age was also entered as a predictor in the regression analyses.

Results
Group Differences

The normal-speed handwriting group ($n = 35$) scored higher than the slow handwriting group ($n = 34$) on all measures (see Table 35.2). MANOVA revealed a significant difference between the two groups on all measures using Wilks's lambda [.59905, $F(10, 58) = 3.88193$, $p < .001$]. Except on the Visual Closure and Visual Discrimination subtests, all of the univariate F test values were significant at the .05 level.

Correlation Among Handwriting Speed, Age, and Test Results

Tables 35.3 and 35.4 present the overall correlation matrixes for the slow and normal-speed handwriting groups, respectively. Age, the ULSD, visual memory, and visual sequential memory were the only four measures that correlated significantly with handwriting speed for both groups of handwriters.

Regression Analysis

Stepwise regression was used to identify the strongest predictors of handwriting speed for each handwriting group. Handwriting speed was selected as the criterion variable; age, the ULSD, the seven visual–perceptual subtests, VMI, and the Vigilance Task were the predictor variables. Given the small number of participants ($n = 34$ in the slow handwriting group; $n = 35$ in the normal-speed handwriting group) relative to the number of predictor variables ($n = 11$), predictors with negligible correlations ($r < .20$) with handwriting

Table 35.2. Means, Standard Deviations, and Results of Univariate *F* Tests on Perceptual–Motor and Vigilance Tests for Slow and Normal-Speed Handwriters

Tests	Slow	Normal Speed	$F(1, 67)$	p
Upper Limb Speed and Dexterity subtest (Bruininks, 1978)			26.71	.0001
M		40.5	48.9	
SD	6.5	7.0		
Visual Discrimination			2.11	.151
M	13.7	14.3		
SD	1.9	1.2		
Visual Memory			12.58	.001
M	9.9	12.2		
SD	3.1	2.4		
Visual–Spatial Relation			10.86	.002
M	13.8	14.9		
SD	1.6	1.2		
Visual Form Constancy			11.28	.001
M	9.5	11.8		
SD	3.4	2.4		
Visual Sequential Memory			9.64	.003
M	11.2	13.3		
SD	3.2	2.4		
Visual Figure Ground			9.01	.004
M	10.1	12.6		
SD	3.7	3.1		
Visual Closure			0.92	.342
M	10.2	11.0		
SD	3.3	4.0		
Visual–Motor Integration			10.49	.002
M	22.8	29.9		
SD	9.1	9.3		
Vigilance			7.87	.007
M	38.5	41.8		
SD	5.4	4.4		

Note. n = 34 for slow handwriters; n = 35 for normal-speed handwriters.

speed were not included in the stepwise regression analysis.

For the slow handwriting group, the best predictors of handwriting speed were age, which accounted for 42.4% variance; visual sequential memory, accounting for 13.1%; and the VMI, accounting for 6.5% [$F(3, 30) = 16.2997$, $p < .0001$]. For the normal-speed handwriting group, only age and the ULSD were found to be

significant predictors. Age accounted for 64.4% of the variance, and the ULSD accounted for 9.95% of the variance in handwriting speed [$F(2, 32) = 46.296$, $p < .0001$].

Discussion

In this study, we found that, as a group, the slow handwriters performed less well than the normal-speed handwriters on all measures (see Table 35.2). For the Visual Discrimination test and the Visual Closure test, however, the difference between the groups was not significant. Perhaps the familiarity of the written text to participants—it contained characters that the children had already learned—taxed less heavily the basic visual-processing abilities of discrimination and closure. Task familiarity has been found to significantly influence handwriting speed (Dixon, Kurzman, & Friesen, 1993). Therefore, visual discrimination and visual closure may play a less important role in copying familiar texts.

Poor coordination or inadequate fine motor skills have often been invoked to explain slow handwriting speeds (Berninger & Rutberg, 1992; Levine et al., 1981; Lindsey & Beck, 1984; Sovik & Arntzen, 1991; Sovik et al., 1982). In this study as well, fine motor skill as measured by the ULSD was strongly correlated with handwriting speed in both groups (see Tables 35.3 and 35.4). However, the regression analysis showed that fine motor skill was an important predictor of handwriting speed only for the normal-speed handwriting group and not for the slow handwriting group. This suggests that two different mechanisms might underlie the handwriting performance of the two groups, with the slow handwriters relying more heavily on visual processing, especially sequential memory and visual–motor integration and the normal-speed handwriters' performance more related to upper-limb coordination.

Table 35.3. Correlation Matrix of Handwriting Speed, Age, Fine Motor Proficiency, Visual–Perceptual Measures, Visual–Motor Integration, and Vigilance for Slow Handwriters

Variable	1	2	3	4	5	6	7	8	9	10	11	12
1. Speed	—											
2. Age	.65***a	—										
3. Upper Limb Speed and Dexterity subtest (Bruininks, 1978)	.49**a	.25	—									
4. Visual discrimination	−.05	−.10	−.05	—								
5. Visual memory	.48**a	.28	.04	.01	—							
6. Visual spatial relations	.25a	.04	−.08	.57***	.25	—						
7. Visual form constancy	.18	.17	−.05	.38*	.46**	.33	—					
8. Visual sequential memory	.38*a	.03	.30	.17	.51**	.28	.18	—				
9. Figure ground	−.12	−.20	.09	.43*	.25	.32	.61***	.23	—			
10. Visual closure	.05	.08	−.14	.39*	.45**	.32	.58***	.35*	.45**	—		
11. Visual–motor integration	.29a	−.02	.18	.09	.31	.37*	.19	.12	.26	.32	—	
12. Vigilance	.31a	.09	.34	.16	.43*	.24	.37*	.31	.55**	.11	.23	—

Note: $n = 34$.
[a] Variables with $r > .2$ were tested as predictor variables in the regression analysis.
$*p < .05.$ $**p < .01.$ $***p < .001.$

The fact that visual sequential memory was the second best predictor for slow handwriters also might suggest that when intervention is required for slow handwriters, occupational therapy should be directed toward enhancing the memory for visual form and sequence. Although the present study examined Chinese handwriting, the importance of visual memory is similar to that reported in two studies on English written language in children with handwriting difficulties. Whereas Myklebust (1973) found these children had difficulties in mentally visualizing letters and words,

Table 35.4. Correlation Matrix of Handwriting Speed, Age, Fine Motor Proficiency, Visual–Perceptual Measures, Visual–Motor Integration, and Vigilance for Normal-Speed Handwriters

Variable	1	2	3	4	5	6	7	8	9	10	11	12
1. Speed	—											
2. Age	.80***a	—										
3. Upper Limb Speed and Dexterity subtest (Bruininks, 1978)	.78***a	.68***	—									
4. Visual discrimination	.09	.16	.33	—								
5. Visual memory	.53**a	.37*	.60***	.31	—							
6. Visual spatial relations	.23a	.19	.01	.08	.15	—						
7. Visual form constancy	.33a	.24	.32	.36*	.46**	.33	—					
8. Visual sequential memory	.45**a	.34*	.54**	.24	.46**	.18	.44**	—				
9. Figure ground	.37*a	.33*	.28	.29	.28	.26	.43*	.30	—			
10. Visual closure	.11	.03	.15	.17	.27	.14	.45**	.19	.38*	—		
11. Visual–motor integration	.42*a	.34*	.43**	.18	.49**	.32	.41*	.24	.51**	.37*	—	
12. Vigilance	.26a	.16	.36*	−.14	.37*	−.24	.04	.26	−.01	.30	.17	—

Note: $n = 35$.
[a] Variables with $r > .2$ were tested as predictor variables in the regression analysis.
$*p < .05.$ $**p < .01.$ $***p < .001.$

Levine et al. (1981) noted their impairment in memory retrieval for visual patterns and sequences. Although it is possible to speculate on the differences between the processing of Chinese (a logographic script) and English (an alphabetic script), Tzeng, Hung, Chen, Wu, and Hsi (1986) found overwhelming support from both a literature review and their own neurological studies of patients with brain damage that there are more similarities than differences in the processing of the two scripts. Both of the scripts, for example, are processed in the left brain hemisphere on the basis of their phonological characteristics.

The finding that handwriting speed was strongly correlated with age for both slow and normal-speed handwriters is consistent with previous studies (Hamstra-Bletz & Blote, 1990; Sovik, 1975; Tseng & Hsueh, 1997; Ziviani & Elkins, 1984). Increased handwriting speed follows naturally from the empirically observed fact that coordinated handwriting movements improve with age and schooling (Meulenbroek & van Galen, 1986; Sovik, 1993).

The finding that the slow handwriters performed more poorly in a laboratory measure of attention than the normal-speed handwriters supports clinical observations of a strong relationship between slow handwriting and teachers' ratings of inattention. This finding also suggests that a possible component of slow handwriting stems from difficulties with maintaining vigilance under unstimulating conditions. Helping parents and teachers to promote an optimal arousal level to facilitate attention span deserves occupational therapists' serious consideration when working with children with slow graphomotor output.

Conclusion

This study was not an attempt to examine the relationship of quality or speed to handwriting performance. Quality and speed are important, and both should be addressed as valid and independent indicators of handwriting performance. This study is perhaps one of the few that examined slow handwriters and found that these children, as a group, were poorer than children with normal speed handwriting in graphomotor output, in level of perceptual–motor skills and proficiencies, and in attention.

Results of regression analyses showed that the slow handwriting group was not just slower than the normal-speed handwriting group: They were qualitatively different in the way they processed written information. The performance of the slow handwriters seemed to heavily depend on visual processing, whereas that of the normal-speed handwriters was motor based. Findings of this study suggest that intervention for slow handwriters should focus on facilitating visual processing, including memory and visual–motor integration, rather than the fine motor training so often emphasized in occupational therapy programs.

Acknowledgments

We thank those participating teachers and children from Tong-man Elementary School and Ji-shin Elementary School. This study was supported through funding awarded to the first author by the National Science Council, NSC 86-2314-B-002-236.

References

Alston, J., & Taylor, J. (1987). *Handwriting: Theory, research, and practice.* New York: Croom Helm.

Amundson, S. J., & Weil, M. (1996). Prewriting and handwriting skills. In J. Case-Smith, A. S. Allen, & P. N. Pratt (Eds.), *Occupational therapy for children* (pp. 524–541). St. Louis, MO: Mosby.

Beery, K. E. (1989). *The Developmental Test of Visual–Motor Integration* (3rd ed.). Cleveland, OH: Modern Curriculum Press.

Bergman, K. E., & McLaughlin, T. F. (1988). Remediating handwriting difficulties with learning disabled students: A review. *B. C. Journal of Special Education, 12,* 101–120.

Berninger, V. W., & Rutberg, J. (1992). Relationship of finger function to beginning writing: Application to diagnosis of writing disabilities. *Developmental Medicine and Child Neurology, 34,* 198–215.

Bruininks, R. H. (1978). *Bruininks–Oseretsky Test of Motor Proficiency.* Circle Pines, MN: American Guidance Service.

Carlson, K., & Cunningham, J. (1990). Effect of pencil diameter on the graphomotor skill of preschoolers. *Early Childhood Research Quarterly, 5,* 279–293.

Cermak, S. (1991). Somatosensory dyspraxia. In A. Fisher, E. A. Murray, & A. C. Bundy (Eds.), *Sensory integration: Theory and practice* (pp. 138–170). Philadelphia: F. A. Davis.

Cornhill, H., & Case-Smith, J. (1996). Factors that relate to good and poor handwriting. *American Journal of Occupational Therapy, 50,* 732–739.

Dixon, R. A., Kurzman, D., & Friesen, I. C. (1993). Handwriting performance in younger and older adults: Age, familiarity, and practice effects. *Psychology and Aging, 8,* 360–370.

Gardner, M. F. (1982). *Test of Visual Perceptual Skills.* Seattle, WA: Special Child Publications.

Gordon, M. (1991). *Instruction Manual for the Gordon Diagnostic System* (GDS) *Model III–R.* DeWitt, NY: Gordon Systems.

Hamstra-Bletz, L., & Blote, A. W. (1990). Development of handwriting in primary school: A longitudinal study. *Perceptual and Motor Skills, 70,* 759–770.

Hamstra-Bletz, L., & Blote, A. W. (1993). A longitudinal study on dysgraphic handwriting in primary school. *Journal of Learning Disabilities, 26,* 689–699.

Johnson, D. J., & Carlisle, J. F. (1996). A study of handwriting in written stories of normal and learning disabled children. *Reading and Writing, 8,* 45–59.

Levine, M. D., Oberklaid, F., & Meltzer, L. (1981). Developmental output failure: A study of low productivity in school-aged children. *Pediatrics, 67,* 18–25.

Lindsey, J. D., & Beck, F. W. (1984). Handwriting and the classroom experience: A recapitulation. *The Pointer, 29,* 29–31.

Maeland, A. F. (1992). Handwriting and perceptual-motor skills in clumsy, dysgraphic, and "normal" children. *Perceptual and Motor Skills, 75,* 1207–1217.

Martlew, M. (1992). Handwriting and spelling: Dyslexic children's abilities compared with children of the same chronological age and younger children of the same spelling level. *British Journal of Educational Psychology, 62,* 375–390.

McHale, K., & Cermak, S. (1992). Fine motor activities in elementary school: Preliminary findings and provisional implications for children with fine motor problems. *American Journal of Occupational Therapy, 46,* 898–903.

Meulenbroek, R. G. J., & van Galen, G. P. (1986). Movement analysis of repetitive writing behaviour of first, second, and third grade primary school children. In H. S. R. Kao, G. P. van Galen, & R. Hoosain (Eds.), *Computer recognition and human production of handwriting* (pp. 273–286). Singapore: World Scientific.

Myklebust, H. R. (1973). *Development and disorders of written language: Vol. 2. Studies of normal and exceptional children.* New York: Grune & Stratton.

Oliver, C. E. (1990). A sensorimotor program for improving writing readiness skills in elementary age children. *American Journal Occupational Therapy, 44,* 111–116.

Rubin, N., & Henderson, S. E. (1982). Two sides of the same coin: Variations in teaching methods and failure to learn to write. *Special Education: Forward Trends, 9,* 17–24.

Sovik, N. (1975). *Developmental cybernetics of handwriting and graphic behavior.* Oslo, Norway: Universitetsforlaget.

Sovik, N. (1993). *Development of children's writing performance: Some educational implications.* In A. F. Kalverboer, B. Hopkins, & R. Geuze (Eds.), *Motor development in early and later childhood: Longitudinal approaches* (pp. 229–246). New York: Cambridge University Press.

Sovik, N., & Arntzen, O. (1991). A developmental study of the relation between the movement patterns in letter combinations (words) and writing. In J. Wann, A. M. Wing, & N. Sovik (Eds.),

Development of graphic skills: Research perspective and educational implications (pp. 77–89). New York: Academic Press.

Sovik, N., Arntzen, O., & Teulings, H. L. (1982). Interactions among overt process parameters in handwriting motion and related graphic production. *Journal of Human Movement Studies, 8,* 103–122.

Thomassen, J. W. M., & Teulings, H. M. (1983). The development of handwriting. In M. Martlew (Ed.), *The psychology of written language: Developmental and educational perspectives* (pp. 179–213). New York: Wiley.

Tseng, M. H., & Hsueh, I. P. (1997). Performance of school-aged children on a Chinese Handwriting Speed Test. *Occupational Therapy International, 4,* 294–303.

Tseng, M. H., & Murray, E. A. (1994). Differences in perceptual–motor measures in children with good and poor handwriting. *Occupational Therapy Journal of Research, 14,* 19–36.

Tzeng, O. J. L, Hung, D. L., Chen, S., Wu, J., & Hsi, M. S. (1986). Processing Chinese logographs by Chinese brain-damaged patients. In H. S. R. Kao, G. P. van Galen, & R. Hoosain (Eds.), *Graphonomics: Contemporary research in handwriting* (pp. 357–374). Amsterdam: North Holland.

van Galen, G. P. (1993). Handwriting: A developmental perspective. In A. F. Kalverboer, B. Hopkins, & R. Geuze (Eds.), *Motor development in early and later childhood: Longitudinal approaches* (pp. 217–228). New York: Cambridge University Press.

Weil, M. J., & Amundson, S. J. C. (1994). Relationship between visuomotor and handwriting skills of children in kindergarten. *American Journal of Occupational Therapy, 48,* 982–988.

Ziviani, J., & Elkins, J. (1984). An evaluation of handwriting performance. *Educational Review, 36,* 249–261.

Ziviani, J., Hayes, A., & Chant, D. (1990). Handwriting: A perceptual motor disturbance in children with myelomeningocele. *Occupational Therapy Journal of Research, 10,* 12–26.

VI
Scholarship of Discovery:
Parental Hopes, Experiences, Perspectives, Routines, and Shifts

CHAPTER 36

Parental Hopes for Therapy Outcomes

Children With Sensory Modulation Disorders

Ellen Cohn, Lucy Jane Miller, and Linda Tickle-Degnen

Ellen Cohn, ScD, OTR/L, FAOTA, *is lecturer, Boston University, Sargent College, 635 Commonwealth Avenue, Boston, MA 02215.*

Lucy Jane Miller, PhD, OTR, *is assistant professor, University of Colorado Health Sciences Center, Department of Pediatrics, Denver.*

Linda Tickle-Degnen, PhD, OTR/L, *is assistant professor, Department of Occupational Therapy, Boston University, Sargent College of Health and Rehabilitation Services, Boston.*

The Individuals With Disabilities Education Act of 1990 mandates family-centered care for children and families with special health care needs (U.S. Department of Education, 1995). This legislation places families at the core of the intervention process and acknowledges the influence of families in their children's development. Numerous authors in the occupational therapy literature have advocated a family-centered care approach (Brown, Humphry, & Taylor, 1997; Burke & Schaaf, 1997; Cohn & Cermak, 1998; Humphry & Case-Smith, 1996; Lawlor & Mattingly, 1998; Miller & Hanft, 1998), arguing that successful intervention requires sensitivity to the perspectives of families. Specifically, providing family-centered services requires that professionals understand the hopes and outcomes desired by families who seek services. Listening to parents' hopes for therapy outcomes is one way to understand the personal meaning that parents attach to the therapy process (Spencer, Davidson, & White, 1997).

The importance of honoring parents' perspectives on outcomes of occupational therapy for their children was highlighted by Dunn (1994) and Parham and Mailloux (1996), and by Bundy (1991) specifically in relation to sensory integration treatment approaches. Parents have provided ardent testimonials that occupational therapy with sensory integration treatment approaches improves quality of life for their family (Anderson & Emmons, 1995; Occupational Therapy Associates, P. C., 1995). Other occupational therapy literature discusses parental views of experiences related to early intervention using other treatment approaches (Case-Smith & Nastro, 1993; Hinojosa, 1990; Hinojosa & Anderson, 1991; Miller & Hanft, 1998).

This study explored parents' hopes for occupational therapy outcomes for children with sensory modulation disorders (SMD), which manifest as an inability to react to sensory stimulation in a manner appropriate to task demands, environmental contexts, social supports, and cultural expectations (Ayres, 1972;

Originally published 2000 in *American Journal of Occupational Therapy,* 54, 36–43.

McIntosh, Miller, Shyu, & Hagerman, submitted; Parham & Mailloux, 1996): Clinically, persons with SMD present as hyporesponsive or hyperresponsive, or as having labile reactions to sensation (Dunn, 1997; Kinnealey, 1973). By understanding parents' priorities for treatment outcomes for children with SMD, occupational therapists can design intervention and research programs that are congruent with parents' hopes and values.

Method

To research parents' priorities for therapy outcomes, we used a qualitative research methodology: a collective case study approach (Stake, 1994). In qualitative research traditions, researchers are urged to locate themselves in the research process to explore their assumptions and use them productively to interpret findings (Maxwell, 1996; Reay, 1996; Riessman, 1994). As researchers, we each brought individual perspectives; however, it was our common perspective as occupational therapists that shaped the study. As clinicians providing occupational therapy using a sensory integration treatment approach, we have frequently heard anecdotal accounts of the importance of focusing on parents' stated outcomes for their children and their families. However, empirical examination of which outcomes are important to parents has not been documented. As parents, we have firsthand experience living with and parenting children; we believe that successful occupational therapy must be linked to the daily functioning of both the child and the family unit and the meaning and hopes parents attach to the therapy process. We are committed to a top-down approach to evaluation (Trombly, 1993, 1995), beginning with identification of parents' beliefs systems, expectations of their children, and image of family functioning.

Data for this study were generated as part of an ongoing program of research measuring the effectiveness of occupational therapy in treating children identified with SMD at The Children's Hospital in Denver, Colorado. Consistent with a top-down approach to evaluation, the pretreatment interview focused on understanding the daily occupations of children and their families and their hopes for therapy outcomes. The pretreatment intake procedure included a thorough semistructured interview of parents, which was videotaped, audiotaped, and transcribed. Additionally, several standardized assessments were administered, including the Sensory Integration and Praxis Test (ages 5–9) (SIPT; Ayres, 1989) or the Miller Assessment for Preschoolers (ages 4–5) (MAP; Miller, 1988); FirstSTEP (ages 4–5) (Miller, 1993); the Short Sensory Profile (SSP; McIntosh, Miller, & Shyu, in press); and the Child Behavior Checklist (CBCL; Achenbach, 1991). Inclusion criteria for the larger research program were scores < −3 standard deviations on the SSP, characteristics indicative of SMD during administration of standardized scales, and concerns related to sensory processing and related daily living tasks on the clinical interview. Based on the results of these evaluations, children were admitted to the research study.

For this study of parental hopes, five videotaped interviews were randomly selected from the 17 videotaped interviews that had been administered at the time of this study. The five videotapes include interviews with eight parents (three couples and two single parents). Table 36.1 presents demographic information about the parents and their children. Two children lived with their adoptive parents and three children lived with their biological parents. The children varied in ethnicity; however, all of the parents were White. Table 36.2 presents standardized scores of the five children on the SIPT or MAP, the SSP, and the CBCL.

Table 36.1. Demographics of Children and Their Parents

Child's Name[a]	Gender	Age	Ethnicity of Child	Parent's Education
Harry	M	6	Asian	College
Monique	F	8	White	Postgraduate
Joanna	F	5	African-American	< High school
Kisha	F	6	Hispanic	High school
Adam	M	4	White	College

[a]Pseudonym.

Interviews

Parent interviews ranged from 45 min to 60 min and began with the question, "Tell me about (child's name). Talk about what is wonderful or special about (child's name)." The interview included 11 structured questions (see Appendix), but because the interview process was flexible, probes were added, wording was modified, and additional queries or explanations were provided as needed to clarify, explore, or extend information pertaining to parents' views, concerns, and hopes for their children.

Data Analysis

We explored the cases collectively, using grounded theory procedures (i.e., constant comparative method) recommended by Strauss and Corbin (1990). Transcripts were subjected to open coding—the naming and categorizing of phenomena—for themes that related to parents' hopes for therapy outcomes. The open codes or categories were compared and contrasted to detect similarities and differences across the five cases. Categories that represent dimensions of overlap with each other were grouped and analyzed using axial coding. This process binds information in new ways, suggesting relationships and variations among categories (Strauss & Corbin, 1990). From this step emerged the two core categories of our analysis, *child-focused* outcomes and *parent-focused* outcomes.

After creating conceptual categories, we analyzed the relationships between the key categories to generate ideas about phenomena (Strauss & Corbin, 1990). Thus, in the selective coding phase of our data analysis, the core categories were refined and validated by selecting and systematically relating the two primary categories to other possible groupings. We then constructed a taxonomy for classifying parental hopes related to outcomes of occupational therapy for their children and themselves.

To confirm that our interpretations reflected the participants' perspectives, we conducted member checks, testing the validity of our conceptual categories. The categories were further refined based on participants' feedback. The final analytic categories were reviewed by a group of experienced occupational therapy researchers and by a group of sociology doctoral students, both of whom were familiar with grounded theory analysis. Both groups reviewed transcripts and confirmed the researchers' open coding and category construction.

Findings and Interpretations

When asked to identify their hopes and expectations for therapy, parents spoke about three outcomes for therapy that focused on changes in their children. In addition, parents identified two outcomes focused on themselves or their families, viewing themselves as both change agents for their children and recipients of service and support. Findings for each of the two core categories, child-focused outcomes and parent-focused outcomes, are detailed below.

Child-Focused Outcomes

Social participation. Parents in the study wanted their children to develop behaviors and skills needed to "fit in," to belong, and to be included at school and in their communities. They hoped

Table 36.2. Results of Children's Scores in Four Standardized Scales

Participant	Sensory Integration and Praxis Tests			Short Sensory Profile			Child Behavior Checklist	
	<–1 SD	±1 SD	>+1 SD	<–1 SD	±1 SD	>+1 SD	<–1 SD	±1 SD
Harry	KIN LTS	SV, FG FI, GRA DC, MAC CPr, OPr SPr SWB PRN	PrVC	TS TSS UR/SS AF LEW	VAS MT		Internalizing Attn Prob Externalizing Aggressive	Withdrawn Somatic Anx/Depres Social Prob Thought Prob Delinquent
Monique	KIN SWB PRN	SV, FG PPr, CPr MFP, LTS FI, GRA SPr DC, BMC PrVC, PPr	MAC	TS UR/SS AF VAS	TSS LEW MS		Anx/Depres Thought Prob Attn Prob Externalizing Delinquent Aggressive	Internalizing Withdrawn Somatic Social Prob
Joanna	GRA SPr BMC SWB MAC PRN	SV, FG LTS KIN CPr, OPr PPr, PrVC DC FI	MFP	TS UR/SS AF VAS LEW	MS	TSS	Thought Prob Attn Prob Social Prob Externalizing Aggressive	Internalizing Withdrawn Somatic Anx/Depres Delinquent
Kisha	KIN GRA BMC PRN	SV PPr, PrVC CPr, OPr MFP, LTS DC, MAC FI SWB	FG	TS UR/SS AF VAS	TSS LEW MS		Anx/Depres Delinquent Thought Prob Attn Prob Social Prob Externalizing Aggressive	Internalizing Withdrawn Somatic
Adama				TS TSS UR/SS AF VAS LEW	MS		Internalizing Withdrawn Somatic Thought Prob Attn Prob Social Prob	Anx/Depres Externalizing Delinquent Aggressive

Note. Sensory Integration and Praxis Tests: BMC = bilateral motor coordination; CPr = constructional praxis; DC = design copying; FG = figure–ground perception; FI = finger identification; GRA = graphesthesia; KIN = kinesthesia; LTS = localization of tactile stimuli; MAC = motor accuracy; MFP = manual form perception; OPr = oral praxis; PPr = postural praxis; PRN = postrotary nystagmus; PrVC = praxis on verbal command; SPr = sequencing praxis; SV = space visualization; SWB = standing and walking balance. Short Sensory Profile: AF = auditory filtering; LEW = low energy/weak; MS = movement sensitivity; TS = tactile sensitivity; TSS = taste/smell sensitivity; UR/SS = underresponsive/seeks sensation; VAS = visual/auditory sensitivity. Child Behavior Checklist: Aggressive = aggressive behavior; Anx/Depres = anxious/depressed; Attn Prob = attention problems; Delinquent = delinquent behavior; Externalizing = externalizing; Internalizing = internalizing; Social Prob = social problems; Somatic = somatic complaints; Thought Prob = thought problems; Withdrawn = withdrawn.
[a]Miller Assessment for Preschoolers: Total score = 2%; Foundations Index = 1%; Coordination Index = 1%; Verbal Index = 1%; Nonverbal Index = 53%; Complex Tasks = 1%.

that their children would learn appropriate ways to behave so they could conform to the cultural norms of their daily living contexts. Comments such as "We'd like her to be able to sit in a classroom situation and learn" or "We want him to be successful in school" highlighted parents' perceptions of the importance of the school context. One mother specifically identified community as a valued context. She stated, "I would like to be able to take him to the grocery store without him high-jumping off my shoulder." Social participation also included relationships with same-age peers, with siblings, and with other children. One parent stated that having friends and "being socially OK" were major concerns. Another noted the difference between her child's inability and her niece's ability to interact with a baby. She expressed her hopes:

Tamara [her niece] has the ability to sit down…and sit by the baby and be real quiet and just ask questions and look at the baby and touch the baby. Joanna's bouncing and jumping, and I'm afraid she is going to fall on the baby. I mean, it's a totally different thing.

Coster (1998) defined the construct of social participation as "active engagement in the typical activities available to and/or expected of peers in the same context" (p. 341). In this study, Coster's construct describes the parents' highest priority for outcomes: that parents hope that their children will be "able to orchestrate engagement in occupations in a given context that are positive, personally satisfying and acceptable to adults in society who are responsible for children" (p. 340). Valued contexts that the parents in the present study identified included school, home, and the community.

Self-regulation. Parents hoped that their children would develop coping mechanisms to self-regulate their behavior. Adam's mother said, "It is a good thing for children to have self-control and regulate themselves." Although Harry's mother hoped that Harry ultimately would be able to regulate his own hyperactive behaviors, she suggested that if Harry could learn to seek help from others, that could be a useful strategy as well. She expressed a desire for Harry to learn to channel his hyperactivity:

I don't expect for [the hyperactivity] to go away, because I think it is so high right now, and it's just part of [him]. But some way to be able to have him know how to channel that, so it can get down to a level that's acceptable, for instance, in school. That would be really nice. Some overflow into being able to feel how he is feeling and whether he's feeling jittery and what to do about that, where he might be flying off the handle. If he could kind of get a grasp on that, verbally or somehow emotionally, so that he can either tell me, tell the teacher, get some help somehow, or be able to do it himself.

Harry's mother yearned for him to recognize how he feels, to develop a range of options to seek the assistance he needs, and to learn how to regulate his own behavior in the valued context of school.

Kisha's mother expressed a desire for Kisha to learn "to be cognizant" of her own behavior to develop self-control. Kisha's mother hoped that the self-control would generalize to other situations.

I would like to see her be able to stop and realize the consequences of her behavior and change her behavior. There are times she is totally out of control, and she is not cognizant of what she is doing. She doesn't understand why I am so upset when she has been screaming for 2 hours. I would like to see her control that. I know she wants to….So once she learns to control one thing, she is going to say, oh, maybe this can apply here.

Perceived competence. Monique's mother linked establishing internal feelings of self-confidence to Monique's ability to regulate her behavior. She hoped that Monique's recognition of her ability to help herself would lead to greater perceived competence in the context of her emergence as a young woman.

> At this point in Monique's life, when she is about to turn 9, she's entering a time in a young woman's life that is one of the most difficult… the more we can understand about her, the more she can help us to help herself. If it gives her some self-confidence or additional tools to work with on her own when she's not around us, she can say, "I can help myself here, and I feel good about myself."

Trombly (1995) defined *competency* as a sense of satisfaction with one's own implementation of the tasks associated with valued roles. These parents hoped that their children would feel satisfaction with themselves. That is, they hoped that their children would get pleasure from what they themselves were able to do and who they were as people. One mother stated,

> What I want for Harry is, like, happiness or contentment or satisfaction with himself…it is bigger than just self-confidence but includes self-confidence…I wish he could get pleasure from what he himself can do and who he is as a person.

Two themes identified in our study were consistent with valued outcomes identified by Anderson (1993) in her study of parental perceptions of the influence of sensory integration therapy for children with autism. The parents in Anderson's study reported that their children made gains in socialization with other children (social participation) and in their ability to express emotions and desires (self-regulation).

Parent-Focused Outcomes

The parents discussed desired changes for themselves, identifying two interrelated roles: provider of support for their children and recipients of validation as parents for themselves. These parent-focused hopes can best be understood when intervention is viewed as a collaborative process, co-constructed by parents and therapists.

Learn strategies to support the child. The parents in the present study saw themselves as providers of support for their children. In this role, they hoped to become collaborators, combining efforts with occupational therapists to assist children. Ruddick (1989) proposed that one of the major tasks of parenting is to "shape children's growth in 'acceptable' ways" (p. 21), *acceptable* being defined by the cultural context of the family. The parents who were interviewed specifically asked for techniques that they could use to help their children calm down or self-regulate. Because Adam was only 4 years of age, his parents indicated that they were seeking tools to soothe him: "I think if we are just able to learn some techniques to help him calm down."

Many of the parents suggested that understanding their children's behavior would help them to support their child's growth. Monique's mother said, "The more we can understand about her, the more she can help us to be able to help herself." Drawing on the metaphor of "living with an alcoholic," Kisha's mother described her frustration in living with Kisha's unpredictable behavior and wanted to understand what triggered Kisha's behavior.

> She's very moody, it's like living with an alcoholic. You never know. That's the scary part. I still have not been able to figure it out, although I am starting to get clues…as to…what triggers it.

Understanding their children's behavior was a dominant theme among the parents and was consistent with Anderson's finding that parents value understanding their children's behavior from a sensory integration frame of reference.

Personal validation. Closely related to receiving support for parenting their children, the parents hoped that therapists would understand the challenges of living with children with SMD. Joanna's mother stated, "I just can't take it anymore," and Adam's mother said, "He is affecting our lives and everybody around us… he's bouncing off the walls and we can't get him to stop…it's exhausting." In a member check interview, Harry's mother declared,

> I want confirmation that I'm not "weird," that Harry isn't "bad," that there are other children like Harry, that his problems are "real" and not just in my head. I want to be accepted and bolstered for what I do for Harry rather than people thinking that I'm a bad mother.

These parents wanted to understand their children. They also wanted therapists to understand their experience of parenting a child with SMD. The parents hoped that this combination of learning tools to help their child, and being understood and accepted themselves, coupled with the child's improvement in social participation, self-regulation, and perceived competence, would ultimately facilitate sustainable family routines.

> We ultimately want to make it easier to live together as a family.…If Harry is getting better, and I am getting tools to help Harry, and I'm getting confirmation that what I'm doing is OK, then the life of our whole family will get better.

Based on interviews with families with a young child who exhibited developmental delays, Gallimore, Weisner, Kaufman, and Bernheimer (1989) hypothesized that the key adaptation task for the family is organizing daily routines so that they are sustainable, meaningful, and congruent

with the individual needs of family members and with family themes. The families in the Gallimore et al. study constructed and sustained meaningful routines to provide proper care, supervision, and stimulation for their children. Embracing a systems perspective, Gallimore and colleagues noted that the well-being of the family depends on the functioning of the whole system as well as the functioning of each family member. Their data showed that intervention with children with special needs can be effective only when the interventions are sustainably integrated into the routines of the family.

In our study, Joanna's mother wanted therapy to improve the consistency of her daughter's behavior. She wanted to be able "to know that I can count on my daughter." As reported above, another parent wanted to take her child to the grocery store, and yet another parent wanted to feel "OK" about her child being near a baby cousin. These are all examples of the parent's desire to see changes in their child's behavior so that family routines can be sustained.

Parental hopes for therapy outcomes are embedded in contexts in which their children live, learn, and play, as depicted by Figure 36.1. The figure also depicts the child-focused and parent-focused outcomes derived from this study, including the following:

- *Child-focused outcomes:* social participation, self-regulation, and perceived competence
- *Parent-focused outcomes:* strategies to support child and personal validation.

Theoretical Validity of Interpretations

To address the theoretical validity of our interpretations, we searched the interviews for themes other than the five identified and for themes specifically related to processing sensation. In

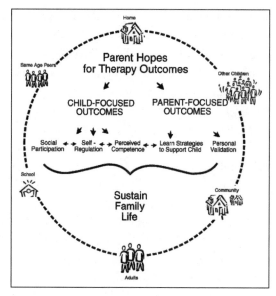

Figure 36.1. Parental hopes for therapy outcomes.

the interview, parents were asked to describe their children's reaction to sensory stimulation, including olfactory, auditory, visual, tactile, taste, and movement stimuli. We selected these questions based on the assumption that because these children were identified as having SMD, we expected that the sensory problems inherent in SMD would be evident in the parental concerns and hopes for their children. However, reexamination of data generated by the question "How does your child respond to sensory stimuli?" revealed that parents' responses were framed in terms of social participation, self-regulation, and perceived competence. For example, Harry's mother noted that his tactile defensiveness interfered with his social relationships with other children.

> He is a child that doesn't like light touch…he is tactile defensive.…When children are around him, they kind of bustle or touch him in the hallway; that's very annoying to him, and it increases his activity level and sometimes increases his aggressiveness. However, he also needs to touch other children. So he constantly

has his hands diddling in the desk of the person next to him.

As a physical therapist, Harry's mother used clinical language (e.g., "tactile defensiveness"), yet she immediately embedded Harry's behavior in the occupational tasks of peer relationships.

She elaborated when she discussed Harry's reactions to auditory stimuli, describing how his sensitivity to such stimuli interfered with his ability to attend a sporting event and have social relationships.

> An overall crowd noise, a background noise, increases his activity level. It makes him angry or more emotionally labile.…A sporting event is pretty difficult for him. He can't go with friends.

Monique's mother also responded to questions about sensory sensitivity by describing functional activities of daily living, such as, "Monique must have the tags cut out of her clothes." She mentioned Monique's preference for cotton and terrycloth clothes but quickly shifted the conversation to behavioral concerns. She explained that Monique fixated on something that she wanted to buy, eat, or do and constantly talked about it. To regulate her own behavior, Monique liked to know what was going to happen next. Although Monique's mother began with information about Monique's sensory processing, she quickly transitioned to concerns about self-regulation and strategies that would help Monique enjoy activities.

Adam's mother also shifted her responses to questions about sensory processing to functional concerns. In response to the question, "Is he sensitive to tags and other things?" Adam's mother talked about his behavioral rigidity.

> I haven't had to take tags out of everything, just the ones that he can feel, he will complain about. Yesterday morning, he went to change his underwear. He looked and he said, "flowers,

Fruit of the Loom," and he gets the other pair of underwear and he puts them right next to each other, "flowers." And then they were OK to put on. Rigidity like that.

Instead of the question about clothing tags eliciting a concern about sensory processing, it evoked a story about Adam's rigid behavior.

These stories illustrate our overall finding that parents of children with SMD are primarily concerned about their children's social behaviors and that sensory concerns are addressed within the context of functional behaviors. Parents rarely talked about their children in terms of the sensory components of function. For example, they did not say, "My child is unable to discriminate tactile input." Instead, the language the parents used embedded performance components (such as tactile discrimination) in the context of everyday occupations.

A thorough review of the five transcripts to search for discrepant data (i.e., data that could not be categorized as social participation, self-regulation, or perceived competence) revealed only one discussion related to the skill of balancing. Monique's father shared that a therapist had told him that his daughter had trouble closing her eyes and balancing at the same time. Although all children had been assessed by an occupational therapist prior to the parent interview, and the therapists' review of findings with parents may have educated parents about their child's clinical issues, the preponderance of parent responses during their interview related to their child's daily occupations.

These findings provide a useful framework for thinking about evaluation, intervention, and outcomes of children with SMD that are meaningful to our consumers. It should be noted that this information relates to only five families with children identified with SMD and may not represent all parents of children with SMD. Further, the multidimensional contributions of temporal,

socioeconomic, and cultural factors on parents' hopes for therapy outcomes were not analyzed for this study and might provide meaningful information related to parents' hopes for therapy outcomes in future studies.

Implications for Practice

The findings highlight the import of understanding parents' realities and the contexts in which children live. Children with SMD have complex and multiple needs extending beyond their sensory processing abilities. This study documents that parents of children with SMD highly value their children's abilities to participate in the contexts in which they live, to self-regulate reactions, and to feel competent.

The study design and findings provide information that will be helpful to occupational therapy practitioners striving to follow recommendations by Coster (1998) and Trombly (1993), who urged therapists to use a top-down approach to the evaluation process, beginning with the occupations the person needs and wishes to perform. Further, our findings imply that these parents seemed to intuitively believe Rogoff's postulate (1990) that, for children, successful management of occupational tasks and participation in society depends on adults and children structuring the environment. Thus, attending to parents' concerns and how they structure their environment to sustain family life is advised.

In practice, the assessments therapists choose and the outcomes they measure are operational definitions for their priorities for change in intervention (Haley, 1994). If therapists begin evaluations with performance components, they may miss meaningful outcomes such as social participation for children and their families. The challenge is to evaluate social participation, self-regulation, and perceived competence in important contexts. Examples of assessments that may be useful for documenting change in the occupational domains mentioned by parents in this study are The School Function Assessment (Coster, Deeney, Haltiwanger, & Haley, 1998), which measures social participation in the school setting; the Child Behavior Checklist (Achenbach, 1991), which measures self-regulation; and the Piers–Harris Children's Self-Concept Scale (Piers, 1984), which measures self-concept. Documenting changes related to parenting occupations is also recommended (see Cohn & Cermak, 1998, for a review of assessments related to the family system).

Given the insights from this research, we recommend that therapists strive to understand issues that are crucial to parents of children seeking occupational therapy services. Knowledge about parents' priorities depends on understanding what behavior, events, persons, or routines mean to those who partake of them. Meanings cannot be assumed. To understand a family's values, goals, and aspirations for their child and themselves, therapists must listen carefully to family members' perspectives. Therapists should ask parents to describe hopes for treatment outcomes and how they will know if therapy is successful. Queries might include, "What are you hoping will be different about your child as a result of therapy?" or "What do you anticipate treatment will do for you or your family?" Using parents' language, rather than clinical language, will help communicate to families that their perspective is respected. Asking parents to describe their family and what they enjoy doing together or asking about family routines may provide valuable insights into the family's experiences. Because parents are the primary decision makers for their children, they should be actively involved in constructing intervention plans. True collaboration involves discovering solutions that best fit families' needs and circumstances. To be effective, intervention must be sustainable within the contexts of family life.

Implications for Research

In addition to using assessments to examine the constructs of social participation, self-regulation, and perceived competence, research is needed to examine the ways in which sensory processing, occupational performance, and performance contexts influence each other and how changes in one domain may or may not lead to changes in another domain. Occupational therapy that uses a sensory integration treatment approach is based on the assumption that enhanced sensory experiences, within the context of meaningful activities, result in more adaptive behaviors (Fisher & Murray, 1991). The parents in this study described hopes for changes in social participation, self-regulation, and perceived competence in their children. Although there is an implicit belief in the profession that occupational performance (social participation), performance components (self-regulation and modulation of sensory stimuli), and performance contexts (home, school, community) are related, it is crucial to recognize that this assumption has not been empirically examined. The relationships are complex and require further exploration and empirical validation. To address the hopes of consumers for intervention and research outcomes, the links must be considered between children's underlying sensory processing difficulties, the impact of difficulties on children's behavior, and the effect that living with SMD and parenting a child with SMD has on the entire family system.

Acknowledgments

We thank the parents and children who participated in this study. We also thank the following: The Denver Children's Hospital Research Institute; R. Hagerman, MD, D. Matthews, MD, and other staff and faculty members at The Children's Hospital, Department of Rehabilitation;

D. McIntosh (research director); J. McGrath (lab coordinator), K. Church, and J. Bonnell for invaluable lab assistance; J. Butler, R. Greer, P. Kenyon, N. Pine, R. Seger, C. Summers, S. Trunnell, and L. Waterford for evaluation and treatment of children; and J. Benzel for administrative support. The study was supported in part by a grant to Sargent College Health and Rehabilitation Sciences, Boston University, from the U.S. Department of Health and Human Services, Health Resources and Services Administration, Maternal and Child Health (MCH) Bureau (MCJ-000-901), and MCH grant # MC J 08941301. In addition, the Wallace Research Foundation provided primary support for the larger research project. This chapter was written in partial fulfillment of the dissertation requirements for the first author's doctor of science degree, Sargent College, Boston University.

Appendix A

Parent Interview

1. Tell me about [child's name]. I especially want to hear about the kinds of things that you enjoy about [child's name], what his or her gifts and talents are, what his or her strong points are.

2. What has led you to seek occupational therapy services for [child's name]? (If necessary: What have you noticed about [child's name] development that concerns you?)

3. Tell me about [child's name] abilities in daily care activities, play, making and keeping friends, following directions, communicating, regulating his or her behavior, activity level, and falling and staying asleep.

4. What do you notice about [child's name] reactions to sounds, reactions to lights and other visual stimuli, reactions to being touched, reactions to smelling things, and reactions to moving in space?

5. Tell me about your pregnancy, delivery, and [child's name] early history.

6. Tell me about [child's name] hospitalizations or medical problems.

7. Tell me about [child's name] previous therapy or treatment.

8. Tell me a little about whom else is in your family. What things do you enjoy together?

9. (If in school) What is school (preschool) like for [child's name]? Is there anything that you would like to see changed about his or her school situation or the way he or she is at school?

10. What kind of toys or outdoor equipment do you have that [child's name] enjoys? What does [child's name] do after school and on weekends?

11. What are your expectations and/or hopes for therapy? (Or, What is it about [child's name] that you are hoping will change?)

References

Achenbach, T. M. (1991). *Manual for the Child Behavior Checklist 4–18* and 1991 Profile. Burlington: University of Vermont, Department of Psychiatry.

Anderson, E. L. (1993). *Parental perceptions of the influence of occupational therapy utilizing sensory integrative techniques on the daily living skills of children with autism.* Unpublished master's thesis, University of Southern California, Los Angeles.

Anderson, E., & Emmons, P. (1995). Sensory integration: The hidden disorder. *Sensory Integration Quarterly Newsletter, 23*(2/3), 8–9.

Ayres, A. J. (1972). *Sensory integration and learning disorders.* Los Angeles: Western Psychological Services.

Ayres, A. J. (1989). *Sensory integration and praxis tests.* Los Angeles: Western Psychological Services.

Brown, S. M., Humphry, R., & Taylor, E. (1997). A model of the nature of family–therapist relationships: Implications for education. *American Journal of Occupational Therapy, 51,* 597–603.

Bundy, A. (1991). Consultation and sensory integration theory. In A. G. Fisher, E. A. Murray, & A. C. Bundy (Eds.), *Sensory integration: Theory and practice* (pp. 318–332). Philadelphia: F. A. Davis.

Burke, J. P., & Schaaf, R. C. (1997). Family narratives and play assessment. In L. D. Parham & L. S. Fazio (Eds.), *Play in occupational therapy for children* (pp. 67–84). St. Louis, MO: Mosby.

Case-Smith, J., & Nastro, M. A. (1993). The effect of occupational therapy intervention on mothers of children with cerebral palsy. *American Journal of Occupational Therapy, 47,* 811–817.

Cohn, E. S., & Cermak, S. A. (1998). Including the family perspective in sensory integration outcomes research. *American Journal of Occupational Therapy, 52,* 540–546.

Coster, W. (1998). Occupation-centered assessment of children. *American Journal of Occupational Therapy, 52,* 337–344.

Coster, W. J., Deeney, T., Haltiwanger, J., & Haley, S. M. (1998). *School function assessment.* San Antonio, TX: Psychological Corporation/ Therapy SkillBuilders.

Dunn, W. (1994). Performance of typical children on the Sensory Profile: An item analysis. *American Journal of Occupational Therapy, 48,* 967–974.

Dunn, W. (1997). The impact of sensory processing abilities on the daily lives of young children and their families: A conceptual model. *Infants and Young Children, 9,* 23–35.

Fisher, A. G., & Murray, E. A. (1991). Introduction to sensory integration theory. In A. G. Fisher, E. A. Murray, & A. C. Bundy (Eds.), *Sensory integration: Theory and practice* (pp. 3–26). Philadelphia: F. A. Davis.

Gallimore, R., Weisner, T. S., Kaufman, S. Z., & Bernheimer, L. P. (1989). The social construction of ecocultural niches: Family accommodation of developmentally delayed children. *American Journal of Mental Retardation, 94,* 216–230.

Haley, S. M. (1994). Our measures reflect our practices and beliefs: A perspective on clinical measurement in pediatric physical therapy. *Pediatric Physical Therapy, 6,* 142–143.

Hinojosa, J. (1990). How mothers of preschool children with cerebral palsy perceive occupational and physical therapists and their influence on family life. *Occupational Therapy Journal of Research, 10,* 144–162.

Hinojosa, J., & Anderson, J. (1991). Mothers' perceptions of home treatment programs for their preschool children with cerebral palsy. *American Journal of Occupational Therapy, 45,* 273–279.

Humphry, R., & Case-Smith, J. (1996). Working with families. In J. Case-Smith, A. S. Allen, & P. N. Pratt (Eds.), *Occupational therapy for children* (pp. 67–98). St. Louis, MO: Mosby.

Individuals With Disabilities Education Act of 1990. Pub. L. 101–476, 20 U.S.C., Ch 33.

Kinnealey, M. (1973). Aversive and nonaversive responses to sensory stimulation in mentally retarded children. *American Journal of Occupational Therapy, 27,* 464–471.

Lawlor, M. C., & Mattingly, C. F. (1998). The complexities embedded in family-centered care. *American Journal of Occupational Therapy, 52,* 259–267.

Maxwell, J. (1996). *Qualitative research design: An interactive approach.* Thousand Oaks, CA: Sage.

McIntosh, D. N., Miller, L. J., & Shyu, V. (in press). Development and validation of the Short Sensory Profile. In W. Dunn (Ed.), *The Sensory Profile: Examiner's manual.* San Antonio, TX: Psychological Corporation.

McIntosh, D. N., Miller, L. J., Shyu, V., & Hagerman, R. (submitted). *Sensory modulation disruption, electrodermal responses, and functional behaviors.* Manuscript submitted for publication.

Miller, L. J. (1988). *Miller Assessment for Preschoolers.* San Antonio, TX: Psychological Corporation.

Miller, L. J. (1993). *FirstSTEP (Screening Test for Evaluating Preschoolers): Manual.* San Antonio, TX: Psychological Corporation.

Miller, L. J., & Hanft, B. E. (1998). Building positive alliances: Partnerships with families as the cornerstone of developmental assessment. *Infants and Young Children, 10,* 1–12.

Occupational Therapy Associates. (1995). *The sensory connection.* Watertown, MA: Author.

Parham, L. D., & Mailloux, Z. (1996). Sensory integration. In J. Case-Smith, A. S. Allen, & P. N. Pratt (Eds.), *Occupational therapy for children* (3rd ed., pp. 307–355). St. Louis, MO: Mosby.

Piers, E. V. (1984). *Piers–Harris Children's Self-Concept Scale.* Los Angeles: Western Psychological Services.

Reay, D. (1996). Dealing with difficult differences: Reflexivity and social class in feminist research. *Feminism and Psychology, 6,* 443–456.

Riessman, C. K. (Ed.). (1994). *Qualitative studies in social work research.* Thousand Oaks, CA: Sage.

Rogoff, B. (1990). *Apprenticeship in thinking.* New York: Oxford University Press.

Ruddick, S. (1989). *Maternal thinking.* Boston: Beacon Press.

Spencer, J., Davidson, H., & White, V. (1997). Helping clients develop hopes for the future. *American Journal of Occupational Therapy, 51,* 191–198.

Stake, R. (1994). Case studies. In N. Denzin & Y. Lincoln (Eds.), *Handbook of qualitative research* (pp. 236–247). Thousand Oaks, CA: Sage.

Strauss, A., & Corbin, J. (1990). *Basics of qualitative research.* Newbury Park, CA: Sage.

Trombly, C. (1993). The Issue Is—Anticipating the future: Assessment of occupational function. *American Journal of Occupational Therapy, 49,* 253–257.

Trombly, C. (1995). Occupation: Purposefulness and meaningfulness as therapeutic mechanisms [1995 Eleanor Clarke Slagle Lecture]. *American Journal of Occupational Therapy, 49,* 960–972.

U. S. Department of Education. (1995). *Seventeenth annual report to Congress on the implementation of the Individuals With Disabilities Education Act.* Washington, DC: Author.

CHAPTER 37

From Waiting to Relating

Parents' Experiences in the Waiting Room of an Occupational Therapy Clinic

Ellen S. Cohn

Ellen S. Cohn, ScD, OTR/L, FAOTA, *is clinical associate professor, Boston University, Sargent College of Health and Rehabilitation Sciences, 635 Commonwealth Avenue, Boston, MA 02215; ecohn@bu.edu.*

Karen is the mother of a 7-year-old girl who received occupational therapy using sensory integration approaches at a private practice in a suburban community. Responding to a question about her experience of taking her daughter to the occupational therapy clinic, Karen said,

> We'd sit in the waiting room and we'd always be reading. Gradually over the weeks, we just started talking. I really enjoyed talking with her [another parent], and it was like a little support group. She would share with me some of the things she was concerned with, and I would share my concerns. So, it was nice to have someone, to have a little support group, while we were there without having to go another night of the week. She had similar concerns.

The analysis of waiting room phenomena came about during a study designed to understand parents' perspectives of outcomes of occupational therapy using sensory integration approaches for their school-age children and their families. As I interviewed Karen and other parents to understand their perspectives, I started to hear a recurring pattern about the waiting room. Many of the parents repeatedly spoke about perceived benefits of sitting in the waiting room and chatting with other parents. Some parents in the study even suggested that I contact other people, now their friends, who they had met in the occupational therapy waiting room. Peggy, a mother of a 6-year-old boy, said,

> The waiting room was very helpful. It was a very helpful, quasi-spontaneous support group, and even though my son was probably the mildest of the group, it was a support group without having to make it happen. It was just very nice moms all there for the same reason, talking about various issues: advocacy issues, insurance issues, life-in-general issues. When you go week after week, you see the same people. It was really helpful.

During the interviews, parents reflected on their experiences and repeatedly spoke of the "unanticipated consequences" of bringing their children to therapy;

Originally published 2001 in *American Journal of Occupational Therapy*, 55, 167–174.

that is, the parents anticipated that the therapy itself would be the main change agent for their children. They did not anticipate benefits for themselves as parents, and the benefits of the waiting room experience were an unexpected finding in this research. Merton (1936), a sociologist, explained that consequences (expected or unexpected) result from interplay between an action and the context of the action. The analysis here examines the context of the action: the waiting room and parents' accounts of their transformative experiences of waiting while their children received occupational therapy. Implications for occupational therapy practice and research are discussed.

By striving to understand parents' perspectives, I recognize the importance of family-centered care in providing services to children with special health care needs and acknowledge the influence of families in children's development. Family-centered care involves meeting family concerns, building on family strengths, respecting family diversity and cultural backgrounds, sharing information, promoting partnerships and collaboration, and encouraging social support (King, King, Rosenbaum, & Goffin, 1999; Lawlor & Mattingly, 1998; Shelton, Jeppson, & Johnson, 1987; Shelton & Stepanek, 1994). Moreover, providing family-centered services requires practitioners to understand what the behaviors, events, persons, and institutions mean to those who participate in them (Cohn & Cermak, 1998; Llewellyn, 1994). Therefore, the study was designed to understand what children's participation in occupational therapy using sensory integration approaches meant to parents.

Method

Participants

I interviewed 16 parents (14 families consisting of 12 mothers and 2 husband-and-wife couples) of children who received occupational therapy using a sensory integration frame of reference at a private clinic in the northeastern United States. Participants were parents of children who had documented conditions of some type of sensory integrative dysfunction as measured by the Sensory Integration and Praxis Tests (Ayres, 1989). The children (4–10 years of age) had participated in at least 32 1-hr therapy sessions and had stopped therapy 1 month to 2 years before the interview. All participating parents were White and in the moderate to affluent socioeconomic status range. A majority of the participants had master's degrees, and except for one participant, all were college educated.

For the children whose parents participated in the interviews, therapy had typically involved a 1-hr session one time per week. Therapy consisted of the "use of enhanced, controlled sensory stimulation in the context of a meaningful, self-directed activity in order to elicit an adaptive response" (Fisher & Bundy, 1991, p. 23). Selected activities incorporated the use of suspended overhead equipment that provided tactile, vestibular, and proprioceptive input to which the child made adaptive responses. Therapists often invited parents into the therapy sessions to observe their children. A minimum of 32 1-hr therapy sessions (approximately 8 months) was the criterion selected to anticipate some type of change. This criterion is based on a review of nine sensory integration efficacy studies with children with learning disabilities (Ayres, 1972, 1978; Carte, Morrison, Sublett, Uemura, & Setrakian, 1984; Densem, Nuthall, Bushnell, & Horn, 1989; Humphries, Wright, McDougall, & Vertes, 1990; Humphries, Wright, Snider, & McDougall, 1992; Law, Polatajko, Schaffer, Miller, & Macnab, 1991; White, 1979; Wilson & Kaplan, 1994). Twenty-four hours of intervention was the modal number of therapy sessions in the reviewed studies. Therefore, it is proposed that the children in the study reported here received enough therapy to anticipate some type of change.

A sample size of 16 was deemed adequate on the basis of two criteria. First, exploratory studies are recommended to use at least eight participants to obtain an adequate amount and range of information (McCracken, 1988). Second, the sample size is consistent with or even slightly larger than that of other qualitative studies recently conducted in the occupational therapy field (Anderson, 1993; Case-Smith, 1997; Case-Smith & Nastro, 1993; Hinojosa, 1990; Hinojosa & Anderson, 1991; Rudman, Cook, & Polatajko, 1997). Recruitment was stopped after the 16th participant because I reached a point at which findings from newly collected and analyzed data became redundant (Strauss & Corbin, 1998).

Parents of children given a primary diagnosis of autism, pervasive developmental disorder, or Fragile X syndrome were not included in the study. Parents of children with these particular conditions may have different concerns about the social–emotional and behavioral manifestations of their children's conditions than parents of children without these conditions. The sample criteria are based on the assumption that they represent a relatively homogeneous subgroup of children who receive occupational therapy in private practice settings using a sensory integration framework.

Procedure

On the basis of chart review, 42 children met the inclusion criteria. Names of parents of 22 children to be invited as potential participants were randomly selected from the total group of those eligible. A letter explaining the study purpose and procedure and offering parents the opportunity to remove their names from the potential participant list was sent to the selected families. Three families requested to have their names removed from the potential participant list, and eight families reported being "too busy" to participate in an interview. Potential participants (those who did

not request to be removed from the list) were called to clarify the purpose and procedure of the study and to determine interest in participating in the study. All participants signed Internal Review Board–approved informed consent forms before the interviews began.

I conducted 1-hr to 2-hr semistructured interviews in each family's home. Questions were adapted to respond to the discussion in the context of each interview. I asked participants to describe a typical day with their child, what about their child led them to seek occupational therapy, and what they had hoped to gain from therapy. I asked whether they saw changes in their child and, if so, to describe an incident that illustrated the change; whether changes they had hoped for had not occurred; and how they came to a decision to stop therapy. After each interview, I wrote reflective memos to record my immediate reactions to the interview. Each interview was audiotaped, transcribed, and checked by thorough review and comparison between the transcript and the original audiotape. In addition, I reviewed each child's clinical chart to document reasons for referral and therapy goals. Throughout the research process, I wrote periodic analytical memos (Miles & Huberman, 1994) to record my evolving thoughts related to the research question and process. After the waiting room phenomenon became apparent, I spent time observing the waiting room.

Data Analysis

Hasselkus (1997) reminded us that as researchers, we are "positioned in relation to that which we are researching" (p. 81), and our particular position becomes the lens through which we make interpretations. Examining this lens is a starting point for all research and enables us to use our reflections productively for insight and analysis. In the spirit of reflexivity, I acknowledge the influences of my own background as both a parent of school-age children and an occupational therapist who has provided occupational therapy using a sensory integration approach. As a parent, I know first-hand the experiences of striving to nurture a child's growth and sense of competence. I share Llewellyn's (1994) view that parenting is an intensely personal yet commonly shared experience. Sharing my parenting experiences, both joys and dilemmas, with other parents provides a powerful source of support and personal validation for the challenges inherent in the occupation of parenting. As an occupational therapist, I try to provide therapy that ultimately makes a meaningful difference for children in the contexts in which they live, learn, and play. I carry an underlying assumption that occupational therapy is effective and can contribute to changes in children and the entire family system. However, I also believe and have documented elsewhere (Cohn & Cermak, 1998) that we have not empirically examined which outcomes of occupational therapy are important to parents who bring their children for intervention.

Using grounded theory procedures recommended by Strauss and Corbin (1998), I reviewed the transcripts to name and categorize the participants' perceptions of valued outcomes. The category of the waiting room immediately emerged after the first interview. As other parents talked about their waiting room experiences, all instances of waiting room talk were compared and contrasted to detect similarities and differences across all the transcripts. The QSR NUD*IST 4.0 (1997) qualitative data analysis software was used to manage and explore the data. To strengthen credibility and ensure that participants' perspectives were accurately represented, I prepared written summaries of each interview and sent the summaries to participants for review. I then contacted each participant by phone to discuss the interview summaries and, on the basis of their feedback, made modifications to the sum-

maries as needed. Finally, I analyzed the summaries along with the interview data. To honor confidentiality, pseudonyms are used throughout this chapter.

The Waiting Room Experience

For this particular group of parents, the waiting room was an important component of their experiences of bringing their children to occupational therapy. *Webster's Third New International Dictionary* (1976) defines *waiting* as staying in place in expectation of, deferring, holding back in expectation, delaying hope, or delaying hope of a favorable change. Waiting is at the crossroads of the present and the future and certainty and uncertainty (Gasparini, 1995). These definitions capture the essence of what the participants were doing while their children received occupational therapy. The participants brought their children to occupational therapy because they hoped for some change, and they held those hopes in abeyance while they sat with other parents. They waited in suspense, week after week, hoping for some change to unfold. The end result was unknown, the future uncertain. Deb, the mother of a first-grade boy, described how she would sit in the waiting room each week and talk with other parents about her hopes: "I sat in the waiting room hoping that there would be hope for him. That he could learn to live with his condition....We wanted him to be normal. We wanted him not to hurt himself or others." Another mother, Lynn, said, "I felt like he [her son] was getting older, and I wanted him to be out in the world doing things that other kids do. There were a lot of us sitting there saying that."

Liminality

The participants' children all had invisible conditions, that is, their sensory integrative dysfunction was not readily visible to the untrained eye. Yet each participant's presence in the waiting room made his or her child's condition and need for intervention obvious to the other parents. In addition to being an assertion of hope, visits to the occupational therapy clinic each week activated feelings of *liminality,* described by Murphy (1987) and Murphy, Scheer, Murphy, and Mack (1988) as a state of waiting. A distinguished anthropologist who developed quadriplegia from the effects of a spinal tumor, Murphy viewed disability as a form of liminality. In Murphy's view, liminality is closely related to sociologist Victor Turner's (1969) idea of rites of passage in which the purpose of the rituals of passage is to involve the community in the transformation of an individual from one position in society to another. This transformation typically occurs in three phases: isolation or separation, ritual emergence or transition, and reincorporation into society. During the transition from isolation to emergence, the person is thought to be in a liminal state, a social limbo in which he or she is left "waiting." Turner (1964/1972) titled one of his essays *Betwixt and Between,* an apt description of the suspended position of a person seeking a change or transformation. By virtue of being in the waiting room, parents moved from a position of parenting a child with an invisible condition to the threshold of waiting for some type of transformation.

A Weekly Ritual

Bell (1992) claimed that ritual activities are set aside from the flow of other daily activities and that the distinction between rituals and day-to-day routines is based, in part, on the beliefs of the social group. I argue here, on the basis of what the participants told me, that the waiting experience in and of itself provided parents with a weekly ritual in which they shared their experiences. This weekly waiting room ritual helped parents to transform their experiences of parenting their

children with sensory integrative dysfunction. The parents shifted from a position of isolation (parenting children with invisible, yet challenging conditions) to a position of shared experience in which others understood their concerns. Two major characteristics of ritual are predictability and sharing of experience. In fact, Durkheim (1915/1965) proposed that rituals provide a means for a group to affirm itself through shared experience. Unlike waiting rooms where there are different persons waiting at each visit, the waiting room experience described here had predictability. The participants repeatedly saw the same parents each week, which provided the opportunity to develop relationships and share common concerns and feelings.

Murphy (1987) observed that persons in a liminal state often put their differences aside and view others in the same position in an egalitarian manner. This nonhierarchical social position offers the potential for linking with other parents and sharing revelations frankly. For the participants in this study, the waiting room was found to have become a contained setting that facilitated interaction, and their experiences were transformed into something other than just "waiting." In the context of the waiting room, participants found affiliation and a refuge from the world of others who could not understand their parenting experience. One mother, Nancy, talked about a parent she met in the waiting room:

> She had similar concerns. It was very nice to have someone to talk to. I think any parent dealing with SI [sensory integration] therapy must experience doubts [about their parenting]. The mothers that I talked to in the waiting room certainly did.

Naturally Occurring Support

Karen, the mother whose interview opens this chapter, told me that over several weeks, parents gradually shifted from reading to talking to each other. Typical waiting room behavior usually involves reading or staring straight ahead. The chairs may be arranged in rows that minimize eye contact and the potential for interaction (Holmes-Garrett, 1990; Rodgers, 1990). The waiting room I observed was more like a family room than a waiting area. Comfortable couches facing a set of movable chairs sat in a sunny, welcoming room, with toys placed in an area behind the couches for the children. Perhaps the furniture and its arrangement coupled with the repetition of this particular waiting room experience invited parents to let go of the usual waiting room rituals of reading and avoiding interactions with others who are waiting. The social rules typical of most waiting rooms were rewritten. Rather than being a place where busy parents avoided each other, the waiting room was transformed into a support network. The parents shared a desire to understand their children; obtain information about their children's conditions and available resources; and receive support, hope, and affiliation. For example, one mother, Marie, said,

> I heard about a tutor through someone in the waiting room....The waiting room was really fun....Because you are in a vacuum, you are worried about things. I had a doctor who I had a really bad experience with....I found out another mother was going to him. He was the pits. So you weren't alone, and everybody else has concerns. Everybody there had questions.

Marie and the other participants described important interpersonal, socially interactive, and supportive features of the waiting room experience. The perceived benefits derived from these spontaneous social supports are consistent with the benefits of social support described by other researchers. Caplan (1974) examined naturally occurring social supports and concluded that a mutual and reciprocal quality exists in the interactions with people who help each other. The mutuality is emphasized by the fact that the support is voluntary and spontaneous. Both the giver and receiver of support are equally, although differently, benefited by the contact. Often, people prefer to receive help from others who have personally experienced the same or similar predicaments because the help appears more authentic.

In a comprehensive examination of parent support groups, Hauser-Cram, Warfield, and Krauss (1997) identified two functions of such groups. One function is to act as a form of intervention for parents who have unusual parenting challenges; another is to help parents be advocates for their children. Both functions assist parents in their parenting occupation. The link between social support and well-being is well documented for parents of children with disabilities. Support, both informal and formal, has been found to enhance well-being and family functioning by acting as a buffer to stress (Dunst & Trivette, 1990; King et al., 1999; Wallander et al., 1989). In related research, Quittner, Glueckauf, and Jackson (1990) suggested that social support mediates the relationship between parenting stress and outcomes. In both the "buffer" model of social support and the "mediator" model, social support is viewed as having a positive impact on family functioning. Furthermore, parent-to-parent programs (Llewellyn, Griffin, & Sacco, 1992; Santelli, Turnbull, Lerner, & Marquis, 1993) provide parents with the valuable opportunity to give as well as receive assistance, which has been found to enhance self-efficacy and self-esteem (Kagan & Shelley, 1987; Zigler & Weiss, 1985). On the basis of their research, many of these authors recommended that centers of care provide practical assistance for information and networking opportunities through such mechanisms as parent newsletters or parent support groups.

Downward Social Comparison

In listening to the words of the participants in this study, another waiting room phenomenon became apparent. In addition to the outward interactions resulting in social support, a quiet, internalized experience simultaneously occurred that resulted from comparing one child with another. Renowned social psychologist Leon Festinger (1954) identified the process of *social comparison* in which people use others both for determining how well they have done and for learning what they should do. In Festinger's view, peoples' attitudes and beliefs are based on particular reference points. Thus, one way in which we attempt to understand human experience or form beliefs is through social comparison. Other people serve as a reference to help us determine how we are supposed to behave and how good we are at a particular type of behavior. By design, the participants' children all had more subtle forms of sensory integrative dysfunction than many of the other children receiving occupational therapy at this particular clinic. The social comparison process offered the participants a unique perspective that influenced their understanding of their children. Deb described her observation this way:

> It was a really good thing for me to see the children that were treated at the clinic. It made me appreciate, help me remember how lucky we were not to have a really stressful [son]. Some of these children, my heart goes out to their parents....It was very therapeutic for me to see the other kids. Not all of them, but most of them at our time were in much worse shape than my son.

Many of the participants shared similar observations. Being better off than others in a similar situation, as described previously, has been identified by social psychologists as a downward social comparison. For example, studies have shown that stress from health problems induces a desire to compare one's health with that of others (Mollerman, Pruyn, & van Knippenberg, 1986; Taylor, Buunk, & Aspinwall, 1990) and that downward social comparisons contribute to well-being and positive feelings (Hakmiller, 1966; VanderZee & Buunk, 1995; Wills, 1981). Numerous participants echoed these findings as they spoke about observing parents with children who had more significant problems than theirs. This observation and downward social comparison process helped the participants reframe their perceptions of their children and helped them accept their situation. For example, the mother of a 5-year-old boy said,

> I always felt like he was borderline whether he needed to be there, because I would talk to other people there or see other children come in and they clearly needed some kind of help. They had bigger issues. So I thought, "Well, my situation isn't so bad. There's nothing really wrong with my son. He just needs help getting himself more cohesive."

Another mother, Johanna, framed her waiting room experience in terms of sympathy. She explained,

> I think I got a lot of sympathy for people whose kids were in much worse condition than my son. Just spending time in the waiting room was an amazing, eye-opening, and heart-wrenching experience....I began to see my situation as a piece of cake compared to other people.

Reframing

The social comparisons that occurred in the waiting room led many of the parents to reframe their assessment of their children or situation. While reflecting on changes that may have occurred from bringing her son to occupational therapy, Johanna described how she reframed her expectations for him: "You know, I think I am less hard on my son. I gave up on the homework [being perfect]. Who cares? It doesn't matter as long as an effort was made. It doesn't have to be perfect." Niehues, Bundy, Mattingly, and Lawlor (1991) and Case-Smith (1997) identified *reframing* as a process of coming to see a person or situation in a new way because one has changed the framework, or lens, through which he or she views the situation. These researchers claimed that reframing is a valuable service provided by occupational therapists working in schools. Case-Smith noted that by educating teachers about the potential relationship between sensory processing and behavior, occupational therapists enabled teachers to view student behaviors in a more positive way and gave them a basis for developing effective teaching strategies. In the present study, therapists' efforts to educate parents about sensory processing may have helped the participants reframe their expectations of their children. Perhaps unknown to the therapists, the comparisons participants made in the waiting room also had a powerful influence on their construction of their own children's behavior. Comparing their children's behavior to others less fortunate enabled the participants to see their children's strengths. They reported a downward social comparison and a positive reframing of their children's behavior. What about the parents whose children have more significant conditions? How do these parents perceive their waiting room experience?

Summary

The participants in this study took their children to therapy with the expectation that somehow occupational therapy would help their children's future. It was surprising to find that the experience of simply sitting in the waiting room may have contributed to the process of expected change. Crossing the threshold into the waiting room moved these parents from the isolation of parenting children with invisible conditions to

the liminal state of waiting or readiness for change. Through their weekly interactions with one another, sharing stories, experiences, parenting challenges, and resources, these parents gave and received naturally occurring support for parenting children with sensory integrative dysfunction. Although family-centered care encourages social support, this study shows us that support not only may come from professionals but also can occur naturally in a waiting room environment. In addition to the natural support parents provided one another while in the waiting room, the parents were reassured by comparing their children with children who were more severely involved. This comparison seemed to play an important role in participants reframing their expectations for their children and for themselves as parents.

Implications for Practice and Research

At the theoretical level, this research echoes the importance of expanding the definition of occupational therapy beyond direct intervention with children to include parents as well. The findings raise our awareness that ritual interactions are complex and may have deeper meaning and consequences than we fully appreciate. Lawlor and Mattingly (1998) suggested that a redefinition of practice includes recognition of how encounters with family members are influenced by the cultural world of practice. As therapists and researchers, we need to pay attention to the entire context surrounding the intervention process, not just the explicit therapeutic encounter.

Findings from this research raise questions about what constitutes family-centered care. An outpatient clinic, by its very nature and no matter how family friendly the staff may be, is not inherently family-centered. Thus, we might ask, How can we provide family-centered care in an outpatient setting? Some practitioners might argue that family-centered care involves parents as active participants in the therapy, collaborating with the therapist and child in the therapy rooms rather than sitting in the waiting room. Although collaboration between professionals and parents is important, we have seen in this sample that the social support available in the waiting room might be another powerful aspect of family-centered care. If the experience of these parents has implications for others, then attending to the broader practice environment can be seen as part of a family-centered approach. We need to understand how parents are making sense of the entire therapy experience, not just interventions focused on children in isolation of their caregivers.

In this study, the waiting room experience emerged as a meaningful and symbolic feature of the entire therapy. Although occupational therapists have viewed occupation and adaptation as an interactive process between persons and environments (Barris, 1986; Barris, Kielhofner, Levine, & Neville, 1985; Frank, 1996; Spencer, 1998), we have not explored how a physical setting, such as a waiting room, might shape naturally occurring activity and social interaction with the symbolic meanings attached to places. Representing the field of humanistic geography, Rowles (1991) invited occupational therapists to consider the existential meaning of environments to their clients.

Hoffman and Futterman (1971) noted that most professionals aim to eliminate waiting room time, especially for busy parents. The insights from this research suggest that occupational therapists should aim to create in their waiting rooms a milieu to foster sharing so that parents can talk to one another. Practitioners in other fields have recommended that waiting rooms provide comfortable seating conducive to interaction; private space that is not shared with other professional practices; parenting information and education resources; a lending library; and beverages, such as water, tea, or coffee (Harman, 1997; Koepke, 1993). Providing an inviting environment in which parents can share with each other may be an important component of family-centered care.

Koroloff and Friesen (1991) noted that members of self-help groups are likely to be White, middle income, and well educated, as were the participants in the present study, and Hauser-Cram, Pierson, Walker, and Tivnan (1991) reported that parent support groups were not universally appealing to all families. These findings remind us that the participants in this study represent a very small homogeneous group of parents of children who are likely to seek occupational therapy services. Although the naturally occurring "support groups" were perceived as a positive benefit of their children's therapy, we must be careful to avoid assuming such a support group will be appealing to all our consumers or appropriate to all settings. Is it possible that the similarity of the families receiving occupational therapy at this particular clinic made sharing in the waiting room easier? Further investigation with a more diverse group of parents may help determine whether these findings have implications for other parents.

The label "support group" was not formally applied to groups of parents in the waiting room. Rather, the group support occurred naturally, not institutionally. Does the naturally occurring phenomenon make a difference? Might it be useful to schedule like children at the same time to enhance the possibility of parents developing naturally occurring support networks, or is the downward social comparison resulting from observing a variety of children a crucial change agent? Moreover, further investigation is necessary to test whether the perception of support exchanged in the waiting room and reframing are at all related to outcomes of perceived well-being and sustainability of family life.

Another possible implication of the research reported here is that the process of change resulting from occupational therapy using a sensory integration approach occurs, to some degree, not only with the children but also with the parents. By reframing their children's behavior and receiving support, parents reconstruct their image of their children and themselves in their parenting occupation and change their beliefs about their children. Some researchers have suggested that parental beliefs may directly affect children (Goodnow, 1988, Murphey, 1992). Research efforts need to further explicate whether parental beliefs are indeed connected to behaviors and child and family outcomes. If a connection can be established, then optimal mechanisms for facilitating reframing should be explored.

Finally, this research illustrates the importance of family-centered care. As we strive to provide meaningful intervention with children and their families, we must attend to the broader context of the therapy experience and carefully listen to how families are interpreting their experiences with intervention.

Acknowledgments

I gratefully acknowledge the support of the parents who participated in this study. Much appreciated for their assistance are Teresa May-Benson, MS, OTR/L, and all the therapists at OTA–Watertown, P.C., Watertown, MA. A special note of gratitude is extended to my dissertation advisors, Linda Tickle-Degnen, PhD, OTR/L, Wendy Coster, PhD, OTR/L, FAOTA, Cathy Riessman, PhD, and Jane Koomar, PhD, OTR/L, FAOTA. I thank Betty Crepeau, PhD, OTR, FAOTA, for memorable and stimulating conversations about rituals.

This research was supported in part by a grant to Boston University, Sargent College of Health and Rehabilitation Sciences, from the Department of Health and Human Services, Health Resources and Services Administration, Maternal and Child Health Bureau (MCJ-000-901). Additional funding was obtained from the American Occupational Therapy Foundation and the Anne Henderson Doctoral Scholarship. This article was written in partial fulfillment of the dissertation requirements for the author's degree of Doctor of Science, Sargent College, Boston University.

References

Anderson, E. L. (1993). *Parental perceptions of the influence of occupational therapy utilizing sensory integrative techniques on the daily living skills of children with autism.* Unpublished master's thesis, University of Southern California, Los Angeles.

Ayres, A. J. (1972). Improving academic scores through sensory integration. *Journal of Learning Disabilities, 5,* 24–28.

Ayres, A. J. (1978). Learning disabilities and the vestibular system. *Journal of Learning Disabilities, 11,* 30–41.

Ayres, A. J. (1989). *Sensory Integration and Praxis Tests.* Los Angeles: Western Psychological Services.

Barris, R. (1986). Activity: The interface between person and environment. *Physical and Occupational Therapy in Geriatrics, 5*(2), 39–49.

Barris, R., Kielhofner, G., Levine, R. E., & Neville, A. M. (1985). Occupation as interaction with the environment. In G. Kielhofner (Ed.), *A model of human occupation: Theory and application* (pp. 42–62). Baltimore: Williams & Wilkins.

Bell, C. (1992). *Ritual theory, ritual practice.* New York: Oxford University Press.

Caplan, G. (1974). *Support systems and community mental health: Lectures on concept development.* New York: Behavioral Publications.

Carte, E., Morrison, D., Sublett, J., Uemura, A., & Setrakian, W. (1984). Sensory integration therapy: A trial of a specific neurodevelopmental therapy for remediation of learning disabilities. *Journal of Developmental Behavioral Pediatrics, 5,* 189–194.

Case-Smith, J. (1997). Variables related to successful school-based practice. *Occupational Therapy Journal of Research, 17,* 133–153.

Case-Smith, J., & Nastro, M. A. (1993). The effect of occupational therapy intervention on mothers of children with cerebral palsy. *American Journal of Occupational Therapy, 47,* 811–817.

Cohn, E. S., & Cermak, S. A. (1998). Including the family perspective in sensory integration outcomes research. *American Journal of Occupational Therapy, 52,* 540–546.

Densem, J. F., Nuthall, G. A., Bushnell, J., & Horn, J. (1989). Effectiveness of a sensory integration therapy program for children with perceptual–motor deficits. *Journal of Learning Disabilities, 22,* 221–229.

Dunst, C. J., & Trivette, C. M. (1990). Assessment of social support in early intervention programs. In S. J. Meisels & J. P. Shonkoff (Eds.), *Handbook of early childhood intervention* (pp. 326–349). New York: Cambridge University Press.

Durkheim, E. (1965). The elementary forms of the religious life (J. W. Swain, Trans.). New York: Free Press. (Original work published 1915)

Festinger, L. (1954). A theory of social comparison processes. *Human Relations, 7,* 117–140.

Fisher, A. G., & Bundy, A. C. (1991). Introduction to sensory integration theory. In A. G. Fisher, E. S. Murray, & A. C. Bundy (Eds.), *Sensory integration: Theory and practice* (pp. 3–26). Philadelphia: F. A. Davis.

Frank, G. (1996). Life histories in occupational therapy clinical practice. *American Journal of Occupational Therapy, 50,* 251–264.

Gasparini, G. (1995). On waiting. *Time and Society, 4*(1), 29–45.

Goodnow, J. J. (1988). Parents' ideas, actions, and feelings: Models and methods from developmental and social psychology. *Child Development, 59,* 286–320.

Hakmiller, K. L. (1966). Threat as a determinant of downward comparison. *Journal of Experimental Social Psychology, 2*(Suppl. 1), 32–39.

Harman, R. D. (1997). Is it a waiting room or a reception area? *California Chiropractic Association Journal, 22*(12), 26–27.

Hasselkus, B. R. (1997). In the eye of the beholder: The researcher in qualitative research. *Occupational Therapy Journal of Research, 17,* 81–83.

Hauser-Cram, P., Pierson, D. P., Walker, D. K., & Tivnan, T. (1991). *Early education in public schools: Lessons from a comprehensive birth-to-kindergarten program.* San Francisco: Jossey-Bass.

Hauser-Cram, P., Warfield, M. E., & Krauss, M. W. (1997). An examination of parent support groups: A range of purposes, theories, and effects. *Research in Social Problems and Public Policy, 6,* 99–124.

Hinojosa, J. (1990). How mothers of preschool children perceive occupational and physical therapists and their influence on family life. *Occupational Therapy Journal of Research, 10,* 144–162.

Hinojosa, J., & Anderson, J. (1991). Mothers' perceptions of home treatment programs for their preschool children with cerebral palsy. *American Journal of Occupational Therapy, 45,* 273–279.

Hoffman, I., & Futterman, E. H. (1971). Coping with waiting: Psychiatric intervention and study in the waiting room of a pediatric oncology clinic. *Comprehensive Psychiatry, 12*(1), 67–81.

Holmes-Garrett, C. (1990). The crisis of the forgotten family: A single session group in the ICU waiting room. *Social Work With Groups, 12*(4), 141–157.

Humphries, T., Wright, M., McDougall, B., & Vertes, J. (1990). The efficacy of sensory integration for children with learning disability. *Physical and Occupational Therapy in Pediatrics, 10,* 1–17.

Humphries, T. W., Wright, M., Snider, L., & McDougall, B. (1992). A comparison of the effectiveness of sensory integrative therapy and perceptual–motor training in treating children with learning disabilities. *Journal of Developmental and Behavioral Pediatrics, 13,* 31–40.

Kagan, S. L., & Shelley, A. (1987). The promise and problems of family support programs. In S. L. Kagan, D. R. Powell, B. Weissbourd, & E. F. Zigler (Eds.), *America's family support programs: Perspective and prospects* (pp. 3–18). New Haven, CT: Yale University Press.

King, G., King, S., Rosenbaum, P., & Goffin, R. (1999). Family-centered caregiving and well-being of parents of children with disabilities: Linking process with outcome. *Journal of Pediatric Psychology, 24*(1), 41–53.

Koepke, J. E. (1993). Health care settings as resources for parenting information. *Pediatric Nursing, 20,* 560–563.

Koroloff, N. M., & Friesen, B. J. (1991). Support groups for parents of children with emotional disorders: A comparison of members and non-members. *Community Mental Health Journal, 27,* 265–279.

Law, M., Polatajko, H. J., Schaffer, R., Miller, J., & Macnab, J. (1991). The impact of heterogeneity in a clinical trial: Motor outcomes after sensory integration therapy. *Occupational Therapy Journal of Research, 11,* 177–189.

Lawlor, M. C., & Mattingly, C. F. (1998). The complexities embedded in family-centered care. *American Journal of Occupational Therapy, 52,* 259–267.

Llewellyn, G. (1994). Parenting: A neglected human occupation. Parents' voices not yet heard. *Australian Occupational Therapy Journal, 41,* 173–176.

Llewellyn, G., Griffin, S., & Sacco, M. (1992). The parent-to-parent model in Australia. *Australian Disability Review, 3,* 42–50.

McCracken, G. (1988). *The long interview.* Newbury Park, CA: Sage.

Merton, R. K. (1936). The unanticipated consequences of purposive social action. *American Sociological Review, 1,* 894–896.

Miles, M. B., & Huberman, A. M. (1994). *Qualitative data analysis* (2nd ed.). Thousand Oaks, CA: Sage.

Mollerman, E., Pruyn, J., & van Knippenberg, A. (1986). Social comparison processes among cancer patients. *British Journal of Social Psychology, 25*(1), 1–13.

Murphey, D. A. (1992). Constructing the child: Relations between parents' beliefs and child outcomes. *Developmental Review, 12,* 199–232.

Murphy, R. F. (1987). *The body silent.* New York: Norton.

Murphy, R. F., Scheer, J., Murphy, Y., & Mack, R. (1988). Physical disability and social liminality: A study in rituals of adversity. *Social Science and Medicine, 26,* 235–242.

Niehues, A. N., Bundy, A. C., Mattingly, C. F., & Lawlor, M. C. (1991). Making a difference: Occupational therapy in the public schools. *Occupational Therapy Journal of Research, 11,* 195–212.

QSR NUD*IST 4.0 [Computer software]. (1997). Thousand Oaks, CA: Scolari, Sage Publications Software.

Quittner, A. L., Glueckauf, R. L., & Jackson, D. N. (1990). Chronic parenting stress: Moderating

versus mediating effects of social support. *Journal of Personality and Social Psychology, 59,* 1266–1278.

Rodgers, B. L. (1990). The intensity of waiting: Life outside the intensive care unit. *Focus on Critical Care, 17,* 325–329.

Rowles, G. D. (1991). Beyond performance: Being in place as a component of occupational therapy. *American Journal of Occupational Therapy, 45,* 265–271.

Rudman, D. L., Cook, J. V., & Polatajko, H. (1997). Understanding the potential of occupation: A qualitative exploration of seniors' perspectives on activity. *American Journal of Occupational Therapy, 51,* 640–650.

Santelli, B., Turnbull, A. P., Lerner, E., & Marquis, J. (1993). Parent to parent programs: A unique form of mutual support for families of persons with disabilities. In G. H. S. Singer & L. E. Powers (Eds.), *Families, disability, and empowerment* (pp. 27–58). Baltimore: Brookes.

Shelton, T. L., Jeppson, E. S., & Johnson, B. H. (1987). *Family-centered care for children with special health care needs.* Washington, DC: Association for the Care of Children's Health.

Shelton, T. L., & Stepanek, J. S. (1994). *Family-centered care for children needing specialized health and developmental services* (3rd ed.). Bethesda, MD: Association for the Care of Children's Health.

Spencer, J. C. (1998). Evaluation of performance contexts. In M. E. Neistadt & E. B. Crepeau (Eds.), *Willard and Spackman's occupational therapy* (9th ed., pp. 291–309). Philadelphia: Lippincott.

Strauss, A., & Corbin, J. (1998). *Basics of qualitative research.* Newbury Park, CA: Sage.

Taylor, S. E., Buunk, B. P., & Aspinwall, L. (1990). Social comparison, stress and coping. *Personality and Social Psychology Bulletin, 103,* 193–210.

Turner, V. (1969). *The ritual process: Structure and anti-structure.* Ithaca, NY: Cornell University Press.

Turner, V. (1972). Betwixt and between: The liminal period in rites of passage. In W. Lessa & E. Z. Vogt (Eds.), *Reader in comparative religion: An anthropological approach* (3rd ed., pp. 338–347). New York: Harper & Row. (Original work published 1964)

VanderZee, K. I., & Buunk, B. P. (1995). Social comparison as a mediator between health problems and subjective health evaluations. *British Journal of Social Psychology, 34*(1), 53–65.

Wallander, J. L., Varni, J. W., Babani, L., DeHaan, C. B., Wilcox, K. T., & Banis, H. T. (1989). The social environment and the adaptation of mothers of physically handicapped children. *Journal of Pediatric Psychology, 14,* 371–387.

Webster's third new international dictionary. (1976). Springfield, MA: Merriam.

White, M. (1979). A first-grade intervention program for children at risk for reading failure. *Journal of Learning Disabilities, 12,* 26–32.

Wills, T. A. (1981). Downward comparison principles in social psychology. *Psychological Bulletin, 90,* 245–271.

Wilson, B. N., & Kaplan, B. J. (1994). Follow-up assessment of children receiving sensory integration treatment. *Occupational Therapy Journal of Research, 14,* 244–266.

Zigler, E., & Weiss, H. (1985). Family support systems: An ecological approach to child development. In R. Rapoport (Ed.), *Children, youth, and families: The action–research relationship* (pp. 166–205). Cambridge, UK: Cambridge University Press.

CHAPTER 38

Parent Perspectives of Occupational Therapy Using a Sensory Integration Approach

Ellen S. Cohn

Ellen S. Cohn, ScD, OTR/L, FAOTA, *is clinical associate professor, Boston University, Sargent College of Health and Rehabilitation Sciences, 635 Commonwealth Avenue, Boston, MA 02215; ecohn@bu.edu.*

Sensory integration approaches are the most widely researched intervention within pediatric occupational therapy (Miller & Kinnealey, 1993). Ayres (1972) reported that occupational therapy using sensory integration approaches, when coupled with special education, was a promising method for improving academic scores of children with learning disabilities. Since then, various authors have investigated Ayres's claim. Ottenbacher's (1982) meta-analysis of eight studies concluded that empirical support exists for the efficacy of occupational therapy using sensory integration approaches, whereas subsequent reviewers have claimed that the evidence in support of sensory integration approaches was inconclusive (Arendt, Mac Lean, & Baumeister, 1988; Daems, 1994; Polatajko, Kaplan, & Wilson, 1992; Schaffer, 1984; Spitzer, Roley, Clark, & Parham, 1997; Vargas & Camilli, 1999; Wilson & Kaplan, 1994). Although much of this research indicates that sensory integration approaches are effective in increasing children's motor, sensory processing, and academic skills, no definitive conclusions can be drawn regarding efficacy.

Many studies regarding the efficacy of sensory integration approaches have relied on measures of performance components for outcome evaluation. Use of perceptual, motor, sensory, and cognitive scales has narrowed the focus of the research. To broaden our understanding of outcomes, researchers have identified the need to understand the outcomes of occupational therapy from the child and family perspective (Bundy, 1991; Butler, 1995; Cohn & Cermak, 1998; Parham & Mailloux, 1996; Roley & Wilbarger, 1994).

In an era when health care reforms mandate that the consumer be included as an active participant in developing the intervention (Christiansen, 1996), understanding the consumers' perspective is crucial (Brown & Bowen, 1998; Simeonsson, Edmondson, Smith, Carnahan, & Bucy, 1995). Parents have provided ardent testimonials that occupational therapy using sensory integration approaches improves the quality of their family life (Anderson & Emmons,

Originally published 2001 in *American Journal of Occupational Therapy,* 55, 285–294.

1995; Occupational Therapy Associates, 1995). These testimonials suggest that parental satisfaction with therapy outcomes is an important domain for outcomes research. Although authors have described parents' points of view related to early intervention (Case-Smith & Nastro, 1993; Hinojosa, 1990; Hinojosa & Anderson, 1991; Miller & Hanft, 1998; Washington & Schwartz, 1996), similar discussions of parents' perspectives on occupational therapy using sensory integration approaches with older children are just emerging.

Using naturalistic program evaluation methods (Lincoln & Guba, 1985), Anderson (1993) explored parental perceptions of the impact of occupational therapy using sensory integration approaches on the daily living skills of children with autism. Parents in Anderson's study reported that their children made gains in several areas: willingness to try new play activities, socialization with other children, and ability to express emotions and desires. Furthermore, these parents reported an increase in their understanding of how sensory processing difficulties affected their children. Related research documented parents' hopes for their children before their children's participation in occupational therapy using sensory integration approaches (Cohn, Miller, & Tickle-Degnen, 2000). The parents in Cohn et al.'s (2000) study spoke about two overarching hopes for change in therapy: changes in their children and changes for themselves in their parenting occupation. Three themes pertinent to the occupation of children—social participation, self-regulation, and perceived competence—were identified, and two themes related to the occupation of parenting emerged—the desire to learn strategies to support their children and personal validation of the parenting experience. Ultimately, parents hoped to be able to sustain their family life.

The study reported here builds on Anderson's (1993) and Cohn et al.'s (2000) foundation by systematically describing parents' perceptions of occupational therapy using sensory integration approaches for their children. Understanding parents' perceptions of outcomes may help therapists to design interventions that are congruent with parents' values and support our attempts to deliver authentic, family-centered care (Lawlor & Mattingly, 1998). In addition, a framework for exploring measures that operationalize these crucial variables for further research can be developed.

Method

To understand parent perspectives of outcomes, I used a collective case study approach (Stake, 1994). I interviewed 16 parents (14 families consisting of 12 mothers and 2 husband-and-wife couples) of children who received occupational therapy using a sensory integration frame of reference at a private clinic in a northeastern U.S. suburban community. Parents of 22 children were randomly selected from a list of 42 children who met the inclusion criteria for participation. These 22 parents received a letter explaining the purpose of the study and offering them the opportunity to remove their name from the potential participant list. Those parents who did not request to be removed from the list were called to schedule interviews. Only 2 families scheduled the interviews to include both mother and father. A majority of the parents lived in single-family homes in suburban communities, and 50% held master's degrees. With the exception of 1 parent, all had college degrees. The sample was homogeneous, as all participants were White and in the moderate-to-affluent socioeconomic range.

The participants were parents of children 4 to 10 years of age who had documented diagnoses of some type of sensory integration dysfunction as measured by the Sensory Integration and Praxis

Tests (Ayres, 1989), who participated in at least 32 1-hr therapy sessions, and who stopped therapy at least 1 month to 2 years before the interview. A minimum of 32 1-hr therapy sessions (approximately 8 months) was the criterion selected to anticipate some type of change. This criterion is based on a review of nine sensory integration efficacy studies with children with learning disabilities (Ayres, 1972, 1978; Carte, Morrison, Sublett, Uemura, & Setrakian, 1984; Densem, Nuthall, Bushnell, & Horn, 1989; Humphries, Wright, McDougall, & Vertes, 1990; Humphries, Wright, Snider, & McDougall, 1992; Law, Polatajko, Schaffer, Miller, & Macnab, 1991; M. White, 1979; Wilson & Kaplan, 1994). Twenty-four hours of intervention was the modal number of therapy sessions in the reviewed studies. Therefore, it is proposed that the children in the study reported here received enough therapy to anticipate some type of change.

Parents of children given a primary diagnosis of autism, pervasive developmental disorder, or Fragile X syndrome were not interviewed for this study. These children may have different social–emotional and behavioral dysfunction than children without these conditions. The sample criteria are based on the assumption that they represent a relatively homogeneous subgroup of children who receive occupational therapy in private practice settings using a sensory integration framework.

Procedure

Interviews were conducted in each family's home and ranged from 1 hr to 2 hr. I asked participants to describe a typical day with their child, what about their child led them to seek occupational therapy, and what they had hoped to gain from therapy. I also asked whether they saw changes in their child and, if so, to describe an incident that illustrated the change. Finally, I asked whether changes they had hoped for had not occurred and how they came to a decision to stop

therapy. Each interview was audiotaped, transcribed, and checked by thorough review and comparison between the transcript and the original audiotape. Throughout the research process, I wrote reflective memos to record my immediate reactions to the interviews, and I wrote periodic analytical memos (Miles & Huberman, 1994) to record my evolving thoughts related to the research question and process. Recruitment was stopped after the 16th participant because I had reached a point at which findings from newly collected and analyzed data became redundant (Strauss & Corbin, 1998).

Data Analysis

To develop new insights, Frank (1997) recommended systematically examining our theoretical concerns and reflecting on our own views. Rather than eliminating our subjective reactions, Frank has encouraged us to use our reflections productively for insight and analysis. In the spirit of reflexivity, I acknowledge the influences of my own background as both a parent of school-age children and an occupational therapist who has provided occupational therapy using a sensory integration approach. As a parent, I know firsthand the experiences of striving to nurture children's growth and sense of competence. My parenting experience has taught me that sustaining the family system is a complex endeavor in which I must continually strive to understand my children's behavior in relation to the challenges in their worlds. As an occupational therapist, I try to provide therapy that ultimately makes a meaningful difference for children in the contexts in which they live, learn, and play. I carry an underlying assumption that occupational therapy is effective and can contribute to changes in children and the entire family system. However, I also believe and have documented elsewhere (Cohn & Cermak, 1998) that we have not empirically examined which outcomes of occupational therapy are important to parents who bring their children for intervention. Further, my interpretations are informed by a recent analysis of parental hopes for therapy outcomes (Cohn et al., 2000).

Using grounded theory procedures recommended by Strauss and Corbin (1998), I reviewed the transcripts to name and categorize changes described by parents. The experience of change is not always a straightforward formulation, and not all parents interviewed had positive or definitive perceptions of the benefits of occupational therapy using sensory integration approaches. Even though some parents questioned the value of intervention, they all reported that their children thoroughly enjoyed occupational therapy and were always eager to attend and that the therapy was a very positive experience for their children. The transcripts were divided into two classifications: positive and questionable perceptions of intervention. A new set of questions emerged from this distinction: For the parents who attributed positive outcomes to occupational therapy, what were the benefits they valued? What was missing for the parents who did not perceive definitive benefits? These questions were explored in the interpretative process. The specific themes in the positive and questionable categories were compared and contrasted to detect similarities and differences across all the transcripts. The QSR NUD*IST 4.0 (Non-numerical Unstructured Data-Indexing Searching & Theorizing) (1997) qualitative data analysis software was used to manage and explore the data.

To strengthen credibility and ensure that participants' perspectives were accurately represented, I prepared written summaries of each interview and sent them to participants for review. I then contacted each participant by phone to discuss the summaries and on the basis of their feedback, made modifications to the summaries as needed. I analyzed the summaries along with the interview data. Further, I rigorously examined the data to search for data samples that might be inconsistent with emerging concepts. Finally, peer examination was used to check categories developed from the data analysis. The transcripts were analyzed by a group of eight occupational therapists, each with more than 5 years of experience providing occupational therapy using sensory integration approaches, to discuss evolving concepts. To honor confidentiality, pseudonyms are used throughout this chapter.

Findings and Interpretation

Before examining parents' perceptions of the outcomes of occupational therapy using sensory integration approaches, we need to understand the reasons why parents seek the services of occupational therapists. A review of participants' responses to the question, "At what point did you decide to seek therapy for your child?," revealed a common concern. All participants worried that their children were not "fitting in" or "keeping up" with their peers. Donna, the mother of a now 7-year-old boy, described her son's rejection from kindergarten: "I applied for him to attend kindergarten at the private school where my other son was attending. It is pretty common for them to just accept siblings, and they didn't [accept him]."

Bonnie worried about her daughter's behavior on the school playground. Her daughter would be pacing the playground by herself rather than playing with other children. During parent–teacher conferences, Bonnie's main concern was always about friendships. Bonnie explained that other parents were concerned about academics, but she was focused on her daughter's social world.

Another mother, Janet, worried that her son "was just so incredibly far behind his classmates. He was so taken up with the basic tasks that he couldn't get on to doing anything fun." During preschool, Jenny's mother noticed that her daughter was "10 steps behind everyone else" in her dance class. She observed that Jenny could not process what the dance teacher was saying. The following year in kindergarten, Jenny's teacher reported that Jenny was "just not getting it." To the teacher, Jenny seemed too scared to move around in her environment.

A few mothers worried that their children's aggression and social problems interfered with social participation. Darcy sought the services of occupational therapy because she had a big "teddy bear" kind of kid who was hurting other children. She was concerned about his relationships with peers:

> He didn't know his own force. He would go to give a person a hug, and he would just about strangle them because he couldn't feel [his own strength]. He didn't mean to hurt his friend because he is not that kind of kid. He was hurting people without realizing because it wasn't hurting him. He didn't feel that he had connected with somebody. He was acting in a way that was unacceptable.

Darcy reflected on the impact of her son's condition. She recalled, "I was a wreck. I couldn't believe we had a bully as a child. It wasn't what I saw as my vision for my child."

These stories echo the words of parents who brought their children for occupational therapy using sensory integration approaches reported by Cohn et al. (2000). The parents hoped that their children would develop behavior and skills needed to "fit in," belong, or be included in school, home, and the community. Coster (1998) defined such hopes and reasons for bringing children to occupational therapy as *social participation:* "active engagement in the typical activities available to and/or expected of peers in the same context" (p. 341). Given that the parents in the present study also brought their children to occupational therapy because they were concerned about their children's social participation, it is not surprising that the most valued and significant changes reported by these parents were changes that opened children and parents to the possibility that their children could succeed in the social world in which they live, learn, and play.

Another similarity to Cohn et al.'s (2000) parental hopes research is that the parents in this study also reported changes that can be categorized as child focused and parent focused. Although these categories were identified in previous research, the distinctions between child-focused and parent-focused benefits emerged in all of the parent interviews in this study as well.

Child-Focused Outcomes

Within the overarching category of child-focused outcomes, the parents' perceptions of the benefits or outcomes of therapy can be categorized into three interrelated constructs: abilities, activities, and reconstruction of self-worth (see Figure 38.1). The constructs are ordered according to their objectivity. That is, improvements in abilities are directly observable, whereas reconstruction of self-worth is more subjective. Conversely, the participants reported that they valued improvements in their children's self-worth more than they valued improved abilities. They viewed their children's improvements in abilities and engagement in activities as contributing to their children's reconstruction of self-worth. Thus, the term *social participation* captures the integration of all three child-focused outcomes valued by parents.

Abilities. Participants spoke about objective and observable changes in their children's abilities. Trombly (1995) defined *abilities* as "skills that one has developed through practice and that underlie many different activities" (p. 962). Trombly gave the example of eye–hand coordination as an ability that "emanates from developed capacities that the person has gained

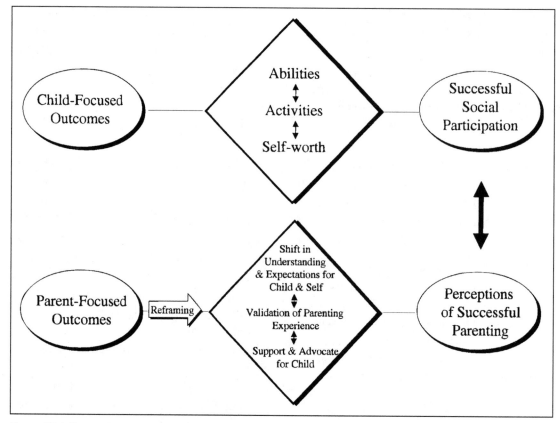

Figure 38.1. Parents' perspectives of therapy outcomes.

through learning or maturation" (p. 962). These abilities can be described and observed as things that occur within the body. All of the participants, even those who questioned the value of occupational therapy, were able to describe concrete, directly observable changes in their children. Ira's mother was able to see that his "fine motor skills" came a long way, and Wilma's mother noticed that her daughter's "balance and coordination" improved: "Her balance is better. Her coordination is better. She does more gross motor things. Her inner coordination is better."

Janet pointed out that her son's condition was not very extreme and that it was hard to know whether therapy helped, but she was clear that he "definitely got much stronger. His physical self is much more together."

Although Randy's mother also questioned whether occupational therapy made her son's or her life easier, she was able to objectively observe that her son's "upper body strength got stronger." Further, she noted a change in her son's "body and spatial awareness." She said that when Randy was small, he was unable to climb through a tunnel because he could not figure out where he was in relation to the tunnel. By the end of therapy, Randy knew where his body was in space. Although Randy's mother described these changes in Randy's abilities, she continued to question whether occupational therapy intervention helped him to "fit into his world," which, as she said, "is what parents really care about."

The participants did not identify deficits in their children's abilities as a reason for seeking occupational therapy; rather, they had focused on problems with social participation. However, abilities were observable outcomes that these parents could easily identify. Even the participants who questioned the value of occupational therapy were able to identify improved abilities. One father who questioned the value of occupational therapy paradoxically stated that therapy helped his daughter's "motor functions, but the correlation [with other areas of performance] was not an obvious one." This father's comments echo the views of other participants who had questionable perceptions of occupational therapy.

Activities. Participants who clearly described benefits of occupational therapy using sensory integration approaches reported that their children used their newfound abilities to enhance participation in activities. The term *activity* used here is based on the World Health Organization's (1999) ICIDH–2 definition, which defines activity in the broadest sense to capture everything that a person does at any level of complexity from simple activities to complex skills and behaviors. The participants' descriptions of various activities can be further categorized into organized activities, play, and personal care.

Organized activities are defined as "uses of time that are purposive, ongoing, structured, and more or less voluntarily chosen (although parental and peer pressures may influence the process of making choices)" (Medrich, Roizen, Rubin, & Buckley, 1982, p. 158). Many of the organized activities mentioned by participants were either sports-related or lessons. For example, Darcy was proud that her son was now accomplished in soccer and loved basketball. She believed that these were activities he never could have done before therapy. Allison's mother hypothesized a link between her daughter's abilities and her participation in dance lessons: "[Allison] really enjoyed OT [occupational ther-

apy]. It might have helped her with her coordination. She wasn't a very coordinated person, but she does ballet now...and she loves [the classes]." Jenny's mother also hypothesized that occupational therapy contributed to her daughter's emerging ability to participate in organized activities, such as gymnastics or swimming lessons:

> Amazingly, she was able to take gymnastics from second through fourth grade...she's so determined with gymnastics. She worked on it and she could finally do a handstand....And she was able to swim in the deep end....She used to jump in and come right back out.

Participants also reported changes in their children's abilities to participate in personal care activities. *Personal care* "refers to those activities that are essential to taking care of one's body, such as eating, dressing, grooming, bathing, and management of oral and toilet hygiene" (Primeau & Ferguson, 1999, p. 485). Rebecca reflected that her son was now able to be independent in dressing himself. She recalled that in the days before he received occupational therapy, dressing himself was a challenge. Diane told a similar story about her daughter: "[Before therapy], it took a long time for her to be able to dress herself and get all that stuff organized in the morning. She's been able to do that for 2 years now."

Play, which some authors argue is the primary occupation of children (Bundy, 1993; Parham & Primeau, 1997; Primeau & Ferguson, 1999), was another activity in which parents reported changes in their children's performance. Donna reflected on her son's advances in play after therapy: "After that first year [of therapy] we went away for the summer, and he just did a lot of running and things that kids do in the summer, and I just thought he had made enormous progress." Diane told a story about her daughter's sheer delight once she was able to master play activities:

> She was finally able to participate on the playground. She was able to do the monkey bars for the first time. She was just so happy....The first time she could ride a bike...was so meaningful for her because she was probably a year behind the other kids.

Reconstruction of self-worth. A third child-focused outcome, reconstruction of the child's self-worth, was highly valued by the participants. On the basis of Harter's (1983) work, Mayberry (1990) defined *self-worth* as a general evaluation of the way we feel about the self-concept domains that are important to us, including competencies that we recognize in ourselves and perceived social acceptance by persons who are important to us. Bonnie was most pleased about her daughter's changed feelings about herself: "I could see she was happier. Psychologically, there was a dramatic change over time....The therapist was tremendous with helping her accept herself....She felt better about herself, and she felt it was helping." Noting changes in her son, Donna reported,

> He would just be so invigorated and a new person. That is what I remember about OT. I would bring one child and would come home with a different child. The experience of having all that physical input made him happy.... I would see it right after a session.

The parents also perceived that occupational therapy enabled their children to take more risks. Linda attributed her daughter's willingness to try new things to therapy: "She has learned how to take more risks. When she was first there, when she came upon something that was hard for her, she just stepped back. She has gotten better at taking risks." Linda talked about changes in her daughter Wilma's sense of self as providing a foundation for the future. Linda suggested that

Wilma was going to have to work hard and that Wilma now knew about making mistakes and persevering. According to Linda, occupational therapy taught Wilma "how to learn" and provided her with the internal experience that she could derive satisfaction in the things she attempted. Therapy became a catalyst for Wilma to imagine the things she might do in the future.

Earlier research reported similar findings (Anderson, 1993; Ayres & Mailloux, 1983), documenting that after occupational therapy using sensory integration approaches, parents of children with autism noted changes in their children's self-worth, illustrated by gains in initiation to seek challenges or take risks. Further, using physical therapy principles, Schoemaker, Hijlkema, and Kalverboer (1994) documented that therapy may have a potent impact on a child's self-worth and willingness to engage in motor activities. These potential changes in self-worth can be interpreted using R. White's (1959) effectance motivation model. White claimed that children will work toward mastery if they believe that their attempts will be successful. Building on White's notion, Harter (1978) proposed that children's perceived competence was related to their previous attempts at mastery within a particular context or domain, and this perceived competence affected children's motivation to participate in activities in that domain. Enhanced willingness to engage in activity is consistent with Ayres's premise that sensory integration may "enable further purposeful activity" (Ayres & Mailloux, 1983, p. 536).

Parent-Focused Outcomes

The parent-focused outcomes are inextricably linked to the children's constructions of self-worth. Perhaps the most robust finding is that participants reported numerous benefits from understanding their children's behaviors from a sensory processing perspective. In defining the consultative role of occupational therapy, Bundy (1991) proposed that *reframing,* a process of enabling others to understand the client's behavior in a new way or from a different perspective, can help consultees understand the client, develop effective strategies for interacting with the client, and provide parents with a basis for more satisfying parenting experiences. Bundy's notion of reframing is based on Toulmin's (1953) argument that reframing is a form of science in which we learn to see data in new ways. Reframing involves "seeing" or "hearing" differently.

As depicted in Figure 38.1, the participants suggested that such reframing facilitated a shift in expectations for themselves and their children, validated their parenting experience, and enabled them to support and advocate for their children. Together, these by-products of reframing ultimately opened participants to the possibility that they could be successful parents and their children could become successful participants in their worlds. As participants understood their children's behavior from a sensory processing perspective, they became more accepting of their children. This acceptance, participants believed, led to improved sense of self-worth in their children. Bonnie's perspective vividly illustrates this perceived connection:

> [OT] helped us accept her needs and it helped her accept her own needs. From that perspective, I think it calmed us all down. It made us less frantic about trying to fit into this mold of a child that doesn't exist. And it made us all more accepting of her behaviors....It helped us try to work with her needs and not just our needs for her....I began to understand her needs. That was important. Psychologically she was getting hurt because she was thinking she was a bad person....My child was incredibly happier as a result, and that was a really important measurement for me. I could see she was happier. [The OT] was tremendous with helping her accept herself.

Shift in understanding and expectations for child and self. All of the participants had a desire for their children to become greater social participants in their worlds; some also imagined that occupational therapy might cure their child's problem. Rebecca hoped that therapy would fix her child's problem, and Darcy hoped that therapy would make her son "normal." Olivia actually used the word *cure* and later in her interview made an analogy to ear infections. She reflected that she had initially hoped for a cure but learned that her son's sensory integration problems were not as clear-cut as an ear infection and that there was no "medicine" to make the condition go away. Rather than viewing their children's condition as something that "needed fixing," the majority of participants described how their expectations for their children and themselves as parents shifted.

Diane found that her knowledge of her daughter's sensory processing enabled her to be more supportive of her daughter: "If she is goofing off with a kazoo, I know it is helping her. [In the past], I might have said, 'Stop it.' The self-calming techniques that kids naturally do, I understand them better." Olivia told a story quite typical of many children with tactile sensitivity:

> One thing that's driving me crazy is when he puts his socks and shoes on and then feels a wrinkle or something, he takes his shoes off again. For him, this is a big problem. It's just driving him crazy. I got to understand that a little better. I take into account that he is not doing it on purpose and that I should be more patient.

Ira's mother claimed that she learned to be aware of the kind of person her son is and be more aware of his concerns. At first, she thought his behaviors were just "typical-boy" behaviors, but now she believes that she is more sensitive to his needs and tries to structure the day to meet them: "[OT] taught me to be more aware of him as a person who is different than what you might expect. And it kind of helped me focus on what he does."

Validation of parenting experience. Cohn et al. (2000) documented that parents seek validation of the challenges inherent in parenting children with sensory integration problems. Many participants concurred that new understandings of their children helped validate earlier experiences. Donna was relieved to understand her son's early experiences from a different perspective: "It kind of clarified his whole nursery school experience, why it was unpleasant for him....When I read his [OT] report I thought, 'That's why nursery school was so tough for him.'" Randy shared similar sentiments:

> The kid was born super sensitive to sound, and it was very helpful when the tests were done. Not just to affirm that I wasn't insane but in trying to understand some of the things that were difficult for him.

These two examples also are reflective of many of the other participants' sentiments.

Support and advocacy for child. Participants used their new understanding of how their children process sensory information to advocate and communicate with school personnel. Olivia said, "[My understanding of my son's sensory processing] gave me a chance to sit down at the beginning of the school year and say, 'This child does have particular concerns.'" Olivia was particularly pleased that the therapists who worked with her son gave her "very useful hints on everyday little problems." She recalled a time when her son was in a holiday play at school. He could not tolerate a headpiece he was supposed to wear, and the therapist gave her good ideas on how to change the costume. Peggy learned to advocate with teachers to allow her child to hold objects in her hand during circle time. She told one teacher that her daughter had trouble sitting on the floor during circle time. The teacher eliminated sitting on the floor altogether so that her daughter would "fit in" with the rest of the class.

Implications for Practice

The findings from this study suggest that the parents who attributed positive outcomes to occupational therapy perceived changes in three domains of their children's functioning: abilities, activities, and sense of self-worth. They described how changes in one domain affected the other areas of functioning. The participants who questioned the benefits of occupational therapy did not describe interrelationships between their children's abilities and their children's broader social world. It is unknown whether these participants understood the therapists' assumption that improvements in abilities might influence engagement in activities and improve self-worth. Conversely, these participants may have understood this assumption of sensory integration theory but just did not observe relationships among improved abilities, activities, and self-worth in their children. The insights gained from the study highlight the importance of striving to understand parents' expectations for therapy and how they are making sense of what is occurring in and as a result of therapy. Parents' perceptions may serve as a powerful indicator of whether therapy has had an impact on aspects of the child's life considered important by the parents.

Although some participants were initially searching for a cure for their children's condition, all reframed their expectations. After their children participated in occupational therapy, many participants envisioned a future for their children that included ongoing acceptance, accommodation, and advocacy. They valued this reframing or reconstruction of expectations for their children and themselves as parents. Similar findings have been reported in the early intervention literature. Parents of younger children who received occupational therapy also valued the support, information, and strategies learned to enhance their parenting (Case-Smith & Nastro, 1993; Hinojosa, 1990; Washington & Schwartz, 1996). All of these studies remind us to consider the broader context in which children live and to design interventions that move beyond "fixing the person" (Brown & Bowen, 1998, p. 56). One way to develop goals and interventions that are congruent with parents' concerns and that move beyond direct intervention is to ask parents and children questions that relate to the social world in which they live, work, and play. Children's everyday life should be the beginning point of our evaluation process.

Moreover, supplementing the use of standardized scales, which predetermine and potentially constrict the constructs we measure, with tools that allow children and parents to identify important life goals and rate their importance may assist us in providing therapy that is more congruent with our consumers' goals. The School Function Assessment (Coster, Deeney, Haltiwanger, & Haley, 1998), which measures social participation in the school setting, and The Pediatric Interest Profiles (Henry, 2000), which describes participation in play activities, are two newly developed tools that attend to participation from the consumer's perspective.

The finding that reconstruction of self-worth was a valued outcome by the participants suggests that it is important for therapists to monitor how our young consumers perceive themselves across the various contexts of their everyday life. Children's experiences of therapy and everyday life is critical to our evaluation of the value of therapy. Willoughby, King, and Polatajko (1996) urged therapists to use psychometrically and conceptually sound measures to monitor the "domains of self-worth" most meaningful to children and families. The All About Me Scale (Missiuna, 1998), which evaluates young chil-

dren's perceptions of their self-efficacy in the performance of fine and gross motor activities, offers therapists a tool to begin to document one dimension of the construct of self-worth. The domains of scholastic competence, athletic competence, self-care competence, behavioral competence, and social competence are also important for occupational therapists to consider when trying to understand a child's perceived self-worth (Willoughby et al., 1996).

Implications for Research

Given the paucity of data on consumers' perspectives on occupational therapy using sensory integration approaches, additional research is recommended. Some participants hypothesized that their children's improved abilities contributed to enhanced participation in activities and reconstruction of self-worth. Based on Coster's (1998) conceptualization, I have categorized these perceived outcomes as "social participation." These hypothesized relationships between abilities and social participation are likely to be complex and require further elaboration and empirical validation. Moreover, further exploration is necessary to understand why some parents did not perceive changes in their children's abilities, activities, and self-worth. Is the lack of perceived change based on children's actual occupational performance, or might parents' lack of perceived change be related to unclear expectations of occupational therapy using a sensory integration approach?

The parent-focused outcomes also require further elaboration and empirical examination. Many questions related to the hypothetical interrelationships among the child-focused and parent-focused outcomes remain. Of particular concern is whether changes in parents' understanding and expectations, validation of the parenting experience, and parents' support and advocacy for their children relate to parents' sense of themselves as successful parents. Do parenting changes, in turn, relate to social participation for their children? Although there is emerging evidence documenting the relationship of parents' beliefs and children's achievement (Goodnow, 1988; Murphey, 1992), research efforts are needed to explicate all of the proposed connections. Further, we have yet to determine whether the outcomes proposed in this study are present in the broader population of consumers of occupational therapy using sensory integration approaches.

The participants were from White, middle- and upper-socioeconomic-status families; thus, the perspectives of other populations remain unknown. Moreover, the school setting is central to children's lives, and the perspectives of teachers were not included in this study. Finally, and perhaps most importantly, the voices of the children themselves were not heard. Therefore, one of the many challenges facing future researchers is to listen to other persons in the world of children as well as to the children themselves. Ultimately, we need a new understanding of therapy that emphasizes the relationship between therapy and the everyday lives of children and families.

Acknowledgments

I extend a special note of gratitude to the parents who shared their time and perspectives. I value and thank my dissertation committee members, Linda Tickle-Degnen, PhD, OTR/L; Wendy Coster, PhD, OTR/L, FAOTA; Cathy Riessman, PhD; and Jane Koomar, PhD, OTR/L, FAOTA, for their insightful critiques. Much appreciated for their assistance are Teresa May-Benson, MS, OTR/L, and all of the therapists at OTA–Watertown, P.C., Watertown, MA.

This study was conducted in partial fulfillment of the requirement for the doctor of science degree at Boston University, Sargent College of Health and Rehabilitation Sciences. It was supported in part by a grant from the American Occupational Therapy Foundation, the Anne Henderson Doctoral Scholarship, and a grant to Boston University from the U.S. Department of Health and Human Services, Health Resources and Services Administration, Maternal and Child Health Bureau (MCJ000-901).

References

Anderson, E. L. (1993). *Parental perceptions of the influence of occupational therapy utilizing sensory integrative techniques on the daily living skills of children with autism.* Unpublished master's thesis, University of Southern California, Los Angeles.

Anderson, E., & Emmons, P. (1995). Sensory integration: The hidden disorder. *Sensory Integration Quarterly Newsletter, 23*(2/3), 8–9.

Arendt, R. E., Mac Lean, W. E., & Baumeister, A. A. (1988). Critique of sensory integration therapy and its application in mental retardation. *American Journal on Mental Retardation, 92,* 401–411.

Ayres, A. J. (1972). Improving academic scores through sensory integration. *Journal of Learning Disabilities, 5,* 24–28.

Ayres, A. J. (1978). Learning disabilities and the vestibular system. *Journal of Learning Disabilities, 11,* 30–41.

Ayres, A. J. (1989). *Sensory Integration and Praxis Tests.* Los Angeles: Western Psychological Services.

Ayres, A. J., & Mailloux, Z. (1983). Possible pubertal effect on therapeutic gains in an autistic girl. *American Journal of Occupational Therapy, 37,* 535–540.

Brown, C., & Bowen, R. E. (1998). Including the consumer and environment in occupational therapy treatment planning. *Occupational Therapy Journal of Research, 18,* 44–62.

Bundy, A. C. (1991). Consultation and sensory integration theory. In A. G. Fisher, E. A. Murray, & A. C. Bundy (Eds.), *Sensory integration: Theory and practice* (pp. 318–332). Philadelphia: F. A. Davis.

Bundy, A. C. (1993). Assessment of play and leisure: Delineation of the problem. *American Journal of Occupational Therapy, 47,* 217–222.

Butler, C. (1995). Outcomes that matter [Editorial]. *Developmental Medicine and Child Neurology, 37,* 753–754.

Carte, E., Morrison, D., Sublett, J., Uemura, A., & Setrakian, W. (1984). Sensory integration therapy: A trial of a specific neurodevelopmental therapy for remediation of learning disabilities. *Journal of Developmental Behavioral Pediatrics, 5,* 189–194.

Case-Smith, J., & Nastro, M. A. (1993). The effect of occupational therapy intervention on mothers of children with cerebral palsy. *American Journal of Occupational Therapy, 47,* 811–817.

Christiansen, C. (1996). Nationally Speaking— Managed care: Opportunities and challenges for occupational therapy in the emerging systems of the 21st century. *American Journal of Occupational Therapy, 50,* 409–412.

Cohn, E. S., & Cermak, S. A. (1998). Including the family perspective in sensory integration outcomes research. *American Journal of Occupational Therapy, 52,* 540–546.

Cohn, E. S., Miller, L. J., & Tickle-Degnen, L. (2000). Parental hopes for therapy outcomes: Children with sensory modulation disorders. *American Journal of Occupational Therapy, 54,* 36–43.

Coster, W. (1998). Occupation-centered assessment of children. *American Journal of Occupational Therapy, 52,* 337–344.

Coster, W. J., Deeney, T., Haltiwanger, J., & Haley, S. M. (1998). *School function assessment.* San Antonio, TX: Psychological Corporation/Therapy SkillBuilders.

Daems, J. (Ed.). (1994). *Reviews of research in sensory integration.* Torrance, CA: Sensory Integration International.

Densem, J. F., Nuthall, G. A., Bushnell, J., & Horn, J. (1989). Effectiveness of a sensory integration therapy program for children with perceptual–motor deficits. *Journal of Learning Disabilities, 22,* 221–229.

Frank, G. (1997). Is there life after categories? Reflexivity in qualitative research. *Occupational Therapy Journal of Research, 17,* 84–98.

Goodnow, J. J. (1988). Parents' ideas, actions, and feelings: Models and methods from developmental and social psychology. *Child Development, 59,* 286–320.

Harter, S. (1978). Effectance motivation reconsidered: Toward a developmental model. *Human Development, 21,* 34–64.

Harter, S. (1983). The development of the self-system. In M. Hetherington (Ed.), *Carmichael's manual of child psychology: Social and personality development* (pp. 275–385). New York: Wiley.

Henry, A. D. (2000). *Pediatric Interest Profiles: Surveys of play for children and adolescents.* San Antonio, TX: Therapy SkillBuilders.

Hinojosa, J. (1990). How mothers of preschool children perceive occupational and physical therapists and their influence on family life. *Occupational Therapy Journal of Research, 10,* 144–162.

Hinojosa, J., & Anderson, J. (1991). Mothers' perceptions of home treatment programs for their preschool children with cerebral palsy. *American Journal of Occupational Therapy, 45,* 273–279.

Humphries, T., Wright, M., McDougall, B., & Vertes, J. (1990). The efficacy of sensory integration for children with learning disability. *Physical and Occupational Therapy in Pediatrics, 10*(3), 1–17.

Humphries, T. W., Wright, M., Snider, L., & McDougall, B. (1992). A comparison of the effectiveness of sensory integrative therapy and perceptual–motor training in treating children with learning disabilities. *Journal of Developmental and Behavioral Pediatrics, 13,* 31–40.

Law, M., Polatajko, H. J., Schaffer, R., Miller, J., & Macnab, J. (1991). The impact of heterogeneity in a clinical trial: Motor outcomes after sensory integration therapy. *Occupational Therapy Journal of Research, 11,* 177–189.

Lawlor, M. C., & Mattingly, C. F. (1998). The complexities embedded in family-centered care. *American Journal of Occupational Therapy, 52,* 259–267.

Lincoln, Y. S., & Guba, E. G. (1985). *Naturalistic inquiry.* Beverly Hills, CA: Sage.

Mayberry, W. (1990). Self-esteem in children: Considerations for measurement and intervention. *American Journal of Occupational Therapy, 44,* 729–734.

Medrich, E. A., Roizen, J. A., Rubin, V., & Buckley, S. (1982). *The serious business of growing up: A study of children's lives outside school.* Berkeley: University of California.

Miles, M. B., & Huberman, A. M. (1994). *Qualitative data analysis* (2nd ed.). Thousand Oaks, CA: Sage.

Miller, L. J., & Hanft, B. E. (1998). Building positive alliances: Partnerships with families as the cornerstone of developmental assessment. *Infants and Young Children, 10,* 1–12.

Miller, L. J., & Kinnealey, M. (1993). Researching the effectiveness of sensory integration. *Sensory Integration Quarterly, 21*(2), 1–7.

Missiuna, C. (1998). Development of "All About Me," a scale that measures children's perceived motor competence. *Occupational Therapy Journal of Research, 18,* 85–108.

Murphey, D. A. (1992). Constructing the child: Relations between parents' beliefs and child outcomes. *Developmental Review, 12,* 199–232.

Occupational Therapy Associates. (1995). *The sensory connection.* Watertown, MA: Author.

Ottenbacher, K. (1982). Sensory integration therapy: Affect or effect. *American Journal of Occupational Therapy, 36,* 571–578.

Parham, L. D., & Mailloux, Z. (1996). Sensory integration. In J. Case-Smith, A. S. Allen, & P. N. Pratt (Eds.), *Occupational therapy for children* (3rd ed., pp. 307–355). St. Louis, MO: Mosby.

Parham, L. D., & Primeau, L. A. (1997). Play and occupational therapy. In L. D. Parham & L. S. Fazio (Eds.), *Play in occupational therapy for children* (pp. 2–21). St. Louis, MO: Mosby.

Polatajko, H., Kaplan, B., & Wilson, B. (1992). Sensory integration for children with learning disabilities: Its status 20 years later. *Occupational Therapy Journal of Research, 12,* 323–341.

Primeau, L. A., & Ferguson, J. M. (1999). Occupational frame of reference. In P. Kramer & J. Hinojosa (Eds.), *Frames of reference for pediatric occupational therapy* (pp. 469–516). Philadelphia: Lippincott Williams & Wilkins.

QSR NUD*IST 4.0 [Computer software]. (1997). Thousand Oaks, CA: Scolari, Sage Publications Software.

Roley, S. S., & Wilbarger, J. (1994, June). What is sensory integration? A series of interviews on the scope, limitations, and evolution of sensory integration theory. *Sensory Integration Special Interest Section Newsletter,* pp. 1–7.

Schaffer, R. (1984). Sensory integration therapy with learning disabled children: A critical review. *Canadian Journal of Occupational Therapy, 51,* 73–77.

Schoemaker, M., Hijlkema, M., & Kalverboer, A. (1994). Physiotherapy for clumsy children: An evaluation study. *Developmental Medicine and Child Neurology, 36,* 143–155.

Simeonsson, R. J., Edmondson, R., Smith, T., Carnahan, S., & Bucy, J. (1995). Family involvement in multidisciplinary team evaluation: Parent and professional perspectives. *Child Care, Health and Development, 21*(3), 1–16.

Spitzer, S., Roley, S. S., Clark, F., & Parham, D. (1997). Sensory integration: Current trends in the United States. *Scandinavian Journal of Occupational Therapy, 4,* 1–16.

Stake, R. (1994). Case studies. In N. Denzin & Y. Lincoln (Eds.), *Handbook of qualitative research* (pp. 236–247). Thousand Oaks, CA: Sage.

Strauss, A., & Corbin, J. (1998). *Basics of qualitative research.* Newbury Park, CA: Sage.

Toulmin, S. (1953). *The philosophy of science: An introduction.* London: Hutchinson.

Trombly, C. A. (1995). Occupation: Purposefulness and meaningfulness as therapeutic mechanisms [1995 Eleanor Clarke Slagle Lecture]. *American Journal of Occupational Therapy, 49,* 960–972.

Vargas, S., & Camilli, G. (1999). A meta-analysis of research on sensory integration treatment. *American Journal of Occupational Therapy, 53,* 189–198.

Washington, K., & Schwartz, I. S. (1996). Maternal perceptions of the effects of physical and occupational therapy services on caregiving competency. *Physical and Occupational Therapy in Pediatrics, 16*(3), 33–54.

White, M. (1979). A first-grade intervention program for children at risk for reading failure. *Journal of Learning Disabilities, 12,* 26–32.

White, R. (1959). Motivation reconsidered: The concept of competence. *Psychological Review, 66,* 297–323.

Willoughby, C., King, G., & Polatajko, H. (1996). A therapist's guide to children's self-esteem. *American Journal of Occupational Therapy, 50,* 124–132.

Wilson, B. N., & Kaplan, B. J. (1994). Follow-up assessment of children receiving sensory integration treatment. *Occupational Therapy Journal of Research, 14,* 244–266.

World Health Organization. (1999). *ICIDH-2: International classification of functioning and disability* (Beta 2 draft). Geneva, Switzerland: Author.

CHAPTER 39

Mothers' Perceptions of Child Care Assistance

The Impact of a Child's Disability

Terry K. Crowe, Betsy VanLeit, and Kirsten K. Berghmans

Terry K. Crowe, PhD, OTR/L, FAOTA, *is director and associate professor, Occupational Therapy Program, Department of Orthopaedics, University of New Mexico, Health Sciences and Services Building, Room 215, Albuquerque, NM 87131-5641.*

Betsy VanLeit, MPA, OTR/L, *was lecturer II, Occupational Therapy Program, University of New Mexico, Albuquerque, at the time of this writing.*

Kirsten K. Berghmans, MS, OTR/L, *is staff occupational therapist, Moriarty Public Schools, Moriarty, NM, and doctoral student in biomedical sciences, University of New Mexico, Albuquerque.*

Originally published 2000 in *American Journal of Occupational Therapy,* 54, 52–58.

Caring for any young child takes an inordinate amount of time, and the demands escalate if the child has a disability (Eiser, 1993). In addition, as children with disabilities grow older and heavier, daily caregiver tasks, such as bathing and dressing, may become even more demanding (Turnbull & Turnbull, 1990). In the words of one parent of a child with multiple disabilities,

> I dreaded getting up in the morning. The thought of another day was just intolerable…[Levi's] feedings took almost 2 hours. Then I played with him, bathed him, dressed him, positioned him. There were lots of doctor visits, getting his medications, washing his diapers. The days would just grind by. There were no weekends. Every day you go through his 8- to 12-hour routine. I never, ever slept through a night. I still don't. I'm up with Levi 1 to 2 hours. I wake up exhausted. (Knowles, 1987, p. 2)

A number of studies have described the time use of mothers of children with special needs. Harris and McHale (1989) reported that two-thirds of the mothers of children with mental retardation indicated that they had experienced difficulty with time demands related to caring for their child. Mothers are often prevented from doing other activities they want to do, including family outings, spending time with other family members, and carrying out household duties (McAndrew, 1976; Widerstrom & Goodwin, 1987). Johnson and Deitz (1985) compared the time use for physical child care (feeding, personal care, transportation) of mothers with preschool children who either had physical disabilities or were typically developing. The authors found that the mothers of children with special needs spent significantly more time engaged in physical child care activities than did the latter. In addition, mothers of the children who were typically developing regularly engaged in activities away from home significantly more often. Similarly, Harris and McHale (1989) found that mothers of children with mental retardation spent significantly more time each day doing child-related activities than did mothers of children who were typically developing.

Interestingly, increased participation in activities with children who were mentally retarded correlated with increased family problems. The authors suggested that "keeping children occupied or entertained by participating in leisure and recreational activities, such as playing or going on outings, may be as demanding and time consuming for mothers as are tasks labeled caregiving" (p. 237).

Crowe (1993) compared the time use of mothers with children younger than 5 years of age. She found that mothers of children with multiple disabilities spent an average of 39.7 hr per week in child care activities, mothers of children with Down syndrome spent 32.8 hr, and mothers of children who were typically developing spent an average of 33.0 hr per week performing child care tasks. Mothers of children with multiple disabilities spent significantly more child care time than did the other two groups. In addition, mothers of children who were typically developing spent more time socializing with other adults than did mothers of children with Down syndrome or multiple disabilities. Indicative of the heavy time demands associated with caring for children with disabilities, Joosten (1979) found that Dutch mothers slept 1 hr less per night if their child had myelomeningocele than if their child was typically developing.

Mothers of children with disabilities have been studied more extensively than fathers (King, King, & Rosenbaum, 1996). In one of the few studies of fathers' child care involvement with children with disabilities and without disabilities, Young and Roopnarine (1994) found that middle-class fathers in two-parent families spent about one-third as much time in child care activities as their spouses. This involvement did not differ whether the child had a disability. The authors also found that the mothers in the study perceived that they received more support from extended family and extrafamilial members than did the

fathers. Interestingly, mothers' self-perceptions of competence in caring for their children were stronger than fathers' self-perceptions. In comparing paternal caregiving in families where the child had a motor impairment, developmental delay, Down syndrome, or typical development, Erickson and Upshur (1989) found that mothers perceived that their husbands performed significantly fewer child care tasks in families when the child had a motor impairment.

Reasons suggested for the paucity of literature on paternal caregiving in families where there is a child with a disability include underestimation of the importance of fathers in childrearing (Lamb, 1983), the assumption that fathers are less affected than mothers by the child's disability (Sabbeth, 1984), and the fact that fathers tend to be less involved in the child's therapeutic care than mothers (Linder & Chitwood, 1984). There is increasing recognition, however, that it is important to focus on paternal involvement in families of children with and without disabilities (LaRossa & Reitzes, 1995; Young & Roopnarine, 1994) because it is apparent that fathers' participation in child care has an impact on the marriage, both parents, and the child (Lamb, 1987; Menaghan & Parcel, 1990; Piburn & Boyce, 1992).

Purpose of Study

Three groups of women participated in this study: mothers of children with multiple disabilities, mothers of children with Down syndrome, and mothers of children who were typically developing. The purpose of this study was to examine and compare perceptions of mothers of children with disabilities and of children without disabilities concerning the amount of time that fathers and other persons spent in child care as well as maternal satisfaction with the reported child care division of labor. *Child care* was defined to include bathing, dressing, or grooming the child; feeding or preparing a meal for the child; participating in the child's school program; transporting the child to child-centered activities; observing the child in therapy or educational activities; and talking with the child's therapist or teacher.

Method

Participants

The participants were 135 mothers of young children who were part of a larger research project that addressed mothers' time use and role perception (Crowe, 1993; Crowe, Clark, & Qualls, 1996; Crowe, VanLeit, Berghmans, & Mann, 1997). Women had to meet the following eligibility criteria: (a) have a child who met the group and age specifications, (b) be part of a two-parent household, (c) not be employed outside the home for more than 20 hr per week, (d) have no more than three children living in the home, and (e) have no foster children.

Group criteria depended on whether the child of focus had a disability. Forty-five mothers had children with multiple disabilities (including 53% neuromuscular disorders, 24% global developmental delays, 7% myelodysplasia or other developmental concerns), 45 mothers had children with Down syndrome, and 45 mothers had children with typical development. A functional checklist was developed to assist in the selection and categorization of children with multiple disabilities because this grouping was not diagnosis dependent. Children in this group had to have difficulty in at least two functional ability areas (mobility, feeding, playing, dressing, toileting, communication) as based on the mothers' perceptions. Children with multiple disabilities had difficulty in an average of 3.1 functional areas compared with children with Down syndrome, who had difficulty in an average of 1.4 functional areas.

To further describe the children of the participants in this study, the Battelle Developmental Screening Test (BDST; Newborg, Stock, Wnek, Guidubaldi, & Svinichi, 1984) was administered to all children. The BDST is a 96-item screening test with items in the domains of personal–social, adaptive, motor, communication, and cognitive development. This test was standardized on 800 children and has reliability and validity backing. The average amount of delay of children with multiple disabilities was 65% (range = 32%–100%). Children with Down syndrome had an average percentage of delay of 44% (range = 0%–78%). One 6-month-old child with Down syndrome had no obvious developmental delay at the time of testing according to the BDST. Children with typical development could have no more than a 15% delay according to the BDST. Sixty-two percent of the children identified as typically developing had no delay, 27% had a 1% to 10% delay, and 11% had an 11% to 13% delay. Three mothers were dropped from the study because their children demonstrated a delay of more than 15%. As a group, the children with typical development had less than 1% delay according to the BDST results.

Children of participants had to be from 6 months of age to 5 years of age. Each of the three groups of participants had children distributed across three age groups as there were 15 children from 6 to 12 months (infants), 15 children from 1 to 3 years (toddlers), and 15 children from 3 to 5 years (preschoolers). A one-way analysis of variance (ANOVA) determined that there were no significant differences between the ages of children in the three groups. Gender of the children was not controlled, but there were no significant differences in the gender distribution (54% boys, 46% girls) among the three groups. The children were predominantly Caucasian, with 4 Asian-American children, 3 African-American children, and 1 child from Saudi Arabia.

Table 39.1 describes demographic characteristics of the families. Statistical tests (ANOVAs) were used to examine differences among groups for number of siblings and parental age and education. Chi-square analysis was used for group effect of family income comparisons. The mothers of children with multiple disabilities were significantly younger than the women in the other two groups, the families of children with Down syndrome had more children, and the fathers of children with Down syndrome were older. The parents of the children who were typically developing were significantly more educated and had a higher income than parents in the other two groups.

Instruments

The two instruments used for this study were the Demographic Background Questionnaire developed by the primary author and the Caregiver's Activity and Recording of Events (CARE) Inventory (Crowe, 1991). Besides descriptive information about the participants and their families, questions about distribution and satisfaction of child care and housework were included in the Demographic Background Questionnaire.

The CARE requires participants to self-chart their daily activities over a 7-day period and has three sections: (a) recording specific activities each 1/2 hr over a 24-hr time frame, (b) indicating which activities were found to be stressful, and (c) charting who was responsible for the target child (i.e., the child recruited for the study on the basis of age and group status).

This chapter focuses on the third section. For each 1/2 hr, the mother was asked to indicate whether (a) someone other than the mother was primarily responsible for the child's care, (b) the child was with her when she was performing various activities, or (c) the child was sleeping. If someone else was identified as responsible for the child's care, the specific person (child's father, grandparent, siblings, school program, babysitter, other) was recorded. The data according to mothers' perceptions regarding the persons responsible for the target children's care were used for data analysis. It is possible that if fathers of children were asked to chart their involvement with target children, their perceptions would be different than the perceptions of the mothers.

Procedure

A faculty member and two graduate students (one occupational therapist and one physical therapist) collected the data. Interrater reliability of scoring of the BDST was established before and during the study. Percent agreement ranged from 88.5%

Table 39.1. Characteristics of Families

Characteristic	Multiple Disabilities		Down Syndrome		Typically Developing		
	M	SD	M	SD	M	SD	p
Number of siblings of target child	1.0	0.8	1.3	0.8	0.8	0.7	.006
Age of mother (in years)	29.6	5.0	33.9	5.1	32.3	4.1	.0001
Years of maternal education	13.8	2.1	14.3	2.3	16.0	2.1	<.0005
Age of father (in years)	31.8	5.2	35.6	5.9	33.2	3.7	.002
Years of paternal education	14.6	2.5	14.9	3.0	17.3	2.7	<.0005
Family income (No. of families)[a]							
<$29,999	20		11		8		
$30,000–$49,999	18		23		19		.005[b]
>$49,999	4		8		16		

Note. N = 45.
[a]Not all families reported income.
[b]p value obtained from χ^2 = 14.64.

to 99% across the course of the study. Procedural compliance was analyzed to ensure that crucial steps were followed for a minimum of 95% of the time during the data collection.

An appointment was arranged within 1 week of a referral of a participant from the community. At the home visit, the participant signed a human subject consent form, the BDST was administered to the target child, and the Demographic Background Questionnaire was collected. Additionally, mothers were trained on how to reliably fill out the CARE by completing a CARE that was based on hypothetical examples of time use. Participants needed to obtain a 100% agreement on the example within two trials. Unless there were special circumstances (e.g., the mother was planning to do something unusual, like take a trip), the mother started the CARE the day after the home visit. A researcher contacted mothers by telephone once during the week to remind them to complete the CARE and to answer any questions. The home visit took between 60 and 90 min. After the inventory was returned, a small honorarium was sent.

Three persons coded the completed CAREs. After training, the coders coded six pilot CAREs, and interrater reliability was more than 93% among all coders. Throughout the coding process, interrater reliability was checked periodically, with a mean percentage of agreement of 95% between Coders 1 and 2 (14 checks) and a mean percentage of agreement of 94.5% between Coders 1 and 3 (9 checks). Number of checks was based on the number of CAREs coded.

Data Analysis

The time that the mothers perceived that the fathers and other caregivers spent with the target child was totaled, and descriptive statistics were calculated. A one-way, between-subjects ANOVA was run on the means of all samples and totals, weekends, and weekdays by group. An analysis was also performed if any time differences spent by the father according to the age of the child existed. The amount of child care that mothers provided and their satisfaction with child care arrangements were tallied, and a correlation coefficient was calculated.

Results

Paternal Time Spent Performing Child Care

All fathers spent similar amounts of time with the target child independent of group status. On average, fathers spent 5.2 hr during the week (Monday–Friday) and 4.6 hr on the weekend providing child care. The mean paternal time spent in child care activities for the entire week was 9.8 hr. Table 39.2 and Figure 39.1 illustrate differences between groups in paternal time spent providing child care. However, no significant differences were found. In addition, fathers did not spend significantly different amounts of time providing care for children according to their age. The large standard deviations indicate wide variations of child care time spent by fathers within groups. Some fathers spent as much as 35.7 hr per week per-

Table 39.2. Time (in Hours) Spent With Target Child by Fathers

Time Spent	*M*	*SD*	Maximum
Weekday			
MD	4.7	4.3	16.1
DS	6.0	4.8	26.2
TD	4.8	3.6	15.0
Weekend			
MD	4.5	4.2	17.8
DS	5.0	3.6	19.3
TD	4.4	3.7	12.8
Total			
MD	9.2	6.6	25.3
DS	11.0	7.3	35.7
TD	9.3	5.6	22.0

Note. MD = multiple disabilities; DS = Down syndrome; TD = typical development. No significance between means by group based on a one-way, between-subjects ANOVA ($p = .05$) was found.

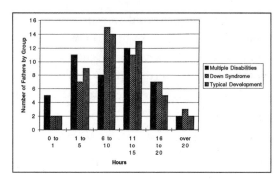

Figure 39.1. Time spent with child by father.

forming child care activities, whereas other fathers spent no time.

Time Spent by Other Than Parents Performing Child Care

CARE data indicate that relatives, childsitters, nurses, school personnel, and others also spent time providing child care to the target child during the week. Mothers of children with multiple disabilities as well as mothers of children with Down syndrome reported a weekly average of 11 hr that their child spent with other caregivers besides the parents. Children who were typically developing spent an average of 7.9 hr per week with other caregivers. No significant differences between groups were found. As with paternal caregiving, there was great variability in the number of hours that others spent providing child care within each group (see Table 39.3).

Maternal Satisfaction With Child Care Division of Labor

Mothers were asked to estimate the percentage of child care that they performed as well as the amount of child care performed by their partners. Figure 39.2 illustrates that the majority of mothers believed that they performed 80% to 100% of all child care. Interestingly, 102 out of 132 women (75.5%) were satisfied with their division of child care labor between mothers and fathers. No significant correlation was found

Table 39.3. Time (in Hours) Spent With Target Child by Others

Caregiver	M	SD	Maximum
Relative			
MD	4.4	6.0	25.3
DS	4.2	5.5	35.7
TD	2.2	3.8	22.0
Childsitter			
MD	0.9	2.8	8.3
DS	2.9	8.6	26.4
TD	1.8	2.6	9.1
Nurse			
MD	0.8	9.0	22.5
DS	0.1	0.6	1.5
TD	0.1	0.5	3.3
School			
MD	4.1	9.0	34.3
DS	3.3	11.0	40.0
TD	2.0	6.2	21.0
Other[a]			
MD	0.6	6.1	16.9
DS	0.4	2.2	7.9
TD	1.7	3.4	12.0

Note. MD = multiple disabilities; DS = Down syndrome; TD = typical development. No significance between means by group based on a one-way, between-subjects ANOVA ($p = .05$) was found.
[a]Other included neighbors, siblings, in-laws, and friends.

between percentage of child care performed and satisfaction of division of labor.

Discussion

In the process of exploring paternal and other child care provider time spent caring for children, it became apparent that mothers did the lion's

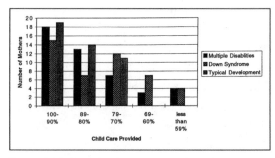

Figure 39.2. Perceived percentage of child care provided by mothers.

share of child care regardless of whether their child had a disability. This is consistent with other general time use studies that have found that women do almost 80% of all child care (Robinson & Godbey, 1997). In addition, it has been found that when men do spend time with children, it tends to take the form of play or helping with homework rather than activities such as feeding or bathing, for which women are responsible (McBride & Mills, 1993). This division of labor has been tracked since the 1960s and does not seem to have changed as women have increasingly entered the workforce. The previously published finding using the same sample as this study (Crowe, 1993) that child care hours increased for mothers of children with multiple disabilities is not surprising, considering the impact of extra child-related activities, such as therapy visits, doctor appointments, and additional time spent helping children perform basic self-care activities. However, it is noteworthy that mothers seemed to be the ones doing this extra work. Paternal hours spent performing child care were not different for the three groups. Similarly, Barnett and Boyce (1995) found that mothers of children with Down syndrome decreased their time in paid employment to compensate for increased child care time demands. Fathers decreased their time spent in social activities (as did mothers), but their paid employment hours did not change. These findings suggest that mothers are the ones who make accommodations in terms of roles and time use to manage the additional responsibilities associated with caring for a child with special needs. It has been suggested that professionals working with families may contribute to this pattern by assuming that mothers will be the family members responsible for these extra caregiving tasks and carrying out intervention activities (Allen & Hudd, 1987).

According to mothers' perceptions, fathers spent approximately one-quarter to one-third of the time as mothers providing child care, independent of the child's group membership (multiple disabilities, Down syndrome, typical development). This is consistent with another study of fathers' child care involvement with preschool-age children with and without disabilities (Young & Roopnarine, 1994), in which fathers spent approximately 35% to 36% as much time as mothers in child care. The authors also reported that mothers believed that they were more committed and competent as child care providers than did fathers, suggesting that mothers felt more comfortable with their more extensive caregiving role than fathers. It is possible that mothers in the current study spent more time performing child care than fathers, partly because they felt more capable of handling the multiple tasks required. In addition, the mothers in this study only worked a maximum of 20 hr outside the home.

Other adults, including relatives, childsitters, nurses, and school personnel, also spent time providing child care in all groups. In fact, this group of extended family and extrafamilial caregivers on the average spent more total time each week with the target child than did the fathers. Children who were typically developing received somewhat fewer hours of child care by others (although not significant) than the children in the other two groups. It is possible that families with children with Down syndrome and multiple disabilities qualified for and required specialized childsitter services (e.g., respite programs) that the families of children who were typically developing did not receive. In addition, children with Down syndrome and multiple disabilities spent approximately 2 hr per week more with relatives than did children who were typically developing. This suggests that perhaps relatives rallied to provide additional support to families in which the child had special needs. On the other hand, as described earlier, mothers picked up most of the additional child care hours associated with caring for a child with multiple disabilities. The fact that other caregivers did not assume these responsibilities could suggest that it was difficult for mothers to find child care providers who were comfortable with or capable of working with children with special needs. In a qualitative study of single mothers caring for children with disabilities or chronic illness, finding competent child care was identified as an important concern (Gabor & Farnham, 1996).

There was tremendous variation in the number of hours that individual fathers and others spent performing child care activities with individual families. This suggests that there is no "best" or typical pattern and that families construct a division and pattern of labor in a manner that meets their particular needs. In fact, most mothers were satisfied with their child care arrangements despite the fact that they performed most of it themselves. Not surprisingly, previous analysis of data from this study found that mothers valued their caregiver role, although many hoped to eventually assume more paid employment or to return to school sometime in the future when their child was older (Crowe et al., 1997).

An ecocultural approach to interpreting the variation of child care configurations for individual families may be helpful in this context. Ecocultural theorists suggest that families actively attempt to establish a daily routine that is sustainable, personally satisfying, and responsive to the needs of their child with a disability (Gallimore, Weisner, Kaufman, & Bernheimer, 1989). Essentially, families find strategies to accommodate and adjust to the demands of daily life when there is a child with special needs (Bernheimer & Keogh, 1995). For some women, that may mean allocating fewer hours to paid employment to spend additional hours providing child care. For some families, moving closer to relatives so that extended family can help with respite may be an option. In some instances, fathers may change their work schedule to be more available to assist with child care. Although, on average, mothers are providing the majority of child care in all families, there are also clearly unique solutions that individual families are using to meet daily demands. Additional qualitative information will be helpful when attempting to understand the time use allocations and levels of satisfaction in families with children who may or may not have special needs.

Limitations

This study was intentionally limited to women who worked fewer than 20 hr per week and were part of two-parent households. In addition, selection criteria excluded women with more than three children. It is possible that women who were working full-time, caring for children without assistance from a partner, or caring for many children would demonstrate different patterns of child care than the women in this study. In addition, most of the participants in this study were Caucasian. Families from other ethnic groups may have different expectations about the involvement of fathers and other family members in child care activities. Finally, this study reports only mothers' perceptions about daily time use patterns and satisfaction. It is possible that paternal perceptions would be different concerning the amount of time spent providing child care by different parties.

Implications for Occupational Therapy

This study highlights the fact that parents of children with disabilities, and mothers in particular, are very busy people. Occupational therapists need to be sensitive to their situation and to avoid adding additional responsibilities (e.g., home therapy programs) that may overburden parents. Mothers especially may not be able to maintain a balance of roles if the parenting role becomes too time consuming, which may negatively affect parental and family relationships, health, and wellness.

In this study, fathers and other child care providers did not change the amount of time they spent in caregiving activities, even when the child had special needs. Instead, mothers performed the additional tasks associated with caring for a child with special needs. Generally, mothers reported that they were satisfied with this arrangement, but therapists need to avoid assuming that mothers will be the responsible party. Every family has its own system of accommodations that they use to manage their daily routine. By listening to and collaborating with parents, it may be possible to identify a division of labor that best meets individual family needs.

Acknowledgments

We thank the women and children who participated in this study; Nancy Wicher, PT, and Edyth Johnson, OTR, who assisted with data collection; and Carolyn Thurman, OTR/L, and Lyda Baker, OTR/L, who assisted in data entry.

This research was supported by the American Occupational Therapy Foundation, the U.S. Department of Education (Office of Special Education and Rehabilitative Services), and the University of Washington James I. Doi Dissertation Support Fund.

References

Allen, D., & Hudd, S. (1987). Are we professionalizing parents? Weighing the benefits and the pitfalls. *Mental Retardation, 25,* 133–139.

Barnett, W. S., & Boyce, G. C. (1995). Effects of children with Down syndrome on parents' activities. *American Journal of Mental Retardation, 100,* 115–127.

Bernheimer, L. P., & Keogh, B. K. (1995). Weaving interventions into the fabric of everyday life: An approach to family assessment. *Topics in Early Childhood Special Education, 15,* 415–433.

Crowe, T. K. (1991). *Time use and role perceptions of mothers with young children: The impact of a child's disability.* Unpublished doctoral dissertation, University of Washington, Seattle.

Crowe, T. K. (1993). Time use of mothers with young children: The impact of a child's disability. *Developmental Medicine and Child Neurology, 35,* 621–630.

Crowe, T. K., Clark, L., & Qualls, C. (1996). The impact of child characteristics on mother's sleep patterns. *Occupational Therapy Journal of Research, 16,* 3–22.

Crowe, T. K., VanLeit, B., Berghmans, K. K., & Mann, P. (1997). Role perceptions of mothers with young children: The impact of a child's disability. *American Journal of Occupational Therapy, 51,* 651–661.

Eiser, C. (1993). *Growing up with a chronic disease: The impact on children and their families.* London: Jessica Kingsley.

Erickson, M., & Upshur, C. C. (1989). Caretaking burden and social support: Comparison of mothers of infants with and without disabilities. *American Journal on Mental Retardation, 94,* 250–258.

Gabor, L. M., & Farnham, R. (1996). The impact of children with chronic illness and/or developmental disabilities on low-income, single-parent families. *Infant–Toddler Intervention, 6,* 167–180.

Gallimore, R., Weisner, T. S., Kaufman, S. Z., & Bernheimer, L. P. (1989). The social construction of ecocultural niches: Family accommodation of developmentally delayed children. *American Journal on Mental Retardation, 94,* 216–230.

Harris, V. S., & McHale, S. M. (1989). Family life problems, daily caregiving activities, and the psychological well-being of mothers of mentally retarded children. *American Journal on Mental Retardation, 94,* 231–239.

Johnson, C. B., & Deitz, J. C. (1985). Time use of mothers with preschool children: A pilot study. *American Journal of Occupational Therapy, 39,* 578–583.

Joosten, J. (1979). Accounting for changes in family life of families with spina bifida children. *Z. Kinderchir, 28,* 412–417.

King, G. A., King, S. M., & Rosenbaum, P. L. (1996). How mothers and fathers view professional caregiving for children with disabilities.

Developmental Medicine and Child Neurology, 38, 397–407.

Knowles, J. (1987, Summer). Caring for a child with special needs. *Advocate,* p. 2.

Lamb, M. E. (1983). Fathers of exceptional children. In M. Seligman (Ed.), *The family with a handicapped child* (pp. 125–146). Philadelphia: Grune & Stratton.

Lamb, M. E. (1987). Introduction: The emergent American father. In M. E. Lamb (Ed.), *The father's role: Cross-cultural perspectives* (pp. 3–25). Hillsdale, NJ: Erlbaum.

LaRossa, R., & Reitzes, D. C. (1995). Gendered perceptions of father involvement in early 20th century America. *Journal of Marriage and the Family, 57,* 223–229.

Linder, T. W., & Chitwood, D. G. (1984, Summer). The needs of fathers of young handicapped children. *Journal of the Division for Early Childhood,* pp. 133–139.

McAndrew, I. (1976). Children with a handicap and their families. *Childcare, Health and Development, 2,* 213–237.

McBride, B. A., & Mills, G. (1993). A comparison of mother and father involvement with their preschool age children. *Early Childhood Research Quarterly, 8,* 457–477.

Menaghan, E., & Parcel, T. (1990). Parental employment and family life: Research in the 1980s. *Journal of Marriage and the Family, 52,* 1079–1098.

Newborg, J., Stock, J. R., Wnek, L., Guidubaldi, J., & Svinichi, J. (1984). *Battelle Developmental Inventory.* Allen, TX: DLM Teaching Resources.

Piburn, D. E., & Boyce, G. C. (1992). *Mother's perception of father's contribution to childcare and its influence on mother's perception of stress in families of children with disabilities.* Logan: Utah State University, Early Intervention Research Institute.

Robinson, J. P., & Godbey, G. (1997). *Time for life: The surprising ways Americans use their time.* University Park: Pennsylvania State University Press.

Sabbeth, B. (1984). Understanding the impact of chronic childhood illness on families. *Pediatric Clinics of North America, 31,* 47–57.

Turnbull, A. P., & Turnbull, H. R. (1990). *Families, professionals and exceptionality: A special partnership* (2nd ed.). Columbus, OH: Merrill.

Widerstrom, S. H., & Goodwin, L. D. (1987). Effects of an infant stimulation program on the child and the family. *Journal of the Division for Early Childhood, 11,* 143–153.

Young, D. M., & Roopnarine, J. L. (1994). Fathers' childcare involvement with children with and without disabilities. *Topics in Early Childhood Education, 14,* 487–502.

CHAPTER 40

Shifts in Parent–Therapist Partnerships
Twelve Years of Change

Jim Hinojosa, Christine T. Sproat,
Supawadee Mankhetwit, and Jill Anderson

Jim Hinojosa, PhD, OT,
FAOTA, *is professor, New*
York University, 35 West 4th
Street, 11th Floor, New York,
NY 10011;
jim.hinojosa@nyu.edu.

Christine T. Sproat, MA,
OT, *is occupational therapist,*
Children's Therapy Center,
Seattle.

Supawadee Mankhetwit,
PhD, OT, *is lecturer,*
Department of Occupational
Therapy, Faculty of Associated
Medical Sciences, Chiang
Mai University, Amphur
Muang, Chiang Mai,
Thailand.

Jill Anderson, MS, OT, *is*
adjunct faculty, New York
University, New York.

Originally published 2002
in *American Journal of*
Occupational Therapy,
56, 556–563.

Hinojosa, Anderson, and Ranum (1988) reported on a national survey that investigated the roles of occupational therapists working with parents of preschool children with cerebral palsy. Although the majority of respondents believed that they were competent in working with parents, they did not believe that the basic professional education in occupational therapy had adequately prepared them. Hinojosa et al. concluded that therapists could benefit from expertise in counseling and training to work collaboratively with parents. The purpose of the present study was to replicate the original study to identify current occupational therapists' attitudes and values in their working relationships with parents of preschool children with developmental disabilities after two decades of legislative support (Individuals With Disabilities Education Act of 1990 [IDEA, P.L. 101–476]; IDEA Amendments of 1991 [P.L. 102–119]; IDEA Reauthorization of 1997 [P.L. 105–117]) and educational efforts (Brewer, McPherson, Magrub, & Hutchins, 1989; Dukewitz & Gowan, 1996; Dunst, Trivette, & Deal, 1988; Filer & Mahoney, 1996; Hinojosa, Moore, Sabari, & Doctor, 1994).

Research (Humphry, Gonzalez, & Taylor, 1993; Judge, 1997; Lamorey & Ryan, 1998; Noojin & Wallander, 1996) and other reports in the literature (Filer & Mahoney, 1996; Lawlor & Mattingly, 1998; L. Thompson et al., 1997) have discussed the value of family involvement in intervention. In family-centered intervention, the focus of intervention is guided by the needs of the entire family (Dunst, Trivette, & Deal, 1994; Filer & Mahoney, 1996; Humphry & Case-Smith, 2001; Malone, 1997; Rosenbaum, King, Law, King, & Evans, 1998). When family-centered care guides intervention, therapists support each family member's natural roles to foster effective intervention. In this approach, family members are valued and considered to be equal to the professionals as members of the intervention team (Brewer et al., 1989; Hinojosa et al., 2001). As Lawlor and Mattingly (1998) pointed out, involving family members in therapy has not been added easily to the therapist's practice, especially when contemporary service delivery systems value therapeutic interventions that account only for the child's specific needs.

The importance of collaborative family–therapist relationships is now readily accepted (Filer & Mahoney, 1996; Humphry & Case-Smith, 2001; Lawlor & Mattingly, 1998). Given this acceptance, researchers need to examine more closely the distinct characteristics of parent–therapist relationships. In a recent study of 10 Australian families receiving early intervention services for their children between 2 and 5 years of age, K. M. Thompson (1998) concluded that involvement with families creates a greater time demand for the professional and often can lessen hands-on time with the children. The mothers in this study reported that the amount of intervention time their children received from therapists affected their children's development. They also believed that increased frequency of service combined with more time reinforcing therapy at home would improve their children's progress. Additionally, they wanted reassurance and feedback from their service providers about their children. Finally, these mothers emphasized the need for informal support within an open and friendly relationship with their children's therapists. These findings corroborate the conclusions of earlier studies (Brown, Humphry, & Taylor, 1997; Case-Smith & Nastro, 1993; Hinojosa, 1990; Humphry & Thigpen-Beck, 1998).

Since the 1970s, legislation has mandated family-centered care for programs and services to children with disabilities (Walker, 1992). Professional efforts within the past 10 years have supported the goal that the education of therapists should include the acquisition of the knowledge and skills needed for family-centered practice (Hinojosa et al., 1994; Humphry & Link, 1990; Schaaf & Mulrooney, 1989). Because research and legislation support the importance of parent–therapist partnerships, it is advantageous to explore the current attitudes and values of occupational therapists working with parents of preschool children with developmental disabilities. The present study replicated a 1987 national survey that examined therapists' relationships with parents of preschool children with cerebral palsy. This study broadened the scope to include the parents of preschool children with developmental disabilities. The purpose of this study was to identify current occupational therapists' attitudes and values in their working relationships with these parents after 12 years of legislative support. Data also were collected on occupational therapists' perceptions of parents' needs and roles.

Method

A mailed questionnaire was used to collect data from a random national sample of 400 occupational therapists. A pilot study was conducted to refine the questionnaire. To examine the roles of occupational therapists working with parents of preschool-age children with cerebral palsy, the questionnaire originally developed by Hinojosa et al. (1988) was revised using current terminology and expanded to address issues for parents of children with a broader range of disabilities. The revised five-page questionnaire consisted of 59 items on (a) demographics, (b) occupational therapists' attitudes toward working with parents, and (c) occupational therapists' roles with parents. Survey items varied and were written using rank order, rating scales, and open-ended questions. Respondents were instructed both in the cover letter and throughout the questionnaire to answer questions only as they related to their practice with parents of preschool children with developmental disabilities. This survey was conducted according to the procedures outlined by Dillman (2000) and Babbie (1990).

Validity and Reliability of the Questionnaire

An expert group of 15 pediatric occupational therapists examined the instrument for face and content validity by completing the survey and a critique form. Thirteen (93%) had practiced for more than 7 years, 12 held master's degrees, and 1 held a doctorate. The critique form asked for their input on the length of time taken to complete the survey, the accuracy of the terminology, the relevance of the questions, and the clarity of the questions and instructions. The therapists reported that the survey took between 15 min and 30 min to complete. On the basis of feedback, some directions were clarified and some were refined to improve clarity and readability. A Cronbach's alpha was used to examine the internal consistency of the pilot data for the first two sections on attitudes and parent–therapist issues. An alpha of .77 was found for these sections, leading to the acceptance of the items as a reliable composite instrument. Test–retest reliability was not determined.

Sample and Procedure

The questionnaire; a cover letter describing the nature of the study; a request form for receipt of results; and a stamped, self-addressed envelope were mailed to a random sample of 400 registered occupational therapists who were members of the Developmental Disabilities Special Interest Section of the American Occupational Therapy Association in 1998. The sample was selected by computer from those members who had stated that they work with children from birth to school age. Follow-up letters were sent through first-class mail to nonrespondents 6 weeks and 12 weeks after the first mailing. At 16 weeks, a final follow-up letter, another survey, and postage-paid return envelope were sent to nonrespondents.

Data Analysis

A total of 327 (81.8%) of the 400 questionnaires were returned. Of these, 125 (31.3%) were unanswered because the respondents did not currently work with preschool children with developmental disabilities, and 3 were returned because of incorrect addresses. Responses from the 199 therapists remaining formed the database of this survey. Respondents represented 46 states. Some did not answer all the questions, and some did not answer questions according to the instructions. Thus, the tables in this chapter are based on varying numbers of respondents. Totals, therefore, also varied with the number of accurately completed responses.

Data were coded and analyzed using the Statistical Package for the Social Sciences, Version 10.0 (SPSS, 2000). Descriptive statistics were used to analyze and report the data. Demographic differences among respondents were analyzed using chi-square analysis for independence at the alpha level of .05. After calculating descriptive statistics for each item in the survey, a one-way analysis of variance (ANOVA) was performed for four demographic variables (i.e., therapist age, place of practice, years in pediatrics, degree attained) to determine whether total scores on the survey differed significantly on the basis of these independent variables.

Results

Data from the survey provided information in five areas: (a) demographic information on the occupational therapists; (b) occupational therapists' attitudes toward working with parents; (c) occupational therapists' perception of the attitudes, concerns, and needs of parents; (d) occupational therapists' roles with parents; and (e) issues, difficulties, and satisfactions that arise from therapists' working relationships with parents.

Demographic Information

All respondents had earned bachelor's degrees. The highest earned academic degree of almost two-thirds was a bachelor's degree (n = 122, 61.2%); more than one-third (n = 72, 36.7%) had earned master's degrees; and 2 (1%) had earned doctoral degrees. More than one-third (n = 75, 38.1%) worked in educational institutional settings, such as preschools or schools; 25 (12.7%) worked in private practices; and 25 (12.7%) worked in home-based therapy situations. Respondents were predominantly female (n = 192, 97%) and ranged in age from 23 to 68 years (M = 37.9 years, median = 38 years, SD = 10.08). Eighty-seven (44%) had worked more than 10 years in pediatrics and were advanced practitioners. More than half (54.9%) indicated that they were parents.

Factors Occupational Therapists Consider Important in Working With Parents

Each respondent ranked his or her agreement with statements on issues related to working with parents (e.g., occupational therapists work most effectively with parents who appear invested in their child's progress, occupational therapists do not have enough time to spend with parents) on a forced-choice Likert scale of 1 *(strongly agree)* to 4 *(strongly disagree)*. Most of the respondents agreed that they worked more effectively with parents who were invested in their child's progress (see Table 40.1). Most also reported that they considered working with parents to be an important aspect of occupational therapy intervention and that its importance has not been overemphasized.

Almost three-quarters of the therapists (72.5%) reported that their basic professional education adequately prepared them to work with parents. More than three-quarters (76.6%) believed that working with parents has a greater impact on a child with disabilities than any other aspect of intervention. The majority (59.4%) believed that therapists do not have enough time to spend with parents. Analyses of responses to two other items were equally distributed (agree, disagree). Those two items were "parents do not

Table 40.1. Therapists' Rankings of Their Views About Working With Parents

View	Strongly Agree		Agree		Disagree		Strongly Disagree		N^a
	n	%	n	%	n	%	n	%	
Occupational therapists work most effectively with parents invested in their child's progress	88	44.4	94	47.5	16	8.1	2	0	198
Work with parents has a greater impact on a child than any other aspect of occupational therapy	57	28.9	94	47.7	44	22.3	2	1.0	197
Basic occupational therapy education adequately prepares occupational therapists to work with parents	28	14.3	114	58.2	47	24.0	7	3.6	196
Occupational therapists do not have enough time to spend with parents	28	14.2	89	45.2	63	32.0	17	8.6	197
Parent's feelings toward their child's disabilities interferes with intervention objectives	11	5.6	77	39.1	89	42.5	20	10.2	197
Parents do not understand the roles of occupational therapists	7	3.6	70	35.9	105	53.8	13	6.7	195
Importance of working with parents has been overemphasized	3	1.5	1	0.5	116	58.3	79	39.7	199
Occupational therapy focus on skill development is more important than working with the parents	0	0	16	8.0	116	58.3	67	33.7	199

[a]N varies according to the number of respondents who answered each question as instructed.

understand the roles of occupational therapists" and "parents' feelings toward their child's disabilities interfere with intervention objectives."

Perceptions of Issues Important to Parents

From a list of common issues relevant to having a child with developmental disabilities, respondents were asked to identify and rank three issues that most commonly arose during their interactions with parents (see Table 40.2). The issue ranked first by 29.7% was parents adjusting to their child's disabilities. The issue ranked second by 26.6% was the child's progress in therapy. The importance of the two highest ranked issues becomes evident when the total number of respondents rating these issues as first, second, and third most common is combined. These combined numbers of respondents indicate that 61.5% selected progress in therapy and 54.7% selected parents adjusting to their child's disability as issues frequently arising during parent–therapist interactions. The distribution of the rank for other issues listed did not indicate that any arose with consistent frequency (see Table 40.2).

Table 40.3 summarizes respondents' perceptions of parental concerns about the child's progress by asking them to rank order six concerns. Ambulation was ranked as the highest parental concern by 96 (49.5%) respondents. A total of 129 respondents selected ambulation as either their first or their second most common parental concern. A total of 114 selected speech and language development as either their first or their second most common parental concern. Almost half (49.5%) selected concerns about the child's future as the least important concern.

Role of Occupational Therapists With Parents

Of the 199 respondents, 170 estimated percentages of time they spent in selected activities with parents from a fixed list (see Figure 40.1). When the percentages of time spent on activities that involved the child's therapeutic program are combined (discussing the child's disability, teaching techniques, home programming, home management, discussing the child's behavior and preschool placement), it appears that the respondents spend two-thirds of their time (66.4%) instructing parents about the care of their child.

Table 40.2. Occupational Therapists' Perceptions of Issues Most Frequently Arising During Parent–Therapist Interaction

| | Perceived Frequency of Issues | | | | | | | | |
| | Most Common | | Second Common | | Third Common | | Total | | |
Issue	n	%	n	%	n	%	n	%	Nª
Parents adjusting to their child's disability	57	29.7	30	15.6	18	9.4	105	54.7	192
Child's progress in therapy	51	26.6	45	23.4	22	11.5	118	61.5	192
Results of the evaluation	34	17.7	19	9.9	11	5.7	64	33.3	192
Parents' individual differences	18	9.3	20	10.4	27	14.0	60	31.1	193
Added services	12	6.3	12	6.3	19	9.9	43	22.4	192
Others	10	5.2	8	4.1	13	6.7	31	16.1	193
Treatment goals	8	4.2	28	14.6	27	14.1	63	32.8	192
Lack of progress in therapy	7	3.6	15	7.8	20	10.4	42	21.9	192
Cause of the child's disability	7	3.6	14	7.3	22	11.5	43	22.4	192
Parental decision	6	3.1	12	6.3	23	12.0	41	21.4	192

ª*N* varies according to the number of respondents who answered the question as instructed.

Table 40.3. Occupational Therapists' Perceptions of Most Important Parental Concerns Related to a Child's Progress

Area of Concern	Concern[a]						N[b]
	1	2	3	4	5	6	
Ambulation	96	33	18	22	13	12	194
Speech and language	28	86	43	19	14	3	193
Concern about the future	24	12	9	19	33	95	192
Reducing negative behaviors	21	21	43	42	32	34	193
Cognitive development	20	30	56	35	39	12	192
Activities of daily living skills	5	16	25	56	61	32	195

[a]Ranked from 1 *(of most concern)* to 6 *(of concern)*.
[b]*N* varies according to the number of respondents who answered each question as instructed.

They estimated that they spent 30% of their time discussing all parent-directed concerns, including parental needs and feelings, play activities, and social and personal discussions.

Respondents rated on a 4-point scale *(not important, somewhat important, very important, essential)* the importance of listed parent-related factors when treating a preschool child with disabilities. They reported that it was essential to explore parental goals, help parents to understand therapists' roles, provide information about the abilities of the child, and instruct parents on home programs. Providing support and information on advocacy programs and support groups were valued but believed to be less essential.

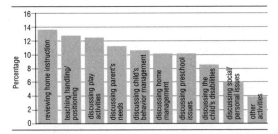

Figure 40.1. Percentage of time occupational therapists spent in selected activities with parents.

Demographic Analysis

Four items on the survey were demographic in nature—degree attained, age of therapist, place of practice, and years of practice in pediatrics. Responses for all survey items that were not demographic in nature were summed, and this total was analyzed for significant differences within each of the four demographic variables using a one-way ANOVA (SPSS, 2000). One of the four demographic items—6 years or fewer or 7 years or more of practice in pediatrics—achieved significance at the .05 level, $F(1, 197) = 4.064$, $p = .019$, indicating a significant difference between the total sum of scores on survey items between these two groups. Respondents with more years of experience reported that working with parents had the greatest influence on a child's progress. No significant differences were found among sums of scores based on age (37 years or older), degree attained, or place of practice, although age was near statistical significance probably because it is highly correlated with the more salient factor of years in pediatric practice.

Occupational Therapists Experienced Difficulties and Satisfactions Working With Parents

Responses to two open-ended questions were analyzed for recurring themes and to gather descriptive data regarding the difficulties and satisfactions the respondents experience while working with parents. The first question asked, "What are the three most difficult issues to deal with that you have experienced in working with parents?" The respondents listed many difficulties from which several consistent themes emerged. Dealing with parent denial was a major theme and viewed as a formidable challenge for therapists. Within this theme, respondents discussed parents' "unrealistic" expectations and their "inability to recognize the needs of their children." Another theme was parental noninvolvement, where respondents reported that parents often expected others to assume care of their child and that they did not follow through with recommendations. Included in this theme were inconsistent attendance to therapy, lack of respect for the therapist's knowledge, and lack of children's progress in therapy. The final theme evolved from social issues that affect the therapeutic process. Respondents discussed parental stress, poor financial resources, unstable family units, poor parenting skills, lack of community resources, limited social interactions with others, and poor parent accessibility as obstacles to working effectively with parents.

Responses to the second question, which asked respondents to identify the most satisfying experiences they had working with parents, supported the notion that therapists find it satisfying to generate change for the child and parent through education and the use of clinical knowledge and skills. The respondents reported satisfaction when the parent placed trust in their professional judgment and, therefore, in the parent–therapist relationship. One of the respondents described fostering a parent–therapist relationship as "parent empowerment." Parent appreciation of the therapist's efforts, the child's observable progress, and parent acceptance of the child's disability were reported as other satisfying experiences.

Discussion

A national survey examined 199 occupational therapists' attitudes and values related to their interactions with parents of preschool children with disabilities. This study replicated an earlier national survey that examined therapists' relationships with parents of preschool children with cerebral palsy (Hinojosa et al., 1988).

In the 1988 study, 85% of respondents reported that they did not believe that their basic professional education had prepared them to work with families. In contrast, almost three-quarters (72.5%) of the respondents in the current study stated that they believed their professional education *did* prepare them to work with families that had a child with a disability. This finding suggests that basic professional education programs are better preparing occupational therapists with the necessary skills to work appropriately with parents of a child with disabilities. As in the prior study, the respondent sample consisted of experienced therapists; 44% had more than 10 years of experience working in pediatrics. It is possible that work experience as well as formal educational training contributed to beliefs that they were prepared and effective at collaborating with family members.

In both studies, respondents reported their beliefs that parents consider their children's progress to be critically important. This finding suggests that therapists are providing services in conjunction with parents' concerns when they focus interventions to address a child's specific deficit and are concerned with the child's progress in deficit areas. In most cases, a child is referred to occupational therapy because of a specific performance skill deficit; therefore, it is reasonable to infer that therapists would implement interventions to address the specific deficits. Further, it is logical that parents are focused on their children's services that assess the identified primary deficits. The current study revealed that respondents maintain that the amount of time therapists spent with a child is as important as the time they spent working with parents and other family members. Yet, more than three-quarters (76%) agreed that the time they spent with parents had a greater impact on a child than any other aspect of intervention.

Therapists' perceptions of issues important to parents have remained the same in the past 12 years; in both studies, respondents reported ambulation followed by speech and language as primary concerns for parents of preschool children with disabilities. As in the prior study, respondents reported that a child's future was of least concern to parents. Given the age group that respondents were asked to consider—preschool children with developmental disabilities—it would make sense that parents focus their concerns on their child developing the ability to walk and talk rather than on their child's future. Lawlor and Mattingly (1998) proposed that parents and therapists have a different sense of time. Based on their analysis of parent narratives, they concluded that parents are more future oriented than therapists. Because these survey data were collected from therapists, it would be appropriate to interview or survey parents of preschool children with disabilities about what issues are important to them. If, in actuality, parents and therapists have different perceptions of time horizons as reported by Lawlor and Mattingly, then therapists may need to reexamine their belief that parents of preschool children are more focused on the more immediate developmental goals for their children as these survey data suggest.

Parents' own ability to adjust to their child's disability and their interest in the progress of their child continue to be the most common issues therapists face in interacting with families. When respondents rated their actual time spent with parents, 66.4% of the time was spent instructing the parent in matters regarding the child's therapeutic program. Thirty percent of therapists' time is spent discussing affective issues, such as parent needs, feelings, and concerns. These findings supported the previous study in reiterating therapists' perceptions of the importance parents place on understanding their child's disability and the progress of their child. During their child's therapy, parents often become more knowledgeable about deficits. The child's progress in deficit areas is one of the central issues therapists discuss with families throughout intervention.

When respondents were asked about the amount of time they spent on specific activities with parents, the results demonstrate that therapists still spend a significant amount of time reviewing home instructions and teaching handling and positioning techniques. Consistently, respondents reported that they spend less time focusing on the child's other needs and the parental needs and concerns. Lawlor and Mattingly (1998) pointed out that it is difficult to maintain the role of expert while trying to connect interventions with the expressed needs of the family. Further, they discussed the fact that the nature of therapeutic intervention requires that therapists focus on problem setting and identification, assessment, treatment options, and treatment efficacy. When working with families, therapists must balance their time and efforts between focusing directly on the child's needs and addressing family member's needs.

As in the prior study, when assessing difficulties and satisfactions in their roles as therapists, respondents reported difficulty with parental denial and unrealistic expectations. They also were dissatisfied when parents did not follow through with recommendations. A relatively new finding from this survey suggests that therapists find difficulty working with parents who face multiple stressors, such as unstable family units, poor parent accessibility, parent stress, lack of financial resources, poor parenting skills, and limited social interactions of parent and family. These issues may affect attendance, consistency of intervention, payment, and carryover of intervention goals. Accessibility to parents, parents under stress, and limited resources challenge therapists' abilities to work in partnership with parents. Although some respondents avoid involvement with family issues in treatment intervention, they are aware that these issues affect the child. Studies indicate that early academic difficulties, attachment disorders, conduct problems, poor social skills, and poor problem-solving abilities often are common for children living in vulnerable families (Keenan & Wakschlag, 2000; Knitzer, 2000; Webster-Stratton, 1998). Helping parents with resources, knowledge, and support necessary to meet their child and family needs is empowering to parents.

Respondents reported satisfaction when parents were actively involved in the child's therapy program and followed their recommendations. They also reported that being appreciated and respected for their knowledge was important to them. Respondents described themselves as feeling more effective when the child has made observable progress and when the parent accepts the child's disability. They also believe that they could be more effective when they provided parents with information and strategies to make decisions and when parents actively participated in their child's intervention program. Parents are better able to meet their own needs and the needs of their child when they are able to exercise some control and decision making about solutions to problems and the resolution of concerns (Cauthen & Knitzer, 1999; Dunst et al., 1994; Galinsky, Shubilla, Willer, Levine, & Daniel, 1994).

The results of this survey suggest positive changes in therapists' perceptions of their preparation and skills for working effectively in partnerships with the parents of a child with a disability. These encouraging changes provide educators and clinicians with an exciting opportunity to further work in partnership with parents in developing effective, collaborative relationships.

Beyond appreciating the importance of family-centered care, educators may wish to focus on teaching strategies for developing collaborative skills. Further, educators may want to address new areas of concern, including dealing with parents who are perceived to be in denial, have unrealistic expectations, or show poor recognition of

their child's needs. We therapists need to better understand these processes by examining what is meant by denial or what determines what is unrealistic. Further, the respondents' comments challenge the profession to expand our knowledge and expertise to support families as they deal with family stress, limited social interactions, and financial constraints.

This study represents the views of experienced occupational therapists treating preschool children with developmental disabilities. The majority of respondents were women who claimed to work mostly with mothers. Because therapists reported working primarily with mothers, the survey results may be most relevant to the relationship between occupational therapists and mothers of preschool children with developmental disabilities.

This study has several limitations. First, the sample, although randomly selected, included a large number of respondents who did not work with preschool children with disabilities. Therefore, although 327 (81.8%) surveys were returned, only 199 formed the database for this study. Sampling error resulted in 125 misidentified therapists who did not currently work in pediatrics. Second, a limitation in terms of the survey development was that test–retest reliability was not done. Finally, the results of this study are limited to therapists' interactions with parents of preschool children; therefore, the findings cannot be generalized to all therapists who work with parents. Even with these limitations, the present study provides evidence that occupational therapists have increasing confidence and skills in working with parents of preschool children with developmental disabilities.

Occupational therapists who work with children with disabilities are in a unique position to facilitate family-centered intervention. This study's findings suggest that occupational therapists recognize the importance of working with parents and that they feel more confident about their skills than they did 12 years ago. At the same time, therapists acknowledge the complexities of developing effective partnerships in the current service delivery systems. The data from this study provide evidence of the positive changes in therapists' knowledge, beliefs, and attitudes toward working with parents that underlie the basis of family-centered care. Research is needed to validate this study's findings and to examine actual practices. Ethnographic studies are needed to enrich our understanding of parent–therapist interactions and validate the findings of this study. Finally, although this study supports the view that occupational therapists may be increasingly competent in working with families, additional research is needed to examine what educational programs are most effective. Occupational therapists need to continue to be creative when working with parents who have children with developmental disabilities. Methods of service delivery, funding and payment, and therapeutic goals need to be adapted to meet each unique family and child's needs.

Acknowledgments

We acknowledge the contributions of Yves Antoine, Felice Blum, Ilaria Borghese, Eunice Lanzas, Carla Pina, Aviva Silber, Harriet Turner, and Melissa Weinberg toward the refinement of the questionnaire and completion of the study. We thank Marie-Louise Blount, AM, OT, FAOTA; Dawn Leger, PhD; and Eileen Francis for editing and assistance. Finally, we thank all the therapists who contributed their time and efforts to complete and return the survey.

References

Babbie, E. R. (1990). *Survey research methods* (2nd ed.). Belmont, CA: Wadsworth.

Brewer, E. J., McPherson, M., Magrub, P. R., & Hutchins, V. L. (1989). Family-centered, community-based, coordinated care for children with special health care needs. *Pediatrics, 83,* 1055–1060.

Brown, S. M., Humphry, R., & Taylor, E. (1997). A model of the nature of the family–therapist relationship: Implications for education. *American Journal of Occupational Therapy, 51,* 597–603.

Case-Smith, J., & Nastro, M. (1993). The effect of occupational therapy intervention on mothers of children with cerebral palsy. *American Journal of Occupational Therapy, 46,* 811–817.

Cauthen, N. K., & Knitzer, J. (1999). *Beyond work: Strategies to promote the well-being of young children and families in the context of welfare reform.* New York: National Center for Children in Poverty.

Dillman, D. A. (2000). *Mail and telephone surveys* (2nd ed.). New York: Wiley.

Dukewitz, P., & Gowan, L. (1996). Creating successful collaborative teams. *Journal of Staff Development, 14*(4), 12–16.

Dunst, C., Trivette, C., & Deal, A. (1988). *Enabling and empowering families: Principles and guidelines for practice.* Cambridge, MA: Brookline Books.

Dunst, C. J., Trivette, C. M., & Deal, A. G. (1994). *Supporting and strengthening families: Methods, strategies, and practices.* Cambridge, MA: Brookline Books.

Filer, J. D., & Mahoney, G. J. (1996). Collaboration between families and early intervention service providers. *Infants and Young Children, 9*(9), 22–30.

Galinsky, E., Shubilla, L., Willer, B., Levine, J., & Daniel, J. (1994, January). State and community planning for early childhood systems. *Young Children,* pp. 54–57.

Hinojosa, J. (1990). How mothers of preschool children with cerebral palsy perceive occupational and physical therapists and their influence on family life. *Occupational Therapy Journal of Research, 10,* 144–162.

Hinojosa, J., Anderson, J., & Ranum, G. W. (1988). Relationships between therapists and parents of preschool children with cerebral palsy: A survey. *Occupational Therapy Journal of Research, 8,* 285–297.

Hinojosa, J., Bedell, G., Buchholz, E. S., Charles, J., Shigaki, I. S., & Bicchieri, S. M. (2001). Team collaboration: A case study of an early intervention team. *Qualitative Health Research, 11,* 206–220.

Hinojosa, J., Moore, D. S., Sabari, J., & Doctor, R. G. (1994). Competency-based training program in early intervention. *American Journal of Occupational Therapy, 48,* 361–366.

Humphry, R., & Case-Smith, J. (2001). Working with families. In J. Case-Smith (Ed.), *Occupational therapy for children* (4th ed., pp. 95–130). St. Louis, MO: Mosby.

Humphry, R., Gonzalez, S., & Taylor, E. (1993). Family involvement in practice: Issues and attitudes. *American Journal of Occupational Therapy, 47,* 587–593.

Humphry, R., & Link, S. (1990). Preparation of occupational therapists to work in early intervention programs. *American Journal of Occupational Therapy, 44,* 828–833.

Humphry, R., & Thigpen-Beck, B. (1998). Parenting values and attitudes: Views of therapists and parents. *American Journal of Occupational Therapy, 52,* 835–842.

Individuals With Disabilities Education Act. (1990). Pub. L. 101–476, 20 U.S.C. § 1400.

Individuals With Disabilities Education Act Amendments. (1991). Pub. L. 102–119, 20 U.S.C. § 1400.

Individuals With Disabilities Education Act Reauthorization. (1997). Pub. L. 105–117, 20 U.S.C. § 1400 *et seq.*

Judge, S. L. (1997). Parental perceptions of help-giving practices and control appraisals in early intervention programs. *Topics in Early Childhood Education, 17,* 457–476.

Keenan, K., & Wakschlag, L. S. (2000). More than the terrible twos: The nature and severity of behavior problems in clinic-referred preschool children. *Journal of Abnormal Child Psychology, 28,* 33–46.

Knitzer, J. (2000). *Promoting resilience: Helping young children and parents affected by substance abuse, domestic violence, and depression in the context of welfare reform.* New York: National Center for Children in Poverty.

Lamorey, S., & Ryan, S. (1998). From contention to implementation: A comparison of team practices and recommended practices across service delivery models. *Infant–Toddler Intervention, 8,* 309–331.

Lawlor, M. C., & Mattingly, C. F. (1998). The complexities embedded in family-centered care. *American Journal of Occupational Therapy, 52,* 259–267.

Malone, D. M. (1997). A rationale for family therapy specialization in early intervention. *Journal of Marital Family Therapy, 1,* 65–79.

Noojin, A. B., & Wallander, J. L. (1996). Development and evaluation of a measure of concerns related to raising a child with physical disabilities. *Journal of Pediatric Psychology, 21,* 483–498.

Rosenbaum, P., King, S., Law, M., King, G., & Evans, J. (1998). Family-centered service: A conceptual framework and research review. *Physical and Occupational Therapy in Pediatrics, 18*(1), 1–20.

Schaaf, R. C., & Mulrooney, L. L. (1989). Occupational therapy in early intervention: A family-centered approach. *American Journal of Occupational Therapy, 43,* 745–754.

Statistical Package for Social Sciences. (2000). SPSS 10.0 [Computer software]. Chicago: Author.

Thompson, K. M. (1998). Early intervention services in daily family life: Mothers' perceptions of the ideal versus actual service provision. *Occupational Therapy International, 5,* 206–221.

Thompson, L., Lobb, C., Elling, R., Herman, S., Jurkiewicz, T., & Hulleza, A. (1997). Pathways to family empowerment: Effects of family-centered delivery of early intervention services. *Exceptional Children, 64,* 99–113.

Walker, D. K. (1992). Building a family-centered early intervention system. In J. J. Gallagher & P. K. Fullager (Eds.). *The coordination of health and other services for infants and toddlers with disabilities: The conundrum of parallel service systems* (Report No. ED-353-705). Bureau of Family Community Health, Massachusetts Department of Public Health. (ERIC Document Reproduction No. ED358587)

Webster-Stratton, C. (1998). Preventing conduct problems in Head Start children: Strengthening parent competencies. *Journal of Consulting and Clinical Psychology, 66,* 715–730.

CHAPTER 41

Constructing Daily Routines

A Qualitative Examination of Mothers With Young Children With Disabilities

Diane Hammon Kellegrew

Diane Hammon Kellegrew, PhD, OTR, *is assistant professor, University of Southern California, Department of Occupational Science and Occupational Therapy, 1540 Alcazar Street, CHP-133, Los Angeles, CA 90033; kellegre@hsc.usc.edu.*

Every day, mothers and children participate in predictable, familiar routines. Daily routines can encompass mundane occupations, such as dressing and bathing, and more symbolic traditions and rituals, such as bedtime prayers and spiritual worship ceremonies. Through the construction of daily routines, mothers provide their children with hundreds of opportunities to practice and develop skills necessary to fully participate in society. In addition, daily routines form a compelling and efficient method of transmitting the practices and values of the culture in which the child is raised. This qualitative study sought to examine factors that influence the ways in which mothers construct daily routines for their young children with disabilities.

The Impact of Daily Routines on Development

Rogoff (1993) and Rogoff, Mistry, Goncu, and Mosier (1993) contended that parents and children collaboratively determine the nature of activities and responsibilities. The child often seeks out tasks and occupations that contribute to the mastery of skills necessary for his or her development. The adult arranges tasks and occupations to foster a child's skill acquisition. The child's development is directly affected by these mutual roles.

Valsiner (1985) asserted that adults selectively regulate children's experiences, essentially "canalizing" the child in directions specified by the parent's goals. Parental goals are in turn shaped by the society's cultural values. Cross-cultural studies support this notion. For example, children of the Kipsigis tribe are canalized in the direction of early independence within the community setting to contribute to activities of the household. Shortly after being weaned, at approximately 2 years of age, young Kipsigi children frequently carry messages to neighbors (Harkness & Super, 1983). In contrast, American middle-class homes tend to restrict children's community explo-

Originally published 2000 in *American Journal of Occupational Therapy, 54,* 252–259.

ration in favor of emphasis on other goals such as school performance (Rogoff et al., 1993). The channeling of a child's occupations therefore creates systematic variations in the opportunities for development.

Ecological paradigms can provide useful models to examine the child's development in the context of family ecology (Bronfenbrenner, 1979). One ecological model, ecocultural theory, uses the daily routines of the home as the unit of analysis (Bernheimer, Gallimore, & Weisner, 1990). Ecocultural theory contends that families are "driven by the task of constructing and sustaining a daily routine" (Gallimore, Weisner, Kaufman, & Bernheimer, 1989, p. 219). This model builds on earlier ecological paradigms proposing that families function as socially constructed systems called the "ecocultural niche" (Weisner, 1984). All activities of the niche, including the daily routines, reflect the cultural values that influence family practices (Weisner, Gallimore, & Jordan, 1993). The niche is affected by distal ecological variables, including the social and political climate, as well as by proximal factors, such as the family's economic status. Ecocultural theory proposes that ecological variables can modify the cultural practices within the niche. For example, a single mother who believes that she should be her child's primary caregiver may need to resort to full-time day care to support her family. Her cultural practices are modified because of her economic needs.

The impact of ecocultural factors on the families of children with disabilities was explored in a longitudinal series of studies called Project CHILD and Project REACH (Weisner, Matheson, & Bernheimer, 1996). The participants were drawn from 102 families of children with disabilities for whom the diagnosis was initially unknown. Predictable patterns of adjustments in daily routines, called *accommodations,* were evident across families (Gallimore et al.,

1989). The patterns of accommodation identified as domains were the following:

1. Family subsistence and financial base
2. Accessibility of health and education services
3. Home and neighborhood safety and convenience
4. Domestic task and chore workload for family
5. Child care tasks
6. Child play groups and peers
7. Marital role relationships
8. Social support
9. Father's role
10. Sources of parental information and goals.

The study findings suggested that the families of children with disabilities accommodated to the constraints and opportunities presented in daily life in a manner similar to families from similar cultural backgrounds with children who were typically developing (Gallimore, Weisner, Bernheimer, Guthrie, & Nihira, 1993). However, parenting a child with a disability correlated with increased accommodations in the domains of child care and service. Parents' perception of the child also influenced the frequency and intensity of family accommodation (Bernheimer, Gallimore, & Kaufman, 1993). In particular, the child with high medical needs or increased behavioral demands required more adjustment of the family's daily routines. Parents perceived the accommodation of their daily routines as either a constraint (negative) or resource (positive) in accordance with the cultural values of the niche members (Bernheimer et al., 1990). Therefore, the valence, or meaning, attached to various forms of daily routine adjustments appeared idiosyncratic to each household.

The literature examining ecocultural theory indicates that the aggregate of a family's daily routines can provide insight into family ecology. However, it is unclear whether examining one domain of routines, such as self-care occupations, also would reflect the spectrum of environmental and cultural influences on the family. In addition, the series of studies that form the foundation for ecocultural theory have relied on reports from parents that describe established home routines. It is not known whether such a retrospective analysis can comprehensively identify factors that influence the emergence of one repertoire of routines over another. This issue is particularly important when considering that daily routines provide opportunities for mothers to channel their child's development. This channeling initially takes place at the point of the child's emerging skill, and refinement of emerging skill takes place over time. Therefore, examination of daily routines as the child's skill emerges and develops might provide additional information about the construction of daily routines.

Intervention Examining Daily Routines

All children benefit from daily routines that promote development. However, the skills acquisition of some children is more sensitized to home routines. For children with disabilities, the daily reinforcement of occupations provides a practice component that can be crucial for both skills acquisition and maintenance (Kellegrew, 1998; Koegel, Koegel, Kellegrew, & Mullen, 1996). Parental support is particularly salient for occupations that take place primarily in the home, such as self-care routines. Younger children also depend more on parental structure of home routines to reinforce emerging skills.

Intervention that draws on the consistent and functional nature of daily routines has a natural appeal for occupational therapy practitioners. I explored the role of daily opportunities for self-care

occupations on the skill performance of young children with disabilities nearing their third birthday (Kellegrew, 1998). Self-care occupations that the mothers valued and that were also goals on the children's individual family service plans were targeted. Using a multiple-baseline, across-subjects design, mothers were asked to provide daily opportunities for their child's emerging dressing or eating occupations and to monitor the child's success. Two mothers adapted their daily routines to provide increased opportunities for their child to engage in the self-care occupation. These two children demonstrated rapid self-care independence in the targeted skill, which was maintained after completion of the intervention study.

The third child in this study demonstrated a marked increase in self-feeding when given increased opportunity. However, the child's caregiver did not continue to provide the child with opportunities to eat independently, and he remained dependent in this area. Despite the mother's knowledge that independent eating was within the child's repertoire, this occupation was not spontaneously integrated into the family's daily routines. The child's ability to perform an occupation did not appear to guide the construction of the family's daily routines as is suggested by the literature (Porn, 1993). This leads to the question, What factors are influential in determining the evolution of daily routines within a family? Understanding the ways in which families construct routines can provide useful information that contributes to increased efficacy in designing and integrating intervention into the daily life of the family.

This research study examined the process through which mothers construct self-care routines for their young children with disabilities. Qualitative methods were used because this form of inquiry is uniquely suited to explore the ways in which people make meaning and negotiate their lives (Carlson & Clark, 1991). This research specifically sought to understand the mother's point of view as she designed and orchestrated everyday routines over time. Ecocultural theory was incorporated as a conceptual framework for the study. The study analysis extended past work with this theory by examining specifically the construction of children's self-care routines as they emerged within the everyday life of the family.

Method

Participants

The participants were recruited from a large early intervention center in a suburban county adjacent to Los Angeles, California. Children whose dressing and eating ability was rated as "emerging" by the occupational therapists and physical therapists at the early intervention program were selected for participation. Six families, including seven children with disabilities and their mothers, were involved in the study. Two of the children were adopted siblings near the same age.

The child participants ranged in age from 28 months to 32 months and had a variety of conditions, including cerebral palsy, developmental delay, severe dyspraxia, and Down syndrome. Four children were girls, and three were boys. The adult participants included six mothers and one maternal grandmother who cared for the child during most of the work day. All families were intact, middle class, and from a Caucasian ethnic background. All fathers worked a traditional work week. Five of the six mothers were full-time homemakers, and one mother worked full-time. Two of the seven children were only children, whereas the remaining families had other siblings (see Table 41.1).

Data Collection

In keeping with a qualitative framework, all data were collected in natural environments, and observations were designed to capture the fluid, complex interactions of everyday life. One researcher (myself) collected all data. Before the start of the study, a pilot project was conducted to hone the interview format and videotaping procedures.

Data were collected in two phases. The first phase involved all six families. Unstructured audiotaped interviews were conducted individually with each mother. Interview topics explored the family's daily routines and ecological challenges, such as economic resources and transportation issues. The mother's values and beliefs regarding child rearing also were explored. Self-care routines were videotaped and gathered for all families during naturalistic observations of mealtime and child dressing routines. Data, in this phase, were gathered over the course of one to two visits per family.

The second phase of data collection incorporated three of the original six families: the

Table 41.1. Description of Participants

| Child (Age) | Condition | Mother | | Father | | Siblings |
		Education	Vocation	Education	Vocation	
Allison (32 months)	Down syndrome	BA	Homemaker	BA	Construction	1 younger
Eliza (28 months)	Spastic cerebral palsy	High school	Manicurist	JD	Attorney	None
Karen (30 months)	Mild cerebral palsy	Some college	Homemaker	Some college	Grocer	1 older
Nathan (32 months)	Down syndrome	BA	Accountant	BA	Accountant	1 older
Paul (28 months)	Down syndrome	BA	Homemaker	BA	Sales	None
Rose (30 months)[a]	Prenatally exposed to drugs	High school	Homemaker	BA	Accountant	3 older
Seth (30 months)[a]	Down syndrome	Same as for Rose	Same as for Rose	Same as for Rose	Same as for Rose	3 older

[a]Rose and Seth are adopted.

families of Paul, Allison, and Nathan. Nathan's grandmother, his primary caregiver during the day, also was included. Phase 2 participants were selected using two criteria: (a) the child's emerging self-care ability was evident and (b) consistent routines requiring the child's self-care independence were not yet an established part of daily life. It was hoped that following these families over time would give insight into the evolution of daily routines that incorporated emerging skills. Each of the three families was observed and videotaped one to four times weekly during mealtime and child dressing routines for approximately 2 months.

Additionally, in-depth interviews of the mothers and Nathan's grandmother were conducted over the 2-month period. Nathan's mother and grandmother were interviewed separately during an initial and an interim interview, and they were interviewed together during the last interview. For all participants, questions from the initial interviews were reexamined to determine changes in perspective across time. Additional queries exploring the caregiver's perception of her child's skills were conducted during the last interview because this emerged as an area of interest during preliminary data analysis. Both phases of the study yielded 72 videotaped observations and 15 interviews for coding and analysis.

Data Analysis

The daily routines of the home were the unit of analysis of interest for this study. However, each home routine can encompass a wide range of elements. In their ecocultural examination of classroom routines, Tharp and Gallimore (1988) contended that the examination of single routines can be best understood by examining activity settings, or the units of activity that involve the interaction between members of the niche in a goal-directed action. The five components of activity settings include the following:

1. Personnel present
2. Values and goals
3. Tasks being performed
4. Meanings, feelings, and motives
5. Cultural scripts that govern the interaction.

Data were aggregated and coded from both phases of the study according to the five components of activity settings. The procedure for coding narrative data and observational data differed. Narrative data included the transcripts of all interviews and the transcripts of approximately 20% of each videotaped routine. Videotaped routines that appeared to most inform the study, as determined by the researcher, were chosen for transcription. The narrative data were grouped according to the basic idea of the communication and then coded into one of the activity setting components by the researcher. Observational data, gathered from the videotapes, were segmented by counter numbers into action units according to the task performed. Activity setting components were coded for each action unit. An experienced graduate student researcher independently cross-checked the accuracy of the coding for 30% of both the narrative data and the observational data.

Coded observational and narrative data from both phases of the study were then examined to determine patterns both within and among families. In particular, the manifestation of routines in response to the child's changing self-care skills was a focus. Two major patterns, accommodation and anticipation, emerged that described the manner in which mothers constructed daily routines. The findings of the study were reviewed for veracity with a researcher experienced in qualitative inquiry.

Results

Personnel Present

The work schedules of the adults had an impact on the number of personnel present during self-care occupations. Five of the six fathers were not present during any of the families' weekday meals. One mother worked full-time. She was not available for her child's breakfast or lunch but dined with her child each evening. The caregivers who were present during the children's meals usually ate at a different time than the children. Only one mother regularly ate breakfast or lunch with her child. The mothers reported that children and adults usually dressed separately. In addition, two of the four families with multiple siblings reported that their child did not dress in the company of a sibling.

Tasks and Activities

Across participants, a similar cooking routine and menu, use of household space, and time use during mealtime occupations were noted. For example, the children's breakfast foods typically consisted of juice, cereal, yogurt, toast, waffles, or eggs. All children were fed at a table, in or near the kitchen. There was slightly less consistency noted in the families' dressing routines. In particular, the gender of the child influenced the clothing choices. Daytime clothing for boys consisted of pull-on pants, T-shirts, socks, and tennis shoes. The girls were occasionally dressed in clothing that was more difficult to put on independently, such as leggings or jumpsuits.

Dressing took place on the floor for four of seven children, and three children were dressed on a high platform such as a changing table or high bed. Children dressed on the floor tended to be more active in the dressing process. For example, they might hand their mother a shoe or retrieve an item of clothing out of a drawer. Children dressed on changing tables or platforms tended to be more passive, as these children did not participate in the dressing process unless prompted by the mother.

All children were more independent in mealtime occupations than dressing occupations, despite the similarity in developmental difficulty for these two self-care domains (Furuno et al., 1994). Most mothers noted that eating occupations were more readily observed by those outside of the immediate family. In contrast, dressing occupations were viewed as private. Paul's mother commented, "Dressing is not a subject that you talk to other moms about. It's a privacy issue, I guess. Even in just talking to my family....No one says, 'Is he dressing?'" The higher value most mothers placed on independent eating skills appeared partially driven by the possibility of public scrutiny. This is illustrated by a conversation between Nathan's mother and grandmother.

> *Grandma:* I can remember the time when I met Connie's friend with her little girl at the restaurant, and she ordered spaghetti for her little girl.
> *Connie:* And you were horrified, I remember.
> *Grandma:* She let her eat it with her hands!
> *Connie:* I remember. In a public place!

Goals and Values

The values mothers placed on self-care routines appeared tied to their goals for their child's future. In essence, these mothers attempted to anticipate the skills their child would need in the near future. For example, Allison's mother was concerned that her daughter was not toilet trained, a prerequisite for admission to a regular preschool that she was considering. As a consequence, this mother identified Allison's self-dressing as a goal, stating, "Maybe if she can dress herself and take her pants off, it would help potty train her."

The interaction between mothers' goals and their perception of future expectations was noted during the construction of daily routines for tasks other than self-care. One mother sought playmates who were typically developing for her adopted daughter who had been prenatally exposed to drugs. She reported, "Rose will be normal. She's going to go to college. We are already saving money." However, she envisioned that her son would require special placement his entire life and subsequently did not view playmates who were typically developing as important for the child, stating "Seth just tags along."

The expressed goals and values of these mothers were modified by the ecological variable of time. "Depending on the time…," "If I have time…," and "When I have time…" were phrases frequently used by all mothers that illustrated the interplay among goals, values, and ecological reality. When the morning routine was more hectic, most mothers increased their assistance, either by feeding a child who was usually independent in eating or by quickly dressing a child without eliciting cooperation.

In addition, the variable of time tended to have a more profound impact on the child whose skills were less independent or slow than it did on the child whose skills were fully independent. For example, Eliza was relatively independent in manipulating feeding utensils but tended to be slow. On days when she had early physical therapy appointments, she was fed. On days without time pressure, she was encouraged to feed herself. In contrast, Karen was independent in self-feeding and would do so in a timely manner. When confronted with time pressure, Karen's mother adapted their daily routine in a way that retained the element of self-feeding independence. Karen ate her sandwich in the car 4 days a week while her mother traveled to pick up an older sibling from preschool.

Lack of time also led to a modification of parenting values. For example, Nathan's mother worked full-time and as a consequence had to rely on her mother, the child's daytime caregiver, to make decisions regarding Nathan's activities. She realized that the grandmother's choices differed from her own. Nathan's mother commented,

> She [the grandmother] doesn't expect him to do anything. She doesn't think he can do certain things, mostly self-help skills. I don't know

that I agree with it. But, I can't be there really to teach him lessons. I've come to the realization that certain things are not worth fighting over. Certain things I am particular about. Those are the things I will fight for.

Motives, Meanings, and Feelings

The motives, meanings, and feelings associated with the enactment of daily routines appeared tied to two components: (a) the mother's perception of the child's skill performance and (b) the mother's child-rearing perspective. Across all families, mothers consistently gauged their child's skill performance to determine the types of routines that might be most appropriate. For example, Nathan's grandmother commented, "He doesn't really play, so he's too young to have a playmate." Her perception of Nathan's play skills led to daily activities that did not include social partners for Nathan.

The skill performance of most young children will vary from day to day, and the children in this study were no different. All of the mothers adjusted the structure of their child's self-care occupations on the basis of variations in their child's cooperation and skill. In essence, these mothers appeared to fine-tune their daily routines and expectations in accordance with their perceptions of their child's abilities at that moment. A comment made by Paul's mother illustrated this point: "Does he feed himself? Yes, he does. But sometimes he does, and sometimes he doesn't. I feel I want to be realistic about the things he does. It's not just black and white."

The mother's child-rearing style and perspective also appeared to contribute to the meaning and motive assigned to everyday events and the subsequent construction of daily routines. For example, Allison's mother displayed a child-rearing style that appeared child centered. This mother explained her strategy for introducing new routines: "When she wants to do something, she tries. She just tries, and that's how I know she's ready. I let her tell me." This child-rearing approach influenced the meaning the mother attributed to the child's behavior and introduction of more demanding expectations for her daughter. In this case, Allison had an expressive language delay that clouded the communication between mother and child. The mother frequently described her daughter's cues as unclear, which had a major impact on the construction of daily routines. Allison's mother commented,

> Like for breakfast, I would make her six things because I didn't think her yes or no were clear. Or I'm not sure she totally understood I was giving her an option. I would make her something, and it started out that she would get down from the table and, like, go and get out the cheese when she wanted cheese.

Another child, Karen, also had an expressive language delay. In contrast to Allison's mother, Karen's mother displayed a child-rearing style that required her children to fit a template of acceptable child behavior, whether the child was actually capable of the task at the moment. This child-rearing style also influenced the meaning, motive, and feeling surrounding the construction of daily self-care routines. Karen's mother stated,

> I just expect things and whether or not she can do them or not, I at least expect her to try. Like I ask her to make the bed, and if Karen at least tries to tug on it, I know she's comprehending that I want her to do something with the bed.

In keeping with this mother's template of acceptable child behavior, child-initiated activities that did not fit within the template were discouraged. In one illustration, Karen's mother stated, "Karen will take the straw and pull it [the paper wrapper] down, and knock the cup over, so I won't give her a straw. I just took it away." Independently using a straw was not important to this mother, therefore, she did not tolerate a

"mess" when the child initiated the activity. However, she did tolerate "messes" when Karen tried to perform other, more valued occupations, such as brushing her teeth.

Cultural Scripts

Cultural scripts describe the shared interactions that occur between niche members as they go about their daily routines (Tharp & Gallimore, 1988). The observation tapes revealed that most scripts between caregiver and child had a sense of continuity and familiarity. Each participant appeared to know the expectations and abilities of the other. For example, when Seth announced that he was finished with breakfast, his mother quickly ran to his chair. He then stood up and jumped into her arms. The mother reported that this was Seth's daily routine and, if she was not fast enough, Seth would jump from the high chair directly to the floor.

Some cultural scripts were quite specific, including exact phrases and behavior. For example, Eliza said, "I have troubles" when experiencing difficulties poking her waffle with a fork. If her mother perceived that Eliza was truly unable to perform the task, she would assist her. If she thought that Eliza might be capable of handling the problem independently, she would reply, "You can do it." Eliza would then proceed to eat her meal independently. When Eliza changed the script to say, "Help, Mommy," her mother responded, "You have troubles?" Eliza then began again, this time with the "correct" response, "I have troubles." This process was repeated five to six times per meal.

Cultural scripts between mother and child could destabilize as expectations during the daily routines evolved. This was clearly demonstrated when reviewing Paul's self-dressing progress during the 2-month observation period. Initially, Paul preferred to play with his mother during the dressing occupation. Later, Paul's mother became much more insistent that Paul cooperate during dressing, thus changing the focus or goal of the dressing time. During the first few days, Paul cooperated but then rebelled and repeatedly tried to reinstate the play-like script. When his mother persisted, Paul's behavior aligned to the new expectation for independent dressing with a new cultural script between mother and child.

Synthesis of Activity Settings

A synthesis of the activity setting analysis identified two processes through which mothers designed and orchestrated daily routines: accommodation and anticipation. The process of accommodation describes the ways in which mothers modified and adjusted routines to adapt to daily challenges. The process of accommodation is set in present time and implies that mothers adjust and adapt to everyday challenges. Accommodations were most often required in response to the child's changing skill ability. For example, most mothers adjusted the level of independence they would require of their child in response to their perception of the child's ability. Eliza's mother evaluated Eliza's request for assistance with her waffle to determine whether she really needed physical assistance or just verbal support. Allison's mother looked to her child for cues about her readiness before initiating more challenging routines. Nathan's grandmother did not request the child to feed himself because she was concerned that he "couldn't really do it." The mother's analysis of the child's present-time skill performance directly contributed to the construction of home routines.

Participants also used a companion process to that of accommodation, best described as anticipation. The process of anticipation is rooted in future time. Mothers anticipated their child's future needs and orchestrated daily routines that would reinforce or develop those skills perceived as beneficial to the child's future success. Because all of these

children were turning 3 years of age, transition from early intervention services to a preschool setting was a consideration for each family. Those mothers considering a regular preschool placement seemed to be more focused on normalization goals, such as appropriate social skills or independent self-care skills. Mothers who had decided on a special education setting expressed more interest in their child's academic daily activities. One mother commented that she did not have to "work on self-care skills" because special education teachers are trained to provide this service.

Discussion

This study examined mothers' construction of self-care routines for their young children with disabilities. For these participants, the creation of routines was a complex enterprise, influenced simultaneously by broad ecocultural variables and a reciprocal relationship unique to each caregiver–child dyad. Ecocultural theory, used as a conceptual framework, examined larger forces that had an impact on the construction of these mothers' routines. Ecocultural theory proposes that families accommodate or adjust their daily occupations in response to environmental variables and cultural influences. Past research using ecocultural theory has primarily focused on broad patterns of accommodation across the aggregate of a family's routines at a fixed point in time. The current study extended the research on ecocultural theory by examining the construction of just one domain of routines, children's self-care occupations, as they emerged across a 2-month time frame. The findings indicate that ecocultural components of daily routines are recognizable, even when examining a single routine.

In support for the basic premise behind ecocultural theory, both cultural values and ecological variables were prime forces in the formation of self-care routines. The cultural component of the routines in particular created similar patterns across families. Cultural practices, embedded in every aspect of these families' lives, reflected a Western orientation (Frank, 1994). Of special note was the solitary nature of the daily meal-time and dressing routines and the distinction between private and public behavior observed in these families. Weisner (1984) commented,

> Western children live in a remarkably private culture....[W]e encourage such privacy early in children's lives by giving them their own rooms and spaces, their own toys and other posses-sions....American children learn how to make behavior and possessions private or at least capa-ble of being kept private as a matter of their choice. (p. 355)

Ecological variables also influenced the overall structure of self-care routines. For these families, middle-class socioeconomic status con-tributed to similar types of resources, including access to early intervention services, adequate transportation, and home ownership. As predicted by ecocultural theory, environmental forces mod-ified the cultural goals and practices of families. On a day-to-day basis, participants most often noted lack of time was a pervasive ecological con-straint. This was in keeping with other research that noted time constraints as a major considera-tion for most families (Brotherson & Goldstein, 1992). In the current study, the time demands of self-care routines were a pivotal factor in the types and consistency of children's self-care occupa-tions. Children who were less competent in self-care skills were less likely to be given oppor-tunities for self-care independence when time was limited. This can be a factor in the self-care development of some children with disabilities who may require more daily practice to achieve skill proficiency.

One finding unique to this study suggests that on a daily basis, mothers make small adjust-ments in the home routines that shape the types of opportunities for skill development offered to their child. This orchestration of daily routines appeared to be a blended process between accom-modation to everyday events and anticipation of future needs. Just as mothers have been noted to fine-tune their speech in response to their child's communication, the mothers of this study fine-tuned or accommodated their expectations for skill development in response to their child's skill performance on any given day. Through this process, they formed an evaluation of their child's ability, taking into account daily fluctuations in skill level. Concurrently, mothers anticipated the skills their child would need in the future. The daily routines that mothers created were those that met two criteria: (a) must be within the child's potential ability and (b) was required to meet a future demand. The joint process of accom-modation and anticipation appeared to have tremendous power to frame the everyday lives of the child with disabilities. Through mothers' con-struction of routines, the young child's emerging skills either were reinforced and strengthened or were ignored.

The findings of this study have implica-tions for occupational therapy intervention. Clark (1993), described occupational storymaking and storytelling as used to elicit therapeutic changes in an adult woman who had survived a stroke. The findings of the current study support the value of adapting occupational storymaking and story-telling for use with the mothers of children with disabilities. Occupational storytelling seeks to elicit a picture of the individual person as an occu-pational being. In many ways, the mothers in this study described their child's skill ability in terms of occupations such as bedmaking, choosing breakfast foods, or playing with peers. Reflected in the storytelling were mothers' perceptions of their child's occupational ability. Storymaking thus can be used to assist the mother in recognizing and interpreting the child's abilities, which in turn can have an impact on the types of daily opportunities for occupation presented.

Additionally, storymaking involves the therapist and client creating stories to be enacted in the future (Mattingly, 1991). In this study, a mother's vision of her child's future played a pivotal role in the types of daily routines constructed. Some mothers had great difficulty envisioning the possibilities available for their child. For some mothers, preschool placement a few months away appeared to be farthest point in the future for which they could picture their child. Other mothers already had conceptualized a view of their child as an adult and had organized daily routines to support this future vision. Intervention that incorporates storymaking can be a promising avenue for mothers and therapists to explore possible futures available to a child. This exploration can alter the types of daily opportunities for skill development presented to the child with disabilities.

There are limitations in the generalizations of these findings. For these families, the upcoming transition from early intervention services to school-based services appeared to make school placement concerns particularly salient. One avenue for future research is to examine whether age-related developmental events, such as the increasing independence associated with adolescence, represent predictable opportunities for parents to shape their child's routines in response to future needs. Future research also might explore whether parents' expectations for future events are significantly influenced by their child's personal characteristics. For example, does the mother of a child with behavior problems appear more astute to the social demands of future settings because she is more aware of her child's limitations? In this study, the children were of similar developmental capacity. Additional inquiry might examine the extent to which a mother's perception of her child's abilities alter her vision of future possibilities.

In keeping with the strong national trend toward family-centered care, the findings of this study support an ecocultural view of the family. Furthermore, these results suggest that intervention for children with disabilities need not be at the level of child skill training (Marfo, Browne, Gallant, Smyth, & Corbett, 1991; Weisner et al., 1996; Young, Davis, Schoen, & Parker, 1998). Indeed, occupational therapy services that strive to promote a clearer maternal understanding of the child's present and future occupational potential can result in the creation of home routines that promote development.

Acknowledgments

I thank Robert Koegel, PhD; Michael Gerber, PhD; and Betsy Brenner, PhD, for their comments on earlier drafts. I also thank the staff and families at the Child Development Center, Simi Valley, CA, for their support and cooperation.

This research was conducted in partial fulfillment for a doctoral degree in educational psychology from the University of California at Santa Barbara.

References

Bernheimer, L. P., Gallimore, R., & Kaufman, S. Z. (1993). Clinical child assessment in a family context: A four-group typology of family experiences with young children with developmental delays. *Journal of Early Intervention, 17*, 253–269.

Bernheimer, L. P., Gallimore, R., & Weisner, T. S. (1990). Ecocultural theory as a context for the individual family service plan. *Journal of Early Intervention, 14*, 219–233.

Bronfenbrenner, U. (1979). *The ecology of human development: Experiments by nature and human design.* Cambridge, MA: Harvard University Press.

Brotherson, M. J., & Goldstein, B. L. (1992). Time as a resource and constraint for parents of young children with disabilities: Implications for early intervention services. *Topics in Early Childhood Special Education, 12*, 508–527.

Carlson, M. E., & Clark, F. A. (1991). The search for useful methodologies in occupational science. *American Journal of Occupational Therapy, 45,* 235–241.

Clark, F. A. (1993). Occupation embedded in real life: Interweaving occupational science and occupational therapy [1993 Eleanor Clarke Slagle Lecture]. *American Journal of Occupational Therapy, 47,* 1067–1078.

Frank, G. (1994). The personal meaning of self-care occupations. In C. Christiansen (Ed.), *Ways of living: Self-care strategies for special needs* (pp. 27–50). Rockville, MD: American Occupational Therapy Association.

Furuno, S., Inatsuka, T., O'Reilly, K., Hosaka, C., Zeisloft, B., & Allman, T. (1994). *HELP checklist (Hawaii Early Learning Profile).* Palo Alto, CA: VORT.

Gallimore, R., Weisner, T. S., Bernheimer, L. P., Guthrie, D., & Nihira, K. (1993). Family responses to young children with developmental delays: Accommodation activity in ecological and cultural context. *American Journal on Mental Retardation, 98,* 185–206.

Gallimore, R., Weisner, T. S., Kaufman, S. Z., & Bernheimer, L. P. (1989). The social construction of ecocultural niches: Family accommodation of developmentally delayed children. *American Journal of Mental Retardation, 94,* 216–230.

Harkness, S., & Super, C. M. (1983). The cultural construction of child development: A framework for the socialization of affect. *Ethos, 11*(4), 221–231.

Kellegrew, D. H. (1998). Creating opportunities for occupation: An intervention to promote the self-care independence of young children with special needs. *American Journal of Occupational Therapy, 52,* 457–465.

Koegel, L. K., Koegel, R. L., Kellegrew, D. H., & Mullen, K. (1996). Parent education for prevention and reduction of severe problem behavior. In L. K. Kogel, R. L. Kogel, & G. Dunlap (Eds.), *Positive behavior support: Including people with difficult behavior in the community* (pp. 3–30). Baltimore: Brookes.

Marfo, K., Browne, N., Gallant, D., Smyth, R., & Corbett, A. (1991). Issues in early intervention: Insights from the Newfoundland and Labrador evaluation project. *Developmental Disabilities Bulletin, 19*(2), 36–65.

Mattingly, C. (1991). The narrative nature of clinical reasoning. *American Journal of Occupational Therapy, 45,* 998–1005.

Porn, I. (1993). Health and adaptedness. *Theoretical Medicine, 14,* 295–203.

Rogoff, B. (1993). Children's guided participation and participatory appropriation in sociocultural activity. In R. H. Wozniak & K. W. Fischer (Eds.), *Development in context: Acting and thinking in specific environments* (pp. 121–153). Hillsdale, NJ: Erlbaum.

Rogoff, B., Mistry, J., Goncu, A., & Mosier, C. (1993). Guided participation in cultural activity by toddlers and caregivers. *Monographs of the Society for Research in Child Development, 58*(8, Serial No. 236).

Tharp, R. G., & Gallimore, R. (1988). *Rousing minds to life.* New York: Cambridge University Press.

Valsiner, J. (1985). Parental organization of children's cognitive development within home environment. *Psychologia, 28,* 131–143.

Weisner, T. S. (1984). Ecocultural niches of middle childhood: A cross-cultural perspective. In W. A. Collins (Ed.), *Development during middle childhood* (pp. 335–369). Washington, DC: National Academy Press.

Weisner, T. S., Gallimore, R., & Jordan, C. (1993). Unpackaging cultural effects on classroom learning: Hawaiian peer assistance and child-generated activity. In R. N. Roberts (Ed.), *Coming home to preschool: Sociocultural context of early education* (pp. 59–60). Norwood, NJ: Ablex.

Weisner, T. S., Matheson, C. C., & Bernheimer, L. P. (1996). American cultural models of early influence and parent recognition of developmental delays: Is earlier always better than later? In S. Harkness & C. M. Super (Eds.), *Parents' cultural belief systems* (pp. 496–532). New York: Guilford.

Young, K. T., Davis, K., Schoen, C., & Parker, S. (1998). Listening to parents. *Archives of Pediatric and Adolescent Medicine, 152,* 255–262.

CHAPTER 42

The Orchestration of Occupation

The Dance of Mothers

Elizabeth A. Larson

Elizabeth A. Larson, PhD, OTR, *is assistant professor, University of Wisconsin–Madison, Department of Kinesiology, Occupational Therapy Program, 2180 Medical Sciences Center, 1300 University Avenue, Madison, WI 53706.*

Orchestration is a useful metaphor for understanding the organizational structure that undergirds occupation. As commonly used, the term *orchestration* is the composition or arrangement of music and the combination of elements so as to achieve a maximum harmonious effect (*Webster's New Collegiate Dictionary,* 1977). The root of orchestration comes from the Greek *orcheisthai,* to dance. Occupational science has initially conceptualized orchestration as the "ideation, composition, execution, ordering, and qualitative aspects of occupation through the course of one's day" (University of Southern California, Department of Occupational Therapy, 1989, Appendix G, p. 6). Like playing music or dancing, daily rounds are arguably rhythmic and cyclic and desirably arranged to maximize harmonious occupational engagement.

To be a useful metaphor for occupational science, orchestration must account for the complex rhythmic, arrhythmic, recursive, nonrecursive, cyclic, linear, and developmental patterns of occupation in daily rounds throughout a person's lifetime. As yet, the intricacies of the orchestration of daily occupations are only beginning to be articulated (Primeau, 1996; Segal, 1996, 2000).

Conceptually, this musical metaphor of orchestration holds promise in fostering study of occupational patterns. For example, in orchestration of music, a desirable harmony supports the melody and has unity, variety, and rhythm that change at intervals (Piston, 1962). These qualities of harmony are also desirable in the composition of daily rounds of occupations. The notes, which could be thought of as representing occupations, are arranged both vertically in relation to one another (co-occurring or enfolded occupations) and in parallel structures (sequenced in daily rounds) coordinated with a central tone or key (life theme or personal values). Two or more notes or occupations can be consonant, producing stable and complete sounds, compatible enactment of occupations, or dissonant, creating restless unresolved sounds, incompatible enactment of occupations. Although a promising and helpful concept for examining occupation,

Originally published 2000 in *American Journal of Occupational Therapy, 54,* 269–280.

the dimensions or processes of orchestration that are related to the engagement in and daily enactment of occupations have not been uncovered in any depth.

Literature Review

Orchestration has been used in the literature largely to refer to complex processes that require anticipation, forethought, sifting of information, decision making, and a coordinated response. From sensorimotor responses to organizational structures, the term *orchestration* has been applied to processes aimed at producing well-designed and coordinated responses within the systematic constraints and affordances from the micro to macro level of systems (Bruenjes, 1994; Craigie, 1985; Eldridge, 1983; Hamilton-Dodd, Kawamoto, Clark, Burke, & Fanchiang, 1989; Harry, 1992; Leviton & Greenstone, 1984; Shandlen & Newsome, 1996; Tharp & Gallimore, 1988; Zelman, McLaughlin, Geld, & Miller, 1985).

These studies examine common processes of orchestration. First, there is an informational dimension where taking in, sifting, and using information leads to choices, decisions, and actions (Craigie, 1985; Hamilton-Dodd et al., 1989; Shandlen & Newsome, 1996; Tharp & Gallimore, 1988; Zelman et al., 1985). This "decision making" involves a balanced consideration of all important factors (Bruenjes, 1994; Hamilton-Dodd et al., 1989; Tharp & Gallimore, 1988; Shandlen & Newsome, 1996; Zelman et al., 1985). This process also involves consideration of the environmental press, or the available constraints and resources (Bruenjes, 1994; Tharp & Gallimore, 1988; Zelman et al., 1985). The social environment is crucial when constructing well-orchestrated responses; this includes making choices that are prioritized, harmonized, and congruent with the individual's personal respon-

sibility within a social group (Bruenjes, 1994; Hamilton-Dodd et al., 1989).

Bruenjes (1994), a nurse, defined *orchestration of health* for middle-aged women as the moderating and encouraging of physical, emotional, spiritual, and environmental factors to achieve a sense of harmony or being "in tune." She concluded that these women orchestrated or "conducted" their health via processes of prioritizing, choices, balancing, selecting moderation, interaction, and responsibility in daily activities. These processes of health orchestration emphasized interpersonal and intrapersonal aspects of the orchestration and may be useful in pointing to potential areas of study in occupation.

Both Primeau's (1996) and Segal's (1996) studies contribute to the understanding of how families orchestrate daily parent–child co-occupations. They uncovered parents' strategies in orchestrating daily occupations. Primeau illustrated both the inclusion and segregation strategies parents used to incorporate parent–child play within daily routines. Inclusion strategies required parents to enfold occupations; segregation strategies meant parents stopped for play breaks during the daily routines. Segal, in studying families parenting children with attention deficit hyperactivity disorder, conceptualized an orchestration strategy of unfolding in which enfolded occupations are separated and performed at different times or by different persons to increase the children's occupational independence and success. Beyond these findings, research also needs to begin to define the processes of occupational orchestration.

Choosing and orchestrating satisfying rounds of daily occupation is believed to be a potent influence on subjective well-being (Primeau, Clark, & Pierce, 1990). Reich and Zautra (1983) intuited that well-being was most likely related to the orchestration of occupations or the freedom to choose desired occupations and avoid undesired ones. However, their research did not bear this out. Having more desires was related to positive subjective well-being, but successfully meeting demands also related to more positive well-being, despite the occupations not being desired ones (Reich & Zautra, 1983). Mothers often make choices of occupations that are geared toward meeting the demands of parenting children—safeguarding the children's health, nurturing their development, and socializing them to be community members—rather than their own needs. Although Reich and Zautra's work discounts a simplistic view of the orchestration of occupation related to free choice of occupations in daily life, it does not illuminate the complexity of orchestration of occupation and subjective well-being.

Besides all the typical daily demands, mothers parenting older children with severe disabilities must often perform physical caregiving and child supervision that is as intensive as parenting infants and toddlers. These mothers often engage in complex nonnormative caregiving routines over extended periods that require careful modifications of daily family routines to successfully accommodate the child with special needs. In addition, these mothers must coordinate daily family schedules with professionals in the educational and health care systems. Mothering a child with special needs requires additional skills, knowledge, and organization. These mothers devote more time to caregiving and household labor, which often results not only in restrictions on their personal choices of occupations but also in limited time for sleep (Bailey & Simeonsson, 1988; Kazak & Marvin, 1984; Leyser & Dekel, 1991; Singer & Farkas, 1989). Research has demonstrated that these additional daily challenges can produce stress and periodic depression (Beckman, 1991; Breslau, Strauch, & Mortimer, 1982; Bristol, Gallagher, & Schopler, 1988; Friedrich, Wilturner, & Cohen, 1985; Goldberg, Morris, Simmons, Fowler, & Levinson, 1990;

Kazak & Marvin, 1984; Shapiro & Tittle, 1990; Sloper & Turner, 1993).

This study's aim was to uncover the complexities of the relationship of subjective well-being and orchestration of daily rounds of occupations for mothers parenting children with disabilities. The findings presented here are one part of this study of mothers' occupations and well-being when parenting a child with a disability, an in-depth analysis of which has been previously published (Larson, 1998). This chapter focuses on how mothers orchestrate daily occupation to meet their maternal aims.

When a phenomenon is particularly complex, it is often helpful to study the extreme case (Patton, 1989). In this case, participants were selected whose daily rounds hypothetically compromise subjective well-being due to constraints on choices of occupations and to the frequent demands of caregiving. Given the ongoing and intensive caregiving and recognized time restrictions for mothers parenting children with severe disabilities, this group of mothers may be described as the extreme case and thereby were an important group of informants to illuminate the relationship of occupations and subjective well-being.

Method

Participants

Six Mexican-origin mothers volunteered to participate in a series of interviews and a daylong participant observation and to complete a well-being scale (Juster, Hill, Stafford, & Parsons, 1988) and the Hassle Scale (Kanner, Coyne, Schaefer, & Lazarus, 1981). Participants were recruited through an agency that provided services to children with disabilities and a local interagency coordinating council. Mothers of Mexican origin were selected because, at the current growth rate,

Latinos were projected to be the largest minority in Los Angeles and the United States by the year 2000 (Vega, 1990).

Participants included three mothers who participated in a pilot study and three additional mothers who were all selected on theoretical grounds to provide variability on dimensions. A balance of mothers at either extreme of certain dimensions (i.e., perceived maternal subjective well-being, marital support, primary language [Spanish or English], generation of residence [first or second]) was sought to provide variability within this group. All of the mothers were parenting children with severe disabilities. Severe disabilities were defined as having a combination of the following characteristics: limited or absent self-care skills, severe cognitive disabilities, physical impairments, bowel and bladder problems, impaired communication skills, or severe behavior problems.

The six participants were from 27 to 42 years of age, with educational attainments varying from ninth-grade education to graduate degrees. Two completed less than high school, three had some college or vocational training, and one was a physician with a master's degree from a Mexican university. Each had two to five children and resided in predominantly Latino areas of Los Angeles. Family incomes ranged from $1,000 to $1,909 monthly (in 1994). All six worked as homemakers, with four also employed outside the home during the study.

The children with disabilities were between 5 and 11 years of age and experienced the onset of disability between birth and 3 years of age. Three had cerebral palsy–spastic quadraparesis, one had spastic quadraparesis, one had blindness and global developmental delay, and one had high-functioning autism. Four attended a classroom for students with severe handicaps, one had a home school program, and one attended a regular education class (see Table 42.1). All names

used here for mothers and children are pseudonyms to protect their identities.

Data Collection

Data were collected through a series of interviews with each participant, a daylong observation, and two scales. The questions generated for the initial interview guide were drawn from reviewed literature, which suggested the potency of daily activity on subjective well-being, the relevance of daily interactions and well-being (e.g., hassles), the interpretive aspects of activity, limits on mothers regarding choice of occupations, and the relevance of the mother's view of the meaning of maternal work as a coping strategy and modifier in stress (Affleck & Tennen, 1991; Bailey & Simeonsson, 1988; Bristol et al., 1988; Crnic, Friedrich, & Greenberg, 1983; Dunst & Trivette, 1986; Harris & McHale, 1989; Margalit & Raviv, 1983; Patterson & McCubbin, 1983; Shapiro, 1989; Singer & Farkas, 1989; Wallander, Pitt, & Mellins, 1990).

The guide for the second interview was reflexively generated from the initial interviews and based on the participants' completion of the two scales. Questions were asked about their view of how their life differed from families without children with disabilities, the process or changes in their life as a result of the child's disability, their definitions of well-being, and the influence of relationships on their well-being.

The Hassle Scale and well-being scale were completed before the second interview and were used as a means to probe for additional information during the second interview. The Hassle Scale was used to examine frequently experienced minor stressors. Participants were asked to comment on items they ranked as moderate or highly stressful. Previous studies of mothers of children without disabilities given the Hassle Scale suggested that contextual hassles were better

Table 42.1. Description of Participants

Characteristic	Consuelo	Jesucita	Juliana	Mariana	Mariza	Marta
Age (years)	39	41	27	33	32	38
Paid and unpaid work	Part-time hospital housekeeper; homemaker	Coordinator of service agency; homemaker	Homemaker; part-time sales	Homemaker; part-time sales	Part-time secretary and college student; homemaker	Homemaker; foster mother
Language	Spanish, some English	English	Spanish, some English	Spanish	English, Spanish	Spanish
Child	Miguel	Sara	Andrew	Carlos	Lucita	Rachel
Age (years)	11	10	8	6	10	5
Child's disability	Cerebral palsy–spastic quadraparesis; global developmental delays secondary to series of seizures at 3 months of age; nonverbal; dependent for care	Spastic quadraparesis; global developmental delays secondary to febrile seizure/ Taiwanese flu; nonverbal; dependent for care	Autism, severe aggression and suicidal behaviors; average intellectual ability but limited social skills; fluent bilingually; independent in self-care	Cerebral palsy–spastic quadraparesis; developmental delays secondary to prematurity; speaks few words in Spanish and English; eats, dependent in other self-care	Blindness secondary to extreme prematurity; global developmental delays; nonverbal; dependent in self-care	Cerebral palsy–spastic quadraparesis secondary to pneumonia; global developmental delays; nonverbal; dependent in self-care
Family members (age in years)	Mother, father, son (11), daughter (8)	Mother, father, daughter (14), son (12), daughter (10)	Mother, father, son (8), son (6)	Mother, father, son (8), son (6)	Mother, daughter (14), daughter (12), daughter (10), son (8), son (7)	Mother, father, daughter (7), daughter (5), son (3)

predictors of psychological well-being than major life events (Chamberlain & Zika, 1990, 1992). The Hassle Scale requests that mothers rank the severity of commonly experienced minor stressors; it has a test–retest reliability ranging from .77 to .79.

The well-being scale was drawn from the Time-Use Longitudinal Panel Study (Juster et al., 1988). It uses a 7-point Likert scale to rank five dimensions of well-being *(life as a whole, income, standard of living, extent achieving success, employment)*. Like with the Hassle Scale, participants were asked to expand on the rankings they chose for each item. This strategy of using the Hassle Scale and well-being scale as interview probes evolved from a pilot study in which the scales fostered more informative discussions about daily stressors and subjective well-being

than mothers otherwise offered. These scales were also useful for triangulation, providing an additional source of confirmation of mothers' daily experience and subjective well-being.

After completing the questions from these two interview guides, a daylong observation was scheduled with each participant. A final follow-up interview or series of interviews were conducted to clarify unanswered or unclear points from the previous interviews and from the observation. Data were recorded through audiotapes and field notes.

A minimum of 22 hr of data was collected with each participant. Each participant was interviewed in her home, except for two interviews that were conducted elsewhere at one participant's request. Mothers participated in three to six interviews that lasted from 2.5 to 4 hr. Field notes from interviews included documentation about the home environment, context of the interview, and interpersonal interactions. Field notes from the daylong observation included the participant's child-care routine, daily rounds of activities, relevant household and community factors, the sequence of events, and the amount of time spent in each occupation. Typically, field notes from the daylong observations were 29 to 66 pages in length, single spaced. From 235 to 541 single-spaced pages of data were generated for each participant.

A native Spanish-speaking translator who was briefed on interview techniques and qualitative methods was present for the three Spanish-speaking participants' interviews and observations. Audiotaped interviews were transcribed in English or Spanish and English, depending on the participant's first language. In addition, the transcriptions of spoken Spanish were translated and included in interview transcripts. The final Spanish and English transcriptions were reviewed by four different bilingual readers who judged the quality of translation and found no systematic problems.

Data Analysis

Data analysis was an ongoing recursive process during data collection. In the research log and in interview transcriptions, theoretical notes were generated that identified major themes and additional points of inquiry that also guided evolving coding strategies. After transcription, typed interviews were exported to a qualitative software analysis program, Ethnograph.[1] This program is a data management system that assisted in the coding and analysis procedures.

An interpretive interactionism approach framed data analysis (Denzin, 1989). This approach begins by bracketing the phenomenon by separating it into key experiential units. Initially, this includes line-by-line coding to simply name findings, which is followed by the examination of findings for key units. Once identified, these units are examined for recurrent essential features and thematically sorted and grouped. Units are then reassembled to construct theory, and the elements are relocated into real-life contexts.

Coding of Spanish–English transcripts and English transcripts was a multistep process that included line-by-line coding, repeated recodings of the entire data set with more refined codes, thematic sorting and grouping of codes that described the recurrent essential features, and a relational analysis. This recursive coding process continued until all data were coded and no new codes emerged.

Following Miles and Huberman (1984), the relational analysis included the generation of metaphors to account for patterns in the data and to connect findings to theory. This multilayered analysis was focused on maternal occupations and uncovered tacit processes that underlie maternal occupations. When describing daily occupations, participants spoke often about how they accomplished their daily occupations and the importance of this to achieving success in maternal work. These orchestration processes were implicit in the participants' descriptions of daily rounds of occupations and were grouped and named by the researcher.

Trustworthiness of data was ensured through a reflective log chronicling the process of research, methodological, and theoretical decisions; repeated and in-depth interactions with participants; triangulation sources for alternative viewpoints, including the field notes and scales; and outside audits by a panel of experts. This panel of experts was composed of three doctoral students who were trained in qualitative methods and who had extensive experience as pediatric occupational therapists

[1]Qualis Research Associates, PO Box 2070, Amherst, MA 01004.

working with ethnically diverse families. Two were fluent in Spanish and English. Emergent findings were presented and critiqued periodically by this group over 1 year. In addition, member checking with a key participant was used to verify the validity of the embrace of paradox metaphor.

Findings[2]

For these participants, their successes in mothering a child with a disability was closely linked to their feelings of subjective well-being. When queried about their subjective well-being, they often responded with "In what respect?" and touched on their emotional state, physical health, capacity to meet the demands of mothering, the family's health, progress toward desired goals, and the satisfaction of basic needs of food and shelter. Prominent in their responses was the link of their mothering to their subjective well-being. The participants consistently linked their well-being to their child's progress; however, when parenting a child with a disability, success in parenting is uneven and difficult.

Life compositions, like musical ones, contain movements that build on occupational themes or motifs, reveal developmental changes in occupations across movements, and support long-term endeavors (Clark, 1993). The occupational motif that guided these participants' current maternal occupations was the metaphor of the embrace of paradox[2] (Larson, 1998). The embrace of paradox included the

> management of internal tension of opposing forces between loving the child as he or she was and wanting to erase the disability, between dealing with the incurability while pursuing

solutions and between maintaining hopefulness for the child's future while being given negative information and battling their own fears. (Larson, 1998, p. 865)

These participants' narratives revealed that, although they embraced their child despite the disability, they also simultaneously rejected the disability, continuing to aspire to a more typical experience of mothering. Aside from these contradictory thoughts about their own child, participants also were torn between the opinions of others regarding the child's future and their own hopes for improvements, solutions, and miracles. Mothers' well-being was bolstered through a positive evaluation of their circumstances, a perception of control in their life, and a sense of optimism that evolved from their embrace of this paradox. Striking an optimistic stance favoring possible progress was vital to continuing ongoing maternal work. Coming to terms with the disability through this stance sustained these participants' maternal work. This occupational motif, the metaphor of the embrace of paradox, guided the mothers' orchestration of daily occupations.

Processes of Orchestration of Occupation

These participants, guided by their occupational motif, used eight thought processes to compose maternally driven and child-sensitive individual occupations and daily rounds of occupations. The orchestration processes included planning, organizing, balancing, anticipating, interpreting, forecasting, perspective shifting, and meaning making (see Table 42.2). These thought processes appeared to undergird and structure the participants' rounds of occupations and were constrained and afforded by the participants' personal and cultural values and the personal resources available to them in the family's ecocultural context (e.g., the husband's or other family members' participation in household work or child care, family finances). After a description of the pro-

---

[2]The findings presented here are only one part of this study of mother's occupations and well-being when parenting a child with disability (see Larson, 1998).

Table 42.2. Processes of Orchestration

Process	Definition
Planning	Method of achieving maternal aims, conceptualizing strategies for design of occupations
Organizing	Configuring of occupations into a functional routine
Balancing	Taking into account the interests, preferences, and desires of family members when organizing occupations; harmonizing, prioritizing, and negotiating with family members to design the occupational form, to synchronize between members, and to sequence occupational rounds
Interpreting	Conceptualization of child's desires, needs, preferences, and wants to design and recompose occupations
Anticipating	Advanced foresight to address demands of temporally proximate and distant occupations and to counter disruption/create positive contingencies in occupations
Forecasting	Prediction of possible futures and embedding of occupations into current daily rounds to move toward those future possibilities
Perspective shifting	Overarching process; revising of perceptions of previous events and their meaning related to ongoing occupational engagement and choice
Meaning making	Overarching process; finding alternative spiritual, optimistic, and meaningful explanations for life circumstances and occupational patterns

cesses of orchestration, an illustration of orchestration within the single occupation of "feeding the child dinner" will conclude the discussion of the findings.

Planning and Organizing in Occupation

The participants frequently spoke of how additional planning or organization, the first two processes in orchestration, were needed to successfully complete all of their daily plans. *Planning,* as used here, is a method to achieve maternal aims by putting intention into action. This includes conceptualizing in advance strategies that make occupations expedient and well designed. *Organizing* is a configuring of occupations into a functional routine and workable sequence.

Planning and organizing occurred on both a small scale at the level of the single occupation and a large scale in daily and weekly routines. For example,

I wash my clothes on Tuesdays or Fridays…and then on Saturdays, iron everything for the whole week. Or if I…didn't have the clothes [done] then I would do it the day before [for the next morning].

Most of the participants found it difficult to organize a routine that addressed all the things they would like to do. As previous research has suggested, time was a precious and fleeting commodity for mothers (Chamberlain & Zika, 1990). "I try to…do everything [each] day that I have to do, but sometimes…24 hours is not enough." Two of the working participants, Jesucita and Mariza, hired child care workers to expand the number of occupations that could be accomplished in the service of the child and family's needs. The greater the time constraints, especially for Mariana when she both worked and parented, the more crucial was organization to meeting all of the mothers' aims:

I would like to get better organized. I lack a little bit of organization. I sometimes feel I cannot do [everything]. There are too many things that I have to do that have accumulated. More than anything I have to do chores because if I [don't], I do not feel good.…I try to do a little of everything. I feel stressed all day, and I sometimes feel like taking a nap.…But I cannot fall asleep.…I am thinking, "I am going to do this, I am going to go there, I am going to go there tomorrow." And I cannot fall asleep.…Because I still cannot get organized.

Later, better organization and quitting paid work led to greater satisfaction for Mariana because she was able to do more of the things she desired:

"Now that I don't work, I give myself the opportunity to think things out [plan], and organize. I am not pressed for time anymore." This change still did not include more rest, personal time, or leisure but rather a greater devotion of time to activities that would promote her son Carlos's independence. In both circumstances, with too little time when working for pay and with sufficient time when working only as a homemaker, Mariana demonstrates the link of the experience of occupation and its orchestration. Inability to fit occupations into an organized routine and complete them daily created a cumulative stress that disrupted rest, whereas greater satisfaction was derived from a well-planned daily round.

Planning was especially important to live life consciously rather than being rushed. For Jesucita, the lack of planning led to feeling that she was living life on automatic pilot:

Go[ing] through a day seems automatic—not even thinking about what I'm gonna do the next day. It's just like, wake up in the morning and go through the series of tasks, the things I need to do, without really thinking: "What am I looking forward to? What am I gonna be doing in the [next] 5 minutes? What's my plan?" I'm just so busy living and doing that I don't often stop to think where I'm going.

Balancing in Occupation

The process of *balancing*, taking into account the interests, preferences, and desires of family members when organizing occupations, required that the participant harmonize, prioritize, and negotiate with the family in orchestrating occupation. One family member can be "out of tune" with the rest, creating stress for the entire family. Again, Jesucita's family demonstrated this:

We're just all so tuned in....It's the kids and I....[My husband]...sometimes he's totally off....[My son] started calling him Mr. Monkey Wrench. That gives you an idea...because some-

times we're all like harmonized [about] what we're gonna do, and he'll come and totally change the plan...it creates a bit of anxiety because they're not sure what's gonna happen after all....I like to plan things....I don't like a lot of changes.

Sometimes the out-of-tune family member was the child with a disability. In both balancing and organizing, the participant frequently chose to work around the child to accomplish necessary occupations, such as those of providing food and shelter. Mariana and her husband sometimes left Carlos with a babysitter for 2 or 3 hr a week so that they could go shopping for groceries or other purchases. Carlos's frequent tantrums in public places, especially when his demands for a new toy or attention were not immediately met, disrupted the shopping and made it difficult for Mariana to make her selections and shop in a timely manner. Not taking Carlos allowed Mariana to more efficiently complete shopping with a minimum of stress.

In the case of Mariza's daughter, Lucita's unpredictable moods sometimes meant that family outings were planned to exclude her. Mariza chose to exclude Lucita on some outings with her other four children so that everyone could enjoy the event:

It's kind of hectic for me. And sometimes...when I don't want to go through that, I leave her with my mom....I don't know how she's gonna react [from day to day]...if she's gonna be comfortable or she's gonna be mad...or upset. I mean, it depends....It's more for [my other children that I leave her with my mom].

The orchestration process of balancing requires that the mother make key decisions about priorities in sequencing and synchronizing occupations. This required selecting dominant occupations among the competing needs of the family members that form the core pattern of daily rounds, arranging consonant enfolded occupations when possible to meet multiple needs simultaneously, and arranging compatible times and series of occupations among family members. Mothers considered their multiple responsibilities of managing the home to provide healthy meals, a clean environment, and acceptable clothing; of fostering their children's growth and development; of creating a harmonious family environment; of managing the family's financial resources; of adding varied, interesting, and enjoyable occupations to the family routine; and of meeting individual and group family member needs when balancing occupations.

Anticipating in Occupation

Often, the participants tailored many of their maternal and household occupations to be responsive to their child, anticipating what procedures were the least disruptive and most sensitive to their child. Marta described how she prepared in the morning by getting out the child's clothing, diaper, and braces, even before waking the child, "I start changing her slowly like this...and I move her feet, I am talking to her or I hold her for a while [before I put her braces on]." Mariza described a similar child-sensitive, child-contingent, highly organized morning routine:

> I change my routine because sometimes Lucita is still asleep, and I don't wake her up until I'm ready....I have everything in the car. So the last thing I want [to do] is change Lucita....I give her a *licuado,* her [breakfast] shake, and then everything is ready, so I just change her, and then comb her hair...put her in the car, and let's go.... And it's working because...it gives me more time to stay...a few minutes in [her] class [and talk to the teacher].

This process of *anticipating* child-sensitive methods for performing an occupation required advanced foresight of the requirements of the occupation that will occur immediately (temporally proximate) or later (temporally distant) in the day. Several participants described how they dress the child for the activities they will do that day:

> I write down on Miguel's calendar where they are going in the afterschool program. I have to [look and] see [what] Miguel's activities [are], the ones he does in the morning. Like if he has sports in the morning, I put on his sports clothes, or if in the afternoon he has a party or something [I dress him for that].

Foresight about the possible contingencies that need to be provided for in daily occupations was wide ranging. Participants anticipated their child's moods and cycles and orchestrated occupations around them. This included knowing the child's fussy time, nap time, play time, or meal time. These mothers provided toys, played music for the child, or "worked" with the child during specific routine times in the day, based on the child's mood and their own schedule.

Participants also anticipated the strategies and methods necessary for their child's safety, comfort, or participation. After Rachel had come home from school with scratches, both accidentally self-inflicted and caused by another child on the bus, Marta began to cross Rachel's arms across her chest and wrap them inside the blanket for travel on the bus to prevent further injuries. Both Marta and Mariza, conscious of past illness, were careful about dressing the children in coats, hats, and blankets when traveling to school. Mariana, to get Carlos to eat, put cards from a game he liked next to him at mealtime as a promise that if he ate well, they would play the game. Juliana, knowing from school personnel that her son tossed out his school breakfast and lunch untouched, insisted that he eat breakfast at home.

Interpreting in Occupation

Interpreting, the fifth of the occupational processes, is the mother's conception of her child's desires, needs, preferences, and wants drawn from the child's nonverbal and verbal cues, which are then used to design occupations. This process may be unique to this group of mothers because the majority of children were nonverbal. "[Lucita] doesn't tell me [how she's feeling]. I really don't know. I have to guess." The ability to understand their own children's needs was crucial to the mother's perception that she was meeting her child's needs. In desiring to be a good mother and to organize occupations that were beneficial to fostering the child's development, promoting the child's independence, and pleasing the child, participants needed to interpret the child's communications and reactions to caregiving and other events. Following are the descriptions of Mariza and Jesucita, respectively, interpreting their child's cues and the relation to occupational selection:

> [When she's in a good mood] she's clapping, she's laughing....But when she's in a bad mood...she starts biting herself. That's when I know she's not comfortable, and she just don't want to be in the chair anymore.

> I usually end up cleaning, picking up...clearing dishes and washing them. And at that same time, I'm on my own with Sara...and she is really fussy during that time. So I have to constantly be running to either put weights on her hands if she's drooling, or bring her, and sit her [wheelchair] next to me at all times, or [get] one of the kids to read to her.

Marta said, "When Rachel hears the noise [of the cellophane package of pork rinds], she starts chewing and...then she says 'uh, uh,' and I put one in her mouth and she eats it." Although these children's cues were often incredibly subtle from a stranger's point of view, these mothers were able

to decipher the child's emotions and wants based on a broad range of subtle nonverbal expressions, physical movements, or limited verbal skills. An exception was Andrew, who was autistic and was able to express his needs verbally.

The ability to interpret was very important to the participants. Difficulty in discerning the child's wants or hurts, especially when visible injuries were unaccounted for, led the participants to thoroughly investigate all incidents with whomever was in charge of the child's care at the time: "When he gets home with a little [injury] I always...call and ask them to please tell me what happened because he cannot." Another difficulty in this respect was assisting other persons to understand their child: "We try to get what he wants. But it is very hard and even harder to make other people understand him."

Forecasting in Occupation

Forecasting, as a process in orchestration, is temporally distinct and distant from anticipating, which occurs within the immediate present. Forecasting is located in the projected future. Based on current circumstances, mothers predicted possible futures for their children. Forecasting included the possible acquisition of self-care skills or learning to talk or walk. Although the children at the time often lacked many of the basic underlying skills to walk or eat independently, their mothers seemed to adhere to the philosophy that the journey toward independence began with a single step. A mother's desires and concerns for the family and the child's future were evident in forecasting.

Unlike children without disabilities whose changing bodies and maturing behavior push the parent along to a revised view of the child, Jesucita experienced her daughter, Sara, as being in a time warp:

> She has cousins that are a year older and a year younger....I see what they're doing. Kids do dif-

ferent things...depending on whatever the fad is. So I wonder what kind of fashion, what kind of clothes [Sara] would like, what kind of movie, TV programs, what would be happening to her. And I start to think, "What was [her sister] doing at that age?"...But I try to picture her, and I miss that....She's going to need new tennis shoes soon. And I'm thinking I'm going to see what other 10-year-olds...are wearing....She used to love clothes.

In this example, the participant made efforts to keep a temporal coherence for the child by dressing her in age-appropriate fashions that the child might enjoy. Forecasting was part of the temporal work the mother does in orchestrating the occupations of maternal work attending to both the present and the future.

Perspective Shifting and Meaning Making in Occupation

As overarching processes, these last two processes of orchestration are different in order from the previous six processes. Perspective shifting and meaning making were part of the participant's reflective interpretation of her behavior as she engaged in occupation and were central to her hopefulness and concern about her child's development. These processes often included the management of "crashes" or disruptions in the mother's plans for her child's care and progress, her persistence in maternal work, the shifting and often spiritual view of her child, and the increased appreciation for the preciousness of human life.

The management of frustrations and the ability to continue on with demands in the orchestration of occupations occurred through the process of perspective shifting and meaning making. After receiving the diagnosis of the child's condition or coming to a full realization of the impact of the child's disability (once the child was medically stable), most of the participants experienced a stage of immobility and inactivity. Once they decided to actively address their child's disability by re-

organizing the household around the child's special needs, finding professional services, and learning to manage the child's care, these mothers rebounded emotionally. This emotional shift was facilitated by changing their view of the difficulty and believing in God and assisted the mothers in moving beyond discouragement and limited engagement in occupations. *Perspective shifting* involved the revision of previous events and their meaning as related to ongoing occupational engagement and choice.

Meaning making, which seemed to frequently occur in tandem with perspective shifting, was the finding of alternative spiritual, meaningful, and optimistic explanations for life circumstances and occupational patterns. For typical families, it is only when subjective well-being is gauged as life meaning that parents have higher levels of subjective well-being than nonparents (Umberson & Gove, 1989). For mothers whose children have disabilities, making sense or meaning making may be even more essential to their subjective well-being.

These two processes were used to come to terms with the impact of the child's disability and accept the altered lifestyle the disability imposed on caregivers, to maintain hope in the face of pessimistic advice, to see the early marital struggle over the disability in a new light, and to love the child despite the disability. These emotional and mental processes had an impact on the participant's selection and engagement in occupation. Although not all "practicing" Catholics, the participants described God and faith as essential to going forward and "not being defeated" in their daily struggle. The reflections of Consuelo, Juliana, and Mariana, respectively, illustrate this:

Faith in God is what keeps us going trying to understand Miguel's reality in a nice way...to understand Miguel is a different path sent by God to know the world better.

I tell [God], "You have a reason for sending him to me." It is hard. It is hard because accepting is one process and living with [him] is another process.

I feel that I have learned to live with what I have, and besides to start forgetting all the bad things and think of the good things....Maybe that is why I feel better, because it is important to learn to solve your problems even if there are certain situations that demoralize you...at the same time.

For Juliana and her family, the occurrence of Sara's disability had a profound spiritual effect on the family, causing the father to take on an active lay ministerial role and the family to return to church and embed spirituality as a daily consideration in their lives: "When Sara almost died, we turned to God. And then I started to realize how far off the road we were. We started again to go to church, to pray."

Although bolstered by faith, daily struggles and roadblocks forced these mothers to let go of the belief that all things were under their control and to organize and plan those things that were:

Well, right now, like my husband says, "I am not going to look far ahead." I do not look that far ahead anymore [to what her son will be as an adolescent]....I say, "He is going to be a troublesome young man, very violent." I know he is going to be violent. But I also say, "If they give him more therapy, I believe he is going to get better."...He may become something. God permitting.

I avoid thinking about it...sometimes...I don't want to think of what's going to happen...whatever happens, happens....If I think I need to do something, I'll do it. But if I don't get what I'm working toward, then I'll just accept it, or [think that] I should have worked harder. There's no sense crying over spilled milk.

Maintaining hope, contrary to others' opinions and sometimes contrary to their own fears,

also required taking another viewpoint. In interactions with both professionals and their own families, participants were sometimes forced to see something better: "I felt bad for [my family] to tell me, 'Well, look at her [Rachel].' Instead of helping me, they discouraged me even more." Despite this discouragement, Marta described how she turned her energies toward finding positive solutions for her daughter's problems. Consuelo articulated the difference in perspective between her and the orthopedic surgeon about her son's dislocated hip:

It bothers me very much because the orthopedist and I could not understand one another. I believe it is because we talk at two different levels. I talk about my son, and he [talks] about his job, or the way he bills....I feel that we talk about two different things, and Miguel is in the middle.

Finding meaning, through faith or a shifted perspective, was also an important step in fostering and allowing these mothers to embrace the paradoxical joy and pain of parenting a child with a disability:

[My husband] would say..."It is not something out of this world....God gave [Andrew] to us like that, that is life....We have to struggle for him." And he is the one who has helped me.

[Carlos] made me understand the good things. I see life from another point of view....To value life and live it to the fullest....And to see the greatness of God....Not just to live life to the fullest, but valuing it more and wanting the best for him and my other son.

As limited as Miguel is...he has filled my life with happiness. He has given me a very different perspective about my life, of living, of love, of patience...the beautiful things I have learned from him.

Consuelo even engaged in myth making surrounding Miguel's disability. For example, she suggested that he does not talk because she dreamed of coaxing him to say sweet things to her about what a wonderful mother she was and, instead of lying, he won't speak. Or that he does not walk here on earth because he walks above the earth being closer to God. Mariza also saw her daughter as a more pure spiritual being who was closer to God.

These last two processes, perspective shifting and meaning making, seemed to have a global influence over daily occupations and the mother's subjective well-being and had a guiding influence over the orchestration of an individual occupation. These findings reflect what other research has suggested about the powerfulness of life meaning in maternal work in relation to maternal subjective well-being (Umberson & Gove, 1989; Zika & Chamberlain, 1992) and occupation.

An Illustration of Orchestration in an Occupation

The inception of occupation differed among and between participants because of individual preferences and values. As illustrated in Table 42.3, the chunk of occupation called "feeding a child dinner" varied among participants in form and components partly because the participants orchestrated the occupation specifically to meet their child's special needs, to be in harmony with their values, to fit within that day's routine, and to fit the family's context.

The differences in each participant's dinner routines is compared in Table 42.3 across all the processes of orchestration of occupation (except for perspective shifting and meaning making, which were more global in their influence on this occupation). This analysis shows commonalities and differences in "feeding the child dinner." Common among all the dining routines was the participation of the mother–child pair, the consumption of food, and emphasis on the healthiness of the diet. Differences appeared in the orchestration processes of planning, organizing, balancing, anticipating, forecasting, and interpreting and were uniquely configured for each family. Differences also appeared in the sequence, strategies, space, number of additional participants, and timing of the dinner routine.

The child's disability also had a decisive influence on the structure of the occupation of "feeding the child dinner" and demonstrated the participant's responsiveness to the child's needs. Low child insistence and high child contentment allowed the participant greater flexibility in the processes of planning, organizing, and balancing. For example, both Lucita's and Rachel's dinner times were highly deferrable, whereas during Carlos's dinner, he was the center of attention, and parents traded off in his supervision so that his mother could clean up after dinner. Anticipating and interpreting were more vital for the mother when the child was nonverbal and had limited communication. Among the children who were nonverbal, participants had developed sophisticated interpretations of their children's gestures, facial expressions, and sounds. Their forecasts were often related to the child's comfort, health, and the mothers' future ability to give care. In these examples, the process of forecasting linked the present and future and embedded the mothers' goals and plans in the daily routines.

Discussion

This research depicts how mothers' orchestration of occupation is related to an occupational motif and includes "ideation, composition, execution, ordering, and qualitative aspects of occupation" (University of Southern California, Occupational Therapy Department, 1989) within a single occupation and throughout a day's round of occupations. Guided by the embrace of paradox, these mothers used eight processes to orchestrate their

Table 42.3. Orchestration in "Feeding the Child Dinner"

Process	Consuelo–Miguel	Juliana–Andrew	Mariana–Carlos	Jesucita–Sara	Mariza–Lucita	Marta–Rachel
Planning	Fed Miguel a diet similar to family's diet. Food was prepared in bite-size pieces.	Food types were planned around Andrew's very limited food preferences (fried chicken or meat).	Food types were selected for Carlos to prevent anemia and maintain a healthy weight.	Fed Sara a diet similar to rest of family. Frequently used nutritional supplements when Sara did not eat meals.	Fed Lucita the same diet as rest of the family with special preparation due to Lucita's lack of chewing.	Fed Rachel a diet similar to rest of family. Food prepared in bite-size pieces.
Organizing	Included additional time in schedule for Miguel's slower eating. Alternately fed Miguel and then ate her own meal. After meal, gave Miguel milk in a cup with a straw.	Children's dinner was ready immediately after school when they were hungry.	Food was ready as soon as children arrived home from school. Had alternate strategies if Carlos would not eat meal. Allowed extra time for feeding Carlos.	Sara ate with the rest of the family. Mother began by feeding Sara and then eating some of her own meal. If Sara didn't eat, Jesucita gave her a liquid food supplement.	Feeding Lucita was deferrable depending on pressing demands, usually after family meal. Combined feeding with other activities such as TV watching. Lucita's meal followed by drinking a bottle lying in bed.	Rachel's feeding was contingent and deferrable; she was fed if hungry when she came home from school or after a short nap.
Balancing	Family began meal together, but Miguel and Consuelo remained until he had finished.	Children fed first. Andrew and his brother continued to "pick" during second mealtime for husband, where couple spend time discussing the day.	Served younger brother first and then spent longer with Carlos, assisting him in eating while she also ate. During second mealtime with husband, Carlos sat with his father and finished a drink.	Once family meal was prepared and served to other family members, focus turned to Sara. Continued feeding Sara for an extended time after rest of family had left the table.	Had family meal with four typical children, Lucita was fed earlier or later, or occasionally with family.	Rachel's mealtime shifted around her own hunger and around family mealtime.
Anticipating	Knew that Miguel will eat what is given, didn't feed him sweets because he didn't like them.	Threatened Andrew with loss of video games or other desired activity if he wouldn't eat.	Devised strategies for Carlos to encourage eating (playing games while eating or immediately after).	Expected that Sara's "gassiness" may slow down feeding.	Knew Lucita's typical routine, when she would be awake and hungry.	Watched Rachel's mood to decide when child was hungry.
Interpreting	Watched Miguel's animated facial expressions to determine reaction to the meal. Asked questions and assumed answers without obvious facial expressions to the contrary.	Andrew was able to express his needs and desires.	Noted that Carlos failed to eat when he was not hungry. Queried child about what food he would like and if he wanted more.	Recognized food as one of Sara's few pleasures. Observed child's drooling and sounds to determine her like or dislike of food.	Watched Lucita's subtle facial expressions and the speed she took food to determine if she was hungry and will eat or whether it will need to be deferred to a later time.	Rachel made "uh uh" sounds or cried, which the mother interpreted as wants, satisfaction, or complaint, depending on the qualities.
Forecasting	Reduced sugar in Miguel's foods by substituting honey to prevent cavities.	Gave Andrew daily vitamins to prevent deficiencies due to poor diet. Concerned about who will make Andrew eat when he grows up.	Concerned about Carlos's weight and amount of food intake. Concerned about anemia.	Concerned about Sara getting too heavy for lifting and caretaking.	Concerned that Lucita was heavy to lift had hopes that she will walk.	No particular concerns were expressed about Rachel's future weight.

daily rounds. These processes provide both an elaboration of the definition of orchestration and demonstration of the variations in the temporal levels at which orchestration occurs. Through the orchestration processes, the temporal horizons of life merge within a single day's occupations. Mothers make sense of their past, design their present, and plan for their future within their daily occupational rounds for themselves and family members.

The temporal horizon is apparent in the orchestration within an occupation, the orchestration of a series of occupations, and the inclusion of occupations within daily rounds aimed at creating future possibilities. Within an occupation, participants were attentive to the manner and methods with which they interacted with their children to produce child-sensitive, child-contingent occupations commensurate with their values of being a good mother. At the molar level of occupation, the participants' selection, sequencing, enfolding, and synchronization of occupations included considering competing demands, including the needs of the child with a disability, the other family members' individual needs, and the needs of managing the entire household at the same time. In some cases, the child with a disability was the predominant consideration in rounds of occupations during some time in their development, depending on the child's demandingness or contentedness. In other circumstances, other family members' needs emerged as the predominant influence on the participants' selection and sequencing of occupations. Long-range considerations also swayed the orchestration of occupation to plan for projected future possibilities and goals for all family members.

As suggested in the initial musical metaphor, orchestration holds great promise for elucidating the complex patterns of occupation in which human beings engage. This study considered how occupations may be arranged in compatible or dissonant ways and how the organization of linking or overlapping occupations affects well-being. In addition, further research may examine how patterns of occupation, such as habitual occupations, counterbalance and support the melodies (priority or dominant occupations) of our lives. Likewise, the musical terms that describe the phrasing of music could be helpful in exploring orchestration. How do persons select coordinated sequences of occupations (phrases) and shifts in occupation (ends of phrases) to create daily routines (formal structure) that include rest and inactivity (places for the performer to breathe)? Lastly, what determines the time signature and tempo of a person's lifestyle—is it leisurely, businesslike, or rushed?

This chapter is a beginning attempt to clarify the intricate configurations of occupations with which persons compose their lives on a daily basis. Future research may ferret out common orchestration processes that are used by the general population or by specific individuals with disabilities, may differentiate between the preconceived orchestration and the daily improvisation or recomposition that occurs in occupational rounds, may uncover the ways orchestration processes are culturally transmitted, may examine the relationship of life span development and orchestration of occupations, may investigate the relationship of characteristics of orchestration and the person's occupational experience, or may explore the influence of occupational rounds configurations to health and well-being. Understanding these intricacies of orchestration of occupations can bolster occupational therapy's knowledge to enhance wellness and to provide therapeutic applications for orchestration and recomposition of occupations after disability.

Acknowledgments

I thank Florence Clark, PhD, OTR, FAOTA, for her encouragement in this research and acknowledge her instrumentality in bringing the concept of orchestration to the forefront in occupational science. This study was completed in partial fulfillment of the requirements for the doctor of philosophy degree in occupational science at the University of Southern California.

References

Affleck, G., & Tennen, H. (1991). Appraisal and coping predictors of mother and child outcomes after newborn intensive care. *Journal of Social and Clinical Psychology, 10,* 424–447.

Bailey, D., & Simeonsson, R. (1988). Assessing needs of families with handicapped infants. *Journal of Special Education, 22,* 117–127.

Beckman, P. (1991). Comparison of mothers' and fathers' perceptions of the effects of young children with and without disabilities. *American Journal on Mental Retardation, 95,* 585–595.

Breslau, N., Strauch, K., & Mortimer, E. (1982). Psychological distress in mothers of disabled children. *American Journal of Diseases of Children, 136,* 682–686.

Bristol, M., Gallagher, J., & Schopler, E. (1988). Mothers and fathers of young developmentally disabled and nondisabled boys: Adaptation and spousal support. *Developmental Psychology, 24,* 441–451.

Bruenjes, S. J. (1994). Orchestrating health: Middle-aged women's process of living health. *Holistic Nursing Practice, 8,* 2–22.

Chamberlain, K., & Zika, S. (1990). The minor events approach to stress: Support for the use of daily hassles. *British Journal of Psychology, 81,* 469–481.

Chamberlain, K., & Zika, S. (1992). Stability and change in subjective well-being over short periods of time. *Social Indicators Research, 26,* 101–117.

Clark, F. (1993). Occupation embedded in a real life: Interweaving occupational science and occupational therapy [1993 Eleanor Clarke Slagle Lecture]. *American Journal of Occupational Therapy, 47,* 1067–1078.

Craigie, F. C. (1985). Therapeutic homework: The use of behavioral assignments in office counseling. *Journal of Family Practice, 20,* 65–71.

Crnic, K., Friedrich, W., & Greenberg, M. (1983). Adaptation of families with mentally retarded children: A model of stress, coping and family

ecology. *American Journal of Mental Deficiency, 88,* 125–138.

Denzin, N. (1989). *Interpretive interactionism.* Newbury Park, CA: Sage.

Dunst, C., & Trivette, C. (1986). Looking beyond the parent–child dyad for the determinants of maternal styles of interaction. *Infant Mental Health Journal, 7,* 69–80.

Eldridge, W. D. (1983). Therapist's use of information and dynamics from extramarital relationships to stimulate growth in married couples. *Family Therapy, 10,* 1–11.

Friedrich, W., Wilturner, L., & Cohen, D. (1985). Coping resources and parenting mentally retarded children. *American Journal of Mental Retardation, 90,* 130–139.

Goldberg, S., Morris, P., Simmons, R., Fowler, R., & Levinson, H. (1990). Chronic illness in infancy and parenting stress: A comparison of three groups of parents. *Journal of Pediatric Psychology, 15,* 347–358.

Hamilton-Dodd, C., Kawamoto, T., Clark, F., Burke, J. P., & Fanchiang, S.-P. (1989). The effects of a maternal preparation program on mother–infant pairs: A pilot study. *American Journal of Occupational Therapy, 43,* 513–521.

Harris, V., & McHale, S. (1989). Family life problems, daily caregiving activities, and the psychological well-being of mothers of mentally retarded children. *American Journal on Mental Retardation, 94,* 231–239.

Harry, B. (1992). Criminal's explanations of their criminal behavior, Part 1: The contributions of criminologic variables. *Journal of Forensic Sciences, 37,* 1327–1333.

Juster, T., Hill, M., Stafford, F., & Parsons, J. (1988). *Longitudinal time panel study 1975–81.* Ann Arbor, MI: Inter-University Consortium for Political and Social Research.

Kanner, A., Coyne, J., Schaefer, C., & Lazarus, R. (1981). Comparison of two modes of stress measurement: Daily hassles and uplifts versus major life events. *Journal of Behavioral Medicine, 4,* 1–39.

Kazak, A., & Marvin, R. (1984). Differences, difficulties and adaptation: Stress and social networks in families with a handicapped child. *Family Relations, 33,* 67–77.

Larson, E. A. (1998). Reframing the meaning of disability to families: The embrace of paradox. *Social Science and Medicine, 47,* 865–875.

Leviton, S. C., & Greenstone, J. L. (1984). Team intervention. *Emotional First Aid, 1,* 57–63.

Leyser, Y., & Dekel, G. (1991). Perceived stress and adjustment in religious Jewish families with a child who is disabled. *Journal of Psychology, 125,* 427–438.

Margalit, M., & Raviv, A. (1983). Mother's perceptions of family climate in families with a retarded child. *Exceptional Child, 30,* 163–169.

Miles, B., & Huberman, A. (1984). *Qualitative data analysis: A sourcebook of new methods.* Beverly Hills, CA: Sage.

Patterson, J., & McCubbin, H. (1983). Chronic illness: Family stress and coping. In C. Figley & H. McCubbin (Eds.), *Stress and the family, Vol. II: Coping with catastrophe* (pp. 21–36). New York: Brunner/Mazel.

Patton, M. Q. (1989). *Qualitative evaluation methods* (10th ed.). Beverly Hills, CA: Sage.

Piston, W. (1962). *Harmony* (3rd ed.). New York: Norton.

Primeau, L. (1996). *Orchestration of work and play within families.* Ann Arbor, MI: UMI Company.

Primeau, L., Clark, C., & Pierce, D. (1990). Occupational therapy alone has looked upon occupation: Future applications of occupational science to pediatric occupational therapy. *Occupational Therapy in Health Care, 6,* 19–31.

Reich, J., & Zautra, A. (1983). Demands and desires in daily life: Some influences on well-being. *American Journal of Community Psychology, 11,* 41–58.

Segal, R. (1996). *Family adaptation to a child with attention-deficit disorder.* Ann Arbor, MI: UMI Company.

Segal, R. (2000). Adaptive strategies of mothers with children with attention deficit hyperactivity disorder: Enfolding and unfolding occupations. *American Journal of Occupational Therapy, 54,* 300–306.

Shandlen, M. N., & Newsome, W. T. (1996). Motion perception: Seeing and deciding. *Proceedings of the National Academy of Sciences, 93,* 628–633.

Shapiro, J. (1989). Stress, depression and support group participation in mothers of developmentally delayed children. *Family Relations, 38,* 169–173.

Shapiro, J., & Tittle, K. (1990). Maternal adaptation to child disability in a Hispanic population. *Family Relations, 39,* 179–185.

Singer, L., & Farkas, K. (1989). The impact of infant disability on maternal perception of stress. *Family Relations, 38,* 444–449.

Sloper, P., & Turner, S. (1993). Risk and resistance factors in the adaptation of parents of children with severe physical disability. *Journal of Child Psychology and Psychiatry, 34,* 167–188.

Tharp, R., & Gallimore, R. (1988). *Rousing minds to life.* Cambridge, UK: Cambridge University Press.

Umberson, D., & Gove, W. (1989). Parenthood and psychological well-being. *Journal of Family Issues, 10,* 440–481.

University of Southern California, Department of Occupational Therapy. (1989). *Proposal for a doctoral dissertation in occupational science.* Unpublished manuscript.

Vega, W. (1990). Hispanic families in the 1990s: A decade of research. *Journal of Marriage and the Family, 52,* 1015–1024.

Wallander, J., Pitt, L., & Mellins, C. (1990). Child functional independence and maternal psychosocial stress as risk factors threatening adaptation in mothers of physically or sensorially handicapped children. *Journal of Consulting and Clinical Psychology, 58,* 818–824.

Webster's new collegiate dictionary. (1977). Springfield, MA: Merriam-Webster.

Zelman, W. N., McLaughlin, C. P., Geld, N., & Miller, E. (1985). Survival strategies for community mental health organizations: A conceptual framework. *Community Mental Health Journal, 21,* 228–236.

Zika, S., & Chamberlain, K. (1992). On the relations between meaning in life and psychological well-being. *British Journal of Psychology, 83,* 133–145.

CHAPTER 43

Mothering Young Children With Disabilities in a Challenging Urban Environment

Judith Olson and Susan Esdaile

Judith Olson, PhD, OTR, *is assistant professor, Occupational Therapy Program, Eastern Michigan University, Ypsilanti, MI 48197; judy.olson@emich.edu.*

Susan Esdaile, PhD, OTR, SROT, *is professor and chair, Department of Occupational Therapy, Wayne State University, Detroit.*

Mothering is a pivotal occupation for many women. In occupational therapy practice with children with cerebral palsy and other developmental disabilities, the occupations of mothering may be unseen as they form a silent backdrop against which therapeutic efforts on behalf of a particular child are provided. What about these mothering occupations, and what do mothers have to say about them? In this qualitative study, we examine mothering occupations as two mothers living in a challenging urban environment have experienced them in relation to their children with disabilities.

Literature Review

Numerous studies published in the occupational therapy and occupational science literature have described mothering occupations in support of therapy and the goals of therapy or as adjuncts to therapy (Barrera & Vella, 1987; Case-Smith & Nastro, 1993; Dunlea, 1996; Hinojosa, 1990; Hinojosa & Anderson, 1991). A smaller number of studies have focused more specifically on mothering itself, and it is these studies that are of particular relevance to our research.

Burke, Clark, Hamilton-Dodd, and Kawamoto (1987) developed the Maternal Role Preparation program to help first-time mothers prepare for the birth of their child. This occupational therapy program directly addressed the maternal skills and habit patterns of women who would be doing the occupations of mothering for the first time. A subsequent article (Hamilton-Dodd, Kawamoto, Clark, Burke, & Fanchiang, 1989), reported the results of this pilot study. The authors did not find the maternal preparation program to be associated with greater observed maternal competence. Dyck (1992) studied the normal occupational behavior of 25 women from a mixed-income suburb of the greater Victoria area in British Columbia, Canada, exploring the nature of mothering occupations as they result from a complex dynamic between the per-

Originally published 2000 in *American Journal of Occupational Therapy, 54*, 307–314.

son and the environment. Dyck found that the occupations of mothering were derived from daily routines that intermeshed home provisioning, practical child care, paid employment, transporting children, and providing children with recreational and extracurricular activities. Hermann's (1990) study of adolescent mothers emphasized the facet of mothering that relates to the developmental level of the person who is mothering and its potential to affect such activities as physical caregiving. She found that the participants engaged in a greater percentage of adolescent activities than mothering activities, although they were mothering young children. Hermann's study supports the developmental nature of occupational performance in general.

Using a feminist approach to the analysis of one mother's construction of her definition of mothering, Pierce and Frank (1992) described the mothering of an infant with multiple disabilities from care in the neonatal intensive care unit through care at home. This story highlighted the need for occupational therapy practitioners to understand a woman's conceptualization of her mothering occupations because this shapes the type of involvement she will have with her child. In a mother–child life history that demonstrated the effect of the dynamic process of adaptation on the life of one mother of a child with serious disabilities, Larson (1996) illustrated the power of maternal values to direct the occupations of the woman's life as she aimed for the maximal development of her child. In a study of time use by mothers of children who were typically developing and mothers of children with either multiple disabilities or Down syndrome, Crowe (1993) outlined eight descriptive categories of the activities comprising the daily lives of mothers: homemaking, child care, recreation, personal care, participation and socialization, employment, education, and rest and sleep. If we use the Yerxa, Clark, Jackson, Pierce, and Zemke (1990) defin-

ition of *occupations* as chunks of meaningful activity that can be named in the lexicon of the culture, these activities can be viewed as comprising mothers' daily occupations.

More recently, Crowe, VanLeit, Berghmans, and Mann (1997) explored the caregiving occupations of mothers of young children as they investigated mothers' perceived occupational roles. They reported that mothers of children with Down syndrome had fewer roles than mothers of children who were typically developing. This finding supports the commonly held view that the occupations of mothering children with disabilities are even more time-consuming and energy-intensive than caring for children who do not. This issue was raised by Esdaile (1994) in a discussion of the mothering occupations of women caring for children with disabilities. Esdaile also highlighted the lack of space and time for mothers' social participation and interest development.

The studies cited have contributed to a growing body of knowledge on the occupations of mothering per se. Our own interest was in exploring, in particular, the occupations of mothers of children with severe disabilities while living in a challenging urban environment. Such knowledge can assist occupational therapy practitioners to be better informed about the occupations of mothers of children with severe disabilities and enhance their therapeutic intervention.

Method

We chose the qualitative method of phenomenology (Barritt, Bleeker, Beekman, & Mulderij, 1985) to study the occupations of mothering because it allows an examination of the complex everyday world of individual experience and how the person constructs meaning from that experience. In phenomenological studies, data are always processed through the subjectivity of the researcher (Dickie, 1997). The researchers' assumptions or "preunderstandings" for this study were as follows:

1. Mothering is an occupation in relation, that is, an occupation that requires a minimum of two persons engaged in joint activities or tasks—the mothering person and one being mothered.
2. The occupations of mothering would be prominent in mothers' descriptions of their lives with young children.
3. Our personal views of research frame our research method.

Our first assumption proceeds from the first author's background as an infant mental health specialist (Olson & Baltman, 1994) and the second author's mother–child interaction research (Esdaile & Greenwood, 1995a, 1995b) that support our strong belief in the importance of relationship. Because mothering occurs within the space between the mothering person and the one being mothered, we chose a definition of mothering that incorporates the work of Glenn (1994) and Barnard and Martell (1995). *Mothering* is defined as a variable relationship constructed within different historical and cultural contexts in which one person, usually an adult female, nurtures and cares for another.

The second assumption is derived from our personal histories as White, middle-class, professional women of middle-European background brought up in heterosexual, Roman Catholic families (Ruddick, 1983). We have studied developmental psychology, taught child development, and practiced as occupational therapy practitioners in the community within a social–educational model focusing on mother–child interactions and co-occupations (Dunlea, 1996). We are mothers ourselves.

Regarding our third assumption, we believe that the phenomenological research method sup-

ports a listening to the experiences of women in their occupational engagement, as opposed to observing or measuring it further. We believe that we can gain an understanding of their lives through this listening and that this understanding will ultimately contribute to better service delivery for our clients.

Participants

This pilot study involved two mothers of young children who had received infant mental health services (Olson & Baltman, 1994) through a home-visiting program. These two mothers volunteered to be interviewed about their daily lives with their infants. They were also interviewed about the infant mental health services that they were provided, which were designed to strengthen the social, emotional, cognitive, and physical well-being of infants within the context of secure, stable, caregiving relationships.

Pseudonyms have been provided for both participants and their children. One mother, Sandra, was a 26-year-old single, Black woman with a 2-year-old daughter, Debbie. Her daughter had been a healthy, developing child until she was diagnosed early in her first year with shaken baby syndrome. Subsequently she was described as having cerebral palsy, blindness, and severe cognitive and language delays.

The second mother, 27-year-old Merion, was also single and Black. Her 4-month-old son, Scott, born with a seizure disorder of unknown origin, was severely and multiply handicapped. He died at 1 year of age. Home visits began shortly after his birth and continued with Merion for 3 months after his death.

Data Collection and Analysis

The first author interviewed each mother twice between 1 and 2 years after the completion of the home visits. The home visits were done by an infant mental health specialist. The interviews were semistructured (see Appendix) and lasted about 1 to 1.5 hr. Open-ended questions encouraged the mothers to describe their daily life with their children and what it was like to experience therapeutic home visits. Interviews were audiotaped and resulted in 58 pages of transcription. The mothers were invited to read the transcriptions and discuss them with the interviewer. One mother elected to do so, and her additional comments were incorporated into the interview data. Thematic analysis of the interview data and the determination of essential themes were done using the selective highlighting approach in which statements or phrases that seemed essential to the experience being described were identified (Van Manen, 1990). Both authors separately and independently determined essential themes, but through negotiation and repeated readings, joint agreement was reached regarding the overarching and supporting themes.

Results

Essential Themes

During the home visits, the mothers reported that most of their discussions centered on the occupations of mothering. From the mothers' stories, we identified one overarching theme—doing "what I got to do." Supporting this overarching theme are the subthemes of (a) mothering as caring, with the separate components of mothering as nurturing and mothering as advocacy, and (b) the impact of support systems (or lack thereof) on the occupations of mothering.

Overarching Theme: Doing "What I Got To Do"

Merion believed that Scott had defined mothering for her: "Before Scott was born, I had two other children. I was a very wild person. Hung out, partied, and everything like that." After Scott

was born, "It's like, you know, take care of family, just go to work, come home, take care of the family, and then go back to work." Mothering meant paying total attention to the needs of a dependent other. Her mothering was only in relation to Scott and his needs. Merion described herself after Scott died:

> Very insecure. When Scott was there, I didn't need nobody....When Scott was living, I did mostly everything myself. Whatever I had to do. But when Scott died, it look like, I just, I didn't know how to do nuthin' no more; I just didn't know.

As she adjusted to Scott's death, Merion extended her notion of mothering on the basis of her experience with Scott to her two older children, although the exact activities within the occupations of mothering were changed. But Merion does not expect that kind of mothering behavior from all mothers: "Like I say, every mother is not going to be like me. Every mother is not going to take on the responsibility....It's not that they are a bad person, they just don't handle it."

Sandra repeatedly acknowledged that mothering is "what I got to do," such as diapering, bathing, and feeding. But she spoke equally often of shared family activities—going out to dinner, sending her daughter to camp, spending a day at the amusement park. For her, mothering was what she had to do daily but doing it in a way that was as normal as possible for herself, for her child, and eventually for her husband. She saw the occupations of mothering as normalizing the experience of caring for a child with severe disabilities.

Mothering as Caring: Nurturing and Advocacy

The mothers described performing different activities in the name of caring. These included routine physical care activities, such as those that Sandra described. Because Debbie had to be fed through a gastrostomy tube, Sandra acquired skills used by professionals, including the ability to handle and care for the feeding pump. Debbie's survival depended on the maternal occupation of feeding.

Feeding was the single most important occupation of Sandra's day, yet she described the tasks of feeding as not at all out of the ordinary, saying that this is "what I must do." This comment was made without regret or hint of burden. These feeding tasks were part of the occupations that were deeply embedded in her daily round of meaningful activities.

Merion also kept to additional daily routines related to her son's survival, such as giving seizure medicine at carefully prescribed times:

> I knew that Scott had to have that first med at 6:00 in the morning, and I knew that if he didn't have that med by 12, he would be having a seizure....So, I had to get up; I had to do what I had to do. If I had to be up till 2:00 in the morning...till 4:00, 5:00 in the morning, that's what I had to do.

Other life-preserving routines had to be followed: "If I had to suction him every hour on the hour, that's what I had to do....I know that if I didn't do it, Scott would not survive." There was no anger or burden in Merion's words. Nor did either of these mothers understand these routines to be motivated by guilt. Rather, Sandra and Merion described these occupations of mothering in a matter-of-fact manner.

Besides nurturing, caring took another form for both mothers. Both found and organized agency services to meet their children's educational needs, acting both as advocates for their children and case managers (Bazyk, 1989; Kolobe, 1991). Sandra described the tasks that were involved. These included telephoning agencies that might have appropriate services for Debbie; writing for information about possible services; and attending meetings, even university-related training sessions, to help her child. For Merion, the case management activities included mobilizing early intervention services for Scott's returns from multiple hospitalizations. Both mothers were proud of their competence in completing these tasks without the assistance of outsiders, such as professional case managers. Both mothers identified these activities of case management and advocacy as components of caring.

These mothers were responsible for scheduling appointments, maintaining medication schedules, and planning a round of activities that included the transportation and personal safety of their children. Providing these linkage services (Broday & Schoonover, 1986) is not unique to mothers of children with disabilities. Mothers of children who are typically developing also describe expending their time and energy on carpooling; arranging play dates; and, often, taking total responsibility for scheduling the child's daily activities.

For mothers of children with disabilities, advocacy tasks are part of mothering (Bazyk, 1989; Traustadottir, 1991). All mothers need to advocate, but this becomes much more difficult in a challenging environment. Sandra must speak out for Debbie's needs to become visible and taken care of by society. Sandra must attend meetings, although she finds it hard to make her needs understood by far-distant politicians. She must read literature, although she does not feel capable of reading and comprehending long text. Sandra ascribed her willingness to participate in this study as a way to become seen and heard. She told us her story with the expectation that we would make sure that others heard and understood what her everyday life has been like. The knowledge that her story might help another mother or a professional working with mothers provided some support for her to continue mothering.

For both Sandra and Merion, caring expanded to include obtaining, maintaining, and using a variety of rehabilitation equipment, such as wheelchairs, braces, prone standers, and bathtub chairs. In conjunction with their occupational therapists and physical therapists, these mothers became knowledgeable equipment consumers. Consumer occupations included collaboration with a professional on possible equipment choices, financial planning to be able to purchase equipment when necessary, and environmental adaptation and negotiation. The simplest physical activity—getting out of the house to reach transportation to a scheduled appointment—required preplanning for Sandra to negotiate a growing child in braces and a wheelchair down a flight of stairs; there was no elevator in her building.

Merion, without readily available transportation, relied on her problem-solving abilities to assure transportation for the many occasions that Scott required unscheduled trips to the hospital. She described one incident in which Scott suddenly stopped breathing and she had no telephone to call for help. She reported that she heard shooting in the street outside her home, which she knew from experience would be followed by police sirens and the imminent arrival of police vehicles. She went into the street and stopped a police car and begged for transportation to the hospital. This anecdote illustrates Merion's motivation to ensure the survival of her child and the problem-solving skills that are essential when mothering a child with serious medical problems. It also illustrates the impact of context on mothering solutions.

Merion reported another incident in which Scott missed a scheduled ophthalmology outpatient appointment because of an emergency hospitalization. Understanding the medical system in which she and her son were located, she knew that rescheduling the missed appointment might mean months on the clinic waiting list. Serendipitously, she met the ophthalmologist in a hospital elevator and convinced him that Scott needed to see him that day, as scheduled, right there in the hospital. Caring solutions that meet a child's special needs often must be made without benefit of preparation.

Mothering as caring extends beyond the life of the one child being mothered into that of the broader community. For both mothers, caring activities extended into this realm. Sandra became the president of the Parent–Teacher Association at her daughter's school, and as such, she attends community-wide meetings that have state and federal government implications not just for her daughter but for other children in the community who have disabilities. She mentors other mothers as they enter the school world with concerns, similar to her own, for the immediate care and future of their children. After Scott's death, Merion became a parent advocate with two community agencies. She credited Scott as the source of her strength, and she understood her current positions as directly connected to her caring for Scott.

Impact of Support Systems on the Occupations of Mothering

The context of mothering for both of these women was deficient in support systems for the occupations of mothering. Both mothers had other family—sisters, brothers, and a mother in Merion's case—but they were not supportive to them in their mothering. Sandra's new spouse, Ralph, although not Debbie's biological father, has been willing to help in the everyday tasks of caregiving, but only since he was laid off from his job. Sandra could not count on her extended family members for support of any kind, even though her brother lived in the same house. In fact, her relatives were afraid of Debbie, and this fear prevented them from being a source of support.

Sandra facetiously commented, "What are they afraid of? Catching something?"

Sandra repeatedly referred to her maternal obligation to find appropriate godmothers for Debbie, an important task that she was finding hard to complete. The first woman Sandra had selected for a godmother changed her mind when Debbie's course of normal development was permanently altered. Her next two choices were unacceptable; one was "strung out on crack," and another had just had a stroke.

The notion of godmother was familiar to the interviewer but her understanding of it was different from Sandra's. In Sandra's culture, the tradition of *othermothering* exists. The othermother concept describes an esteemed relationship between an older woman and a younger girl. Collins (1990) has written that African and African-American communities have acknowledged the problems related to investing one person, the mother, with total responsibility for mothering. Consequently, othermothers "assist blood mothers by sharing mothering responsibilities" (Collins, 1990, p. 119). Behar (1993) described a similar relationship in certain Hispanic cultures called *comadre*. It is our speculation that Sandra's concern about a godmother for Debbie was connected to this tradition of othermothering. Given the lack of social and financial support in Sandra's life, the need for an othermother is particularly relevant.

Discussion

Context

It is a tenet of occupational therapy that context influences a person's occupations (Dunn, Brown, & McGuigan, 1994; Kielhofner, 1995; Nelson, 1988). Both levels of context—the *microsystem* level, which includes the physical location and the interpersonal relationships therein, and the *macrosystem* level, which includes those general-

ized "patterns of ideology and organization of the social institutions common to a particular culture or subculture" (Bronfenbrenner, 1979, p. 8)—affect mothering occupations. The caregiving activities that comprise the occupations of mothering are not often seen because the context in which they are performed is the home, considered a private domain. It becomes easy for society not to consider these caregiving occupations as valuable because they are not easily translatable into the language of the macrosystem that deals with such concepts as paid work. If the microsystem caregiving activities could be seen, however, this invisibility and consequent lack of valuation of caregiving occupations might change. This sentiment was echoed by Sandra, who wanted the mental health therapists to come to her home at "any time. Sometimes she [the infant mental health worker] would call and say, 'Is this a bad time?' And I would answer, 'This was the time.'" Sandra wanted the therapist to see her struggles with hair combing, for example, as well as share her child's laughter during bathing. She wanted to be seen in her everyday caregiving occupations and be acknowledged by society for what she was doing.

In this study, mothering occupations were also affected by macrosystem factors, which for these mothers included poverty, violence, and abuse. Both were living in an inner city in the poorest neighborhoods where there was a proliferation of intervention agencies but little money and other resources. Merion reported,

> I really didn't have the money to stay at the hospital, and there would be days and days that I would stay. There would be days when I would go without eating....I really didn't have the money, but had to stay. I had to borrow money.

Eventually, Sandra married Ralph, who supported their family while she continued her maternal occupations. However, when Ralph was laid off, they were forced to reorganize their lives. Ralph took on certain occupations of mothering while Sandra worked outside the home. For this family, economics influenced the distribution of maternal occupations between the parenting partners.

When Merion was growing up, violence was not just outside her door but inside her own home. Her mother had been in an abusive relationship when Merion was young. In fleeing this abusive situation, Merion's mother had abandoned her children. Merion, who admits to resentment toward her mother for this abandonment, now feels that she understands the circumstance that forced her mother to such extreme behavior.

At the time of this study, several years after the diagnosis of shaken baby syndrome was made, Sandra was able, without guilt or self-recrimination, to discuss the fact that her daughter had been a victim of violence at her then-boyfriend's hands. However, she had sought mental health intervention when, in her daughter's third year, she found herself frequently crying, feeling bad, and hoping that Debbie would somehow become normal again. She worried that these feelings would interfere with her "doing for Debbie." Sandra felt guilty for having left her child with her boyfriend only to return home and learn that the child was in the hospital in very serious condition. She needed help to grieve for her child's lost normalcy while simultaneously caring for Debbie, who was severely handicapped.

Mothering and the Practice of Occupational Therapy

We believe that the occupations of mothering deserve the attention of occupational therapy practitioners. These occupations contribute to maternal health that is essential to child development. Although this was a pilot study and included only two participants, we heard in the mothers' stories the potential for connecting the occupations of mothering children with severe physical disabilities to the practice of occupational therapy in these areas: co-created mothering occupations centered on a child's demand for preservation; the influence of the macrosystem (environment) on the occupation of mothering (Bronfenbrenner, 1979); and practice dilemmas (Lawlor & Mattingly, 1998) created, in part, by the macrosystem.

In identifying mothering as "doing what I got to do" in relation to their particular child, participants' occupations of mothering were co-created with another (their child) as a specific network of activities comprising the mother's everyday life. Ruddick (1983) has written that a child has three demands: preservation, growth, and acceptability. Our two participants told us that when mothering a child with severe disabilities, preservation determines mothering occupations. The fabric of a mother's life, that is, the round of activities that comprise her day, are determined by a particular relationship with an individual child. However, mothering occupations are not formed exclusively by the complex interactions that comprise our personal histories. There is the additional influence of environmental forces, such as the isolation described by Rossiter (1986) and echoed by the two mothers in our pilot study.

Rossiter (1986), although not specifically studying mothers of children with disabilities, explored the influence of support systems on the occupations of mothering young children. She argued that the condition of feeling isolated that mothers experience when caring alone for their children inside their homes, outside of the view of society, strongly influences the occupations of mothering. We support this notion and propose further that mothering young children without disabilities is not antithetical to mothering young children with severe developmental disabilities. In fact, there may be more similarities than differences.

Sandra's need to be seen in her occupations of mothering is a reaction to the invisibility she believes surrounds both herself and her child. Rossiter (1986) described this same invisibility with mothers of very young children without disabilities. She presented the factors that isolate mothers: ceasing to leave home to go to a workplace; eliminating previous participation in social events outside of the home; and, primarily, being confined to their own household. The macrosystem, that is society, supports and even constructs this isolation, to some degree, if it values paid work over caring for young children or if it does not provide adequate transportation or other services to facilitate mothers leaving their households. Rossiter concluded that the separation and invisibility of the occupations of mothering cut mothers off from social supports and relegated their problems to their individual struggles.

In the clinical practice of occupational therapy in pediatrics, we meet persons like Sandra and Merion daily. Sandra told us that it was important for her to be seen. She stated that the occupational therapists who had treated her daughter before the study saw her daughter's physical limitations and her needs for therapy and equipment but did not see Sandra as a mother having needs as well.

Lawlor and Mattingly (1998), who identified the "who's the client" practitioner dilemma within the family-centered intervention approach, explained that, within a clinic culture–medical model of service delivery, the client is easily defined as that person actually receiving hands-on treatment. What, then, becomes of the occupational needs of other family members, particularly the mother?

Pawl (1995) speculated that a parallel process to the development of object permanence exists for young children. That is, young children must believe that they exist in the minds of their care-

givers, even when out of their mother's sight. This knowledge, that they exist for the other, provides young children with feelings of safety and security. We believe that occupational therapy practitioners offer mothers a comparable opportunity to be seen and held in the mind of another, namely the therapist's mind, as mothers do their occupations of mothering. However, this requires a broadening of our understanding of the term *client* to include associated clients (Fearing, Clark, & Stanton, 1997).

Finally, our tacit knowledge (Mattingly & Fleming, 1994) of the nature of the real work of occupational therapy as practiced within our current health care system, that is, the macrosystem, is another connection raised by these pilot data (Lawlor & Mattingly, 1998). If narrowly defined real work is only that work that can be reported in meetings or for reimbursement purposes, then Sandra's issues might remain unrecognized as legitimate occupational therapy work. It is our contention that the occupations of mothering are also the real work of occupational therapy.

Limitations

Data were collected with only two participants, both from the same geographical location. This location—an inner-city context—contributed greatly to the shaping of the participants' lives and occupations. Mothers from other locations would describe different contextual factors, and these, too, require study to increase understanding of how context influences the occupations and experiences of mothering. Additionally, although our data consist of detailed descriptions of the experiences of two mothers, the themes that emerged may not generalize to others in their peer group and beyond.

Some may see a limitation in our relying on what these participants told us based on their recall after a period of time has passed. Although memory does degrade over time, we accept a mother's own reconstruction of her story as valid for her and do not believe that a need exists for corroborating evidence from other sources, such as medical charts (Brown, Lumley, Small, & Astbury, 1994).

Conclusion

In this study, the preliminary overarching theme that we identified was that the occupations of mothering young children with severe developmental disabilities in a challenging urban environment involved an acceptance of doing what had to be done. However, what had to be done was created by the mother's relationship with one particular child at one specific historical period of that child's life. These factors intersected with the woman's own beliefs about what she must do in the context in which she and her child lived. Therefore, the context of these women's lives and the caring occupations that took multiple forms were the interrelated subthemes. Further research is needed to increase our understanding of mothering occupations per se and, in particular, mothering children with disabilities in challenging environments.

Acknowledgments

We thank Deborah Weatherston, MA, from the Infant Mental Health Program of the Merrill-Palmer Institute, Wayne State University; and the mothers who were interviewed, for their participation in this study. We also thank Virginia Dickie, PhD, OTR, FAOTA, for her help in the preparation of an earlier draft of this chapter.

This study was supported by a Blue Cross/Blue Shield of Michigan Student Education Grant, 1995–1996, to the first author.

Appendix
Interview Questions

1. Thinking back on how the infant mental health visits began, tell me about how they started.
2. Tell me about that first visit.
3. What was your daily life like with _____ before the visits started?
4. What kinds of things did you do during your visits?
5. What was it like having this person come?
6. What was it about this worker, or these visits, that made you want them to continue?
7. Tell me about your daily life with _____ during the time of the visits.
8. Tell me about your life with _____ now.
9. Looking back on all the visits and thinking about them now, how do you remember them?
10. How has this experience—of being interviewed about your infant–parent visits—been for you?

References

Barnard, K., & Martell, L. K. (1995). Mothering. In M. Bornstein (Ed.), *Handbook of parenting* (pp. 3–26). Mahwah, NJ: Erlbaum.

Barrera, M., & Vella, D. (1987). Disabled and nondisabled infants' interactions with their mothers. *American Journal of Occupational Therapy, 41,* 168–172.

Barritt, L., Bleeker, H., Beekman, T., & Mulderij, K. (1985). *Researching educational practice.* Grand Forks: University of North Dakota Press.

Bazyk, S. (1989). Changes in attitudes and beliefs regarding parent participation and home programs: An update. *American Journal of Occupational Therapy, 43,* 723–728.

Behar, R. (1993). *Translated woman.* Boston: Beacon.

Broday, E. M., & Schoonover, C. B. (1986). Patterns of parent-care when adult daughters work and when they do not. *Gerontologist, 26,* 372–380.

Bronfenbrenner, U. (1979). *The ecology of human development.* Cambridge, MA: Harvard University Press.

Brown, S., Lumley, J., Small, R., & Astbury, J. (1994). *Missing voices: The experience of motherhood.* Oxford, UK: Oxford University Press.

Burke, J., Clark, F., Hamilton-Dodd, C., & Kawamoto, T. (1987). Maternal role preparation: A program using sensory integration, infant mother attachment, and occupational behavior perspectives. *Occupational Therapy in Health Care, 4*(1), 9–21.

Case-Smith, J., & Nastro, M. (1993). The effects of occupational therapy intervention on mothers of children with cerebral palsy. *American Journal of Occupational Therapy, 46,* 811–817.

Collins, P. H. (1990). Black women and motherhood. In P. H. Collins (Ed.), *Black feminist thought* (pp. 115–137). New York: Routledge & Kegan Paul.

Crowe, T. (1993). Time use of mothers with young children: The impact of a child's disability. *Developmental Medicine and Child Neurology, 35,* 621–630.

Crowe, T., VanLeit, B., Berghmans, K., & Mann, P. (1997). Role perceptions of mothers with young children: The impact of a child's disability. *American Journal of Occupational Therapy, 51,* 651–661.

Dickie, V. (1997). Insights from a focused autobiography. *Occupational Therapy Journal of Research, 17,* 98–104.

Dunlea, A. (1996). An opportunity for co-adaptation: The experience of mothers and their infants who are blind. In R. Zemke & F. Clark (Eds.), *Occupational science: The evolving discipline* (pp. 227–246). Philadelphia: F. A. Davis.

Dunn, W., Brown, C., & McGuigan, A. (1994). The ecology of human performance: A framework for considering the effect of context. *American Journal of Occupational Therapy, 48,* 595–607.

Dyck, I. (1992). The daily routines of mothers with young children: Using a socio-political model in research. *Occupational Therapy Journal of Research, 12,* 16–34.

Esdaile, S. (1994). A focus on mothers, their children with special needs, and other caregivers. *Australian Occupational Therapy Journal, 41,* 3–8.

Esdaile, S., & Greenwood, K. (1995a). Issues of parenting stress: A study involving mothers of toddlers. *Journal of Family Studies, 1,* 153–165.

Esdaile, S., & Greenwood, K. (1995b). A survey of mothers' relationships with their preschoolers. *Occupational Therapy International, 2,* 204–219.

Fearing, V., Clark, J., & Stanton, S. (1997). The client-centered occupational therapy process. In M. Law (Ed.), *Client-centered occupational therapy* (pp. 67–88). Thorofare, NJ: Slack.

Glenn, E. N. (1994). Social constructions of mothering: A thematic overview. In E. N. Glenn, G. Chang, & L. R. Forcey (Eds.), *Mothering: Ideology, experience, and agency* (pp. 1–29). New York: Routledge & Kegan Paul.

Hamilton-Dodd, C., Kawamoto, T., Clark, F., Burke, J., & Fanchiang, S. (1989). The effects of a maternal preparation program on mother–infant pairs: A pilot study. *American Journal of Occupational Therapy, 43,* 513–521.

Hermann, C. (1990). A descriptive study of daily activities and role conflict in single adolescent mothers. In J. A. Johnson & E. J. Yerxa (Eds.), *Occupational science: The foundation for new models of practice* (pp. 53–68). New York: Haworth.

Hinojosa, J. (1990). How mothers of preschool children with cerebral palsy perceive occupational and physical therapists and their influence on family life. *Occupational Therapy Journal of Research, 10,* 144–162.

Hinojosa, J., & Anderson, J. (1991). Mothers' perceptions of home treatment programs for their preschool children with cerebral palsy. *American Journal of Occupational Therapy, 45,* 273–279.

Kielhofner, G. (1995). *A model of human occupation: Theory and application* (2nd ed.). Baltimore: Williams & Wilkins.

Kolobe, T. H. A. (1991). Family-focused early intervention. In S. Campbell (Ed.), *Clinics in physical therapy: Pediatric neurologic physical therapy* (pp. 397–432). New York: Churchill Livingstone.

Larson, E. (1996). The story of Maricela and Miguel: A narrative analysis of dimensions of adaptation. *American Journal of Occupational Therapy, 50,* 286–298.

Lawlor, M., & Mattingly, C. (1998). The complexities embedded in family-centered care. *American Journal of Occupational Therapy, 52,* 259–267.

Mattingly, C., & Fleming, M. (1994). *Clinical reasoning.* Philadelphia: F. A. Davis.

Nelson, D. (1988). Occupation: Form and performance. *American Journal of Occupational Therapy, 42,* 633–641.

Olson, J., & Baltman, K. (1994). Infant mental health in occupational therapy in the neonatal intensive care unit. *American Journal of Occupational Therapy, 48,* 499–505.

Pawl, J. (1995). The therapeutic relationship as connectedness: Being held in another's mind. *Zero to Three, 15,* 1–5.

Pierce, D., & Frank, G. (1992). A mother's work: Two levels of feminist analysis of family-centered care. *American Journal of Occupational Therapy, 46,* 972–980.

Rossiter, A. (1986). *From private to public: A feminist exploration of early mothering.* Toronto, ON: Women's Press.

Ruddick, S. (1983). Maternal thinking. In J. Trebilcot (Ed.), *Mothering: Essays in feminist theory* (pp. 213–230). Lanham, MD: Rowman & Littlefield.

Traustadottir, R. (1991). Mothers who care. *Journal of Family Studies, 12,* 211–228.

Van Manen, M. (1990). *Researching lived experience.* Albany: State University of New York Press.

Yerxa, E., Clark, F., Jackson, J., Pierce, D., & Zemke, R. (1990). *An introduction to occupational science, a foundation for occupational therapy in the 21st century.* Binghamton, NY: Haworth.

CHAPTER 44

Maternal Management of the Home as a Developmental Play Space for Infants and Toddlers

Doris Pierce

Doris Pierce, PhD, OTR/L, *is associate professor, Department of Occupational Therapy, Creighton University, 2500 California Plaza, Omaha, NE 68178.*

The relatively unrecognized work that mothers do in managing the play objects and play spaces of infants and toddlers in the home is critical to child development. Conditions in the home affect infant and toddler development through the degree to which opportunities to learn from interactions with the physical environment are provided (Piaget, 1962; Wohlwill & Heft, 1987). Mothers are the stage managers behind the play scene in the home. They are constantly engaged in infant and toddler positioning for play, toy selection, play space set-up, monitoring for safety, and controlling access to areas of the home. It is work that requires judgment, decision making, and ongoing manipulations of the physical environment (Ruddick, 1982).

An understanding of this work is also important for its own sake because it provides depth to our knowledge of the daily occupational experiences of mothers. Much of unpaid maternal work has remained relatively invisible in Western culture, including caregiving for children (Daniels, 1987; Primeau, 1992). Research on mothering has focused primarily on the mother's skills in social–emotional interactions with the infant and in meeting certain standards for infant hygiene and health (Wachs, 1990). The indirect caregiving and developmental support inherent in the management of the objects and spaces of infant and toddler play has not been studied.

The research presented here focuses on the little-studied spatial dimension of occupation. The mother's use of the spaces and objects of childhood play to facilitate her infant's development is one illustration of a primary human mode of adaptation—material culture. Humans have evolved, in part, through the creation of a complex culture that depends on the sophisticated use of objects, such as tools, clothing, vehicles, shelters, electronic devices, and even toys. Play is the way that children become culturally competent in the material world (Bruner, 1972).

An understanding of this maternal work may also support interventions with young children and their mothers. Knowing how the mother typically

Originally published 2000 in *American Journal of Occupational Therapy, 54,* 290–299.

manages the play objects and spaces of the developing infant or toddler can provide insights for intervening on behalf of an infant at risk for developmental delays, a mother with a newly acquired disability, infants in institutional settings, or mothers with needs for supported acquisition of maternal work patterns.

Method

Design

This chapter on how mothers stage the home play opportunities of infants and toddlers reports one aspect of the findings from a study of infant–toddler spatial and temporal development (Pierce, 1996). The study's primary purpose was to produce a substantive theoretical description of developmental progressions in infant interactions with spatial and temporal aspects of the home physical environment from 1 month to 18 months of age. *Substantive* refers to a level of description that is detailed enough to support practitioners' use of the theory yet not so detailed that it is not applicable in a variety of settings (Glaser & Strauss, 1967). During analysis of the developmental progressions in how infants and toddlers were playing with the usual objects and spaces of the home, it became evident that a description of the central role that mothers played in creating, maintaining, and organizing the infant home was required.

Theoretical validity was ensured in the study through a rigorous longitudinal design, which drew on grounded theory (Glaser & Strauss, 1967) and natural history (Goodall, 1986). Grounded theory is the deliberate development of categorical descriptions of phenomena through in-depth qualitative examination of data. This approach relies heavily on comparisons of extremes of likeness and difference in the data, extensive coding, search for negative cases, and memoing to generate a robust description. Natural history is an ethological approach that depends primarily on intensive longitudinal observation of persons in natural contexts and has been used effectively in the study of nonhuman primates.

Participants

Participants in the study consisted of three groups: a pilot sample of 4 infants and their mothers, a comparative sample of videotaped wild chimpanzee infants and mothers, and a primary sample of 18 Caucasian infants who were typically developing and their mothers. Because of literature indicating that maternal and paternal perspectives on infant play are considerably different, the study focused solely on maternal reports. Caucasian mother–infant dyads were used in the interest of obtaining a relatively homogeneous sample. The mothers were enrolled as potential participants before their infants were born. Participants were selected from the Los Angeles, Orange, and San Bernardino counties of California. The resulting sample was stratified so that the nine male infants were evenly spread across socioeconomic levels, as were the nine female infants.

Data Collection

In the primary sample, data were collected monthly in the home, beginning at 1 month of infant age and continuing through 18 months of age. Data included written observation records, maternal interviews, and videotapes of the infants at play. The 313 observation records addressed types of play observed, methodological issues and researcher reflections on research process, and early points of analysis. The 313 maternal interviews averaged 45 min in length (approximately 6,000 total pages of transcription) and focused on changes in the infant's and toddler's object play interests, use of home space, play sequencing, developmental changes in play, and maternal supports to play. Infants and toddlers were videotaped (180 hr total) in independent interaction with the usual objects and spaces of the home, yard, and neighborhood.

Data Analysis

Data analysis began concurrently with data collection and continued after data collection was completed. A unique feature was the use of a computer-assisted video analysis system modeled on a prototype developed for Jane Goodall's video archive at the University of Southern California. Computer support for the qualitative analysis of video data provided the researcher with critical capabilities, including computer control of video decks, rapid and targeted negotiation through the volume of video data, on-screen clip logging and coding, and joint analysis of video and text data.

Data analysis also included extensive memoing throughout the study, compilation of an audit trail to document the emergence and construction of the theoretical description, and regular peer debriefing sessions. Coding scheme development, a critical process in the grounded theory approach (Glaser & Strauss, 1967), went through several phases, including a cross-species comparison and application to the pilot sample.

Each dyad's entire data set (observation record, maternal interview, videotape from each of 18 home visits) was initially coded in developmental sequence, using interfaced video coding and text analysis software. A comparative analysis path was used to maximize important contrasting factors through a deliberate sequence in which the data set of particular mother–infant dyads was coded. For example, a male infant's data set might be selected for analysis after completing a female infant's, or data from an infant with multiple siblings might be examined after that of an infant without siblings. Further coding was selective, seeking fuller development of aspects of the theoretical description. For instance, the developmental sequence in infant and toddler negotiation of the space of the home was analyzed. A final written synthesis of the primary topics of the theoretical description detailed developmental progressions and relations between theoretical categories.

The topics addressed in the theoretical description of infant and toddler spatiotemporal development in the home included progressions in infant development from 1 month to 18 months of age: in gaze and visual play, in ranging over the spaces of the home, in stationary and mobile object play, in temporal organization of play, and in maternal management of the home play context. How participants' socioeconomic status (SES), birth order, maternal employment, or other conditions influenced infant and toddler development was not analyzed.

This chapter reports only the portion of the study data that describes the mother's spatial management of the infant's home play space. The results are reported in two sections, each of which begins with a review of pertinent literature. The sections are (a) the maternal work of managing play objects in the home and (b) the maternal work of organizing and maintaining the home space to support infant development.

Maternal Work of Managing Play Objects in the Home

The study demonstrated that much of the maternal thinking and practices of managing infant play revolve around the play objects. Examining how this work is carried out, and the situations in which it is especially influenced or prevented by broader social factors, makes visible a type of work little examined or appreciated. Yet, this is work on which infant development depends.

Toys, Cookware, Furniture, and Other Playthings: Material Culture of Infant Play

In contrast to other animals, human adaptation requires a multiplicity of physical objects for everyday life: tools, shelters, furniture, vehicles, clothing, and more. In anthropology's history, material culture approaches have often been used to explore meaning in non-Western cultures through examination of the artifacts of daily life (Hodder, 1989). Toys and other household play objects are the material culture of childhood. Play is a central mode of developing in the child the required skills for using the infinite variety of physical objects that are a part of human culture (Bruner, 1972).

Over history, toys have changed dramatically, reflecting changing attitudes toward children and play (Cross, 1997; McClary, 1997). The toy industry expends millions of dollars a year in persuading parents to purchase play objects for their children (Miller, 1998). The cultural messages to be found in commercial toys are value-laden and powerful. Children of today's Western cultures are typically supplied with a greater number of objects specifically intended as playthings than were children at any other point in history.

By watching the 18 infants in their homes, it was easy to see that not all, or even most, of the things they played with were commercial toys. Once the perspective is broadened to a conception of playful interactions with physical objects, rather than commercial toys, the picture of infant and toddler play changes completely. Infants and toddlers spend much of their time playing with furniture, family clothing, steps and stairs, cookware and plasticware, telephones and televisions, doors and windows, and many other everyday objects of family life.

Supporting Infant Play in the Home Is Supporting Infant Development

Appreciation of the importance of a mother's provision of developmental play opportunities through her management of play objects in the home requires one to acknowledge the dependence of typical development on play experience.

Play is the primary occupation of the waking child. Infants and toddlers are in a uniquely concrete and externally represented mode of play and development compared with older children who are more able to mentally manipulate concepts (Piaget, 1952, 1962). This makes the mother's work of providing opportunities to physically manipulate and explore objects of the home environment crucial to her child's development.

Current research on infant play development primarily uses the traditional methods of psychology: a laboratory setting, spatial freedom restricted, standard sets of objects presented, and quantitative analysis of behaviors performed according to a predetermined set of categories. Play development has been documented in the increasing specificity with which infants tailor actions to objects (Palmer, 1989; Rochat, 1989; Ruff, 1984) and movement through relatively broad play stages (Belsky & Most, 1981; Zelazo & Kearsley, 1980). Positive relationships have also been found between development and object complexity and variety in the home (Bradley & Caldwell, 1984; Wachs, Uzgiris, & Hunt, 1971). The degree to which toys produce an observable change or response when acted on by a child has shown a positive relationship with development (Wachs, 1978, 1990; Yarrow, Morgan, Jennings, Harmon, & Gaiter, 1982). Little research has described self-directed infant action (Haith, 1990; Hendricks-Jansen, 1996).

Especially pertinent to this study's focus on the development of interactions with the physical environment of the home is the infant's development of spatial cognition. Piaget (1952) proposed that an infant's spatial cognition develops from a newborn undifferentiated perception, to physically relating objects to each other around 10 months of age, to an increasingly sophisticated internal representation of objects and their relations by 18 months of age. In his ecological theory of perception, Gibson (1986) claimed that the child acquires an understanding of the physical world directly through interactions with the environment, which has been supported by research (Acredolo, 1990; Benson & Uzgiris, 1985; Bremner, 1989; Wellman, 1985). Theoretical perspectives on infant development are beginning to show some attention to a more active, mobile, and spatially contexted view of the infant (Belsky, 1995; Bronfenbrenner, 1995). An examination of mothers' work in providing play experiences that support the infant's or toddler's development of spatial cognition in the home deepens our understanding of the developmental context of infant experience.

Selecting Play Objects

The mothers in the study managed the objects that they considered to be primarily meant for the child's play in very different ways. Many were avid consumers of commercial developmental toys:

> [My mother is] a neuropsychologist. But when I was little, my mom...[made] sure that I had every developmental toy. It's funny because Rick...didn't as much do that. His belief on children and having developmental toys isn't as strong as mine. But I know where it comes from, it comes from the fact that my mom always, I mean, I had everything. [Interview, Belle, 8 months]

Other mothers did not believe that commercial toys were important in the infant's life. Often, this group had limited finances to spend on play objects:

> The mother was pretty direct about saying that the baby doesn't really have any toys, that things have been tight, and her children mainly just play with household objects and use their imaginations. They had just gotten a baby swing at a garage sale, which seemed to be very exciting for everyone, since the baby seemed to like being in it. [Observation record, Julie, 2 months]

The mothers put considerable thought into the purchase of play objects. First-time mothers tended to have vague ideas about what they "ought" to buy and depended heavily on the toy industry's design, labeling, and marketing. They had a strong preference for brightly colored objects for infants. More experienced mothers based their judgments more on what they saw in the developing infant's or toddler's skills and often had a store of outgrown infant toys from a previous child that could be readily brought into the play space. The experienced mothers tended to offer toys with better developmental timing, whereas the new mothers needed time to problem solve what type of toy would be of interest at that point:

> That's a question I ask myself, "What would you like?" That's a big part of it, but if I want it to last, partly it's on the basis that if I've read something that says children this age [would benefit from a certain toy]. Like I'm looking for the right-size blocks that she can hold in her hands. She's supposed to like that right now. I guess it's on the basis of, "Oh, she likes this, maybe she'd like that because it's similar." There's a rattle I've seen that I thought she might like because it's kind of like the one that she loves so much. I'm still kind of perplexed as to what she's going to like. [Interview, Alison, 5 months]

Some mothers also recognized when infants were developing beyond interest in the play objects available to them. This recognition usually came about when the mothers found that the toys no longer engaged the infant, thereby limiting the mothers' freedom to do other household work in the infant's vicinity. The mother's dependence on toys to occupy infants was especially true for infants without siblings. If the available play objects did not hold the infant's attention, the mother might not be able to do the dishes or the laundry or to take a shower. This motivation to engage the infant, combined with a desire to support the infant's development, propelled many mothers on regular excursions to local toy stores. Mothers saw fresh toys as a boon to their efforts to juggle competing task priorities.

By 8 months of age, the infants had entered a period of development where novel objects were desired in quantities. This stage could be quite challenging, especially for mothers who were not financially able to purchase many toys. Some mothers met the challenge by offering household objects for play. Other mothers preferred that the infants play with commercial toys, attempted to encourage this, and supplied a larger number of objects within the infant's reach. However, once the infants were independently ranging over the home landscape, they sought out and explored objects constantly. Anything reachable held possibilities as a plaything. The degree to which the mother allowed access to the spaces and objects of the home restricted or expanded the developmental opportunities available to the infant or toddler.

Where mothers supported and took cues from the infant's self-directed object choices, the play emphasis moved at this age from commercial toys to more household objects: climbing under and over furniture; thrashing magazines; carrying objects around; pulling things out of containers and storage sites, such as toy boxes, shelves, and drawers; playing with family clothing and shoes; and simply enjoying going up and down halls and in and out of rooms. At this point, kitchen cupboards became a primary play site. They were the most frequently used play site in the study, although the type of play there changed as the child matured. The cupboards offered a multiplicity of objects for interaction as well as a proximity to the mother's household work, such as washing the dishes or cooking, which she needed to do within visual range of her infant. Some mothers encouraged cupboard play, rearranging

the contents to better fit the infant's or toddler's interests and safety. A few mothers discouraged cupboard play. Cupboard play is a good example of the degree to which the mother shapes developmental play opportunities in the home and the interactive dynamic between the occupations in which the mother and infant or toddler are simultaneously engaged.

As the infant matured past 1 year of age into toddlerhood, many mothers began to focus on selecting play objects that they believed taught important concepts, such as shape-sorters, picture and talking books, puzzles, and many other educational toys. These sorts of play objects appeared to be most preferred and prevalent in the upper-SES homes. Educational toys were most often used in a socially interactive type of play and rarely as independent object play initiated by the infant.

Routes Whereby Play Objects Came Into the Home

The routes whereby objects specifically intended for play come into the home were interesting in the degree to which they illustrate the mother's involvement in these choices, the influence of the broader culture, and cases in which the mother has more limited control. The primary route of entry was purchases at the toy store by the mother. Often, these shopping trips included the father and other members of the family. Toy marketing greatly influenced the mothers' choices. Six of the 18 infants in the study also received developmental toys every 6 weeks from a toy club promoted in a popular parent magazine.

A number of ritual events introduced, or imported, playthings and infant care equipment into the home. The mother appeared to have less influence over these choices but was also supported in her work of managing the home space for the infant and toddler through these events, which included baby showers, gift-giving holidays, the infant's first birthday, and gift-giving from visiting extended family members.

The five mothers of first-born infants each had at least one baby shower. Groups hosting showers for these mothers were largely female, made up of relatives, friends, coworkers, and church groups. The gifts differed with group make-up but generally included infant clothing, small toys, safety devices, and infant-positioning equipment. Most of the shower gifts had an air of practicality, as if the mothers were being provided with new job tools. The mothers' remarks on insights gained from the gifts, or how surprisingly useful they had been, demonstrated that these baby shower gifts embodied a passing on of important knowledge from expert infant caregiver to novice. The association of this event with the mother's first child, rather than an infant's birth, further supports an interpretation of this event as a modern-day initiation and support ritual for the new mother.

Holidays also function as toy import events, especially the traditional gift exchange celebrations of Christmas and Hanukkah. Infant and toddler gifts on these occasions were usually commercial toys. In the lower SES homes, fewer new toys generally appeared. Some mothers reported intergenerational differences of opinion about the appropriateness of toys, especially in the realm of gender-stereotyped gifts for girls. For example, one mother did not like the small pink plastic vacuum cleaner that her toddler had received from her grandmother, although the child was taking great delight in pushing it all around the house.

Another primary import event was the infant's first birthday. The types of gifts given varied with economic level. With only one exception in 18, birthday gifts included at least one large, wheeled push toy or riding toy. Girls often received a baby doll. Birthday and holiday gifts, unlike shower gifts, were given almost entirely by

relatives and were intended for play, in contrast to the more practical objects given at showers to support the mother's child care work.

Extended family members also introduced objects for the infant and toddler. Visiting relatives often brought gifts, such as a stuffed animal or infant toy, which served as a catalyst for shared play with these rarely seen relatives. Female relatives frequently made cloth comfort objects (e.g., baby quilts, afghans, cloth books, stuffed animals) as gifts. Maternal aunts would pass outgrown toys and child care equipment from one household to another, as different children in the extended family were ready for them. Two maternal grandmothers passed the mothers' cherished infant play objects on to female infants. To the mothers of infant girls, the symbolism of this heirloom gift-giving was a recognition of shared feelings about raising a daughter and symbolized the cyclic repetition of relational patterns across family generations.

The routes via which play objects enter the home demonstrate the primary influences of the culture on the mother's provision of infant and toddler play objects in the home. The toy industry, community members, and immediate and extended family play a role in determining the types and number of play objects the mother makes available to the infant and toddler. Viewing this maternal work within the contexts of toy shopping and gift-giving events makes evident the degree to which the work is integrated, supported, and valued by the culture.

Making Play Objects Available Within the Home

The ways in which the mothers arranged objects to make them available to their infants and toddlers varied both among mothers and across their infants' development. Set-up in the early months of infant age often included a blanket on the floor or some sort of infant-positioning device, such as a bouncer, and a few objects close at hand. Once the infant was competently crawling, mothers no longer routinely placed objects out for play. Rather, they positioned infants near toy boxes and toy shelves. Later, they verbally directed infants to where the objects were stored. For mobile infants and toddlers, mothers used barriers to enclose the infants within a designated play area:

> The big key is: Is the room child safe and blocked off? And then I'll just let her have at it. And...if I need her to be occupied while I'm in the kitchen...I might direct her to here to there....Sometimes, I might open a cupboard and just go, "Hey, look at this".... [Interview, Leslie, 14 months]

With the fully mobile toddler, set-up work shifted to time spent in arranging the home environment to support independent play. Mothers rearranged kitchen cupboards, displayed toys on low shelves, and brought toy storage containers into use in the family living area. A few of the mothers used novelty-maintaining strategies—storing objects out of sight and rotating boxes of them in and out of the play area every few weeks. Mothers spent time daily, often at naptime and bedtime, picking up the variety of objects with which the infant had been playing and placing them in their designated storage sites. A few of the mothers would display the current favorite play objects at infant eye level—on a low coffee table or shelf—where the infant or toddler was likely to come on them and begin self-initiated play. Mothers with multiple children used a less infant-focused style, storing all toys together. This approach provided a greater variety of object choices but less easy access and less accurate developmental fit.

The two single mothers in the study who resided with their parents had less control over how play objects were made available to their infants and toddlers than did mothers living in their own homes. This resulted in a different play experience. For example, at 13 months, one of the toddlers living in his grandparents' home was videotaped playing for 20 min at a coffee table in a living room full of knick-knacks on other tables and shelves. All of his permitted and accessible play objects were on that table. Although he could walk, his independent play was restricted to the table site or to a nearby playpen. In both cases, these mothers spent more time than did the other mothers in redirecting and repositioning their infants away from objects that were within reach, but taboo for play, and the play spaces were more restricted.

Maternal Work of Organizing and Maintaining the Home Space to Support Development

In addition to managing play objects in the home, the mothers managed home and yard spaces within which their infants and toddlers played daily. The spatial configurations of these play spaces, and the work routines through which the mothers maintained their layout and organization, were regularly reconceptualized to fit the developing child's rapidly emerging mobility and ever-present quest for novel objects.

Research on the Impact of the Home Physical Environment on Infant Development

There is limited research on the influence of the physical environment on child development, most of which has focused on institutional environments such as schools, playgrounds, and clinics (Goodnow, 1995; Wohlwill & Heft, 1987). Several studies have shown the negative effects on development of restrictions in floor freedom through use of playpens and other infant care equipment (Ainsworth & Bell, 1974; Wachs, 1979). Theorists have proposed that the consistent feedback available from the physical environment, in contrast to the more variable responses of the social environment, are important for the development of sensorimotor schemata (Piaget, 1952), for learning about what the environment affords (Gibson, 1986), and for development of a concept of the self through relations to the physical world (Neisser, 1991).

Homes of the Study

Because the participants' homes were all located in the greater Los Angeles area, suburban tracts, or apartment complexes, they reflected typical home layouts favored by commercial builders in the United States: a kitchen, an adjacent living room, and bedrooms and a bathroom down the hall or up the stairs. More expensive homes had additional shared family spaces: a den, a television room, or a family room. The larger homes of the highest SES families had multiple spaces to which infants typically were not allowed access: home offices, formal living and dining rooms, pool areas, detached garages, laundry rooms, and live-in housekeeper's quarters. Homes of lower SES families were smaller in size, less safe, more crowded with persons and objects, had fewer objects specifically for play, and lacked outdoor space. Homes of higher SES families were expansive, toy-stocked, and complete with manicured lawns.

Despite wide variations in home space, the determining factor in the infant's experience of the physical environment was clearly the mother's control of the home space. Children in higher SES homes did not necessarily have more play space than those in lower SES homes because much of the higher SES home was often blocked off by baby gates or forbidden by the mother, and a designated playroom held most of the toys.

Mothers in lower SES homes allowed access to the largest percentage of the home space and used the greatest flexibility in constructing that space to fit the infant. Possibly, the pressure of the smaller spaces produced this effect. Two mothers in small homes restructured their home layouts by switching the living room furniture with the infant bedroom furniture, thus facilitating access to play objects, and doubling the available play space in the kitchen and den areas.

The mothers all changed their home space management routines as the infant developed to accommodate the infant's increasing independence in negotiating and exploring the home play space. The homes of single children were managed in a way that was more tailored to that infant's current developmental interests compared with the play spaces of multichild homes, which offered a cafeteria of access and play object choices across developmental levels. Each home play space was unique. However, the greatest concentration of play objects was nearly always adjacent to the kitchen, the mother's primary household work area.

Safety and Order

The modern Western home is a space poorly fit to, and relatively unsafe for, infants and children. It is replete with sharp edges, is made up of multilevel hard surfaces, includes dangerous temperature extremes, holds many small indigestible objects, and is supplied with electricity throughout. The home is also isolated from the wider culture, thereby reducing the number of adults available for child care and the number of playmates for interaction. In contrast, for example, children in Kpelle society (Lancy, 1996) play on the "mother ground," a village gathering place between homes, and infants are carried on their mothers backs until they are mobile. Kpelle rarely engage in conversation or play with children before the "age of sense" at around 7 years.

The mothers in the study controlled infant play space out of concerns for the infants' and toddlers' safety and desires to maintain an orderly home. They went to great lengths to create a safe play space with such devices as baby latches, plug protectors, coffee table corner pads, toilet locks, and "choke size" measuring devices. Mothers regularly used their own bodies to closely guard the infant attempting a daring feat, positioned themselves between the infant and unsafe objects and blocking access to forbidden areas, moved toys onto safer surfaces, and carried infants away from unsafe places. Mothers in the lower SES homes expressed more concerns over infant safety and appeared to exercise more caution and restraint of the infant's play than did mothers in higher SES homes.

Mothers were teaching their infants by 8 months of age about areas of the house that they were not permitted to enter. They taught the infants that certain objects were forbidden and that others could only be used in specific areas. Most infants learned that they only might attempt the stairs alongside an adult. Extreme differences in maternal attitudes about safety were especially evident as the infant or toddler acquired climbing skills. Some mothers forbade this type of play, whereas others cheered their youngsters on.

The Los Angeles area climate supports infant use of outdoor space year-round. The mother managed the yard as play space, but the yard was more strictly supervised than the indoor space. Infant passage through doors to the outside was supervised by an adult. In some homes in the lower SES levels, outdoor private space was limited or nonexistent. Mothers with family yards kept larger toys there, such as riding toys, sandboxes, and swing sets. Although the mothers differed greatly in the degree to which they were concerned with safety issues and control of infant access, all addressed these issues:

> As I was leaving, mother admitted that her neighbor had had to stop his car the day before because Bruce was in the middle of the street. His mother was working on the new computer. She said, "He is so fast now!" Evidently, Bruce does not yet have a sense of boundaries to his

home setting. Or, he does, but violated them. [Observation record, Bruce, 14 months]

Furnishing and Positioning in Play Space

Mothers also used a variety of devices designed to carry, position, or contain infants, such as slings, baby backpacks, bouncers, carriers, car seats, swings, playpens, and strollers. Most were present in all of the homes, with slightly fewer devices in the homes of lower SES families. Often, there was an area of the house that functioned as a parking lot for all of the positioning devices not in use.

The mothers reported that when positioning an infant in holding equipment, they were considering several aspects of the infant's experience. A primary consideration was whether the positioning would successfully occupy the infant and free the mother for nearby household work. They placed infants to maximize their view of the mother and surrounding spaces. Access to objects of interest for gaze and contact was also considered. Sometimes, infants were repositioned from one piece of equipment to another to produce a fresh, attention-sustaining perspective. Infants with siblings close in age were more often placed in holding equipment to keep them safely stable or out of reach. Playpens were observed to be used in situations in which siblings threatened the infant's safety or in situations of small spaces filled with available objects forbidden to infants and valued by adults. The number and variety of infant care devices in these homes and the thought that the mothers invested in providing and making use of them demonstrate that the spatial management of the infant through infant care equipment is a critical component of the Western mother's infant-care practices.

Spatial Ties to Family Members

A constant feature across all mother–infant dyads was the existence of a spatial tie between mothers and infants—the two appeared to be linked in space. For some dyads, this tie seemed due to the infant or toddler following the mother, and in others, it was the mother who followed. However, both mother and infant seemed aware of the distance between them, as if an unseen rubber band stretched between them, increasing in tension as the distance increased, pulling the two back toward each other. The degree to which the infant or toddler led and the mother followed appeared to determine the degree to which the infant was self-directed and exploring to the extreme bounds of the home play space. Child-directed dyads tended to occur in single-child families with mothers who did not work outside the home. Mothers with multiple children, or who did not wish to range over the home space with the infant or toddler, tended to have infants or toddlers who remained more stationary in their play. The infant's spatial tie to the mother was extended to siblings to a lesser degree. An audible sibling in another room increased the tendency of the infant to leave the mother and seek out the sibling.

Discussion

The primary value of these findings is that they ground our understanding of infant development and maternal caregiving in Western cultures in the context of the home physical environment. Too often, infant and toddler development is cast in the languages of psychology and toy marketing, creating a knowledge base that is a blend of lab experimentation in emerging infant subskills and exposure to commercial persuasion by the toy industry. The description presented here makes visible the behind-the-scenes work of mothers by detailing their daily judgments, decisions, and actions as they create play opportunities for infants and toddlers in the home. It makes real the ways

in which developmental opportunities of infants and toddlers at play are created, maintained, and managed in their homes.

The mothers in this study supported and shaped infant and toddler play in the home through their management of home space and its play objects. Each mother was unique in how she went about this work and the environment within which she operated. Yet, there are striking similarities in the dynamic practices of these mothers. They used care and judgment in selecting and offering both commercial and household play objects. More ritualized cultural routes, over which mothers had less control, imported play objects into the home. The mothers spent time setting up objects for play and maintaining their storage and level of novelty. They continuously reconstructed their work routines to fit the developmental changes in the child, allowing increasing spatial freedom and independence in play object selection. All were required to be on guard as they attempted caregiving in environments filled with objects dangerous to young children. These are the general practices that mark the maternal work of managing play objects and spaces of the Western home in this Caucasian sample.

An understanding of how mothers facilitate infant and toddler development through management of home play space can support interventions that target either infant development or mothering. For instance, adapting the home play space for infants graduating from neonatal intensive care units within the restrictions imposed by medical technology is critical to the support of development (Missiuna & Pollock, 1991). For a new mother with physical limitations, her therapist's knowledge of how infants typically play in the home space will provide various strategies that can support her desire to actively nurture her infant's play. Such understanding of human occupation supports insightful practice.

This study brings to light several theoretical points regarding occupation. One point concerns the degree of interpretation of cultural values and individual construction of daily occupational choices in the mothers. The influence of the culture can be seen in

- The effects of consumerism and toy industry advertising on the mother's thinking regarding appropriate play objects,
- Cultural routes for importing toys into the home environment,
- The difficulties of single mothers still in their family home in exerting control over the home play setting,
- The impact of the nuclear family structure and home layout on infant and toddler play, and
- The mother's need for engaging play objects for the child to complete other household work expected within the culture.

Within these cultural demands, however, the mothers exerted a high degree of choice, creativity, and individual variation in how they constructed the play opportunities of the infant in the home.

Another point concerns the phenomenon of co-occupation. The mother's occupations of managing the home play objects and spaces for the infants are not solitary, or even parallel or shared, but a dyadic interplay between the occupations of the mother and those of the infant and toddler. Thus, the mother's occupations require and affect the child's occupations. Co-occupations can be face-to-face interactions, such as a mother and infant turn-taking in peek-a-boo play. They can also occur in alternations linked only in time and space, such as the daily pattern of the toddler carrying toys from the toy box all over the house and the mother returning them to the toy box at the end of the day. The co-occupational nature of maternal work and infant and toddler play is especially indicated by the way in which one person's occupations influences those of the other: The child's emerging mobility changes the mother's management patterns, and the mother's actions in choosing toys and allowing access shapes the child's play opportunities. Co-occupation in an important concept in light of the number of situations in which a linked pattern of occupations is key to treatment, such as that between client and therapist or client and caregiver.

Possibly the most important theoretical point made here about occupation is the description of the spatial dimension of a type of occupation. The spatiality of occupation is a neglected phenomenon in occupational therapy despite the evidently spatial nature of many of the field's central constructs. Habits, activities of daily living, tool use, activity analysis, and function are all spatially constructed, and all of our actions are spatial in their embodiment. Occupations depend on what is afforded by the physical environment (Gibson, 1986). Occupations are grounded in that uniquely human mode of evolution: the creation of a rich material culture. Routines, another central construct of the field, are mapped onto specific objects and spatial locations at which each step in the routine sequence occurs.

Perhaps the profession's lack of research into the spatial aspect of occupation is due to the largely decontextualized nature of our practice. We tend to work with clients in spaces that are separate from the spaces in which acquired skills are to be used. As occupational therapy moves into more contextually intact, community-based practice (Dunn, Brown, McClain, & Westman, 1994), greater theoretical attention to the spatial dynamic of therapeutic occupations can be expected. In the future, we will select, modify, and understand the client spaces in which we are working with much greater theoretical ease and, thus, greater power (Pierce, 1998).

Summary

This study of the behind-the-scenes work done by mothers to facilitate infant and toddler development by creating, furnishing, and maintaining play space in the home explores the spatial dimension of occupation, unearths the intriguing concept of co-occupation, reveals some aspects of the expression of culture and individuality within this type of occupation, and grounds our work with mothers and children in a substantive description of the home as a primary developmental space. By making visible mothers' important indirect work in support of infant and toddler play, our perspective on maternal and infant occupations, and on occupations in general, is both deepened and transformed.

Acknowledgments

I thank the occupational science faculty members of the University of Southern California, especially Diane Parham, PhD, OTR, FAOTA. I thank the American Occupational Therapy Association and the American Occupational Therapy Foundation for the 1993 Dissertation Grant Award, without which a study of this size could never have been undertaken.

References

Acredolo, L. (1990). Individual differences in spatial cognition. In J. Colombo & J. Fagen (Eds.), *Individual differences in infancy: Reliability, stability, prediction* (pp. 45–76). Hillsdale, NJ: Erlbaum.

Ainsworth, M. D. S., & Bell, S. M. (1974). Mother–child interaction and the development of competence. In K. J. Connolly & J. S. Bruner (Eds.), *The growth of competence* (pp. 97–188). New York: Academic.

Belsky, J. (1995). Expanding the ecology of human development: An evolutionary perspective. In P. Moen, G. Elder, & K. Luscher (Eds.), *Examining lives in context: Perspective on ecology of human development* (pp. 545–562). Washington, DC: American Psychological Association.

Belsky, J., & Most, R. (1981). From exploration to play: A cross-sectional study of infant free-play behavior. *Developmental Psychology, 17,* 630–639.

Benson, J. B., & Uzgiris, I. C. (1985). Effect of self-initiated locomotion on infant search activity. *Developmental Psychology, 21,* 923–931.

Bradley, R. H., & Caldwell, B. M. (1984). The relation of infant's home environments to achievement test performance in first grade: A follow-up study. *Child Development, 55,* 803–809.

Bremner, G. (1989). Development of spatial awareness in infancy. In A. Slater & G. Bremner (Eds.), *Infant development* (pp. 123–142). London: Erlbaum.

Bronfenbrenner, U. (1995). Developmental ecology through space and time: A future perspective. In P. Moen, G. Elder, & K. Luscher (Eds.), *Examining lives in context: Perspectives on the ecology of human development* (pp. 619–647). Washington, DC: American Psychological Association.

Bruner, S. J. (1972). Nature and uses of immaturity. *American Psychologist, 44,* 1–11.

Cross, G. (1997). *Kids' stuff: Toys and the changing world of American childhood.* Cambridge, MA: Harvard University Press.

Daniels, A. K. (1987). Invisible work. *Social Problems, 34,* 403–415.

Dunn, W., Brown, C., McClain, L., & Westman, K. (1994). The ecology of human performance: A contextual perspective on human occupation. In C. B. Royeen (Ed.), *AOTA Self-Study Series: The practice of the future: Putting occupation back into therapy* (pp. 1–56). Rockville, MD: American Occupational Therapy Association.

Gibson, J. J. (1986). *The ecological approach to visual perception.* Hillsdale, NJ: Erlbaum.

Glaser, B. G., & Strauss, A. L. (1967). *The discovery of grounded theory.* New York: Aldine.

Goodall, J. (1986). *The chimpanzees of Gombe: Patterns of behavior.* Cambridge, MA: Belknap.

Goodnow, J. (1995). Differentiating among social contexts: By spatial features, forms of participation, and social contracts. In P. Moen, G. Elder,

& K. Luscher (Eds.), *Examining lives in context: Perspectives on the ecology of human development* (pp. 269–302). Washington, DC: American Psychological Association.

Haith, M. M. (1990). Progress in the understanding of sensory and perceptual processes in early infancy. *Merrill–Palmer Quarterly, 36*(1), 11–27.

Hendricks-Jansen, H. (1996). *Catching ourselves in the act: Situated activity, interactive emergence, evolution, and human thought.* Cambridge, MA: MIT Press.

Hodder, I. (1989). *The meaning of things: Material culture and symbolic expression.* Boston: Unwin-Hyman.

Lancy, D. (1996). *Playing on the motherground: Cultural routines for children's development.* New York: Guilford.

McClary, A. (1997). *Toys with nine lives: A social history of American toys.* New Haven, CT: Linnet.

Miller, G. W. (1998). *Toy wars.* New York: Random House.

Missiuna, C., & Pollock, N. (1991). Play deprivation in children with physical disabilities: The role of the occupational therapist in preventing secondary disability. *American Journal of Occupational Therapy, 45,* 882–888.

Neisser, U. (1991). Two perceptually given aspects of the self and their development. *Developmental Review, 11,* 197–209.

Palmer, C. F. (1989). The discriminating nature of infants' exploratory action. *Developmental Psychology, 25,* 885–893.

Piaget, J. (1952). *The origins of intelligence in children.* New York: International Universities Press.

Piaget, J. (1962). *Plays, dreams, and imitation in childhood.* New York: Norton.

Pierce, D. E. (1996). Infant space, infant time: Development of infant interactions with the physical environment, from 1 to 18 months (Doctoral dissertation, University of Southern California, 1996). *Dissertation Abstracts International, 57,* AAG9705160.

Pierce, D. E. (1998). The Issue Is—What is the source of occupation's treatment power? *American Journal of Occupational Therapy, 52,* 490–491.

Primeau, L. A. (1992). A woman's place: Unpaid work in the home. *American Journal of Occupational Therapy, 46,* 981–988.

Rochat, P. (1989). Object manipulation and exploration in 2- to 5-month old infants. *Developmental Psychology, 25,* 871–884.

Ruddick, S. (1982). Maternal thinking. In B. Thorne & M. Yalom (Eds.), *Rethinking the family: Some feminist questions* (pp. 76–94). New York: Longman.

Ruff, H. (1984). Infant's manipulative exploration of objects: Effects of age and object characteristics. *Developmental Psychology, 20,* 9–20.

Wachs, T. D. (1978). The relationship of infants' physical environment to their Binet performance at 2 1/2 years. *International Journal of Behavioral Development, 1,* 51–65.

Wachs, T. D. (1979). Proximal experience and early cognitive–intellectual development: The physical environment. *Merrill–Palmer Quarterly, 25,* 3–41.

Wachs, T. D. (1990). Must the physical environment be mediated by the social environment in order to influence development? A further test. *Journal of Applied Development Psychology, 11,* 163–178.

Wachs, T. D., Uzgiris, I. C., & Hunt, J. McV. (1971). Cognitive development in infants of different age levels and from different environmental backgrounds: An exploratory investigation. *Merrill–Palmer Quarterly, 17,* 283–317.

Wellman, H. M. (1985). *Children's searching: The development of search skill and spatial representation.* Hillsdale, NJ: Erlbaum.

Wohlwill, J. F., & Heft, H. (1987). The physical environment and the development of the child. In D. Stokols & I. Altman (Eds.), *Handbook of environmental psychology* (pp. 281–328). Malabar, FL: Krieger.

Yarrow, L. J., Morgan, G. A., Jennings, K. D., Harmon, R. J., & Gaiter, J. L. (1982). Infants' persistence at tasks: Relationships to cognitive functioning and early experience. *Annual Progress in Child Psychiatry and Development,* pp. 217–229.

Zelazo, P. R., & Kearsley, R. B. (1980). The emergence of functional play in infants: Evidence for a major cognitive transition. *Journal of Applied Developmental Psychology, 1,* 95–117.

CHAPTER 45

Stigma and Its Management

A Pilot Study of Parental Perceptions of the Experiences of
Children With Developmental Coordination Disorder

Ruth Segal, Angela Mandich, Helene Polatajko, and Joanne Valiant Cook

Ruth Segal, PhD, OTR,
*is assistant professor,
Department of Occupational
Therapy, New York
University, 35 West 4th
Street, New York, NY 10012;
rs108@nyu.edu.*

**Angela Mandich, PhD, OT
(reg),** *is assistant professor,
School of Occupational
Therapy, University of
Western Ontario, London,
Ontario, Canada.*

**Helene Polatajko, PhD,
OT (reg),** *is professor and
chair, Department of
Occupational Therapy,
University of Toronto,
Toronto, Ontario, Canada.*

**Joanne Valiant Cook,
PhD, OT (reg),** *is associate
professor, School of
Occupational Therapy,
University of Western
Ontario, London, Ontario,
Canada.*

Originally published 2002
in *American Journal of
Occupational Therapy, 56,*
422–428.

The new International Classification of Functioning, Disability, and Health (ICIDH–2; World Health Organization [WHO], 2001) presents a framework for organizing and describing human functioning and its restrictions. The final draft of this framework consists of two parts: (a) functioning and disability and (b) contextual factors. Each part consists of two components: Functioning and disability consists of (a) body functions and structures and (b) activities and participation, and contextual factors consist of (a) environmental factors and (b) personal factors. This framework is based on the concept that *impairment,* which is defined as problems in body function or structure, may affect an individual's ability to perform activities and to participate fully in life (WHO, 2001). The manner and extent of the impact on activities and participation depend on the impairment, individual characteristics, and the social context.

The sociological, analytic framework of stigma and its management (Goffman, 1963) can elucidate the interactions between impairment and participation. Goffman (1963) defined *stigma* as "possessing an attribute" (p. 3) that makes one different from what others expect one to be and is, therefore, "deeply discrediting" (p. 3) of the person.[1] The discredited attribute may be of the body; of one's character; or of one's race, ethnicity, or religion. Goffman clarified that the attribute not necessarily is discrediting in and of itself but depends on the situation in which persons are interacting. In this chapter, Goffman's conceptualization of stigma situations and their management is used to demonstrate the interactions among impairment, activity, and participation in the case of children with developmental coordination disorder.

Developmental coordination disorder affects about 6% of children between 5 and 11 years of age (American Psychiatric Association [APA], 1994). The

---

[1]The uses of Goffman's (1963) *Stigma: Notes on the Management of Spoiled Identity* in this chapter have been partial and purposive. Therefore, this case study is not intended to give readers a comprehensive review of his framework.

symptoms of developmental coordination disorder may include marked delays in achieving milestones of motor development, dropping things, clumsiness, poor performance in sports, or poor handwriting. If any of these symptoms interferes with a child's performance of daily activities, a diagnosis is warranted (APA, 1994). Observations of school-age children with developmental coordination disorder during organized and free play show that these children spend less time in formal and informal team play than children without the disorder (Smyth & Anderson, 2000).

Physical activity play in the form of free and team play is important for children's social life (Blatchford, 1998; Humphreys & Smith, 1987; Pellegrini & Smith, 1998). In a summary of the literature on physical activity play, Pellegrini and Smith (1998) indicated that exercise play (i.e., gross locomotor movement in the context of play) seems to increase in the late preschool years and peak during primary school years. For example, Blatchford (1998) found that in Britain, 84% of the 11-year-old boys and 36% of the 11-year-old girls played soccer during break time in school. Rough-and-tumble play with peers, a form of free physical activity play, seems to peak around 8 to 10 years of age (Pellegrini & Smith, 1998).

In his longitudinal qualitative and quantitative study of British children's experiences during break time, Blatchford (1998) described how friendships develop in conjunction with physical activity play when children begin their first year in school at 7 years of age. He stated that at the beginning of the year, children play during break time with different groups of children and in various physical play activities. However, as the year progresses, the play groups become more stable in the games played and in the children who belong to the groups. Blatchford concluded that "games are a main medium through which groups come together and friendships are formed" (p. 82). Additionally, rough-and-tumble play seems to

have the social function of establishing and maintaining dominance relationships among boys (Humphreys & Smith, 1987; Pellegrini, 1995; Pellegrini & Smith, 1998).

According to Goffman (1963), participation in society or social groups is possible when groups perceive individuals as possessing all the qualities required for participation. The conglomerate of these qualities creates a stereotype. The group measures every individual who wishes to belong to a social group against this stereotype. Each social situation and group has a set of required characteristics that comprise the stereotype. Individuals who do not possess all of these characteristics are said to have disqualifying attributes. As long as these attributes are not known about or visibly evident in a social situation, individuals who possess them are said to be "discreditable persons." If these disqualifying attributes are known about or visible to others in social situations, these individuals become "discredited persons" (Goffman, 1963).

The discredited and discreditable statuses are Goffman's (1963) distinctions that allow for analysis of stigma situational conditions (see Table 45.1). It is important to note that a person may be discredited in one social situation but not in another. For example, individuals must be a certain height to join professional basketball teams. That is, in such social situations, individuals who are "too short for basketball" are discredited; however, the attribute of being "too short for basketball" is not discrediting in other social situations, such as dodgeball or soccer.

Individuals who possess disqualifying attributes that are visible and, therefore, known about become discredited persons in many situations, regardless of their actual ability to participate fully in social situations. The exclusion of persons with physical disabilities from educational settings and work situations regardless of their ability to participate in and perform all required activities is well recorded in the literature (e.g., Frank, 2000).

Table 45.1. A Summary of Goffman's Analytic Conceptualization of Stigma and Its Management

	The Situational Condition	
Attributes of the Situational Condition	**The Discredited Person**	**The Discreditable Person**
Visibility of stigmatizing attribute	Known and/or visible	Potentially knowable or visible
Stigma management technique	Tension management of unease in social contacts	Information control of personal biography
Participation	Restrictions in terms of acceptance and accessibility in physical and social environments	Contingencies: Potential for stigma in the physical and social environment

Note. Adapted from *Aspects of Stigma: Goffman's Stigma—Understanding the Experience of Impairment, Disability and Handicap*, presented by J. V. Cook, 1998, at the 12th International Congress of the World Federation of Occupational Therapists.

When individuals possess disqualifying attributes that are nonvisible, their ability to manage the flow of information about these attributes is crucial for their social participation (Goffman, 1963). One form of managing stigma refers to the process of hiding an attribute when it disqualifies the individual from participating in a social group and revealing it when the attribute is necessary for group participation. Failing to hide the attribute makes it known to the social group, and the social situations become similar to those when the attribute is visible. Successful management of nonvisible disqualifying attributes means that the attributes remain unknown to the social group. In such situations, participation is contingent on individuals' ability to control the flow of information about their disqualifying attributes. For example, persons with mental illness tend to hide their illness when applying for a job; however, they need to declare its existence if they wish to participate in a support group for persons with mental illness who hold a job.

The management of stigma is hard work because persons with nonvisible disqualifying attributes tend to monitor carefully the activities in which they participate so that their disqualifying attributes will not become evident (Goffman, 1963). In the case of developmental coordination disorder, the disqualifying attribute of poor motor coordination needs to be managed for the children to be accepted by their peers. A small qualitative study of parental perceptions of the social lives of their children with developmental coordination disorder is presented here. Findings demonstrate how children manage their disqualifying attribute and the consequences of these management strategies for the children's social participation.

Method

A qualitative interview research design was used in this pilot study (Kvale, 1996; Marshall & Rossman, 1995). Six families with children with motor coordination problems were recruited from an occupational therapy clinic that specializes in teaching children with motor difficulties to perform activities and occupations of their own choice successfully. At the time of this research, the children were no longer clients of the clinic. The pilot project was approved by a university Research Ethics Board, and the approved letters of information and consent forms were sent to potential participants. Only those parents who signed the forms were included in the study. To protect the participants' confidentiality, all names have been replaced with pseudonyms.

Five of the 6 families were dual-parent families. The single-parent family consisted of a mother and two children. The number of children in the families ranged from two to four. Five families lived in an urban area, and 1 lived in a rural area. In two cases, both parents participated in the interview. Five of the 6 children with developmental coordination disorder were boys, ranging in age from 9 to 11 years of age; the girl was 10 years of age. Parents of 5 of the children reported that the children had other comorbid conditions. All 6 children had been given the diagnosis of developmental coordination disorder by a pediatrician. The children whose parents participated in this study were not evaluated by the researchers for the overall presentation of their motor coordination difficulties. Therefore, the findings reflect parental perceptions of when and where the children's motor coordination difficulties become a discrediting attribute.

Each family was interviewed once for 1 hr to 1.5 hr by the first author. Five interviews took place at the participants' homes, and one occurred in a small interview room at the work setting of one of the authors. The first interview question was a "grand tour" inquiry about the family story (Spradley, 1979). The subsequent "mini-tour" questions (Spradley, 1979) covered the following issues: (a) the social life of the children, with a particular focus on peer relationships; (b) the children's experiences at school; and (c) family life and daily routines. The focus in this chapter is on the children's social life.

All interviews were audiotaped and transcribed verbatim by a professional transcriber. The transcripts were checked for accuracy by the interviewer. The transcripts were fully coded, using the grounded theory approach to analysis (Glaser & Strauss, 1967; Strauss & Corbin, 1998). The initial step of open coding, when the data are fractured and labeled with concepts, revealed that the parents' main concerns revolved around their children's social life. The axial coding, when each coding category is analyzed internally for processes and consequences, revealed that parents related their children's motor difficulties and interests to their social experiences. Finally, organizing the categories into a coherent and meaningful whole was done with the aide of Goffman's

(1963) framework of stigma and the ICIDH–2 (WHO, 2001).

Findings and Analysis

During the interviews, the parents talked extensively about their children's social life. The findings are presented in two analytical themes: stigma situations and shaping participation.

Stigma Situations

Persons with an attribute that may discredit them in interaction with others face potential stigma situations. That is, stigmatization—the nonacceptance of the person—can occur if the context of the interaction leads to discovery of the discredited attribute. The disqualifying attributes of children with developmental coordination disorder—their motor coordination difficulties—is not a discrediting attribute in every social situation: Parents who mentioned that their children had fine motor difficulties did not describe related stigma situations. Stigma situations occur in those social circumstances when the motor difficulties interfere with participation and lead to nonacceptance or rejection. In the following quote, Jennifer, mother of an 11-year-old boy with developmental coordination disorder, described a festive school activity in which her son's motor difficulties became evident:

> May Fair is sort of a celebration of spring, and Michael's class…had to dance around the May pole. It's like a form of folk dancing, and everyone holds [a ribbon attached to the top of] a tall pole.…And what happens is…that they weave around each other [and] create a pattern on the pole. And, and it's gorgeous, but if you screw up where you are in the…pattern, the whole group wants to kill you, and it's obvious you've screwed up the pattern.…[During one song] the boys were still, and the girls were weaving in and out, but the other song required him to go in

and out of each others' skipping while the music is going with the thing [ribbon] in their hand, which is difficult for Michael. He couldn't even skip, he was just running, trying to keep up, the other children were skipping. And at the end of it…Mike and Tanya were the two that were twisted. Michael would not budge.…Tanya was yelling and screaming at him that he had to move.…Finally, Tanya bit the bullet and went around, and it was done. The applause came.

By participating in this activity, Michael's inability to skip at 11 years of age became evident. Additionally, his inability to coordinate himself relative to the others in the group interfered with the group's successful execution of the weave. According to Jennifer, it was evident to her and the other parents that Michael was the cause of the unsuccessful execution of the weave. She also described how the audience was very tense and hesitant with the applause. In this stigma situation, Michael was not rejected for the same reason that he participated: It was a school activity in which all the children had to participate. Therefore, Michael could not choose to avoid participation as a way of managing his stigma.

Donna described the refusal of peers to include her 10-year-old daughter with developmental coordination disorder in their physical activities:

Well, at school I think they sort of almost treat her like a younger sibling. You know, they don't treat her as an equal…as their social equal or their intellectual equal or any way of an equal. The kids in her class, it is just kind of, well Nancy is different. They like her, and some of the children are really very nice and kind to her and that they will try to help her out with things and stuff like that, but they treat her more like a younger child than a child their own age. And, they don't include her in things, like if they are doing skipping and things like that. They just say, "Well, you won't be able to do it." They won't even let her try. She gets excluded from a lot.

Here, Donna reported that her daughter's motor difficulties are known to her peer group and that they exclude her from activities that they believe she would not be able to perform. Similarly, Jane, the mother of a 10-year-old boy with developmental coordination disorder, said that classmates will exclude her son when they engage in sports. She added, "He doesn't fit in, and he doesn't feel that he fits in. So he ostracizes himself. And then quite often, they [classmates] will, if they are in the sports."

In terms of stigma management in these cases, these children had difficulties hiding their stigmatizing attribute of motor difficulties. In the first case with the May pole, the stigma situation was related to a school activity in which the child did not have the leeway to exercise a stigma management technique. Embarrassment to the child and his family was the consequence of this stigma situation. In the second case, the peer group was aware of the girl's motor difficulties and excluded her from activities that they thought she could not perform competently. Exclusion from physical activity play was the result of the stigmatizing attribute of motor difficulties becoming known to the peer group. In the last case, the mother suggested that her son's exclusion from physical activity play is the result of both the child's and the peer group's attitudes and behaviors.

Shaping Participation: Avoiding Stigma Situations

Other parents' reports of their children's social life described situations in which the children did not participate in activities in which they could not perform competently. Although these children avoided stigma situations as described previously, it was not clear that their choice always constituted clear examples of stigma management techniques.

Mary described her 9-year-old son with developmental coordination disorder in one social situation as being "literally on the periphery" of physical activity games:

> He is in cubs. At the beginning of the year, he didn't participate in anything, and they do a lot of not competitive games, but physical games, and he just would not. We would go and pick him up, and he would be standing at the wall, smiling, laughing, running along the side where his friends are.

In this case, the child, Johnny, found a way to be part of the group without participating in the physical aspect of the game and making his motor difficulties interfere with the group activity.

The success of this stigma management strategy may be attributed to both Johnny and his peers. Stigma is a situational attribute, that is, persons are stigmatized when their discrediting attribute is visible or known about *and* the group members reject them. Johnny's peer group was different from those of other children in this study. In the following quote, Mary described that Johnny's peers made sure that he could play tag again and that Nick, a peer, used his own strength and wishes to construct a playful experience:

> He's [Johnny] got one friend at school who wants him to play tag. This little kid, Nick, is a soccer player, and he runs like the wind, but he likes to be "It." Johnny will cry and cry and cry [because he could not run fast enough, and he was It most of the time]. At some point this fall, the teacher had to ban all the boys in the class from playing tag partly because Johnny was crying so much. She just got fed up and said no one was playing tag, but this little Nick latched on to Johnny.…So whenever Johnny was It, he would run slowly past Johnny so that Johnny could catch Nick and then Nick would be It, and then everybody is happy again. But she banned them at one point for 2 weeks. None of them could play. And then she told me that after a few days, some of them came back and asked her if they could play, and she said OK, and then a few

more and then a few more, and then they came to her and said, "Can Johnny play again?" She said he hasn't asked. So they went and got Johnny, and they asked him. They told him to go and ask her, and she said OK, but no more crying. [Johnny said,] "OK." Now he does play tag, occasionally. He still prefers his tractors.

Mary described a social environment that is accepting of Johnny and his motor difficulties. In the second quote, Nick was the enabler of smooth and competent games of tag that everyone enjoyed. However, when these special enabling conditions did not exist, as described in the first quote, when Johnny did not participate in the physical aspect of the game, his behavior did not seem to create a stigma situation.

In spite of this accepting and supportive social environment, Mary said that Johnny "does play tag, *occasionally* [italics added]," indicating that Johnny's choices are comparable with his motor abilities. Other parents discussed their children's interests when describing their social lives. For example, Barbara said the following about her 9-year-old son with developmental coordination disorder:

> He never wanted to play baseball. Like, when kids would get together just for fun and play baseball, he would avoid that. He hates baseball and gym. Phys. ed. stuff. He was so hesitant on climbers that [that] was one of the goals that [the occupational therapist] worked with him on. He really wanted to be able to do the fire pole because he really felt that all his friends did the fire pole and everybody…I don't know if they teased him that he couldn't…or if he just never went near it because he knew he wouldn't, you know. But, he's not a sports person at all.

Here, Barbara indicated that not only does her son not like sports activities, but he also avoids participating, even if the purpose of the game is fun. When she talked about her son's possible motivation for asking to learn to do the fire pole in occupational therapy, she described a possible situation in which her son had to decide how to manage his motor difficulties. She suggested that he may have failed to hide it and was laughed at (i.e., a stigma situation) or that he may have avoided it because he knew he could not do it (i.e., a stigma management technique).

In the following quote, Heather, a single mother of a 12-year-old boy with developmental coordination disorder, suggested that her son had no interest in physical activities:

> So, Alex is the one friend that will come over quite frequently, and he'll have sleepovers with and because Alex has sort of his unusual interests too, they will spend a lot of time just walking around together talking, and you think, "What are you doing?" You know, but, [it's] unusual for little boys. You know, they don't play ball, they walk around or they spend time in their room, and they come out with these amazing drawings, or one day they made this fish out of cards that was huge and very complicated.

In this case, Heather described her son as having unusual interests that make him different from her own perceptions of what boys of her son's age usually do (i.e., fulfill the stereotypical image). Heather did not describe any stigma situations or indicate that her son's choices may be related to his awareness of his motor difficulties. However, his interests and choices protected him from getting into situations that may reveal his disqualifying attribute of motor difficulties, as Heather said, "Socially, he has always been a recluse, really. He's never had a lot of friends."

Later in the interview, Heather described how her son could not master riding his bicycles and lost interest in them until the opportunity to master that activity in the safe environment of the occupational therapy clinic occurred. Once he mastered that activity, his interest in riding his bicycles increased, and he rides to visit friends whom he did not seek before.

Discussion

Physical activity play is important for children's social life in terms of acquiring and maintaining friends and belonging to peer groups (Blatchford, 1998). Such activities may be difficult for children with motor coordination problems to master, and this difficulty appears to reduce their participation in activities (Smyth & Anderson, 2000). The findings from this small qualitative study demonstrate that parent perceptions of their children's social life concur with the research findings. Additionally, they indicate that their children's social life may be influenced by the children's interests and their motor coordination difficulties.

In terms of stigma management, parents reported that the children seem to suffer the social consequences of stigma that Goffman (1963) described. As he stated, "The central feature of the stigmatized individual's situation in life…is a question of what is often…called acceptance" (p. 8). Acceptance by others is what the individual with a discrediting attribute strives for, but acceptance often is withheld when the attribute is visible or known about. Thus, the individual faces two possibilities: situations in which he or she must manage stigmatization or situations which are to be avoided to avoid stigmatization. When the children's motor difficulties are known, they often are excluded from (stigmatized) or they avoid participating in (a form of stigma management) physical activity play. Because physical activity play is an important facet of social life and friendship in middle childhood (Blatchford, 1998), the social life of children with developmental coordination disorder is limited. For example, Donna, whose daughter was excluded by her peer group, said that her daughter played with younger children. And Mary, who described her son as being on the periphery of the game, said that her son's social group has been growing as his motor skill has improved.

In terms of the ICIDH–2 (WHO, 2001), parental descriptions indicate that children's impaired performance of physical activities in the context of play in middle childhood may lead to participation restriction. These restrictions are the results of interactions among impaired function (the impaired motor performance), the physical features of the environment (physical activity play), and the social and attitudinal world (the way social groups and friendship evolve in middle childhood). Parents identified accepting peer groups (i.e., social environment) and skill enhancement as factors that mitigated the restrictions on participation.

Perhaps the most significant findings of this study related to the occupational therapy interventions. In the clinic, the children set their own goals. That is, they chose the occupation or the activity that they wanted to work on in therapy. It seems that the children selected physical activities or occupations, such as throwing a ball, going down the fire pole, or riding bicycles. That is, children with developmental coordination disorder who had the opportunity to master the performance of a desired activity or occupation in a safe environment took advantage of this opportunity.

Some parents described the consequences of mastering such new activities and occupations. Mary indicated that her son's improved motor skill actually increased the size of his social group. Heather stated that her son became more adventurous in going to visit friends who live further away from his home as a consequence of his acquired ability to ride his bicycles. Although Heather did not relate the bicycle riding to changes in her son's social life, she talked about it in terms of an increased repertoire of activities and occupations (i.e., visiting friends). These findings indicate an important direction for future research in the area of the effectiveness of occupational therapy interventions, that is, looking at whether and how interventions are effective in the natural environment of the therapy recipients and, in particular, increasing their social inclusion in peer groups.

Conclusion

In this chapter, portions of Goffman's (1963) framework of stigma were used to elucidate the social processes leading from impairment to participation in the case of children with developmental coordination disorder. In particular, the use of his conceptual model to analyze the findings of this study contributes to our understanding of children's behavior as these children deal with their negatively valued difference from other children. The consequences of stigmatization and stigma management techniques adopted by children with a disability need to be incorporated into our theories and conceptual models of practice. Although the findings of this study are tentative, they illustrate the potential for occupational therapy interventions to enhance the social life of children and the significance of using activities that are relevant to the children's lives.

Acknowledgment

This research was supported by a grant from the Social Sciences and Humanities Council (SSHRC, internal competition, 01/1997–12/1999), University of Western Ontario, London, Ontario, Canada.

References

American Psychiatric Association. (1994). *The diagnostic and statistical manual of mental disorders* (4th ed.). Washington, DC: Author.

Blatchford, P. (1998). *Social life in school: Pupils' experience of breaktime and recess from 7 to 16 years.* Bristol, PA: Palmer.

Cook, J. V. (1998, June). *Aspects of stigma: Goffman's stigma—Understanding the experience of impair-*

ment, disability, and handicap. Paper presented at the 12th International Congress of the World Federation of Occupational Therapists, Montreal.

Frank, G. (2000). *Venus on wheels: Two decades of dialogue on disability, biography, and being female*. Los Angeles: University of California Press.

Glaser, B., & Strauss, A. (1967). *The discovery of grounded theory*. Chicago: Aldine.

Goffman, E. (1963). *Stigma: Notes on the management of spoiled identity*. Englewood Cliffs, NJ: Prentice Hall.

Humphreys, A. P., & Smith, P. K. (1987). Rough-and-tumble play, friendship, and dominance in school children: Evidence of continuity and change with age. *Child Development, 58*, 201–212.

Kvale, S. (1996). *InterViews: An introduction to qualitative research interviewing*. Thousand Oaks, CA: Sage.

Marshall, C., & Rossman, G. B. (1995). *Designing qualitative research* (2nd ed.). Thousand Oaks, CA: Sage.

Pellegrini, A. D. (1995). *School recess and playground behavior: Educational and developmental role*. Albany: State University of New York Press.

Pellegrini, A. D., & Smith, P. K. (1998). Physical activity play: The nature and function of a neglected aspect of play. *Child Development, 69,* 577–598.

Smyth, M. M., & Anderson, H. I. (2000). Coping with clumsiness in the school playground: Social and physical play in children with coordination impairments. *British Journal of Developmental Psychology, 18,* 389–413.

Spradley, J. P. (1979). *The ethnographic interview*. New York: Harcourt Brace Jovanovich College.

Strauss, A., & Corbin, J. (1998). *Basics of qualitative research: Techniques and procedures for developing grounded theory* (2nd ed.). Thousand Oaks, CA: Sage.

World Health Organization. (2001). *International classification of functioning, disability and health: Final draft*. Geneva, Switzerland: Author.

CHAPTER 46

Adaptive Strategies of Mothers With Children With Attention Deficit Hyperactivity Disorder

Enfolding and Unfolding Occupations

Ruth Segal

Ruth Segal, PhD, OTR,
is assistant professor,
Department of Occupational
Therapy, School of Education,
New York University, 35
West 4th Street, 11th Floor,
New York, NY 10012-1172;
rs108@is2.nyu.edu.

Because occupations occur in the stream of time, according to Clark et al. (1991), their study cannot be divorced from the study of time use. Hall (1983) described monochronic and polychronic ways of using time as cultural phenomena. Monochronic time use means scheduling occupations in sequence to be performed one at a time. This process consists of separating occupations, allotting them periods of time, and temporally locating them in the designated temporal slots. Each temporal slot is dedicated to the performance of a single occupation. Monochronic time use is clock-centered; schedules regulate engagement in occupations. When the performance of an occupation involves interactions with others, schedules regulate the time allotted for personal interactions (Hall, 1983).

Polychronic time use is person-centered; the relative importance of persons determines the relative importance of occupations and influences the time it takes to complete them (Hall, 1983). Scheduling is impossible when polychronic time is used. For example, Hall (1983) presented a hypothetical situation of a "monochronic" woman who shows up for her appointment with a "polychronic" hairdresser only to find that the hairdresser chose to "squeeze into" her schedule relatives and personal friends who just dropped in. Therefore, the haircuts for relatives and friends are completed before the customer's haircut.

Polychronic and monochronic time use systems coexist in North American society (Hall, 1983). The public sphere tends to be monochronic in nature, whereas the private sphere of the family tends to be polychronic (Hall, 1983; Zerubavel, 1981). This difference in time use within society may be attributed to gender, the number of the occupations, or the nature of the occupations. In her study of how housework and child care are shared in dual-earner families, Hochschild (1989) observed that only women tended to do two or more occupations at a time. Hall (1983) suggested that for mothers to perform all the

Originally published 2000
in *American Journal of*
Occupational Therapy, 54,
300–306.

occupations expected of them, they must use polychronic time because "how else can one raise several children at once, run a household, hold a job, be a wife, mother, nurse, tutor, chauffeur, and general fixer-upper?" (p. 52).

Lastly, Bateson (1996) suggested that the occupation of caring for a child cannot be regulated by schedules; therefore, other occupations have to be done whenever they can fit with child care. She named this phenomenon of doing more than one thing at a time "enfolded occupations" and described it as "[consisting] of all that can be done while caring for a child" (p. 7).

Ecocultural Theory and Time Use as Adaptive Strategy

In their ecocultural theory, Gallimore, Weisner, Kaufman, and Bernheimer (1989) suggested that parents strive to raise their children according to their values. Such socialization of children requires that parents mediate the effects of their environment. Parental mediation activity consists of using perceived environmental resources to overcome perceived environmental constraints. Time is an environmental feature that can be perceived as a resource or as a constraint.

The amount of time that persons and their families have at their disposal is limited by their participation in work and school (Zerubavel, 1981) and their need for sleep (Fraser, 1987). Families and individuals may use this disposable time to their advantage by organizing occupations in ways that improve their life opportunities and enhance their quality of life (Frank, 1996). The actions taken to organize and reorganize occupations are adaptive strategies (Frank, 1996). They mediate the effects of limited disposable time. In Primeau (1998), enfolding play with children with housework was the adaptive strategy that some parents used to increase the amount of time they spend with their children.

Time Use and Families With Children With ADHD

Children with attention deficit hyperactivity disorder (ADHD) may exhibit one or more of the following symptoms: short attention span, impulsive behavior, and hyperactivity (American Psychiatric Association, 1994). These symptoms are associated with impaired occupational performance in areas such as self-care, schoolwork, and personal responsibility (e.g., chore performance, homework) (Barkley, 1998).

Interventions with children with ADHD consist of medications, counseling, and parent education, especially about special needs (Barkley, 1998; Kelly & Aylward, 1992; Hinshaw, 1994). Additionally, parents may be instructed to simplify their children's occupations and routines by breaking them into smaller tasks and directing the children to take one step at time (Kelly & Aylward, 1992). Such adaptations to the children's daily routines may require parents to increase the time they spend with their children.

The purpose of this study was to describe the daily experiences and adaptations of families with children who have ADHD in the context of schedules, routines, and occupations and, in particular, how maternal experiences and perceptions of their children's abilities and limitations inform the mother's selection and use of adaptive strategies of time use.

Method

Participants

The 17 families who participated in this study were recruited from a national support group for children with ADHD and their families and from an occupational therapy and physical therapy clinic. Three of the families had 2 children with ADHD, thus the total sample of children with ADHD was 20.

Families consisted of 12 dual-parent families and 5 single-parent families (mothers with their children). Nine of the mothers, including the five single mothers, were employed. Socioeconomic status was described by 9 families as upper-middle class (annual income ranged from $50,000 to more than $100,000), by 4 families as middle class (annual income ranged from $15,000–$50,000), and by 4 families as lower-middle class (annual income ranged from $15,000–$50,000). One mother was Hispanic, and the rest of the parents were of European descent. Three families had one child, and 14 had two to four children.

Of the 20 children with ADHD, 14 took Ritalin™, a short-acting medication (3–5 hr) that helps to reduce the symptoms of ADHD. Its most common side effects are insomnia and loss of appetite. The medication's regimen commonly covered school hours and 2 to 3 hr after school (8:00 a.m.–4:00 p.m. or 5:00 p.m.), ensuring that the children's physiological needs for food and sleep were addressed. Such a regimen also meant that during most of the time spent with their families, the children's symptoms were not controlled by medication.

Data Collection

Data were collected with one to four interviews per family. Of the 38 interviews conducted, 9 were with both parents, 1 was with a father, and 28 were with mothers. In the first interview, parents were asked, "Tell me the story of your family." Most responded by providing a detailed account of the development of their children with ADHD, the manifestations of their children's ADHD, how the diagnosis was made, the children's qualities and strengths, and the challenges they face as parents of children with ADHD.

In the second, more structured interview, parents were asked to describe what happened at their home from the time the first person got up until the last person went to sleep as well as how each occupation was performed, who was engaged in performing various occupations, who supervised the children's occupational performance, and how the children were encouraged to engage in their occupations.

All the interviews were audiotaped, yielding a total of 2 to 5 hr per family. The audiotapes were transcribed verbatim by a professional transcriber. The researcher verified the accuracy of the transcription by listening to the audiotapes while reading the transcriptions. Data were also collected via field notes, which described the parents' nonverbal behaviors during the interview (Spradley, 1979).

Data Analysis

Each interview was analyzed as soon as it was transcribed, following the grounded theory guidelines suggested by Strauss and Corbin (1990). Data analysis, therefore, began as soon as the transcript of the first interview was available. Data were coded into meaningful conceptual units (e.g., categories, themes), then each category was examined for conditions, context, strategies, and consequences (as perceived by the parents) (Strauss & Corbin, 1990).

It was clear from the analysis of the first interviews that the difficulties children with ADHD had in completing their own occupations interfered with their families' schedules, routines, and occupations. Subsequent data analysis focused on these disruptions in family life. The intent was to identify and describe when and under what conditions these disruptions occurred and what strategies were used to overcome or prevent them (Strauss & Corbin, 1990).

Trustworthiness and credibility were ensured through triangulation of the data collection methods (i.e., unstructured interviews, semistructured interviews, field notes), through a field journal, and through negative case analysis

(Krefting, 1991; Lincoln & Guba, 1985). Trustworthiness was further enhanced by two additional rounds of data analysis: (a) treating the data as a set of 17 separate family cases and (b) dividing the data into two subsets—the family story transcripts and the daily schedules and routine transcripts. A time lapse of about 1 month between each round of data analysis, a code–recode approach (Krefting, 1991), permitted the researcher to compare subsequent findings with previous findings.

This chapter discusses only the theme of maternal time use as an adaptive strategy. Most of the data were derived from the second interviews, in which mothers described their daily schedules, routines, and how occupations were performed. In the following sections, pseudonyms were used for all persons and locations.

Findings and Interpretations: Enfolding and Unfolding Occupations

Participants described maternal time use strategies as crucial for enabling the occupational performance of their children with ADHD. Mothers tended to use two adaptive strategies—enfolding and unfolding. *Enfolding* occupations is doing more than one occupation at a time (Bateson, 1996). *Unfolding* consists of removing chunks of activities from previously established sequences of enfolded occupations (Segal, 1995). Unfolding leads to a more monochronic time schedule. Mothers using unfolding focused solely on supporting their child's participation in occupations and excluded the performance of overlapping occupations inherent in enfolding. In using unfolding, mothers either chose to perform the previously co-occurring occupations at another time (temporal unfolding) or assigned them to another person at the original time (unfolding by inclusion) (Segal, 1995).

Enfolding Occupations

Enfolding occupations was used by almost all the mothers in this study at some point during the day. Some used this strategy carefully. For example, one mother enfolded the occupation of supervising her children's dressing with the occupation of her own dressing. To facilitate the performance of these occupations, she engaged her children by presenting dressing to them as a play occupation:

> I've gotten to where I kind of have a contest who gets dressed first, who can get dressed the fastest, and, of course, I'm always last. I have more to put on than them. They are pretty good. John is usually first which . . . sometimes that bothers Sherry. Sometimes if he's asleep when I wake up, I'll wake her up first so that she gets her chance to be first, too. [Cathy, an employed widowed mother of a 10-year-old boy with Tourette syndrome and ADHD and an 8-year-old daughter with ADHD]

Before giving a different meaning to the dressing activity, this mother described the arguments she used to have with her children to continue with their dressing because she could not enlist their attention or cooperation.

Another mother enfolded the occupation of monitoring her son's sleep with her leisure occupation of quilting because she found that interrupted quilting did not disturb her as much as interrupted sleep:

> By 9:00 it's my time....[I go to sleep at] 11:30 or 12:00; I like to have a good solid time [to quilt] because sometimes, Jeff [the child with ADHD] wakes up with nightmares. So if I go to bed early, he'll wake up and then I'll have to wake up anyway. So, until he is really solidly asleep, you know, I don't go to bed until then. [Mary, a married, stay-at-home mother of three boys 9, 7, and 4 years of age. The 7-year-old has ADHD]

Enfolding occupations was most commonly used when mothers perceived that there was no other alternative, as in the following example of a family in which the father does not help with either dinner or the child's homework:

> From the time we get home, usually, we start homework of some sort or another. He's supposed to have done some when he's at the sitter's and the Y[MCA]. But there's always some that has to be done. So while I'm working making dinner he's trying to read to me or he's trying to do spelling or multiplication tables or something like that when I'm doing dinner. . . . When [my husband] gets home from work . . . he becomes a couch potato, and he kind of watches TV or works on crafts. [Julie, an employed, married mother of a 9-year-old son with ADHD]

Julie also talked about her family's financial difficulties and how it limits her ability to get hired help.

In the mornings, enfolding occupations was common even among families that used the unfolding strategy in the afternoons and evenings. The following example is given by a mother who paid a tutor to help her daughter with homework while she was preparing dinner:

> [I put the timer on for 10 min and] I'm just putting her in the front bathroom, and I close the door and I say, "You cannot come out until you are dressed." And I do that with her brother too because he will play around. . . . Then I put [the timer] on for another 10 min and in that time she's got to make her bed, brush her teeth, and do her hair. Ideally, if they got all this done, then they'd have some play time. But it rarely works out. They are usually dragging their feet, and then I end up by having to yell. . . . In between all this, I'm trying to get dressed. [Jenny, a married, stay-at-home mother of a 7-year-old daughter with ADHD and a 5-year-old son]

Although the father was commonly at home in the morning, he did not take part in the morning routine.

The following mother described her enfolded occupations in the mornings, although her husband was home. In the afternoons, however, the husband was very involved with their children, making sure that the mother had time to prepare dinner. This family could not afford to pay for hired help.

> [My husband]. . . . if he doesn't have a job, he's still in bed. So it's me. I went to get dressed, and I warned him [the child with ADHD] before I went "Jimmy, I'm going to go to the bathroom, I'm going to get dressed. I don't want to stop getting dressed to come out." And of course I did, so I had to split them up. I sent him to the kitchen because he had the TV on in there. But at least he sat quietly. [Mary, a married, stay-at-home mother of a 7-year-old son with ADHD and a 4-year-old daughter]

Supervising the children's morning routine and occupational performance seemed to be the mothers' responsibility; hired help and other family members were not commonly involved at this time of the day. The mothers tended to facilitate the children's occupational performance through reminders, using timers, or reframing the activity.

Temporal Unfolding: The Reconstruction of Maternal Occupations

Temporal unfolding occurred when mothers reconstructed their own occupations so that they would be able to focus on enabling their children's occupational performance. This adaptive strategy left the mother as the only or main person who was working with the child with ADHD. This strategy was more common among families with limited financial resources and support systems, when the size of the family unit was small (i.e., single mothers), or when the spouses were not involved with the children. Typically, maternal needs were not considered when mothers decided to use temporal unfolding.

This mother described how she solved the problem of her daughter's morning tantrums by addressing only the child's needs. The mother performed her own hygiene, grooming, and dressing after she returned home from driving her daughter to school.

> She does not do well if you wake her up. She also does not do well if you try to hurry her. So I try to always make sure there's time in the mornings. My needs go last. I'll go to the bathroom when I can and brush my teeth and wash my face after I've already said hello to her. Then typically I'll not get dressed. I'll put a coat on or I'll put on sweats and take her to school. I don't worry about how I look because to me, it is more important for her to have as much time as possible in the morning. [Jennifer, a married, stay-at-home mother of two daughters 9 and 4 years of age, whose older daughter has ADHD]

This employed mother chose to temporally unfold the morning routine by doing her own dressing and preparing everything for the day before she woke up her children:

> My weekdays start about 4:45 in the morning. I get up, take my shower, get everything ready for the day. Pull their snack packs, put their ice packs in there, put them by the door—just get it organized. Around 6:30 to 6:45 in the morning, I wake them up. I usually dress them—at least once because they will take something off and throw it around the house. I do this individually [for] each of the children.

> I come downstairs and we normally eat breakfast. We are out of the house somewhere around 7:30, if I'm lucky, and they remember to leave everything at the door. . . . [We] get home around 6:45 to 7:00 in the evening. Right away . . . normally on the weekend, I cook enough so I just pull out a portion; defrost it in the microwave and heat it up. That's their first meal of the night. [Angela, a divorced,

working mother of a 6-year-old son and a 4-year-old daughter, both with ADHD]

Angela also performed most of the homemaking occupations after the children went to sleep. To manage this complete temporal unfolding of homemaking and child care, Angela had to limit her own sleep to 4 or 5 hours a night.

Unfolding by Inclusion: Decreasing the Number of Maternal Occupations

Mothers delegated occupations or chunks of activity to another person to strategically eliminate occupations in their routines and, therefore, enhance their ability to meet their children's needs. Similar to temporal unfolding, this strategy leads to more monochronic maternal time use. In this strategy, another family member or hired help steps in to complete one of the previously enfolded occupations. The intention is to reduce the mother's stress and burden and to enable the children's occupational performances. This strategy was available to families with the financial means to pay for help or with friends or members who actively assisted in child care or homemaking.

In the following example, the father participates in homemaking occupations, which frees the mother to focus on her son's needs and abilities:

> As soon as we get home, it's accomplishing homework. . . . I'm usually the person that does the homework with him while [my husband] is either fixing our dinner or cleaning up [after dinner]. [Susan, a married, employed, mother of a 7-year-old son with ADHD and a 20-year-old son who does not live at home. Her husband took partial retirement to be able to participate equally in raising their child]

According to both parents, this paternal involvement increased their quality of life as a family and as individuals.

The following family has a housekeeper who prepares breakfast 5 days a week:

Father: We all get up at about 6:45. That's everybody simultaneously at once.

Mother: If there is any difficulty, I have a kitchen timer that I set. The goal that we work toward is that he is dressed and his bed is made . . . [that] he puts away his pajamas and is ready to come downstairs to eat breakfast at 7:00.

Father: Right. He comes down, and the housekeeper fixes him breakfast. [Joan and James, employed, married parents of a 7-year-old son with ADHD]

Joan viewed timer use as a process to train the child to be independent in his occupations of dressing and making his bed. Once the child becomes independent, parental supervision will not be needed, and their morning routine will be unfolded.

The next example describes the morning routine as consisting of temporal unfolding, enfolding, and unfolding by inclusion:

I get up probably between 6:45 and 7:00 or 7:15. . . . I'll get dressed and everything and then I'll . . . either wake my daughter up or she's already up and tell her "get dressed." [temporal unfolding]. . . . A lot of times she's already up and getting dressed in her eclectic-looking outfits. . . . My son, Paul, a lot of times he's still asleep. I'll come downstairs, I'll feed the cat, I'll take my medicine, and then I'll go to work [enfolding]. My husband sets his alarm for about 7:30, I think. And so if my daughter's not up, he'll wake her up. Usually, I've gotten her up though. Then he'll give her breakfast, give her her medicine, and take her to school, and then he gives my son his medicine [unfolding by inclusion]. [Cynthia, an employed mother of a 7-year-old daughter and a 5-year-old son, both with ADHD. She takes medicine for depression]

It is possible for Cynthia to engage the father in the morning routine because the night shifts that he worked ended at 2:00 a.m.

This mother also uses temporal unfolding, enfolding, and unfolding by inclusion to complete her morning routine and make sure that her son is ready for the school bus. In this case, however, she delegated some of the supervision of her son's dressing to her own mother:

I usually get up, by choice, at about 5:30 or 5:45. . . . I get the paper; I have a little . . . breathing room when I am alone. I make my coffee, I pack my lunch. If I need to get something ready for him to take to school, I get that ready. . . . He's usually up about 6:00, 6:30. I ideally try to get some kind of breakfast into him. I am doing this and at the same time I'm making my bed, getting ready for work, taking my shower. . . . But my mother does help out a great deal. She sees that he is dressed. [Deanne, a widowed employed mother of a 10-year-old boy with ADHD. They live with Deanne's mother]

In the following morning routine, the level of supervision and the type of unfolding used varies according to the children's ages. The occupational performances of the two older children do not require supervision, permitting the mother to engage in her own spiritual occupation. The mother supervises the occupational performance of her 11-year-old son with ADHD while the father supervises the 5-year-old:

The alarm goes off between 5:30 and 5:45 in the morning, and I get up no later than 5:00 to 6:00. I get up my 16-year-old and my 14-year-old because they have to be at a class at 6:30 in the morning. I get them up, and while they are getting ready and showering and so forth, I usually spend the time from 6:00 to 6:30 [reading] scriptures. I want that connection. And I usually say a prayer, by myself. They leave at 6:30 and then I get Clark up . . . the one with the learning problem.

So, I get Clark up and his clothes are all ready and I bring him into my bedroom because his little brother is still asleep, and while he is getting ready and feeding his fish and so forth, I come downstairs, I make his lunch, and I make breakfast. He comes down about 6:45 and he empties the dishwasher, which is his chore, and then he sits down and he has his breakfast. Then he has to wash his face, brush his teeth, comb his hair, bring all of his books down, and then at 7:00 we start practicing the piano. And we practice from 7:00 to 7:30.

At 7:00 my husband gets up and gets the 5-year-old up. He gets him breakfast, bathed, and ready for school. At 7:15 my other two boys come home. They eat their breakfast.

At 7:40 everybody leaves for school. My husband takes them to school. I get ready. I get into some old clothes and I go walking and I walk 2.5 miles. [Brenda, a married mother of four boys (16, 14, 11, and 5 years of age), whose 11-year-old has ADHD]

In terms of strategies of time use, this mother temporally unfolded her own morning routine and spiritual occupation from the occupation of supervising the morning routine of her 11-year-old son. She enfolded breakfast and lunch preparations with the supervising occupation and unfolded from her routine the supervision of the 5-year-old's occupational performance by delegating to the father.

Certain conditions, circumstances, and consequences influenced the use of enfolding, temporal unfolding, and unfolding by inclusion. Generally, enfolding occurred during the morning routine, regardless of the availability of financial and human resources. Mothers in families with limited financial and human resources tended to enfold occupations in the afternoons as well. Unfolding commonly occurred in the afternoons and evenings. Temporal unfolding was common among families with limited financial and human resources. Unfolding by inclusion was common among families that could afford the financial and human resources required for using it. Temporal

unfolding tended to increase, and unfolding by inclusion to lighten, the burden on the mothers.

Discussion

Maternal Time Use as an Adaptive Strategy

Enfolding occupations, or polychronic time use, has been described as the most person-oriented style of time use (Bateson, 1996; Hall, 1983). However, this style does not seem to function well for families with children with ADHD. The simultaneous performance of several occupations along with supervision of the occupational performance of the children with ADHD was commonly related to conflicts with the children and to work left undone. The mothers used unfolding to limit the number of occupations they were performing at a given time and to change polychronic time use to monochronic time use. They reported that these adaptations allowed them to be more child-centered.

This difference may be attributed to the difficulties that children with ADHD have performing occupations and their tendency to continuously move from one unfinished task to another. The mothers in this study reported that they needed to supervise their children very closely to keep them engaged in their occupations. If the children became engaged in a new occupation, redirecting them to the original task meant interrupting them in their current endeavors, which could become a conflict. In terms of Frank's (1996) concept of adaptation, the use of unfolding, an adaptive strategy, enhanced the quality of life of families by limiting the opportunities for conflicts with the children.

Strategies of Time Use, Adaptation, and Ecocultural Theory

The assumptions of ecocultural theory are as follows: (a) Families actively mediate the effects of their environment, (b) the setting for this mediation activity is in the construction of activity settings and daily routine, and (c) the mediation activity consists of using perceived resources to offset the effects of perceived constraints (Gallimore et al., 1989). Activity settings consist of "who is present, their values and goals, what tasks are being performed, why are they being performed (the motives and feelings surrounding action), and what scripts govern interactions, including those that shape and constrain the child's participation" (Gallimore et al., 1989, p. 217). One can assume that the construct of activity setting is similar to the construct of occupations (Segal, 1998).

The use of temporal unfolding may be interpreted as perceiving time as a resource that can be allocated to different occupations. For example, the 8 hours that are commonly allocated to sleep may be used for other occupations such as getting dressed and getting lunches ready. As indicated earlier, the decision to use temporal unfolding was related to the perception that the family does not have the financial and human resources to use for unfolding by inclusion. Such actions of using perceived resources to overcome perceived constraints is predicted by the ecocultural theory.

Unfolding by inclusion, on the other hand, may be interpreted as viewing time as a constraint. The perception is that there are too many occupations to be completed in a 24-hr day; therefore, some of the occupations must be delegated to someone else. As discussed earlier, choosing unfolding by inclusion was related to the perception that the family has the financial and human resources to support the use of this strategy. As Gallimore et al. (1989) discussed, the perception of what constitutes a resource and what constitutes a constraint differs among families. In this study, for example, although dual-parent families with higher incomes tended to use unfolding by

inclusion, at least two single-mother families with lower incomes used this strategy as well.

Implications for Occupational Science and Occupational Therapy

The findings indicate that enfolding and unfolding occupations were used as adaptive strategies among mothers with children with ADHD. Children's ages, the nature of the children's special needs, and financial and human resources influenced what adaptive strategies could be used and the effects of their use. The shift from polychronic time use, in which enfolding occupations are common, to monochronic time use, in which unfolding occupations are common, actually facilitated the mothers' ability to be oriented toward the person (their children with ADHD) and their occupations. This contradicts the few discussions in the literature about monochronic and polychronic time use (Bateson, 1996; Hall, 1983; Zerubavel, 1981). Although Hall (1983) suggested that in monochronic time, persons are relatively unimportant, in this study, unfolding occupations allowed the mothers to fully attend to their children with ADHD while they were performing their occupations. That is, the one-on-one interactions that are typical in monochronic time use became advantageous for raising children with ADHD. Additional studies of the organization of occupations among families with children of different ages and different special needs would contribute to a more complete understanding of time use as an adaptive strategy.

The finding that human and financial resources influence human choice is important for occupational science research as well as for clinicians. In particular, when purposeful use of enfolding or unfolding occupations are suggested, therapists need to discuss with parents the feasibility of using these strategies. Therapists must carefully discuss with the main caregiver what happens during stressful interactions with the children. If it seems that a change in the organization of occupations is needed, then unfolding or enfolding can be suggested. Before they suggest using an adaptive strategy, therapists must explore what resources are available to the family.

Acknowledgments

I thank Gelya Frank, PhD, for our discussions and her valuable advice during and after my dissertation work.

This chapter was supported by the American Occupational Therapy Foundation Center for Research on Adaptation and Occupation (1992–1995) at the Department of Occupational Science and Therapy, University of Southern California. Principal investigator: Florence Clark, PhD, OTR, FAOTA.

References

American Psychiatric Association. (1994). *A diagnostic and statistical manual of mental disorders* (4th ed.). Washington, DC: Author.

Barkley, R. A. (1998). *Attention-deficit hyperactivity disorder: A handbook for diagnosis and treatment.* New York: Guilford.

Bateson, M. C. (1996). Enfolded activity and the concept of occupation. In R. Zemke & F. Clark (Eds.), *Occupational science: The evolving discipline* (pp. 5–12). Philadelphia: F. A. Davis.

Clark, F. A., Parham, D., Carlson, M. E., Frank, G., Jackson, J., Pierce, D., et al. (1991). Occupational science: Academic innovation in the service of occupational therapy's future. *American Journal of Occupational Therapy, 45,* 300–310.

Frank, G. (1996). The concept of adaptation as a foundation for occupational science research. In R.

Zemke & F. Clark (Eds.), *Occupational science: The evolving discipline* (pp. 47–55). Philadelphia: F. A. Davis.

Fraser, J. T. (1987). *Time, the familiar stranger.* Amherst: University of Massachusetts Press.

Gallimore, R., Weisner, T. S., Kaufman, S. Z., & Bernheimer, L. P. (1989). The social construction of ecocultural niches: Family accommodation of developmentally delayed children. *American Journal on Mental Retardation, 94,* 216–230.

Hall, E. T. (1983). *The dance of life: The other dimension of time.* Toronto, Ontario: Anchor.

Hinshaw, S. P. (1994). *Attention deficit and hyperactivity in children.* Thousand Oaks, CA: Sage.

Hochschild, A. (1989). *The second shift.* New York: Avon.

Kelly, D. P., & Aylward, G. P. (1992). Attention deficits in school-aged children and adolescents. *Pediatric Clinics of North America, 39,* 487–512.

Krefting, L. (1991). Rigor in qualitative research: The assessment of trustworthiness. *American Journal of Occupational Therapy, 45,* 214–222.

Lincoln, Y. S., & Guba, E. A. (1985). *Naturalistic inquiry.* Newbury Park, CA: Sage.

Primeau, L. A. (1998). Orchestration of work and play within families. *American Journal of Occupational Therapy, 52,* 188–195.

Segal, R. (1995). *Family adaptation to a child with attention-deficit hyperactivity disorder.* Unpublished doctoral dissertation, University of Southern California, Los Angeles.

Segal, R. (1998). The construction of family occupations: A study of families with children who have attention deficit/hyperactivity disorder. *Canadian Journal of Occupational Therapy, 65,* 286–292.

Spradley, J. P. (1979). *The ethnographic interview.* Toronto, Ontario: Harcourt Brace Jovanovich.

Strauss, A., & Corbin, J. (1990). *Basics of qualitative research: Grounded theory procedures and techniques.* Newbury Park, CA: Sage.

Zerubavel, E. (1981). *Hidden rhythms: Schedules and calendars in social life.* Los Angeles: University of California Press.

Index

Note. References in **boldface** type indicate tables. References in *italic* type indicate figures.

A

Abilities, 445–447
Academic performance, 183
Acceptance, 538
Accommodation, 477, 484
Achievement leisure occupations, 362, 368–369, 371, 372
Activity settings, 480
ADHD. *See* attention deficit/hyperactivity disorder (ADHD)
Adolescents, 360–372, 507
Adultcentrism, 38
Adults, 396–397, 398
Advocacy, 17
Advocates, 450, 510
Affect, 201, 203, *203*
Affective skills, 5
Airway vulnerability, 8
Anticipation, 484, 497–498
Asperger syndrome, 351–357
Aspiration, 8
ASQ. *See* Conners Abbreviated Symptom Questionnaire (ASQ)
Assessment of Motor and Process Skills (School AMPS), 88–92
Athletics, 368–369, 371
Attachment patterns, 5–6
Attention, 216, 219
Attention deficit/hyperactivity disorder (ADHD)
    adaptive approaches, 302–310
    classroom seating, 268–276
    criteria, 144–145
    described, 289
    mothers' adaptive strategies, 541–550
    weighted vests therapy, 289–299
Attention seeking, 398
Attention span, 410

Attractor state, 66
Auditory processing, 355
Auditory system, **100**
Authority, 39–41
Autism spectrum disorders, 130–139, *135*, **136**
Awareness
    assessment, 111–112
    defined, 110
    evaluation, 114
    example, 162

B

Baby showers, 524
Balancing, of activities, 496–497
Battelle Developmental Screening Test (BDST), 457
Behavior problems, 49–50
Behavioral distress, 241
Behavioral impairment, 54
Birthdays, 524
Bottle-feeding, 9
Brain tissue, in children, 51
Breastfeeding, 9–10
Bruininks-Oseretsky Test of Motor Proficiency (BOTMP), 121, 143
Burn patients, 242–251

C

Canadian Model of Occupational Performance (CMOP), 3–7, *4*, 11–12, 306
Canalization, 476–477
Cardiopulmonary impairment, 54
Caregivers
    attachment patterns, 6
    child care assistance, 455–463
    as clients, 18
    feeding infants with CHD, 10–11
    interactions with disabled children, 254
    time use, 301–310

Caregiver's Activity and Recording of Events (CARE) Inventory, 458
Categorization, 109, 114
Cerebral palsy, and playfulness, 255–265
Chairs, *vs.* therapy balls, 268–276
CHD. *See* congenital heart disease (CHD)
Child care assistance, 455–463
Child-sensitive methods, 497
Children
   communication, 37–47, 41–42
   focus on abilities, 38
   research adaptations, 42–44
Chinese Handwriting Speed Test (CHAST), 406
Choices, children's, 539
Classification. *See* categorization
Classroom assessment, 88–92
Classroom seating, 268–276
Clients, pediatric, 18
CMOP. *See* Canadian Model of Occupational Performance (CMOP)
Co-occupation, 529
Code of Ethics, 380–382, **381**
Cognitive impairment, 54
Cognitive orientation to daily occupational performance (CO-OP), 165
Cognitive performance, 122
Cognitive skills, 5
Collaboration, 424, 465–474
Communication, 37–47, 264
Communication impairment, 55
Community reentry, 56
Competence, perceived, 420
Competencies, 38–39, 420
Congenital heart disease (CHD), 7–12
Congestive heart failure, 8
Conners Abbreviated Symptom Questionnaire (ASQ), 122
Construction of routines, 478–486
Consultative model, 209–214
Control parameters, 67
Cues
   general nature, 165
   interpretation, 498
   learning ability, 160
   in play, 263
Cultural scripts, 483–484
Culture, 485, 529
Cyanosis, 8

D
Daily routines
   impact, 476–478
   mothers' orchestration, 490–503
   mothers with disabled children, 478–486, 509–510
   time constraints, 485
Decision-making, 263–264
Deductive reasoning, 109, 114–115
Deductive Reasoning test, 110–116
Deep pressure, 215–216, 290–291
Deficit areas, 471–472
Delegation, 546–548
Development
   after TBI, 52–53
   home as play space, 518–530
   impact of daily routines, 476–478
Developmental coordination disorder (DCD)
   assessment, 141–153
   criteria, 145, 161
   described, 532–533
   learning, 159–166
   and stigma, 533–539
Developmental Coordination Disorder Questionnaire (DCDQ), 142–153
Developmental delay, 194–207
Developmental processes, 61–62, 62–68
Developmental stages, 42
Developmental Test of Visual-Motor Integration (VMI)
   described, 121–122, 184, 185, 406–407
   limitations, 191
Developmental Test of Visual Perception (DTVP), 172–173
Dewey, John, 230
Diffuse axonal injuries (DAI), 50
Direct-indirect intervention, *vs.* consultative model, 209–214
Discredited persons, 533–534
Distraction, 219, 221, 226
Division of labor, 456, 459–460
Downward social comparison, 434
Draw-A-Person test, 173
Drawing, 78–86, 191
Dropouts, 368–369, 371
DST. *See* dynamic systems theory
Dynamic assessment, 108–109
Dynamic system models, 62–68
Dynamic systems theory (DST), 323–324, 328

E
Early intervention
   case study, 18–20
   current practice, 15–16
   developmental perspective, 69

TBI patients, 56
theoretical foundations, 60–61
Ecocultural niche, 477
Ecocultural theory
assumptions, 548–549
described, 477, 484
and time use, 542
Education, of therapists, 471, 473
Education for All Handicapped Children Act of
1975 (EHA), 376, 377
Educationally related services, 376–377
Embrace of paradox, 493
Emergent behavior, 64–68
Emotional shift, 499
Enfolding occupations
described, 542, 544
examples, 544–545, 548
and families with ADHD children, 548
Environment
CMOP context, 5–6
maternal management of, 518–530
and mothers' routines, 485
ESP. *See* Evaluation of Sensory Processing (ESP)
ETCH. *See* Evaluation Tool of Children's
Handwriting (ETCH)
Ethical dilemma, 380–382, **381**
Evaluation of Sensory Processing (ESP), 96–106
Evaluation Tool of Children's Handwriting
(ETCH), 281, 343–344
Exclusion, 496
Executive functions, 110
Expectations
parental, 450–451
parental shift after occupational therapy, 449–450
parents' identification of, 424
Experience, 63–64
Experience Sampling Method, 363
Eye-hand coordination, 172

F
Faith in God, 499–500
Families. *See also* fathers; mothers; parents
accommodations by, 302
as clients, 18
involvement in therapy, 16
Family-centered therapy
case study, 18–20
challenges, 15–21
characteristics, 465–466
Fathers
participation in caregiving, 546, 547–548
performing child care, 459–460, 461

Feedback, 231
Feeding
CMOP framework, 4–7
concerns with CHD, 7–12
developmental process, 64, 66
handicapped children, 501, **502**
independent, 478
by toddlers, 328–337
Feeding difficulties, 8
Fine motor skills
handwriting speed, 405
interventions, 169
school occupational performance, 90–91
Forecasting, 498
Fragile X syndrome, 315–325
Framing, 263
Friendship frames, 399
Fun Scale, 245, *245,* 249–250
Function, 168–169
Functional play, 328–337
FXS. *See* fragile X syndrome

G
Gifts, 524
Glasgow Coma Scale (GCS), 49, **50**
Goal Attainment Scaling (GAS), 210
Goals, 210, 481–482
God, 499–500
Graded motor practice, 169–170
Graphomotor skills, 75, 78–86
Grip
categorization, 83–84, *340,* 340–341
drawing accuracy, 84–85
forms, **76,** 76–77, *77*
graphomotor skills, 75, 78–86
handwriting, 339–349
Grounded theory, 519

H
Hands-on occupation, 232–238
Handwriting
background, 23
children's, 339–349
in first-grade students, 278–287
intervention approaches, 85–86
proficiency issues, 404–405
speed study, 405–410
Hassle Scale, 491–492
Health, orchestration of, 489
Hebrew Handwriting Evaluation (HHE), 122
Helping, 395–396, 399
Holidays, 524

Home environment, 518–530, 526
Hyperactivity, 126

I
IDEA. *See* Individuals With Disabilities Education
    Act of 1990 (IDEA)
Identity, 532–539
Imitation, 63–64, 65
In-hand manipulation, 172
Individuals With Disabilities Education Act of
    1990 (IDEA), 52, 377, 415
Inductive reasoning, 109
Infant feeding, 4–12
Infant mental health, 16–18
Infants
    affective development, 10
    development through play, 518–530
    play development, 254–265
    socialization, 9–10
Informants, 38–39
Informed consent, 43
Intention, 62–64
International Classification of Functioning,
    Disability and Health (ICIDH), 532
Interpreting, 498
Interpretive interactionism approach, 493
Interviews, on children, 44–45
Invisibility, 514
Isolation, 391, 514

K
Kinesthesis, 278
Kinesthetic Acuity subtest (Runway task), 280–287
Kinesthetic Perception and Memory subtest
    (Pattern task), 280
Kinesthetic Sensitivity Test (KST), 280–287
Kinesthetic training, 278–287

L
Labor, division of, 456, 459–460
Learned helplessness, 194–195
Learning
    development of intention, 63–64
    motor skills, 159–166
    and occupation, 230–231
    task association, 232–238
Legible word productivity, 270
Leisure occupations, 361–372
Liminality, 432
Limitations, social, 391
Loewenstein Occupational Therapy Cognitive
    Assessment (LOTCA), 122

M
Mastery motivation, 329
Material culture, 520–521
Maternal work. *See* mothers
Meaning making, 499–501
Medicaid, 376–382
Medically related services, 376–377
Medication, 289–290
Memory, 232–238, 409–410
Mental retardation, 130–131. *See also* fragile X
    syndrome
Metacognition, 110
Miller Assessment for Preschoolers (MAP),
    118–127, **124–125**
Mobility, 194–207
Monochronic time use, 541
Mothering, 508
Mothers
    of ADHD children, strategies of, 541–550
    adolescent, 507
    caring for children with disabilities, 301–310
    daily routines, 478–486, 490–503, 509–510
    demands on therapists, 466
    home as play space, 518–530
    and infants with CHD, 10
    occupations of mothering, 506–515
    perceptions of child care assistance, 455–463
Motivation, 330–331
Motor impairment, 53
Motor performance, 120, 278–279
Motor skills, 141–153, 159–160
Movement Assessment Battery for Children
    (Movement ABC), 143, 162
Multisensory approaches, 24–31, **27–28**

N
Nasogastric feeding, 9
Natural history, 519
Neurodevelopmental treatment (NDT), 259–261
Nondidactic developmental guidance, 17
Nonlinear relationships, 64
Nonverbal children, 498

O
Observational Scale of Behavioral Distress
    (OSBD), 244
Occupation
    aspects, 231–232, 232
    CMOP context, 5–6
    orchestration of, 488–503
    play as, 240
Occupational engagement, 398–400

Occupational form, 231–232, *232*
Occupational meaning, 335–336
Occupational performance
  determining factors, 4–5
  fragile X syndrome, 315–325
  satisfaction in mothers of disabled children,
    301–310
  in toddlers, 329–330
Occupational repetition, 371–372
Occupational storymaking, 485–486
Occupational therapists, 45–46
Occupational therapy
  children's choices, 539
  intensity *vs.* outcome, 170–178
  medical *vs.* educational orientation, 376–377,
    377
  reasons for seeking, 444–445
Occupational Therapy Code of Ethics. *See* Code of
  Ethics
Occupations. *See also* leisure occupations
  in children, 61–62
  consumer, 511
  of mothering, 506–515
  mothers as advocates, 510
Offenders, young, 362–372
Olfactory system, **101**
Oral aversion, 9
Orchestration, of occupation, 488–503
Organized activities, 447
Organizing, 495–496
Orthopedic impairment, 53
OSBD. *See* Observational Scale of Behavioral
  Distress (OSBD)
Other-mother concept, 512
Oucher scale, 244–245, 249–250
Outcomes
  child-focused, 417, 419–420, 445–448, *446*
  parent-focused, 420–421, 448–450
  parents' expectations, 415–424
Outdoors, 527
Oxygenation, 8

P
Pain, 241–242, 250
Paper, 23
Parent reports, 142–153
Parents
  experiences in an OT waiting room, 428–437
  hopes for therapy outcomes, 415–424
  perspectives of occupational therapy, 441–452
  reasons for seeking occupational therapy,
    444–445

therapist partnerships, 465–474
time use, 455–456
and toddlers' development, 330–331
Passive leisure activities, 362
Pattern tasks, 280, 282
Payment system, 376–382
Peabody Developmental Motor Scale—Fine Motor
  (PDMS-FM)
  described, 89, 171
Pediatric Evaluation of Disability Inventory
  (PEDI), 173
Peer interaction, 170, 178
Peer relationships, 395–396, 399
Pencil grasp. *See* grip
Perceptual-motor training, 23
Performance components, 168–169
Persistence, 328–337
Personal care, 447
Perspective shifting, 499–501
Pervasive developmental disorders (PDD),
  215–216. *See also* autism spectrum disorders
Physical activity, 533, 535–539
Physical environment, 518–530
Physical skills, 5
Piaget, Jean, 38–39
Planning, 495–496
Play
  deprivation in disabled children, 391
  duration and fragile X syndrome, 319
  effects of sensory integration therapy, 447–448
  exercise, 533
  fine motor skills, 170, 178
  interaction characteristics of disabled children,
    397–398
  intervention techniques, **259**
  as occupation, 240–241
  space for infants and toddlers, 518–530
  as therapy, 250
  by toddlers, 328–337
Play objects, 520–525
Playfulness, 254–265
Polychronic time use, 541
Positioning devices, 527
Postconcussion syndrome, 54
Power, 39–41
Preschoolers. *See also* infants; toddlers
  powered mobility, 194–207
  as research subjects, 43
  screening tools, 119–120
  service delivery comparisons, 209–214
  TBI patients, 56–57
  visual-motor skills, 182–189

Prior experience, 16, 17
Prioritizing, 496–497
Privacy, 43, 485
Project Bien Estar, 302–310
Proprioception system, **101**
Psychoanalytic intervention, 17
Psychology, 60–61
Psychosocial impairment, 54
Purkinje cells, 291
Purposeful activity, 240

Q
Questioning techniques, 44–45

R
Reading disability, 144
Reciprocity, 395, 399
Reconstruction of self-worth, 448, 451
Referrals, 51
Reframing
    defined, 449
    by parents, 434–435
    parents' observation, 449–450
Rehabilitation services, 51–52
Reorganization, 66–68
Respiratory distress, 8
Ritalin, 543
Rites of passage ritual, 432
Ritual, 432
Routines
    impact of, 476–478
    mothers with disabled children, 478–486,
        509–510
    time constraints, 485
Runway task training, 280–287

S
Safety, 526–527
Schneck and Henderson's grip scale, **76,** 76–77,
    77, 83–84
School, 393–401
School AMPS, 88–92
School function, 322–323
School Function Assessment (SFA), 88, 319
School reentry, 55
School services, 376–382
Screening tools, criteria, 118–119
Seating, classroom, 268–276
Self-care function, 177
Self-concept, 448
Self-feeding, 328–337, 478
Self-organization, 64
Self-regulation, 419

Self-stimulation
    in children with PDD, 216
    and weighted vests, 219, *220,* 221, *222–225,*
        226
Self-worth, reconstruction of, 448, 451
Sensation avoidance, 323
Sensitivity, 119
Sensorimotor impairment, 53–54
Sensorimotor performance, 23
Sensory Approach-Avoidance Rating, 318
Sensory integration
    autism spectrum disorders, 130–139, *135,* **136**
    fine motor skills, 169
Sensory integration therapy
    deep touch-pressure, 290–291
    handwriting performance, 23
    parents' perspectives, 441–452
Sensory modulation, 269, 275–276
Sensory modulation disorders (SMD)
    defined, 290
    described, 415–416
    parents' hopes for outcomes, 415–424
    and social behaviors, 422–423
Sensory processing
    Asperger syndrome, 351–357
    children with ADHD, 289
    evaluation, 94–106, **100–104**
    fragile X syndrome, 315–325
    measurement, 317
Sensory Profile
    and Asperger syndrome, 352–353
    and autism spectrum disorders, 131–138, *135,*
        136
    described, 96
    validity, 95
Sensory Rating Scale (SRS), 95
Serotonin, 291
Sharing, 263
Short Sensory Profile (SSP), 317
Siblings, 335–336
Social comparison, 434
Social context, 5, 393–401
Social function, 177
Social interaction, 352, 391–401
Social leisure occupations, 362
Social participation, 417, 419
Sociocultural niches, 65
Spatial cognition, 521–522
Spatial ties, 527–528
Specificity, 119
Spiritual effect, 499–500
Spirituality, 7
Stereotypes, 533

Stigma, 532–539
Storymaking, 485–486
Stress, 11, 491–492
Stressors, 472–473
Subsystems, in organization, 64
Support, 17, 420, 450
Support systems, 428–437, 511–512
Swallowing, 8

T
Tactile Defensiveness and Discrimination Test-
    Revised (TDDT-R), 317–318
Tactile system, **101–103**
Temporal unfolding
    examples, 545–546
    time as resource, 549
    users of, 548
Test of Playfulness (ToP), 255–265, **256**
Test of Visual-Perceptual Skills—Non-Motor
    (TVPS), 406
Therapists, 465–474
Therapy balls, 268–276
Time constraints, 485, 495–496
Time-out leisure, 362
Time Perception Inventory (TPI), 305–306
Time use
    of mothers of ADHD children, 541–550
    of mothers of disabled children, 455–456
    satisfaction in mothers of disabled children,
        301–310
    by young offenders, 362–372
Time Use Analysis (TUA), 306
Time-Use Longitudinal Panel Study, 492
Time use strategies, 302
Toddlers, 328–337, 518–530
Toglia category assessment, 110–116
Total Inventories, 95
Touch Inventories, 95
Toys
    availability to child, 524–525
    in infant play, 520–521

selection, 522–524
Traumatic brain injury (TBI), 49–57, **57**
Tripod grip, 84–85, *340*, 340–341

U
Unfolding by inclusion
    described, 546–548
    time as constraint, 549
    users of, 548
Unfolding occupations, 544. *See also* Temporal
    unfolding
Upper Limb Speed and Dexterity (ULSD), 406

V
Validation, 421, 450
Vestibular system, **103–104**
Vigilance, 410
Vigilance Task of the Gordon Diagnostic System,
    407
Vineland Adaptive Behavior Scales-Daily Living
    Skills (VABS), 318–319
Vision skills, 404–405
Visual Aural Digit Span Test (VADS), 122
Visual-Motor Integration (VMI), 406–407
Visual-motor skills, 182–189
Visual perception, 172
Visual system, **104**

W
Waiting rooms, 428–437
Weighted vests, 216–228, 289–299
Writing implements
    diameter, 77–78
    grip formation, 81–82, *82*
writing skill, 85
Writing skills, 77
Writing tools, 23

Y
Yards, 527

About the Editor

Charlotte Brasic Royeen, PhD, OTR, FAOTA, is dean, Doisy School of Allied Health Professions, Saint Louis University. She has been in pediatric occupational therapy for over 25 years. She has authored over 60 peer-reviewed journal articles, given over 100 scholarly presentations, and edited or authored 18 books. In 2003, she presented the Eleanor Clarke Slagle Lecture and received the Outstanding Contributor Award from the Nebraska Occupational Therapy Association.